Essentials of
OPHTHALMOLOGY

Essentials of OPHTHALMOLOGY

Comprehensive Review for Undergraduates and Quick Review for Postgraduates

Dadapeer K
MS DNB (Ophthalmology)
Associate Professor
Department of Ophthalmology
Hassan Institute of Medical Sciences
Hassan, Karnataka, India

Forewords
Premkumar D
Raviprakash D

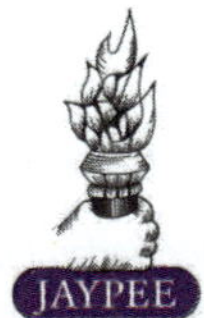

JAYPEE BROTHERS MEDICAL PUBLISHERS
The Health Sciences Publisher
New Delhi | London

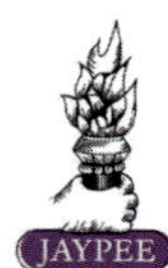

Jaypee Brothers Medical Publishers (P) Ltd

Headquarters
EMCA House
23/23-B, Ansari Road, Daryaganj
New Delhi 110 002, India.
Landline: +91-11-23272143, +91-11-23272703
+91-11-23282021, +91-11-23245672
E-mail: jaypee@jaypeebrothers.com

Corporate Office
4838/24, Ansari Road, Daryaganj
New Delhi 110 002, India.
Phone: +91-11-43574357
Fax: +91-11-43574314
E-mail: jaypee@jaypeebrothers.com

Overseas Office
J.P. Medical Ltd
83 Victoria Street, London
SW1H 0HW (UK)
Phone: +44 20 3170 8910
E-mail: info@jpmedpub.com

EU GPSR Authorised Representative
Logos Europe, 9 rue Nicolas Poussin
17000, La Rochelle, France
Phone: +33 (0) 6 67 93 73 78
E-mail: contact@logoseurope.eu

Website: www.jaypeebrothers.com
Website: www.jaypeedigital.com

Inquiries for bulk sales may be solicited at: jaypee@jaypeebrothers.com

Essentials of Ophthalmology—*Comprehensive Review for Undergraduates and Quick Review for Postgraduates*

First Edition: **2015**
Reprint: 2026
ISBN 978-93-5152-908-8

Printed at SDR Printers

Dedicated to

Love of my life

My wife

Dr Shama Taj KR

Foreword

It is with genuine pleasure that I take advantage of this opportunity to write the foreword for this wonderful book *Essentials of Ophthalmology*, which is the work and effort of Dr Dadapeer K.

One thing about him that always impressed me most was his simplicity, which is also reflected in his book. The simplicity and clinical value of the book can easily be recognized. It is the result of his past experience and intimate knowledge of the subject.

This book has been written as a course material for undergraduates. The aim is to provide students with complete and up-to-date material in simple language and lucid style, with additional material to help them to tackle potential new questions.

Gist boxes have been prepared with a great deal of effort, which will make simple for students to memorize the essentials with least effort. The references of the book have been taken from the recent editions of standard national and international medical publications and authors. Content is formatted to be student-friendly in such a way that reader can easily understand, retain and reproduce the facts. Text has been profusely illustrated with color diagrams, flowcharts and tables, hence helping the students assimilate the facts for long retention.

Lastly, I heartily congratulate the author for his excellent piece of work, which will surely help the students and wishing all the success.

Premkumar D MD (Medicine)
Former Registrar
Rajiv Gandhi University of Health Sciences
Bengaluru, Karnataka, India

Foreword

It gives me immense pleasure to write this foreword for *Essentials of Ophthalmology* by Dr Dadapeer K who has been my student for years. Having known Dr Dadapeer K throughout his student days, he has always had an inquisitive bent of mind with flair of ingenuity and original research. This book is a standing proof for the same.

Today there has been a veritable explosion in scientific information and advances in the field of ophthalmology. As such, it becomes imperative for student of the subject as well as practicing consultants to keep abreast of upcoming trends and ideas. In the melee, it is of utmost importance that a student of the subject remains well-versed with basic concepts and clinical aspects, which forms the backbone of any medical practice. This book bridges the lacuna between these extremes.

This book has been set in a design that is simple and convenient for the reader. Every topic has been dealt with in detail keeping in view of essential concepts and recent advances. Each topic has been divided into subgroups, which offers the quick glance into required data. Tables, charts and illustrations at appropriate places provide a lucid and comprehensive understanding of the subject.

This book would prove to be an invaluable asset for undergraduates and postgraduates for comprehensive study and quick review of ophthalmology.

Wishing all the success for this book ... Happy reading.

Raviprakash D MS (Ophthalmology)
Ex-Director
Bangalore Medical College and Research Institute
Bengaluru, Karnataka, India

Preface

This book is written as comprehensive review for undergraduates and quick review for postgraduates. The book aims to present ophthalmology in a simplified, yet in a comprehensive manner covering all the topics with a lot of clinical photographs and illustrated diagrams. It has the following key features, thus making it an easy-to-use guide for the students:

- Important notes and interesting facts in each chapter
- Gist boxes at the end of each chapter providing summary and important points in each chapter
- Frequently asked questions at the end of each section.

I hope that the book will be a useful guide for the medical students of ophthalmology. Efforts have been made to check for the accuracy of the matter and to correct the mistakes, if any. I will be happy to receive constructive comments, which will help in betterment of the book.

Dadapeer K

Acknowledgments

My wholehearted expression of gratitude to one and all who have contributed in many ways for completion of this book. I affectionately thank my parents Mr and Mrs Karimsab, my uncle and aunt Mr and Mrs Emamsab, my father-in-law and mother-in-law Mr and Mrs Abdul Razak, and my sister-in-law Ms Heena Kousar and brother-in-law Mr Waris for their constant support and encouragement.

My special thanks to my wife, Dr Shama Taj KR, Assistant Professor of Microbiology, SS Institute of Medical Sciences and Research Centre, Davangere, Karnataka, India, for her constant support, encouragement and cooperation without which this book would have never been a reality. I also thank her for authoring a Section on Ocular Microbiology.

I would like to extend my heartful thanks to Dr Pratap VGM, Dr Dilip HR, Dr Gayathri V (Residents in Ophthalmology, Aravind Eye Care Hospital, Madurai, Tamil Nadu, India), Dr Lakshmi (Resident in Ophthalmology, AJ Institute of Medical Sciences and Research Centre, Mangaluru) for all the help in taking the photographs and preparing the book.

I thank Dr Lakshmi BR, Dr Sahana Mainpur, Dr Shwetha S, Dr Farah Zeba, Dr Divya Mishra, Dr Chaitra CM, Dr Archana K, Dr Anuraj, Dr Arpitha, Dr Ashish, Dr Nehla Tahim, Dr Moorthy TN and Dr Ashitha S for helping me in proofreading the book.

I thank colleagues of my department Dr Kavitha CV, Dr Pavana Acharya, Mr Radhakrishna, Mr Nagesh and Mr Ishidhara Kumar (Ophthalmic Officer, Government Hospital, Alur, Hassan, Karnataka) for their help rendered to me.

I would like to thank Dr Ramamurthy D (Chairman, The Eye Foundation and Vice-President, All India Ophthalmic Society), Dr Ravikumar BC (Professor of Dermatology, Hassan Institute of Medical Sciences, Hassan), Dr Gangadhar (Professor of ENT, Shimoga Institute of Medical Sciences, Shimoga, Karnataka), Dr Praveen G (Associate Professor of Community Medicine), Dr Niranjan (Associate Professor of Medicine), Dr Devraja R (Consultant Hepatologist), Dr Sudhanava (Associate Professor of Physiology), Dr Deepak (Associate Professor of Pharmacology, Hassan Institute of Medical Sciences), Dr Pradeep Kumar (Associate Professor of Ophthalmology, Shimoga Institute of Medical Sciences), Dr Sandhya (Professor of Ophthalmology, Sri Siddhartha Medical College), Dr Rakesh (Consultant Ophthalmologist, CSI Mission Hospital, Hassan), Dr CV Andrews (Professor of Ophthalmology, Jubliee Mission Medical College & Research Institute, Thrissur, Kerala), Dr Prakash HM (Associate Professor of Pathology, Vinayaka Mission Medical College, Salem, Tamil Nadu), Dr Niranjan (Associate Professor of Biochemistry, Mahatama Gandhi Medical College and Research Institute, Puducherry), Dr Kavitha (Consultant Ophthalmologist, Vasan Eye Care, Bengaluru), Dr Narendra Shenoy (Consultant Ophthalmologist, Udupi Eye Center, Udupi, Karnataka), Dr Shailaja Shenoy (Associate Professor of Ophthalmology, Kasturba Medical College, Manipal, Karnataka), Dr Venkat (Consultant Ophthalmologist, Globe Eye Foundation, Bengaluru, Karnataka), Dr Prashanth CN (Associate Professor of Ophthalmology, Dr BR Ambedkar Medical College, Bengaluru), Dr Rajashekar (Associate Professor of Ophthalmology, Karnataka Institute of Medical Sciences, Hubballi, Karnataka), Dr Nadeem (Assistant Professor of Ophthalmology, Raichur Institute of Medical Sciences, Raichur, Karnataka), Dr Shenoy (Associate Professor of Ophthalmology) and Dr Dinesh (Assistant Professor of Ophthalmology, Adhichunchanagiri Institute of Medical Sciences, Bengaluru, Karnataka), for their support.

I am grateful to the positive feedback and Foreword written by Dr Premkumar D, Former Registrar, Rajiv Gandhi University of Health Sciences (RGUHS), Bengaluru.

I thank my teacher and guide Dr Raviprakash D, Former Director, Bangalore Medical College and Research Institute, Bengaluru, for his encouragement and for writing Foreword.

I am thankful to Professor Chandrashekar Shetty (Former Vice-Chancellor, RGUHS), Professor Sriprakash KS (Former Vice-Chancellor, RGUHS) for their support and encouragement.

I am thankful to my teacher Dr Jyothi Swarup (Professor of ENT, Sri Siddhartha Medical College, Tumakuru, Karnataka) and my postgraduate teachers Dr Ramesh TK, Dr Sriprakash KS, Dr Shivakumar, Dr Prabha AR, Dr Shivaprasad Reddy, Dr Dakshyani, Dr Suresh Babu and Dr Nagaraju (Bangalore Medical College and Research Institute, Bengaluru) for being an endless source of inspiration and guidance.

I affectionately thank my friends and relatives for their constant support and encouragement.

I extend my deeply felt gratitude to Shri Jitendar P Vij (Group Chairman), Mr Ankit Vij (Group President), Tarun Duneja (Director-Publishing), Mr Venugopal Vishumurthy [Associate Director-South (Sales & Marketing)], Mr Vasudev (Commissioning Editor) and staff of Bengaluru Production Unit and all other technical staff of M/s Jaypee Brothers Medical Publishers (P) Ltd, New Delhi, India.

Contents

Section 3: Conjunctiva

Section 4: Optics and Refraction

Section 5: Cornea

Section 8: Lens

Section 9: Glaucoma

Section 10: Vitreous

Section 11: Retina

Section 12: Optic Nerve

Section 13: Lacrimal System

Section 14: Orbit

Section 15: Strabismus

Section 16: Neurophthalmology

Section 17: Intraocular Tumors

Section 18: Ocular Trauma

Section 19: Community Ophthalmology

Section 20: Systemic Ophthalmology

Section 21: Ocular Pharmacology and Ocular Therapeutics

Section 22: Ocular Microbiology

How to use the book?

Dear Readers...

I have made my sincere efforts to make reading of this book enjoyable by including few special characters. The few highlights of the book are as below.

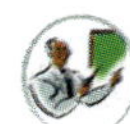

This indicates Important Notes. This needs to be remembered as this will be asked most frequently in the theory, clinical and postgraduate entrance examination.

This indicates Interesting Facts. This is important from the point of view of clinical and postgraduate entrance examination.

This indicates you need to refer this topic in another chapter.

*One star indicates Frequently Asked Question for short answer.

**Two star indicates Frequently Asked Question for short essay.

***Three star indicates Frequently Asked Question for long essay.

I hope you will find these useful while reading.

Wishing you a happy reading.....

Dadapeer K

SECTION 1

Human Eye

1.1 Introduction to Human Eye
1.2 Anatomy of Eye
1.3 Embryology and Congenital Anomalies of Eyeball
1.4 Physiology of Eye and Vision

CHAPTER

1.1 Introduction to Human Eye

Eyes are the important sensory organs responsible for vision. The eyes are broadly classified into simple eyes and compound eyes. Simple eyes are the ones, which have a single lens that focuses the light onto the retina. The eyes of humans and vertebrates are simple eyes. Compound eyes have multiple lenses and they are found in insects.

> The carnivorous animals, which hunt other animals usually have eyes in front of the head and have depth perception to have a three-dimensional (3D) image to catch the prey.
>
> The animals, which are vegetarians and become prey to the carnivore animals, have eyes on the sides of head to have a wider field of vision, so that they can watch for the hunter.

With the evolution of life on earth, the eye has undergone evolution from the simplest eye present in microbes, which can detect only presence or absence of light to the human eye, which has got visual acuity, color vision, contrast sensitivity and depth perception. Eyes are developed to adapt to the requirements of the organism.

HUMAN EYE

Human eye consists of a complex optical system consisting of a transparent lens, which focuses light onto the retina. The human eye is also called 'simple eye'. Retina converts light impulses into neural impulses that travel along the optic nerve to reach the visual cortex, which processes the visual impulses and enables us to see.

Human Eye is Similar to Camera

- Like aperture of the camera, pupil of the eye allows light into the eye.
- Like lens of the camera, which captures light from an object and focuses onto the imaging sensor, lens of the eye focuses light onto the retina.
- Like imaging sensor of the camera, which converts the pattern of light into video signal, retina converts light impulses into neural impulses, which are processed in the visual cortex.

GIST BOX 1.1

- Eyes are the important sensory organs responsible for vision.
- Human eye consists of complex optical system that include a transparent lens, which focuses light onto the retina. The retina converts light impulses into neural impulses that travel along the optic nerve to reach the visual cortex, processes the visual impulses and enables us to see.

CHAPTER

1.2 Anatomy of Eye

Eye consists of eyeball proper and appendages of the eye. Eyeball proper is called globe or bulbus oculi. The appendages of the eye include eyebrows, eyelids, lacrimal apparatus, conjunctiva and extraocular muscles (Fig. 1.2.1).

EYEBALL

Each eyeball is an oblate spheroid structure filled with fluid and enclosed by three layers. Eyeball is kept distended by the pressure exerted on the layers of the eyeball by the fluid inside and it is called intraocular pressure. Each eyeball is placed in a bony cavity situated one on either side of the nose called orbit. Each eyeball is suspended in the orbit by extraocular muscles and fascial sheaths.

Poles of Eyeball

Since eyeball is not a perfect sphere, but an oblate spheroid structure, eyeball has got two poles:

1. Anterior pole.
2. Posterior pole, which corresponding to the central point on the anterior and posterior curvatures of the eyeball respectively.

Equator of Eyeball

Equator of eyeball is the part of eyeball lying midway between anterior and posterior poles of the eyeball.

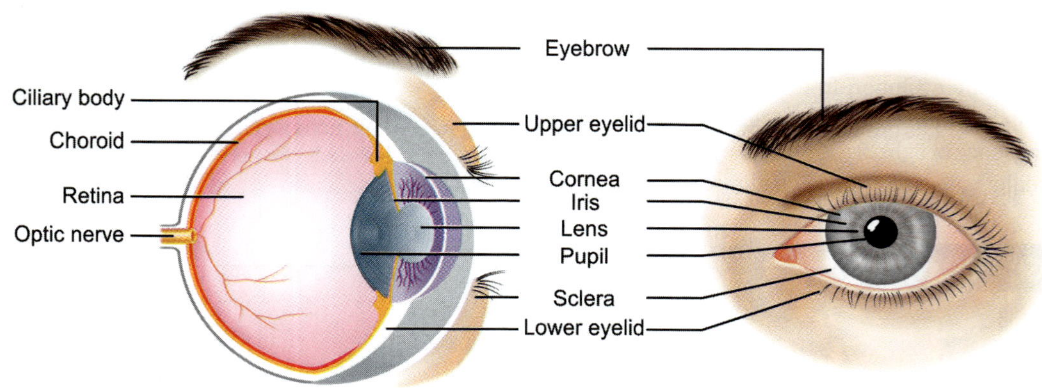

FIG. 1.2.1: Parts of human eye

Optic Axis of Eyeball

An imaginary line passing through the anterior and the posterior poles of the eyeball is called optic axis. The optic nerve leaves the eyeball 3 mm nasal to the posterior pole along the axes of the orbit. The optic axes of the two eyeballs are parallel to each other and the axis of the eyeball make an angle between the axes of the orbit and optic nerve follows the direction of the axis of the orbit (Fig. 1.2.2).

Layers of Eyeball

Eyeball is enclosed by three layers, which are as detailed below.

Outermost fibrous layer: It is constituted by the opaque sclera and the transparent cornea. Cornea accounts for anterior one sixth of the outermost layer and sclera accounts for the remaining five sixths of the outermost fibrous layer. Cornea being transparent is an essential component of optical system of the eye and it refracts light into the eye. Sclera is the tough layer responsible for protection of intraocular contents.

Middle vascular layer: It is constituted by iris, ciliary body and choroid.

Inner neural layer: This layer of the eye is called retina, which converts light impulses into neural impulses that travel along the optic nerve to reach the visual cortex (Fig. 1.2.3).

Segments of Eyeball

The eyeball is divided into two segments:

1. Anterior segment.
2. Posterior segment.

Anterior Segment

Anterior segment includes anterior one third of the eye extending from cornea to the lens including cornea, anterior chamber, iris, pupil, posterior chamber and lens.

Posterior Segment

Posterior segment includes posterior two third of the eye including the structures behind the lens. It includes anterior hyaloid membrane, vitreous humor, choroid, retina and optic disk.

Chambers of Eyeball

The eyeball consists of three chambers:

1. Anterior chamber.
2. Posterior chamber present in the anterior segment.
3. Vitreous chamber present in the posterior segment.

Anterior Chamber

Anterior chamber is a fluid-filled space filled with aqueous humor. It is bounded anteriorly

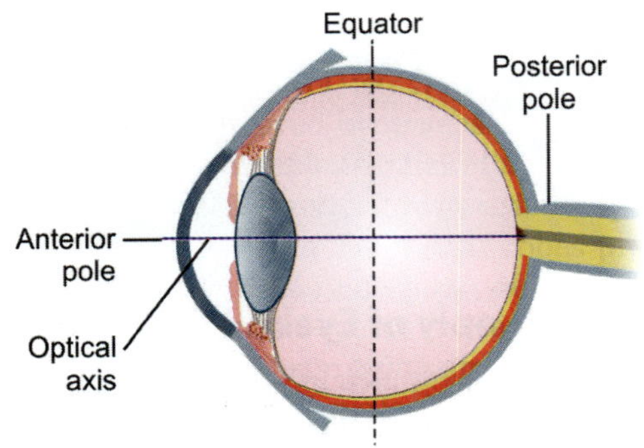

FIG. 1.2.2: Optical axis of the eyeball

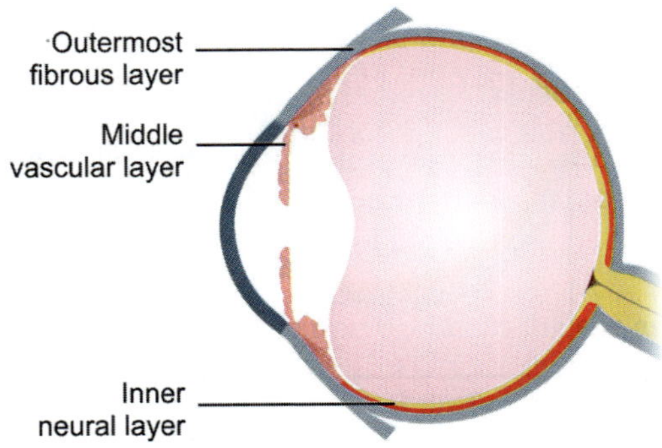

FIG. 1.2.3: Layers of eyeball

by the posterior surface of cornea and a small portion of the sclera, and posteriorly by iris, lens and a small portion of ciliary body. The normal depth of the anterior chamber in the center is about 2.5–3.5 mm. The volume of aqueous humor in anterior chamber is 0.25 mL.

Posterior Chamber

Posterior chamber is a fluid-filled triangular space filled with aqueous humor. It is bounded anteriorly by posterior surface of iris and posteriorly by lens, zonules, ciliary body, and anterolaterally by a part of ciliary body. The volume of aqueous humor in posterior chamber is 0.06 mL.

Anterior and posterior chambers communicate with each other through pupil and the aqueous humor, which is produced in the posterior chamber, is drained through the angle of the anterior chamber.

Vitreous Chamber

Vitreous chamber is situated between the lens and the retina, and filled with inert, transparent gel-like structure called vitreous. Vitreous accounts for 75–80% of the entire volume of the eye with a volume of 4.5 mL and being a transparent structure vitreous forms a part of refractive medium of the eye (Fig. 1.2.4).

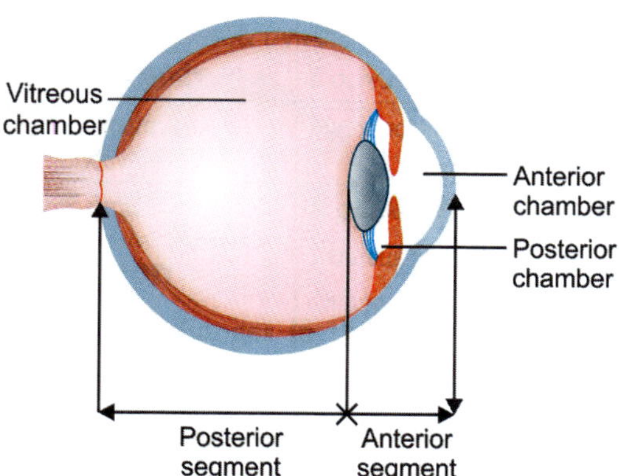

FIG. 1.2.4: Chambers and segments of the eye

Blood Supply of Eyeball*

The blood supply of the eye is from the ophthalmic artery—a branch of internal carotid artery. Ophthalmic artery supplies the blood to eye by two systems:

1. Retinal system.
2. Ciliary system.

Retinal System

Retinal system consists of central retinal artery, which supplies the inner six layers of the retina and central retinal vein that drains blood from inner six layers of the retina.

Ciliary System

Ciliary system consists of anterior ciliary arteries, long posterior ciliary arteries and short posterior ciliary arteries:

1. The anterior ciliary arteries are seven in number, derived from muscular branches of ophthalmic artery and supply the episclera, sclera and limbus.
2. Long posterior ciliary arteries are two in number, they anastomose with anterior ciliary arteries near the root of the iris to form the circulus arteriosus major and supply the ciliary body, ciliary processes and iris.
3. Short posterior ciliary arteries about 20 in number arising from ophthalmic artery and supply the choroid, and optic nerve head. The venous drainage is by anterior ciliary veins and vortex veins.

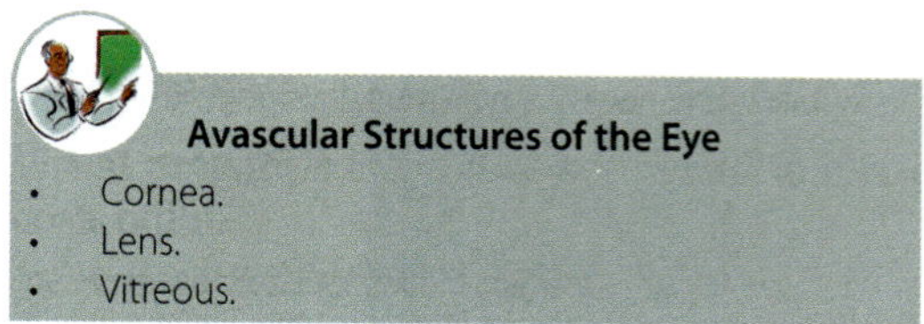

Avascular Structures of the Eye

- Cornea.
- Lens.
- Vitreous.

Nerve Supply of Eyeball

1. The sensory nerve supply of the eye is from short- and long-ciliary nerves, branches of nasociliary nerve arising from ophthalmic division of trigeminal nerve.

> The sensory nerve supply is limited to the cornea, sclera, iris and ciliary body, hence the diseases affecting them are painful; whereas lens, vitreous, choroid and retina do not have sensory nerve supply, hence the diseases affecting them are painless.

2. The sympathetic supply of the eye supplies the dilator pupillae via nasociliary nerve.
3. The parasympathetic supply of the eye supplies the ciliary muscle and sphincter pupillae via branches of oculomotor nerve.

Dimensions of the Adult Human Eye (Table 1.2.1)*

TABLE 1.2.1: Dimensions of eyeball or globe

Dimensions	*Measurement*
Axial length/Anteroposterior diameter	24 mm
Volume	6.5 mL
Circumference at the equator	75 mm
Weight	7.5 g
Vertical diameter	23 mm
Horizontal diameter	23.5 mm

> The axial length of the eyeball at birth is 16.5–17 mm; by 18 months of age, it reaches 20 mm and the adult size of 24 mm is attained by 13 years of age.
>
> Normally, the newborn infant is hypermetropic by +2 D at birth and becomes emmetropic by 10–12 years of age.

APPENDAGES OF EYE

Appendages of eye include eyebrows, eyelids, conjunctiva and lacrimal system.

Eyebrows

Eyebrows are symmetrical collection of hair follicles along the superciliary arch. They separate the eyelids from forehead and form a part of protective mechanism of the eyes.

Eyelids

Eyelids are the mobile skin folds that cover the eye, protect the anterior surface of eye from injury, spread the tear film over the cornea during blinking and take part in tear film drainage by acting over the lacrimal pump.

Conjunctiva

Conjunctiva is a transparent, thin mucous membrane, which lines the anterior surface of globe up to limbus and posterior surface of eyelids. It provides protection to globe as it lines the anterior surface of eyeball and takes part in immune function and defensive mechanisms of eye against microbial organisms by secretion of antibacterial proteins.

Lacrimal System

Lacrimal system consists of secretory part including main lacrimal gland and accessory lacrimal glands, which secrete tears and drainage part including punctum, canaliculi, lacrimal sac and nasolacrimal duct, which drain tears.

ORBIT

Orbits are quadrangular pyramidal bony cavities situated in the skull placed one on either side of the root of the nose between the anterior cranial fossa superiorly and maxillary sinuses inferiorly. Eye and appendages of the eye along with muscles, vessels and nerves of the eyes are situated within the orbit.

VISUAL PATHWAY

Visual pathway is the path along which the visual sensations from retina reach the visual cortex. It involves the optic nerve, optic chiasm, two optic tracts, lateral geniculate body, optic radiation and visual cortex.

GIST BOX 1.2

- Eye consists of eyeball proper and appendages of the eye. The appendages of the eye include eyebrows, eyelids, lacrimal apparatus, conjunctiva and extraocular muscles.
- Each eyeball is an oblate spheroid structure filled with fluid and enclosed by three layers. The three layers of the eye include outermost fibrous layer constituted by transparent cornea and opaque sclera, middle vascular layer constituted by iris, ciliary body and choroid, and the innermost neural layer constituted by retina and optic nerve.
- The eyeball is divided into anterior and posterior segments. The anterior segment includes anterior one third of the eye extending from cornea to the lens. The posterior segment includes posterior two third of the eye including the structures behind the lens.
- The eyeball consists of three chambers, i.e. anterior and posterior chamber present in the anterior segment and vitreous chamber present in the posterior segment.

CHAPTER

1.3

Embryology and Congenital Anomalies of Eyeball

EMBRYOLOGY OF EYE**

Human eye develops from the following:

- Neuroectoderm
- Surface ectoderm
- Mesoderm.

The development of eye begins in the 4th week on 22nd day along with the development of central nervous system (CNS). The anterior part of neural tube, which forms diencephalon of forebrain shows thickening on either side that becomes depressed to form optic sulcus. The optic sulcus is converted into optic vesicle appearing as an outpocketing from the forebrain (Figs 1.3.1 to 1.3.3).

Failure of formation of optic vesicle from neuroectoderm results in anophthalmos.

Each optic vesicle grows and comes in contact with the surface ectoderm. The surface ectoderm, which overlies the optic vesicle thickened to form lens placode by 27 days of gestation. As the optic vesicle reaches the surface ectoderm, it invaginates to form the optic cup. The optic cup is a double-walled structure and it is attached to the forebrain by optic stalk. The optic cup shows asymmetric growth and leaves a deficiency along the inferior surface of optic cup called the 'fetal fissure' or 'choroidal fissure' or 'embryonic fissure'. The hyaloid artery enters through the fetal fissure and it provides nourishment for the developing lens (Figs 1.3.4 to 1.3.6).

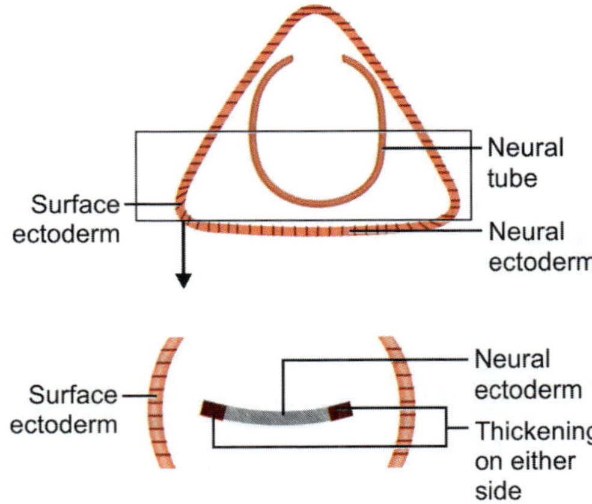

FIG. 1.3.1: Thickening of neural ectoderm

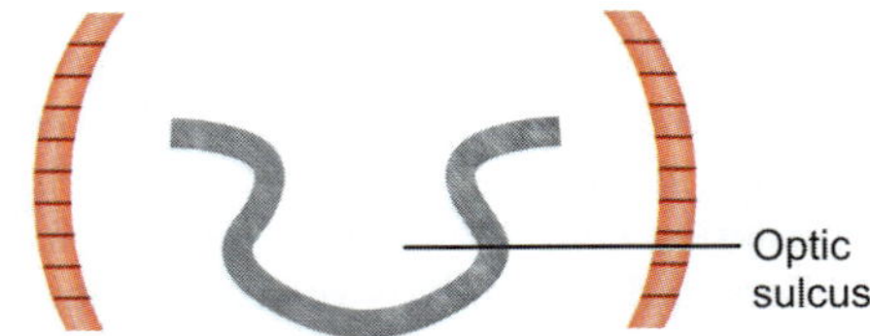

FIG. 1.3.2: Formation of optic sulcus by depression of the thickened neural ectoderm

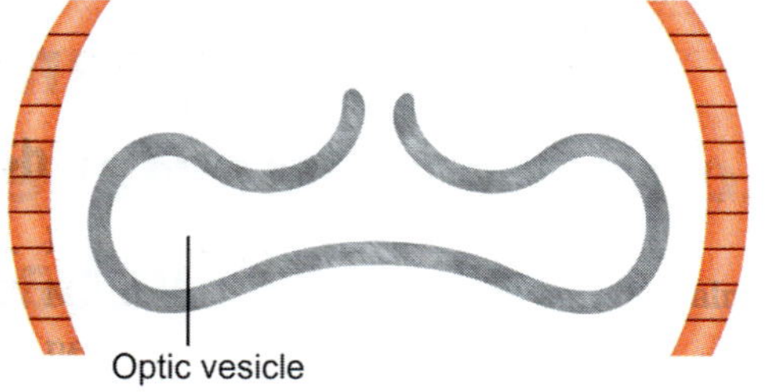

FIG. 1.3.3: Formation of optic vesicle

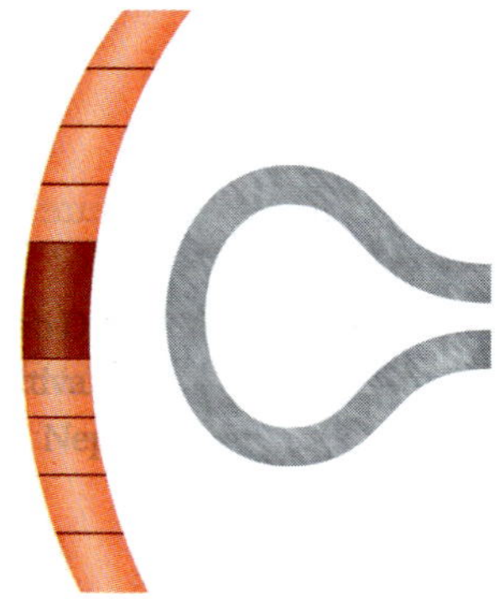

FIG. 1.3.4: Formation of lens placode by thickening of surface ectoderm

> Failure of fusion of the fetal fissure results in typical coloboma. Persistence of hyaloid vasculature results in the formation of persistent hyperplastic primary vitreous.

The fetal fissure closes by 6th week of gestation, this fusion of the fetal fissure results in the formation of future pupil. With closure of the fetal fissure, hyaloid system undergoes involution. The lens placode gets separated from surface ectoderm and it is converted into lens vesicle by 33 days of gestation. The lens vesicle is lined by a single layer of cuboidal epithelium. The posterior cells elongate to form primary lens fibers and fill the lens vesicle resulting in the formation of embryonic nucleus by 40 days of gestation.

The mesoderm, which surrounds the neural tube is carried into optic cup. The mesoderm differentiates into vascular mesoderm and fibrous mesoderm. Fibrous mesoderm in the anterior part forms cornea along with the surrounding surface ectoderm; sclera and extraocular muscles in the posterior part. Vascular mesoderm forms stroma of iris in the anterior part, stroma of ciliary body and choroid in the posterior part (Fig. 1.3.7).

> Retinal detachment occurs because of separation of the neurosensory retina from the pigmented epithelium of retina as these are embryologically derived from different layers of the optic cup.

The outer layer of optic cup acquires small pigment granules and it forms the pigmented epithelium of retina, epithelium of cili-

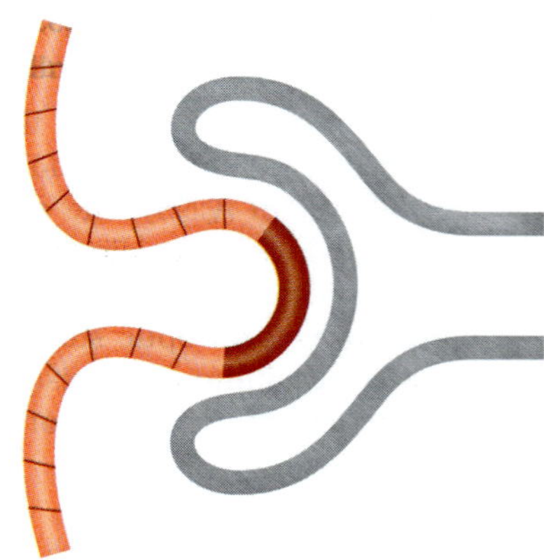

FIG. 1.3.5: Formation of optic cup

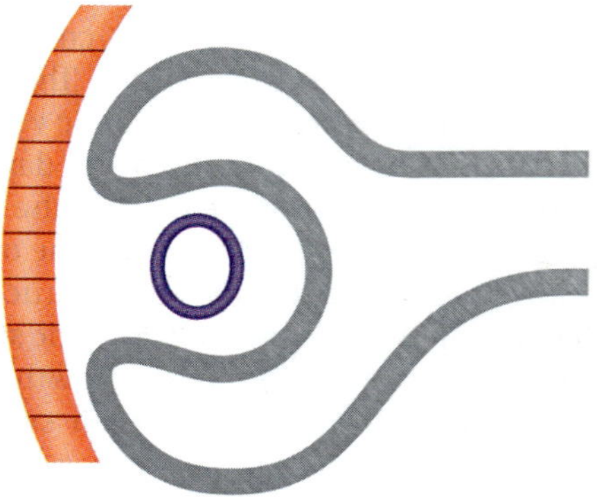

FIG. 1.3.6: Formation of lens vesicle

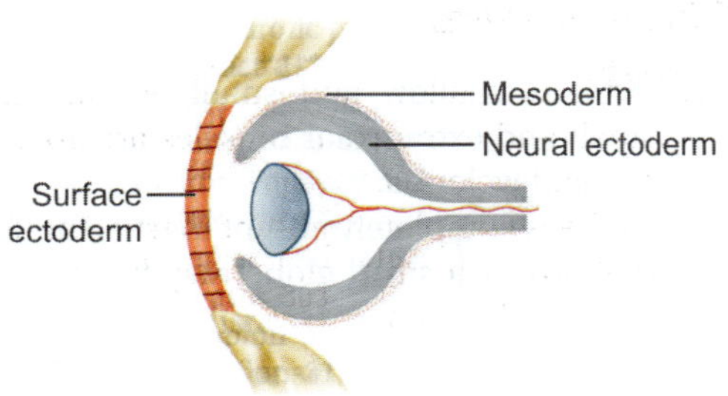

FIG. 1.3.7: Formation of lens with hyaloid vasculature

ary body and epithelium of iris. Inner layer of the optic cup forms the neural layer of retina.

The optic stalk, which connects the optic vesicle to forebrain is filled by axons of retinal ganglion cells and forms the optic nerve. Neuroectodermal cells and mesenchymal cells surrounding the optic stalk give raise to glial cells, and sheaths of the optic nerve respectively (Fig. 1.3.8).

The embryology of development of individual structures and appendages of the eye, and the respective congenital anomalies are described in respective chapters.

The eye develops from ectoderm including neuroectoderm, surface ectoderm and mesoderm.

Neuroectoderm gives rise to sensory retina, retinal pigment epithelium, pigment epithelium of iris, epithelium of ciliary body, optic nerve and muscles of iris (sphincter and dilator pupillae).

Surface ectoderm gives rise to lens, epithelium of cornea, conjunctiva, eyelids and lacrimal passages, lacrimal gland.

Mesoderm gives rise to all the layers of cornea except epithelium, sclera, stroma of iris and ciliary body, ciliary muscle, optic nerve sheath, extraocular muscles, blood vessels, bones of the orbit, connective tissues of the lids and orbit.

Eye develops from ectoderm and mesoderm; no part of the eye or appendages of the eye develop from endoderm.

CONGENITAL ANOMALIES OF EYEBALL

Cyclopia

1. Cyclopia is a rare congenital malformation characterized by single palpebral fissure and single midline orbit. It results from defective development or arrest of development of anterior end of neural plate.
2. It is usually associated with severe degree of malformation of brain such as holoprosencephaly characterized by failure of complete separation of the two hemispheres of the brain.
3. Cyclopia is characterized by gross deformation of the orbit resulting in formation of midline pseudo-orbit and absence of nasal cavity. The midline pseudo-orbit may contain one eye or two fused eyeballs. The presence of two fused eyeballs in a single orbit is called 'synophthalmia'.
4. Cyclopia can be seen in trisomy 13 or Patau syndrome.
5. Cyclopia is usually not compatible with life.

Cyclops was described as a one-eyed giant in ancient Greek mythology.

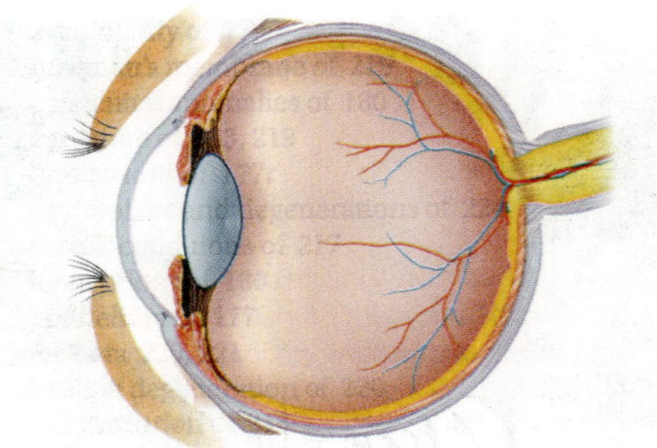

FIG. 1.3.8: Formation of lens with hyaloid vasculature

Anophthalmos*

Definition

Anophthalmos is unilateral or bilateral absence of eyeball because of failure of formation of optic vesicle from neuroectoderm (Fig. 1.3.9).

Etiopathogenesis

Anophthalmos may occur as either idiopathic or sporadic condition, seen in association with:

1. Syndromes such as trisomy 9, trisomy 13, Klinefelter's syndrome, Crouzon's syndrome, Goldenhar syndrome.
2. Infections such as congenital toxoplasmosis, rubella, cytomegalovirus, herpes simplex (TORCH) infections.

Anophthalmos can be of three types, which are as follows:

1. Primary anophthalmos is because of failure of formation of optic vesicle with normal development of the anterior neuroectoderm and normal development of the forebrain.
2. Secondary anophthalmos is because of failure of formation of optic vesicle associated with anomalous anterior neural tube and anomalies involving the forebrain.
3. Degenerative anophthalmos is because of degeneration of the normally formed primary optic vesicle.

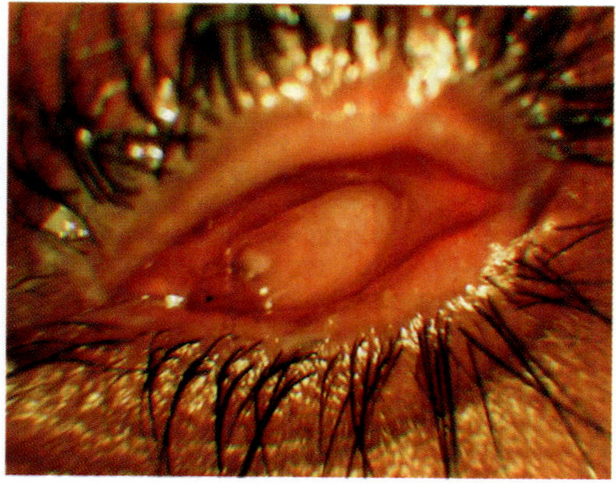

FIG. 1.3.9: Anophthalmos

Clinical Features

1. Orbit is shallow and small, eyelids are small and extraocular muscles are absent or maldeveloped.
2. Globe is completely absent in true anophthalmos or a small globe may be seen in microphthalmos.

Investigations

Computed tomography (CT) scan or magnetic resonance imaging (MRI) is done to find out the associated anomalies of the forebrain.

Treatment

Restoration of the vision is not possible; treatment is mainly aimed at correction of the cosmetic disfigurement by orbit reconstruction and prosthesis as in unilateral cases and visual aids in bilateral cases.

Microphthalmos*

Microphthalmos is a congenital anomaly of the eyeball characterized by axial length of less than 16 mm at birth or less than 22 mm in adults (Figs 1.3.10A and B). It is because of arrest of growth of the eyeball during gestation. Microphthalmos are the following types.

Simple microphthalmos or nanophthalmos: It is a type of microphthalmos characterized by small, but normal eyeball. However, the eye will be hypermetropic because of shorter axial length.

Microphthalmos associated with other ocular malformations and systemic anomalies: It is small and abnormal eyeball associated with ocular malformations, e.g. colobomas or systemic conditions such as trisomy 13, congenital TORCH infections, fetal alcohol syndrome.

Microphthalmos associated with cyst of the eyeball: It is caused by defective closure of the posterior part of the embryonic fissure and proliferation of the neuroectodermal tissue resulting in the formation of a cyst.

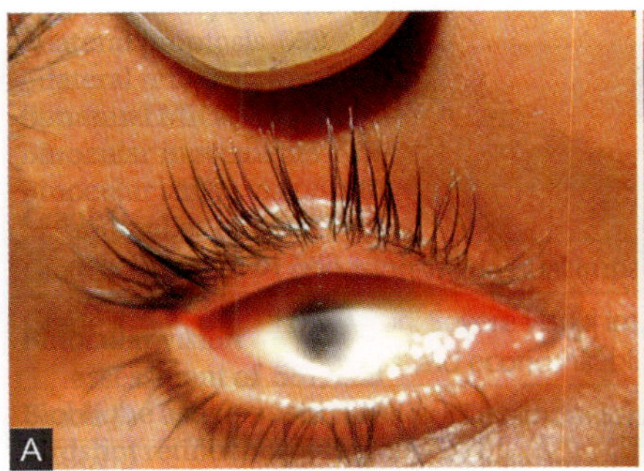

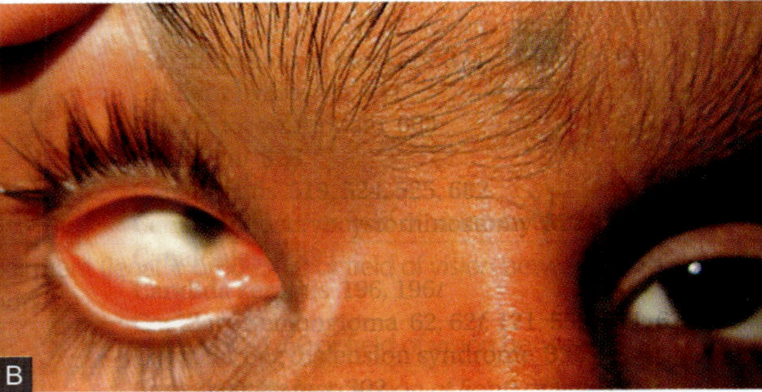

FIGS 1.3.10A and B: Microphthalmos of right eye

Investigations are aimed at finding out the associated ocular malformations and systemic anomalies. Treatment is similar to anophthalmos. Patients with nanophthalmos will have good visual acuity.

Megalophthalmos*

1. Megalophthalmos is a rare congenital anomaly of the eyeball characterized by axial length of more than 30 mm. It is inherited usually as an X-linked recessive condition.
2. It is probably because of defective growth of the optic cup allowing more space for the development of structures of the anterior segment.
3. It shows megalocornea, deep anterior chamber, iridodonesis, phacodonesis and ectopia lentis.
4. High pathological myopia and cataract are usually associated with it.
5. It has to be differentiated from buphthalmos—a condition characterized by marked enlargement of the eyeball seen in congenital or infantile glaucoma (Table 1.3.1).

TABLE 1.3.1: Differences between megalophthalmos and buphthalmos

Megalophthalmos	*Buphthalmos*
Normal clear, but enlarged cornea	Hazy enlarged cornea because of corneal edema and breaks in the Descemet's membrane
Bilateral non-progressive X-linked recessive condition	Unilateral or bilateral progressive condition
Normal intraocular pressure	Elevated intraocular pressure

Congenital Cystic Eye

Congenital cystic eye is a rare congenital anomaly characterized by the presence of cyst due to failure of involution of the primary optic vesicle. It should be differentiated from microphthalmos with cyst, which occurs because of defective closure of the embryonic fissure.

Congenital cystic eye is usually non-hereditary unilateral condition with cyst located under the upper eyelid. Treatment is by excision of the cystic eye and cosmetic correction by implantation of prosthesis.

GIST BOX 1.3

- The development of the eye begins in the 4th week on 22nd day along with the development of the central nervous system.
- The eye develops from ectoderm including neuroectoderm and surface ectoderm and mesoderm.
- Anophthalmos is unilateral or bilateral absence of eyeball because of failure of formation of optic vesicle from neuroectoderm.
- Microphthalmos is a congenital anomaly of the eyeball characterized by axial length of less than 16 mm at birth or less than 22 mm in adults.
- Megalophthalmos is a rare congenital anomaly of the eyeball characterized by axial length of more than 30 mm.

CHAPTER

1.4 Physiology of Eye and Vision

PHYSIOLOGY OF EYE

Eye is the organ of vision and the physiology of eye includes the study of structures, which enables the eye to do this function. Human eye is an image-forming eye in which the light travels through the transparent optical medium of the eye and forms an image on the retina. Transparent structures of the eye including tear film, cornea, aqueous humor, lens, vitreous humor, which constitute optical system of the eye, focus the light onto light-sensitive layer of the retina. The retina converts light impulses into neural impulses, which travel along the optic nerve to reach the visual cortex that processes the visual impulses and enables us to see.

Optical System

Optical system of the eye includes:

1. Tear film is the liquid layer covering the cornea and conjunctiva. It is also called precorneal film or preocular film. It provides a smooth optical refractive surface for the light rays entering the eye.
2. Cornea is the transparent part of the outer fibrous layer and it is the major refractive surface of the eye. The refractive power of the cornea is 44 D, which account for three fourth of the total refractive power of the eye.
3. Aqueous humor is transparent, colorless fluid present in the anterior and posterior chamber of the eye. Being clear and transparent, it forms part of optical medium of eye along with providing essential nutrition and oxygen, and washing away the metabolic waste products from avascular structures of the eye such as cornea, lens and anterior vitreous.
4. Lens is transparent structure situated between the iris and vitreous forming the second major refractive surface of the eye with refractive power of 16 D.
5. Vitreous humor is an inert, transparent, gel-like structure situated between the lens and the retina accounting for 75–80% of the entire volume of the eye with a volume of 4.5 mL. Being transparent, it forms part of refractive media of the eye (Table 1.4.1).

TABLE 1.4.1: Refractive indices and refractive powers

Optical system of the eye	*Refractive index*	*Refractive power*
Tear film	1.35	
Cornea	1.37	44 D*
Aqueous humor	1.33	
Lens	1.39	16 D
Vitreous humor	1.33	

*D, diopter

Retina and Visual Pathway**

1. The photoreceptors including rods and cones are the end organs of vision. Rods are situated in the periphery and are basically responsible for night and peripheral vision. Cones are situated in the center of the retina and are responsible for central and day vision.
2. The visual impulses from rods and cones relay in bipolar cells, which represent first-order neuron of the visual pathway.
3. The visual impulses from first-order neuron are passed onto the ganglion cells, second-order neuron of the visual pathway.
4. The axons of second-order neurons pass through the optic disk to form optic nerve. The axons come out of the globe through lamina cribrosa of sclera, situated in the posterior part of the globe in the retrobulbar space. The axons become myelinated once they come out of the globe and form the optic nerve.
5. Optic nerve passes through the optic canal and enters the cranial cavity. The optic nerves from right and left sides join together above the body of the sphenoid bone to form the optic chiasm.
6. In optic chiasm, axons of the nasal part of the retina from both sides decussate and crossover to the opposite side, whereas axons from the temporal part of retina continue on the same side and continue as optic tract. As a result of crossing of nasal fibers and uncrossing of temporal fibers from both sides, the right side optic tract consists of nasal fibers of left eye and temporal fibers of right eye, and the left side optic tract consists of nasal fibers of right eye and temporal fibers of left eye.
7. The optic tract of each side terminates in lateral geniculate body of corresponding side respectively. Lateral geniculate body represents third-order neuron of the visual pathway. Few axons from the optic tract end in superior colliculi and the pretectal area, which represent the afferent limb of the pupillary light reflex and responsible for light reflex.
8. Lateral geniculate body, the third-order neuron of visual pathway, gives rise to optic radiations, which terminate the visual areas of occipital cortex.
9. Optic radiations representing the superior visual field run in the temporal lobe and those representing the inferior visual field run in the parietal lobe to reach the visual cortex.
10. Primary visual cortex has representation from the contralateral visual hemifield. The central foveal region is represented in posterior part and the peripheral regions are represented in anterior part. The fovea has over-representation in the visual cortex (fovea, which accounts for 0.01% of retina has representation occupying about 8% of the visual cortex) because of high density of ganglion cell in the fovea.

Rods and cones are the end organs of vision. Retina consists of about 120 million rods and 6 million cones.

A rod cell has low-activation threshold and responds to single quantum or photon of light, hence responsible for night vision or scotopic vision. However, as many rod cells converge onto a single second-order neuron, the acuity of rod vision is less when compared to cone cells, where each cone cell connects with a single second-order neuron. A cone cell has high-activation threshold, hence responsible for day vision or photopic vision.

Cones are present in highest density in fovea, the center of the retina and are responsible for central vision and rods, which are situated in the periphery of retina, are responsible for peripheral vision.

PHYSIOLOGY OF VISION

Physiology of vision includes the processes by which the light impulses focused onto the retina are converted into electrical signals or neural impulses, which travel along the visual pathway to the visual cortex.

Rods and cones are the end of vision and they contain pigments called visual pigments. Light rays in the visible spectrum falling on rods and cones initiate photochemical changes called phototransduction.

Rhodopsin Cycle*

The rhodopsin cycle consists of photodecomposition of rhodopsin and its regeneration. The visual pigment, rhodopsin consists of a protein peptide 'opsin' along with 11-cis-retinal, the aldehyde of vitamin A. The light falling on the rods results in conversion of 11-cis-retinal to all-trans-retinal, which gets dissociated from opsin. This process of conversion of 11-cis-retinal to all-trans-retinal is called photodecomposition or bleaching.

The all-trans-retinal is converted into all-trans-retinol and transported to retinal pigment epithelial cell. The all-trans-retinol is converted back to 11-cis-retinal from vitamin A in the retinal pigment epithelium cells and again transported back into the outer segment of rod cells. In the outer segment of the rod cells, 11-cis-retinal unites with opsin to form the rhodopsin. This process of photodecomposition and regeneration of rhodopsin is called rhodopsin cycle.

Vitamin A is stored in retinal pigment epithelium. It is converted into all-trans-retinal, which in turn is converted into 11-cis-retinal by enzyme isomerase. Hence, the deficiency of vitamin A leads to night blindness.

Compared to the rhodopsin cycle, which occurs in rods, the changes that occur in cones are poorly understood. Cones may depend on enzymes within the cones and the Müller's cells for regeneration of the visual pigment.

The photochemical reactions occurring in rods and cones convert the light impulses into electrical impulses; the photochemical reactions are initiated by metarhodopsin II. Metarhodopsin II activated rhodopsin results in decreased cyclic guanosine monophosphate (GMP) in the photoreceptor resulting in hyperpolarization and genesis of electrical impulse.

The visual impulse is transmitted to the ganglion cells via horizontal cells, amacrine cells and bipolar cells as electrical impulse.

The bipolar cells are the first-order neurons of the visual pathway and depending on the response they can be on bipolar cells or off bipolar cells. The on bipolar cells depolarize and respond positively, thereby stimulating the ganglion cells; whereas the off bipolar cells hyperpolarize and respond negatively, thereby inhibiting the ganglion cells. The off cells enhance the visual contrast along with the horizontal cells.

The ganglion cells are the second-order neurons of the visual pathway and they transmit visual impulse as action potentials. The visual information from retina to visual cortex flows as two parallel streams as magnocellular (M) and parvocellular (P) pathway. The 'M' pathway is formed by 'M' ganglion cells and carries visual information regarding movement of image in the visual field and gross analysis of the image. The 'P' pathway is formed by 'P' cells and carries visual information regarding the fine details of the image and color vision.

The axons of the second-order neurons pass through the optic disk to form the optic nerve. The optic nerves from right and left sides join together to form the optic chiasm. In optic chiasm, the axons of nasal part of retina from both sides decussate and crossover to the opposite side, whereas the axons from the temporal part of the retina continue on the same side and continue as optic tract. The optic tract of each side terminates in lateral geniculate body of each side respectively. Few axons from the optic tract end in superior colliculi and the pretectal area, which represent the afferent limb of the pupillary light reflex and responsible for light reflex.

Lateral geniculate body represents third-order neuron of the visual pathway. It consists of six layers, with layers one and two receiving visual information from magnocellular pathway and the remaining from three to six layers receiving visual information from parvocellular pathway.

The optic radiations arising from the lateral geniculate body terminate in the visual cortex. Analysis of the visual information takes place in the visual cortex. The visual cortex is divided into primary visual cortex called Brodmann's area 17 and secondary visual cortex called Brodmann's area 18 and 19. The secondary visual cortex is the visual association area responsible for identifying complex perception of shape and forms of the objects. The light entering the eye elicits four different types of sensations in the visual cortex.

Light sense: It represents the ability to appreciate light of different intensities because of visual adaptation, which includes dark adaptation and light adaptation.

Dark adaptation: It is the ability to appreciate light of low intensity or to see in dark. Rods are responsible for dark adaptation. The normal dark adaptation time is about 20 minutes.

Light adaptation: It is brought by cones. The normal light adaptation time is about 5 minutes.

Humans have low night vision compared to nocturnal animals, e.g. cats, owls. Some nocturnal animals exhibit the presence of a cellular layer behind the retina called tapetum lucidum, which reflects the light back into the retina making the eyes of these animals to glow in night.

Form sense: It represents ability to distinguish the shape of the objects. The measurement of ability to distinguish the shape of the objects is called visual acuity. Visual acuity is a measure of central vision and hence it is a function of the cones. It is highest in the fovea, where the cones are found in highest density.

The hunting carnivore animals including human beings have a specialized part of the retina called fovea. Fovea is characterized by the presence of tightly packed cone cells and absence of rods and other layers of retina except the internal limiting membrane. This arrangement in fovea gives it high acuity because of absence of the layers of the retina, which would interfere with the optics.

Unlike human beings, the birds belonging to raptor species, e.g. eagles, have two foveae in each eye and hence have better acuity of vision than human beings.

Contrast sense: It is the ability to distinguish the changes in the luminance level. Contrast sensitivity is decreased in the diseases of the eye such as cataract, glaucoma, optic nerve diseases, refractive errors and diabetic retinopathy.

Color sense: It is the ability to distinguish different colors. Humans have trichromatic color vision, the ability to identify colors by three primary wavelengths.

Theories of Color Vision**

Trichromatic theory: It was proposed by Young-Helmholtz and states that color vision is because of presence of three different kinds of cones, 'L' cones absorbing red light (565 nm), 'M' cones absorbing green light (545 nm) and 'S' cones absorbing blue light (440 nm) and the remaining colors are produced by mixture of the primary colors such as red, green and blue.

Opponent theory: It was proposed by Ewald-Hering and states that the three opposing color pairs are formed because of linking together of the cones. The three opposing color pairs are blue-yellow, red-green and black-white color. The excitation of one member of the pair inhibits activity of the other.

Modern opponent theory or stage theory: This theory involves both the trichromatic theory and opponent theory in two stages. The first stage is similar to the trichromatic theory and states the presence of three different kinds of cones. The second stage includes the opponent theory and states the linking together of the cones into opponent signals.

GIST BOX 1.4

- Eye is the organ of vision.
- Light travels through the transparent optical medium of eye and forms image on retina. The transparent structures of eye including tear film, cornea, aqueous humor, lens, vitreous humor, which constitute optical system of eye focus light onto the light-sensitive layer of the retina.
- The retina converts light impulses into neural impulses, which travel along the optic nerve to reach the visual cortex that processes the visual impulses and enables us to see.

FREQUENTLY ASKED QUESTIONS (FAQs)

*Short Answers

1. Mention the layers of the eye.
2. Mention the blood supply of eye.
3. Dimensions of the adult human eye.
4. Rhodopsin cycle.
5. Anophthalmos.
6. Microphthalmos.
7. Megalophthalmos.

**Short Essays

1. Embryology of human eye.
2. Visual pathway.
3. Theories of color vision.

BIBLIOGRAPHY

1. Daw N. How Vision Works: The Physiological Mechanisms Behind What We See. New York: Oxford University Press; 2012.
2. Garzozi HJ, Barkay S. Case of true cyclopia. Br J Ophthalmol. 1985;69(4):307-11.
3. Gupta P, Malik KP, Goel R. Congenital cystic eye with multiple dermal appendages: a case report. BMC Ophthalmol. 2003;3:7.
4. Koregol MC, Bellad MB, Nilgar BR, et al. Cyclopia with shoulder dystocia leading to an obstetric catastrophe: a case report. J Med Case Rep. 2010;4:160.
5. Kumar R. Textbook of Human Embryology. New Delhi: IK International (P) Ltd.
6. Maria DL, Srivastava SK, Sankholkar PS. Bilateral congenital anophthalmos (a case report). J All India Ophthalmol Soc. 1967;15(6):241-2.
7. Purves D, Augustine GJ, Fitzpatrick D, et al. Neuroscience, 2nd edition. Sunderland (MA): Sinauer Associates; 2001.
8. Steven WS. The Scientist and Engineer's Guide to Digital Signal Processing.
9. Tsai CK, Lai I, Kuo HK, et al. Anterior megalophthalmos. Chang Gung Med J. 2005;28(3):191-5.
10. Tsitouridis I, Michaelides M, Tsantiridis C, et al. Congenital cystic eye with multiple dermal appendages and intracranial congenital anomalies. Diagn Interv Radiol. 2010;16(2):116-21.

SECTION 2

Eyelids

2.1 Anatomy of Eyelids
2.2 Congenital Anomalies of Eyelids
2.3 Diseases of Eyelid Margin and Eyelashes
2.4 Inflammations and Infections of Eyelids
2.5 Diseases of Eyelid Position and Movement
2.6 Tumors of Eyelids

CHAPTER

2.1 Anatomy of Eyelids

DEFINITION

Eyelids are defined as the mobile skin folds that cover the eye.

FUNCTIONS OF EYELIDS

- Protect anterior surface of eye from injury
- Spread the tear film over the cornea during blinking
- Take part in tear film drainage by acting over the lacrimal pump.

SURFACE ANATOMY

Each eye has got an upper eyelid and lower eyelid. The upper eyelid extends superiorly to the eyebrow and the lower lid extends inferiorly to join skin of the cheek. Both eyelids end as eyelid margin bearing a row of eyelashes.

Palpebral aperture is the elliptical space between the upper and lower eyelid. Palpebral aperture measures vertically about 10 mm and horizontally about 30 mm. Upper and lower eyelids meet medially at medial canthus and laterally at lateral canthus. The upper eyelid has a skin crease formed by insertion of fibers of levator aponeurosis.

The eyelid margin is a 2 mm broad strip and it is divided into a lacrimal portion and ciliary portion. The lacrimal portion does not have eyelashes and glands. The ciliary portion consists of a posterior border and anterior border. The intermarginal area between the anterior and posterior borders of the lid is divided by gray line into posterior part on which meibomian glands open and anterior part bearing eyelashes. Gray line is used as a reference point during surgical procedures to split the lid.

Normally upper eyelid covers 2 mm of cornea and lower eyelid touches the inferior limbus when the eye is open in primary position (Fig. 2.1.1).

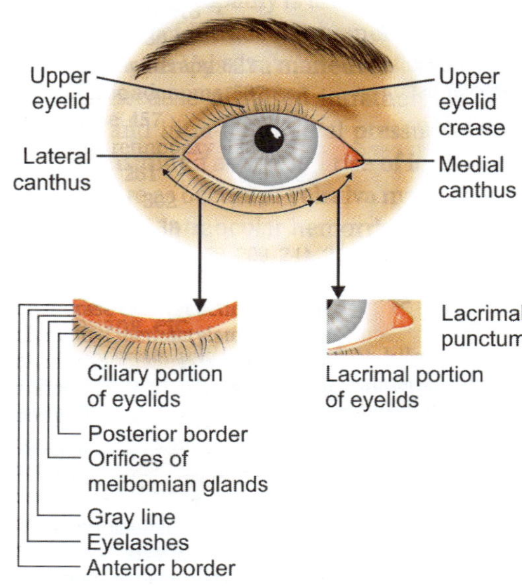

FIG. 2.1.1: Surface anatomy of eyelids (*Note:* Absence of meibomian glands and eyelashes).

GROSS ANATOMY

Layers of Eyelid (Figs 2.1.2 and 2.1.3*)

- Skin
- Subcutaneous tissue
- Striated muscle layer
- Submuscular connective tissue
- Fibrous tissue layer
- Smooth muscle layer
- Conjunctiva.

Skin is the outermost layer of the eyelids and it is the thinnest layer in the body. It does not have a subcutaneous fatty layer.

Layer of loose subcutaneous tissue lies below the skin and it gets distended easily by blood in case of injuries to head, and by fluid in cardiac failure, which presents as puffiness of face.

Striated muscle layer consists of orbicularis oculi. In addition to it levator palpebrae superioris (LPS) is the other striated muscle, which is present only in the upper eyelid.

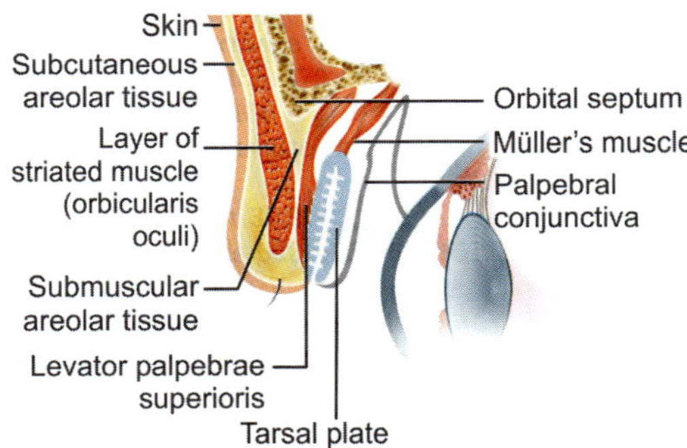

FIG. 2.1.2: Structure of upper eyelid

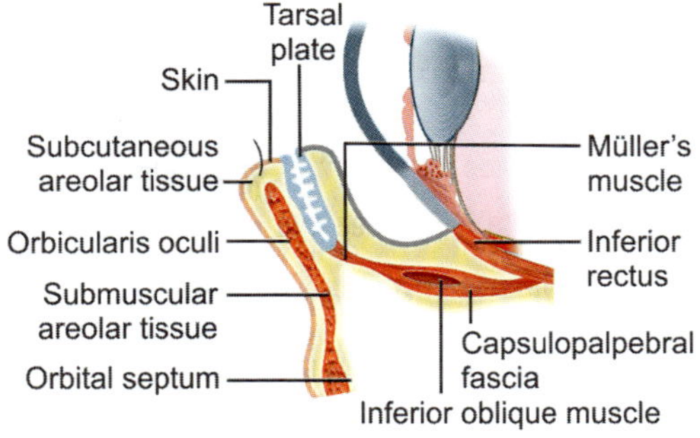

FIG. 2.1.3: Structure of lower eyelid

Submuscular areolar tissue lies between the orbicularis oculi and fibrous layer. Nerves and vessels of lid lie in this layer.

Fibrous tissue layer consists of central thick tarsal, peripheral thin septum orbitale, medial and lateral palpebral ligaments formed by tarsal plate. Tarsal plates give firmness to eyelids and they contain meibomian glands or tarsal glands.

Smooth muscle layer consists of Müller's muscle.

Palpebral conjunctiva lines the inner surface of the eyelids.

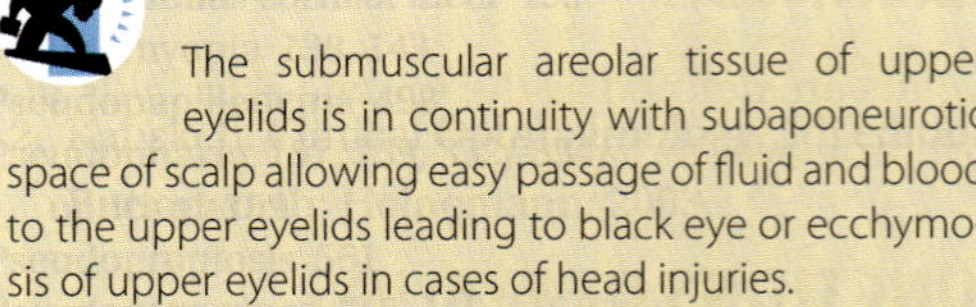

The submuscular areolar tissue of upper eyelids is in continuity with subaponeurotic space of scalp allowing easy passage of fluid and blood to the upper eyelids leading to black eye or ecchymosis of upper eyelids in cases of head injuries.

Since, the nerves supplying the eyelids lie in submuscular areolar tissue, anesthesia for surgeries of eyelids is given in this plane.

Blood Supply

The eyelids are supplied by medial and lateral palpebral arteries, which are branches of dorsal nasal, and lacrimal arteries. The venous drainage is posteriorly into cavernous sinus through ophthalmic veins and anteriorly venous drainage reaches facial, and superficial temporal veins.

Lymphatic Drainage

These are arranged in two sets pre- and post-tarsal. Lateral half drains into preauricular lymph nodes and medial half drains into submandibular lymph nodes.

Nerve Supply

Sensory nerve supply is branches of trigeminal nerve. Upper eyelid is innervated by superior trochlear, supraorbital and lacrimal nerves. Lower eyelid is supplied by infraorbital nerve.

Motor nerve supply is by oculomotor nerve, facial nerve and sympathetic innervations.

GLANDS OF EYELIDS (Fig. 2.1.4)*

Meibomian Glands

They are modified sebaceous glands located in the tarsal plate. They secrete meibum (lipids), which forms the lipid layer of tear film.

Glands of Zeis

They are modified sebaceous glands, which open into the follicles of the eyelashes.

Glands of Moll

They are modified sweat glands that open into the follicles of eyelashes.

Sebaceous Glands

They are present in caruncle and in the hairs of the eyebrows.

Wolfring Glands

These are accessory lacrimal glands situated in the tarsal conjunctiva.

MUSCLES OF EYELIDS (Fig. 2.1.5)*

Orbicularis Oculi

Origin: Nasal part of frontal bone, frontal process of maxillary bone and medial palpebral ligament.

Insertion: By three parts, orbital portion is inserted into skin that encircles eye, palpebral part into eyelids and lacrimal part into lacrimal sac.

Actions: Orbital part causes voluntary closure of the eyelids and palpebral part causes involuntary blinking of eyelids. Lacrimal part is called Horner's muscle that takes part in lacrimal tear drainage.

Nerve supply: Branches of facial nerve.

Paralysis of facial nerve causes lagophthalmos (inability to close eyelids), because of affection of orbicularis oculi.

Levator Palpebrae Superioris

The LPS is present only in upper eyelid.

Origin: At the apex of the orbit above the annulus of Zinn.

Insertion: Inserted into the skin of lid, anterior surface of the tarsal plate and conjunctiva of superior fornix.

Actions: Elevation of upper eyelid.

Nerve supply: Oculomotor nerve.

Paralysis of oculomotor nerve causes ptosis because of affection of LPS.

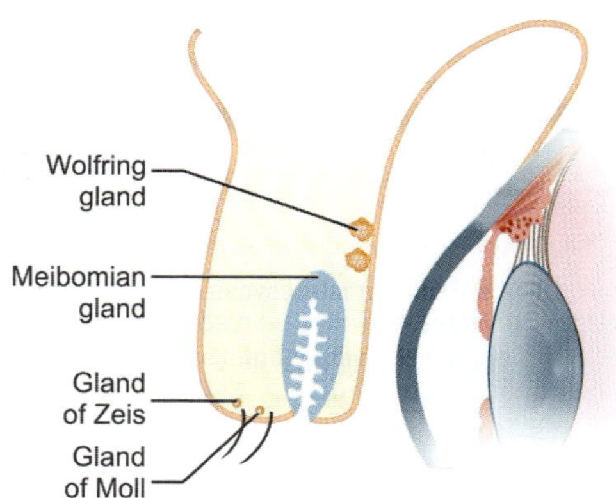

FIG. 2.1.4: Glands of eyelid

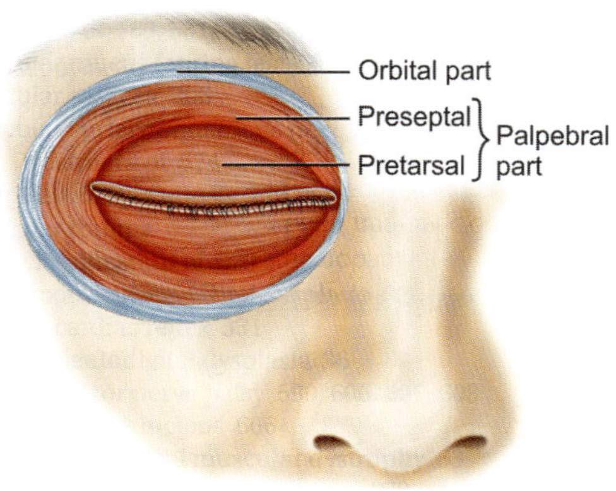

FIG. 2.1.5: Orbicularis oculi

Müller's Muscle

Müller's muscle is a smooth muscle present in both upper and lower eyelids with opposite actions in upper and lower eyelids.

Origin: It arises from LPS muscle fibers in upper eyelid and from inferior rectus muscle in lower eyelid.

Insertion: Inserted into tarsal plate.

Actions: In upper eyelid it causes elevation of upper eyelid and in lower eyelid it causes retraction of lower eyelid.

Nerve supply: Sympathetic nerves.

Paralysis of sympathetic nerve supply as in Horner's syndrome causes ptosis in upper eyelids and inverse ptosis in lower eyelids.

RETRACTORS OF EYELIDS

1. The levator aponeurosis complex is called superior transverse ligament or Whitnall's ligament and Müller's muscle are retractors for upper eyelid.
2. Capsulopalpebral fascia, which is the extension of inferior rectus muscle is called inferior transverse ligament or Lockwood's ligament and Müller's muscle are retractors for lower eyelid.

Capsulopalpebral fascia: It is the retractor of the lower eyelid and it is analogous to levator aponeurosis complex of the upper eyelid. It arises from inferior rectus and it divides into two divisions to enclose inferior oblique muscle. After enclosing inferior oblique muscle the two divisions fuse to form Lockwood's ligament and inserts into inferior border of tarsal plate.

GIST BOX 2.1

- Eyelids are the mobile skin folds that cover the eye. Each eye has got an upper eyelid and lower eyelid.
- The upper eyelid extends superiorly to the eyebrow and the lower lid extends inferiorly to join skin of the cheek. Both eyelids end as eyelid margin bearing a row of eyelashes.
- Upper and lower eyelids meet medially at medial canthus and laterally at lateral canthus.
- Layers of eyelid: Skin, subcutaneous tissue, striated muscle layer, submuscular connective tissue, fibrous tissue layer, smooth muscle layer and palpebral conjunctiva.
- Glands of eyelids: Meibomian glands, glands of Zeis, glands of Moll, sebaceous glands and Wolfring glands.
- Muscles of eyelids: Orbicularis oculi and Müller's muscle are present in both upper and lower eyelid, whereas levator palpebrae superioris is present only in upper eyelid.

CHAPTER

2.2 Congenital Anomalies of Eyelid

EMBRYOLOGY

The development of eyelids starts at 7th week of gestation. Lateral and medial frontonasal processes form the upper eyelid. Frontal and maxillary processes form the lower eyelid. The two lid folds fuse at 9th week of gestation. These two get separated by 5th month of gestation leading to the formation of palpebral aperture enclosed between upper and lower eyelids.

Congenital anomalies of the eyelid occur between 2nd and 5th month of gestation because of failure of fusion of the lid folds during 2nd month or due to failure of separation of the lid folds during the 5th month of gestation or because of arrest in the development of the muscles of the eyelid during this period.

In all cases evaluation should be done to find out the presence of systemic anomalies or syndromes. Most cases require plastic reconstruction of the eyelids. Visual prognosis depends on the associated ocular features.

CRYPTOPHTHALMOS*

Cryptophthalmos is a rare congenital anomaly resulting from failure of eyelid formation. It is characterized by the presence of continuous sheet of skin covering the eyeball extending from forehead to cheek (Fig. 2.2.1).

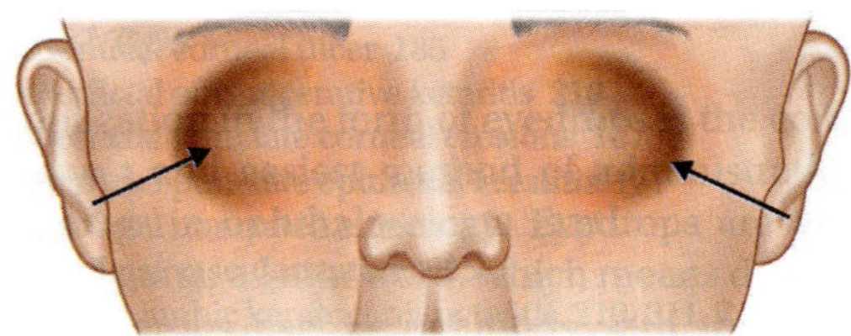

FIG. 2.2.1: Cryptophthalmos (*Note:* Absence of eyelids and presence of continuous sheet of skin extending from head to cheek).

Types of Cryptophthalmos

Complete cryptophthalmos is associated with malformed eyeball with anterior segment agenesis, hence no visual prognosis is present following reconstruction of the eyelids.

Incomplete cryptophthalmos is associated with normal eyeball, hence visual prognosis is better following plastic eyelid reconstruction.

> *Cryptophthalmos syndrome (Fraser syndrome):* Autosomal recessive syndrome characterized by cryptophthalmos associated with syndactyly and genital malformations.

CONGENITAL LID COLOBOMA

Congenital lid coloboma is a congenital anomaly characterized by full thickness defect of the eyelid resulting from failure of fusion of lateral and medial frontonasal processes in the upper eyelid, frontal and maxillary process in the lower eyelid (Fig. 2.2.2).

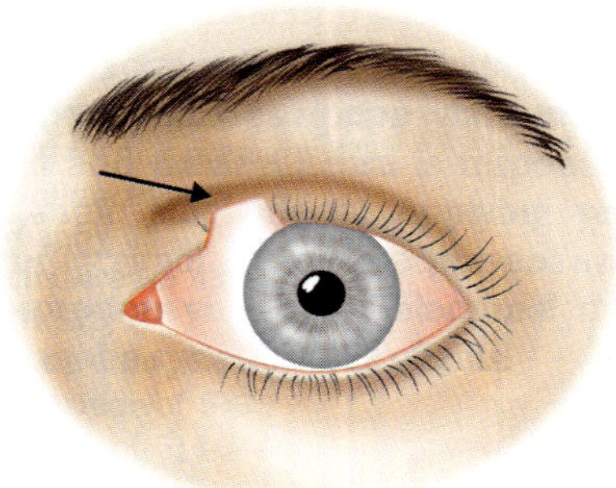

FIG. 2.2.2: Lid coloboma (*Note:* Full thickness defect of the upper eyelid).

Goldenhar syndrome: It is a rare congenital syndrome in which congenital lid coloboma is associated with vertebral column anomalies, preauricular skin tags and limbal dermoid.

Treacher Collins syndrome: It is a congenital syndrome in which lid coloboma is associated with hypoplasia of malar bones.

EPICANTHUS

Bilaterally symmetrical vertical fold of skin covering the medial canthus with concavity laterally is called epicanthus. It is normal in oriental race, in others it is normally seen in newborns, which disappears by the age of 2 years as the nasal bone develops. It causes pseudoesotropia or apparent convergent squint (Fig. 2.2.3).

Prominent epicanthus is seen in infants with Down syndrome.

TELECANTHUS

Telecanthus is a congenital condition in which the distance between two medial canthi is more because of abnormally long medial canthal tendons.

BLEPHAROPHIMOSIS

Blepharophimosis is a congenital condition characterized by the presence of small palpebral aperture (Fig. 2.2.4).

Blepharophimosis Syndrome

Blepharophimosis found in association with telecanthus, epicanthus and ptosis is called blepharophimosis syndrome.

EURYBLEPHARON

Euryblepharon is a condition characterized by elongated horizontal palpebral fissure width

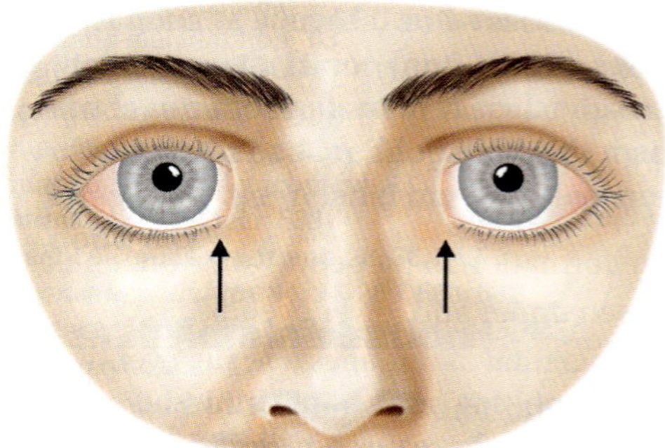

FIG. 2.2.3: Epicanthus (*Note:* Vertical fold of skin covering the medial canthus).

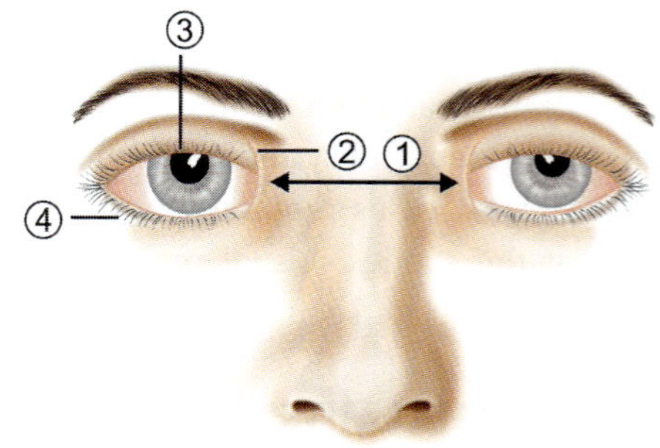

FIG. 2.2.4: Blepharophimosis syndrome (1, telecanthus—increased distance between two medial canthi; 2, epicanthus; 3, ptosis; 4, blepharophimosis).

because of increased horizontal eye length and decreased vertical eyelid skin leading to the appearance of ectropion (Fig. 2.2.5).

EPIBLEPHARON

Epiblepharon is a congenital disorder commonly seen in Mongoloid population characterized by the presence of abnormal horizontal fold of skin near medial canthus leading to misdirection of the eyelashes directed toward the globe. Treatment is by wedge excision of the horizontal fold of skin (Fig. 2.2.6).

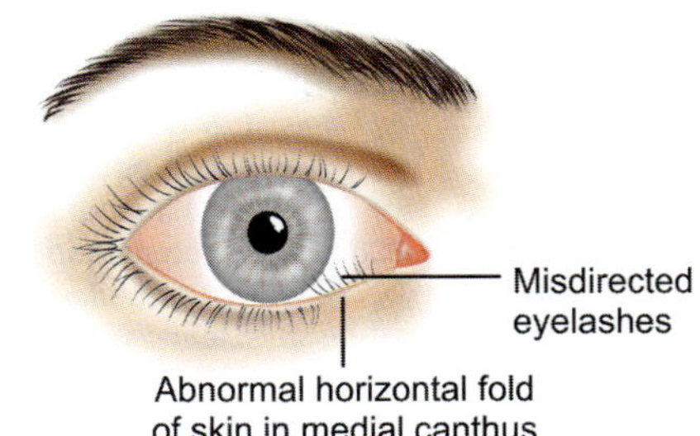

FIG. 2.2.6: Epiblepharon

DISTICHIASIS*

Distichiasis is a rare congenital disorder characterized by the presence of a posterior row of eyelashes directed toward the globe. The posterior rows of eyelashes arise abnormally from meibomian glands. Clinical features and treatment are similar to trichiasis (Fig. 2.2.7).

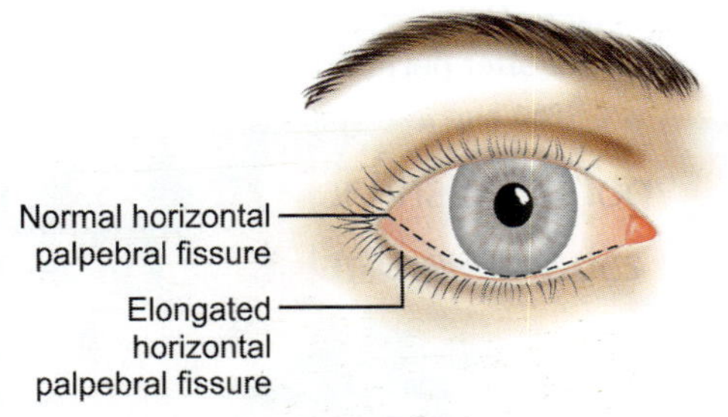

FIG. 2.2.5: Euryblepharon

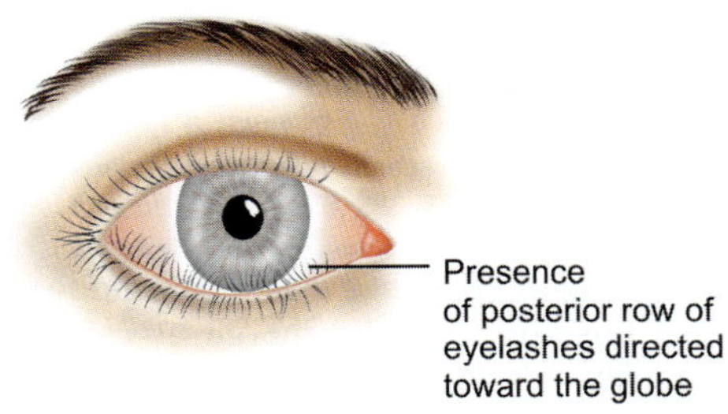

FIG. 2.2.7: Distichiasis

Congenital ectropion, congenital entropion and congenital ptosis are discussed in the respective chapters.

GIST BOX 2.2

- Congenital anomalies of the eyelid occur between 2nd and 5th month of gestation; because, failure of fusion of the lid folds during 2nd month, due to failure of separation of the lid folds during the 5th month of gestation or because of arrest in the development of the muscles of the eyelid during this period.
- Cryptophthalmos is a rare congenital anomaly resulting from failure of eyelid formation. It is characterized by the presence of continuous sheet of skin covering the eyeball extending from forehead to cheek.
- Congenital lid coloboma, epicanthus, blepharophimosis, euryblepharon, epiblepharon, distichiasis are the common congenital anomalies seen in eyelids.

CHAPTER

2.3 Diseases of Eyelid Margin and Eyelashes

TRICHIASIS**

Definition

Misdirection of eyelashes toward the globe with normal position of eyelid margin is called trichiasis (Figs 2.3.1A and B, Fig. 2.3.2).

Etiology

1. Congenital causes are distichiasis and epiblepharon.
2. Acquired causes are the diseases of eyelids, which lead to scarring such as ulcerative blepharitis, trachoma, hordeolum externum, Steven-Johnson syndrome, ocular cicatricial pemphigoid, thermal and chemical burns, post-traumatic or post-surgical scars.

Clinical Features

Symptoms: Foreign body sensation, watering because of rubbing of the eyelashes against conjunctiva or cornea.

Signs: Examination shows one or more eyelashes, which are misdirected and rubbing against the globe. Superficial corneal opacities with superficial corneal vascularization and recurrent corneal erosions may be seen.

Differential Diagnosis

- Distichiasis
- Epiblepharon
- Pseudotrichiasis.

Treatment

1. Removal of the misdirected eyelashes by epilation. Epilation is usually temporary procedure and the eyelash will grow back again.
2. Destruction of the misdirected eyelashes by electrolysis, cryosurgery or laser ablation will offer permanent treatment.

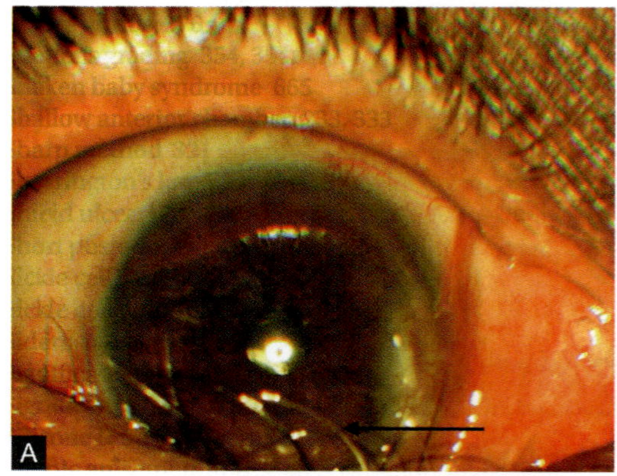

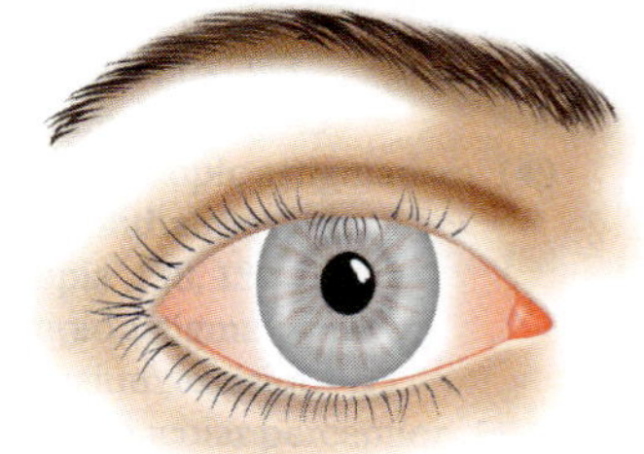

FIGS 2.3.1A and B: Trichiasis. **A.** Inward misdirection of eyelashes of lower eyelid with normal position of eyelid margin; **B.** Inward misdirection of eyelashes of upper eyelid with normal position of eyelid margin.

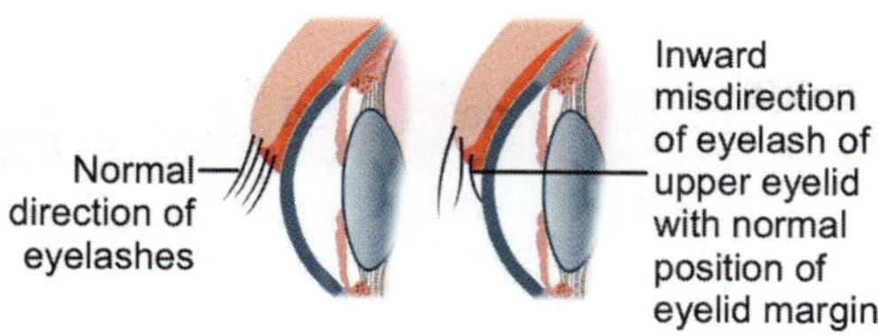

FIG. 2.3.2: Trichiasis—cross section view

3. Full thickness wedge resection of the lid segment is required, if the trichiasis is excessive involving more than half length of the lid margin.

*Distichiasis**: It is a rare congenital disorder characterized by the presence of a posterior row of eyelashes directed toward the globe. The posterior rows of eyelashes arise abnormally from meibomian glands. Clinical features and treatment is similar to trichiasis.

Epiblepharon: It is a congenital disorder commonly seen in Mongoloid population characterized by the presence of abnormal horizontal fold of skin near medial canthus leading to misdirection of the eyelashes directed toward the globe. Treatment is by wedge excision of the horizontal fold of skin.

*Pseudotrichiasis**: Misdirection of the eyelashes because of abnormal position of eyelid margin as in entropion is called pseudotrichiasis. Treatment is by treating the underlying cause for abnormal lid margin position (e.g. entropion).

ENTROPION**

Definition

Inward turning of the eyelid margin is called entropion (Table 2.3.1).

Etiopathogenesis

Entropion results due to overaction of inward forces (protractors), i.e. orbicularis oculi or due to underaction of outward forces (retractors), i.e. levator aponeurosis complex in upper eyelid and capsulopalpebral fascia in lower eyelid acting on the eyelids.

Hence, treatment requires weakening of overacting muscles or strengthening the underacting lid retractors.

Clinical Types of Entropion*

Congenital Entropion

Congenital entropion is due to disinsertion of lid retractors or weak tarsal plate or because of hypertrophy of orbicularis oculi. It usually affects lower eyelid.

*Senile Entropion**

Senile entropion is due to weakening or dehiscence of lid retractors, horizontal lid laxity and overriding of the preseptal orbicularis. It usually affects lower eyelid (Figs 2.3.3A and B, Fig. 2.3.4).

Clinical Tests in Senile Entropion

Senile entropion is the most common form of entropion and it usually affects the lower eyelid, whereas cicatricial entropion usually affects the upper eyelid.

Clinical tests in senile entropion is done to find out the underlying cause:

- Pinch test and snap test: The skin of the lower eyelid can be pulled out by more than 1 cm and when the pulled out skin of the eyelid is released it will take some time to go back to its position indicating lid laxity.
- Dehiscence of lower lid retractors is identified by the presence of deep inferior fornix, a white subconjunctival line in the inferior fornix caused by the detached retractors and little or no movement of the lower eyelid on down gaze.

Spastic Entropion

Spastic entropion is due to spasm of orbicularis oculi due to ocular irritation caused by chronic irritative conditions of conjunctiva or cornea.

Cicatricial Entropion

Cicatricial entropion is due to cicatricial contracture of palpebral conjunctiva and tarsal plate because of scarring and fibrosis seen in conditions such as trachoma, Steven-Johnson syndrome, chemical injuries, and ocular cicatricial pemphigoid.

TABLE 2.3.1: Comparison between ectropion and entropion

Features	*Entropion*	*Ectropion*
Definition	Inward turning of the eyelid margin	Outward turning of the eyelid margin
Symptoms	Symptoms are because of pseudotrichiasis	Symptoms are because of epiphora
Pathogenesis	Entropion results due to overaction orbicularis oculi or due to underaction of levator aponeurosis complex in upper eyelid and capsulopalpebral fascia in lower eyelid	Ectropion results due to underaction of orbicularis oculi
Congenital	Usually affects lower eyelid caused by disinsertion of lower lid retractors; it is treated by tucking of the lid retractors and reconstruction of lid crease	Caused by shortening of skin of the eyelid and it is treated by skin grafting, and reconstruction of the eyelid
Senile	It is due to weakening or dehiscence of lid retractors, horizontal lid laxity and overriding of the preseptal orbicularis	It occurs due to age-related laxity of the eyelid tissues associated with loss of tone of orbicularis oculi muscle
Cicatricial	Cicatricial entropion is caused by scarring and fibrosis of palpebral conjunctiva, and tarsal plate	Cicatricial ectropion is caused by scarring of skin of the eyelid
Mechanical	Mechanical entropion is seen in conditions in which posterior globe support to eyelids is absent, e.g. enophthalmos, phthisis bulbi	Mechanical ectropion is seen in conditions in which the eyelids are pushed out by conjunctival mass or by proptosis

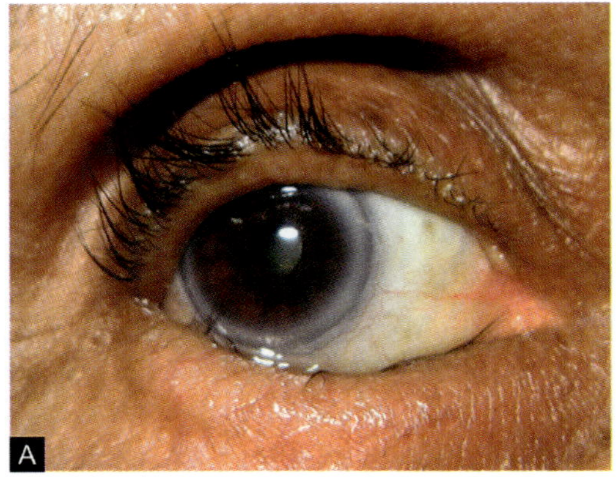

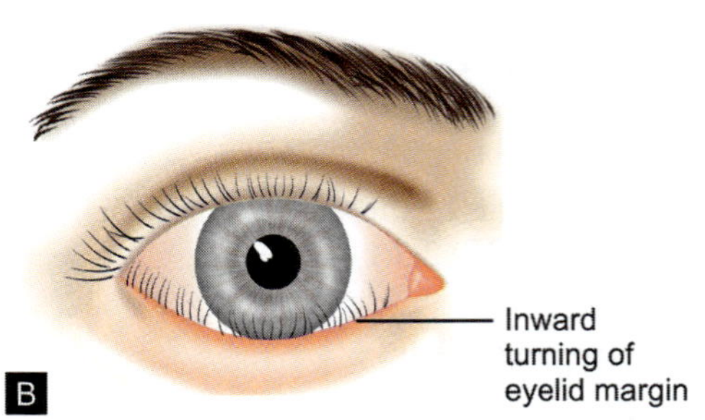

FIGS 2.3.3A and B: Entropion. **A.** Photograph; **B.** Diagrammatic representation.

Mechanical Entropion

Mechanical entropion is seen in conditions such as enophthalmos and phthisis bulbi. This type of entropion is due to lack of support to the lids given by the globe.

Symptoms

Symptoms are due to pseudotrichiasis, because of rubbing of the eyelashes against conjunctiva or cornea and they are similar to trichiasis. For example, foreign body sensation, watering.

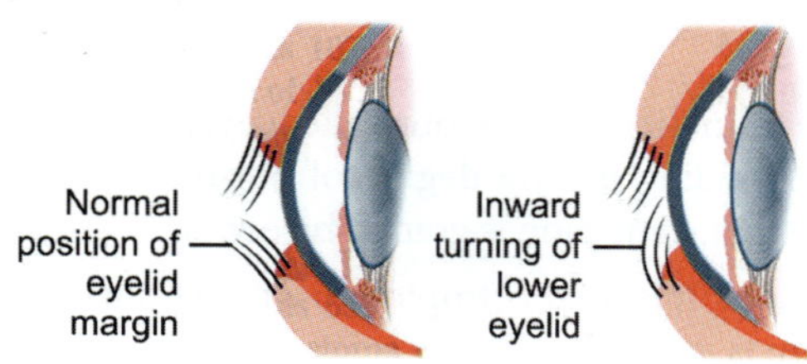

FIG. 2.3.4: Entropion—cross section view

Signs

Examination shows pseudotrichiasis, i.e. misdirected eyelashes within rolled eyelid margin. Depending on the degree of in rolled eyelid margin entropion is graded below.

Grade I: It is mild entropion in which only posterior lid border is in rolled.

Grade II: It is moderate entropion in which posterior lid border and intermarginal strip are in rolled.

Grade III: It is severe entropion in which posterior lid border, intermarginal strip and anterior lid border are in rolled.

Treatment*

1. Congenital entropion is treated by tucking of the lid retractors and reconstruction of lid crease, if required.
2. Senile entropion is treated by:
   a. Horizontal lid shortening in cases with horizontal lid laxity by excision of full thickness trapezoid area of lid at the lateral canthus.
   b. Severe cases are treated by strengthening of the lid retractors by plication or tucking called Jones operation.
   c. In patients with significant overriding of preseptal orbicularis, orbicularis muscle is cut in the center and the two flaps of the muscle are overlapped, and sutured to the lower border of the tarsal plate called modified Wheeler's procedure (orbicularis bracing).
   d. In old debilitated patients lid everting sutures are used as temporary procedure called Quickert procedure.
   e. Spastic entropion is treated by treatment of the underlying disease causing irritation of the conjunctiva or cornea. Some cases may require injection of botulinum toxin into the orbicularis oculi muscle as a temporary procedure.
3. Cicatricial entropion is treated by:
   a. Treating underlying disease causing scarring, fibrosis and surgery is contraindicated during acute phase.
   b. Mild entropion is treated by resection of skin and muscle.
   c. Moderate entropion is treated by resection of skin muscle and tarsal plate.
   d. Severe entropion is treated by replacing the scarred tarsal plate. Tarsoconjunctival graft is used in upper eyelid and sclera graft or autogenous ear cartilage is usually used in lower eyelid.
4. Mechanical entropion is treated by treatment of the underlying cause.

ECTROPION**

Definition

Outward turning of the eyelid margin is called ectropion (Figs 2.3.5A and B, Fig. 2.3.6, and refer Table 2.3.1).

Etiopathogenesis

*Clinical Types of Ectropion**

Congenital ectropion: It is rare condition usually seen in association with congenital anomalies such as blepharophimosis syndrome, Down syndrome. It is usually because of shortening of the skin.

Senile or involutional ectropion: It is the most common type and it affects lower eyelid. It occurs due to age-related laxity of the eyelid tissues associated with loss of tone of orbicularis oculi muscle.

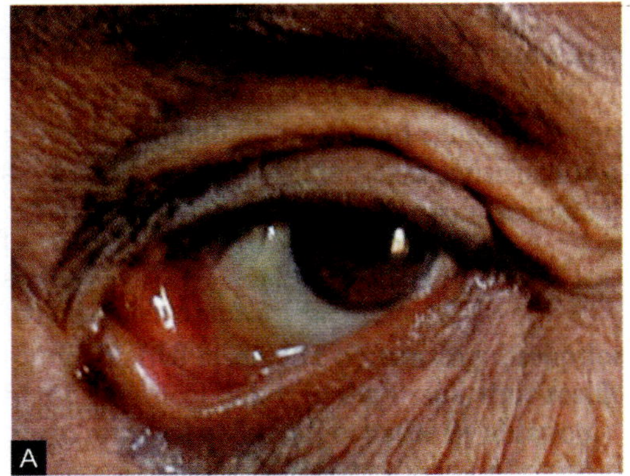

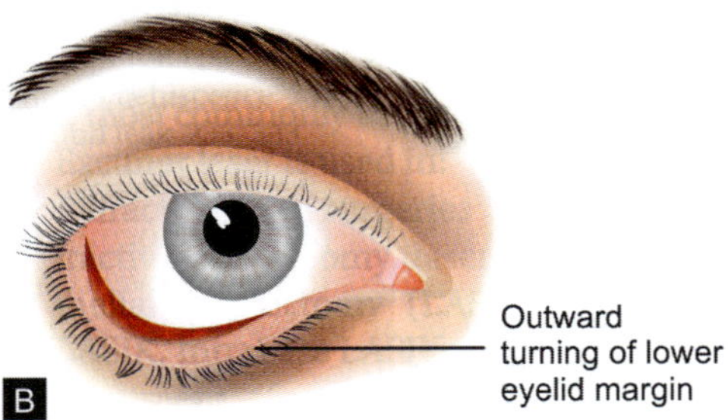

FIGS 2.3.5A and B: Ectropion. **A.** Photograph; **B.** Diagrammatic representation.

Paralytic ectropion: It is seen in paralysis of facial nerve.

Cicatricial ectropion: It is due to scarring of the skin resulting from thermal injuries, chemical injuries, mechanical injuries to the face involving the eyelids and surrounding area.

Mechanical ectropion: It affects lower eyelid in conditions in which the eyelids are pushed out by conjunctival mass or in proptosis.

Symptoms

Symptoms are watering because of disruption of drainage of lacrimal tears because of the eyelid falling away from the globe. Other symptoms include chronic irritation because of long-standing exposure of conjunctiva resulting in chronic conjunctival inflammation and keratinization.

Signs

Examination shows out-rolled eyelid margin. Depending on the degree of out-rolled eyelid margin, ectropion is graded below.

Grade I: It is mild ectropion in which only punctum is everted.

Grade II: It is moderate ectropion in which palpebral conjunctiva is exposed.

Grade III: It is severe ectropion in which conjunctival fornix is exposed.

Treatment

Congenital ectropion is treated by skin grafting and plastic reconstruction of the eyelid.

Senile ectropion is treated by:

1. Mild degree of senile ectropion is treated by tarsoconjunctival resection below the punctum to cause inversion of the punctum.
2. Moderate degree of senile ectropion is treated by horizontal lid shortening.
3. Severe degree of senile ectropion is treated by horizontal lid shortening combined with tarsoconjunctival resection below the punctum to cause inversion of the punctum (Byron smith's modification of Kuhnt-Szymanowski procedure).

Paralytic ectropion is treated by tarsorrhaphy in similar lines as of treatment for lagophthalmos.

Cicatricial ectropion treatment is done once the causative disease is treated and it has led to formation of scar. It is treated by:

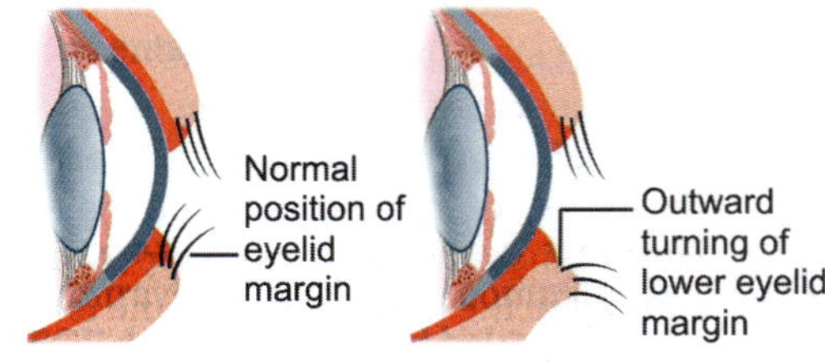

FIG. 2.3.6: Ectropion—cross section view

1. Mild degree of ectropion is treated by excision of the scar and suturing in V-Y pattern (V-Y operation) or by Z-plasty.
2. Severe degree of ectropion requires excision of the scar and skin grafting.

Mechanical ectropion is treated by treatment of the underlying cause.

SYMBLEPHARON**

Definition

Adhesion between palpebral and bulbar conjunctiva (Figs 2.3.7A and B) resulting in adherence of the eyelid to the globe is called symblepharon.

Etiopathogenesis

Chemical burns, cicatricial conjunctivitis such as ocular pemphigoid, Steven-Johnson syndrome involving both palpebral and bulbar conjunctiva simultaneously. Because of healing of raw surfaces on the palpebral and bulbar conjunctiva, adhesions result leading to formation of symblepharon.

Symptoms

Because of adhesions patient will have:

1. Inability to close the eyelids completely leading to exposure of a part of conjunctiva or cornea.
2. Restriction of the eyeball movements leading to diplopia.

Signs

On examination, a fibrous adhesion between the palpebral and bulbar conjunctiva is made out.

Types of Symblepharon

Anterior symblepharon: Adhesion between the bulbar conjunctiva and the palpebral conjunctiva at the eyelid margin.

Posterior symblepharon: Adhesion between the bulbar conjunctiva and the palpebral conjunctiva at the fornix.

Total symblepharon: Adhesion between the bulbar conjunctiva and the palpebral conjunctiva of whole of the eyelid.

Complications

1. Prolonged exposure of conjunctiva will lead to dryness, chronic conjunctivitis and keratinization.
2. Exposure keratitis because of prolonged exposure of cornea.
3. Watering because of epiphora, if symblepharon involves the medial lacrimal portion of the eyelid.

Treatment

1. Excision of the fibrous adhesion and closure of the raw surfaces by conjunctival or mucous membrane graft.
2. Application of soft contact lenses or sweeping by a glass rod coated with ointment to prevent the healing of two raw surfaces together can be employed as a prophylactic measure in the acute stage of the underlying disease causing symblepharon.

ANKYLOBLEPHARON

Definition

Fusion of the upper and lower eyelid margins is called ankyloblepharon.

Etiology

Ankyloblepharon is congenital because of webs of skin between the eyelid margins. Acquired causes include chemical burns or lid injuries simultaneously involving both the lid margins healing of which leads to formation of adhesions and fusion of the lid margins.

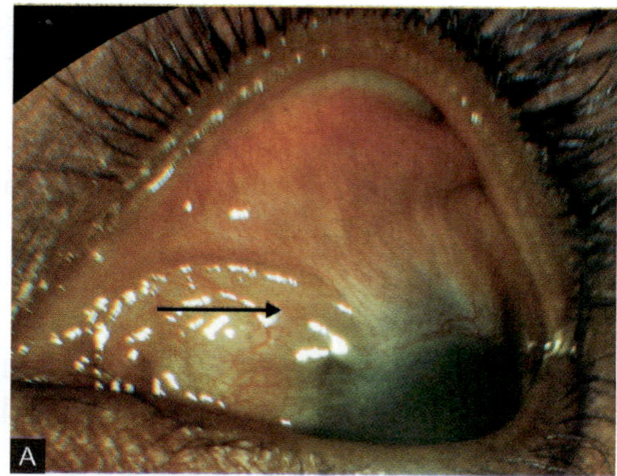

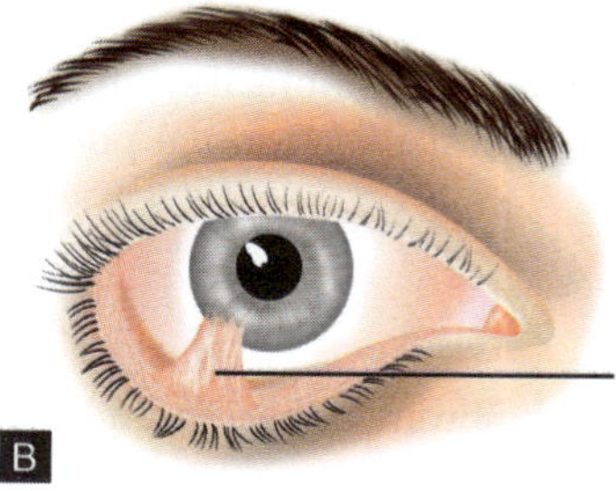

FIGS 2.3.7A and B: Symblepharon. **A.** Photograph; **B.** Diagrammatic representation.

Symptoms

Symptoms are decreased visual acuity when involving the central portion of the eyelid margin thereby obstructing the optical area. Cosmetic disfigurement because of decrease in the palpebral aperture width on the affected side (Fig. 2.3.8).

Signs

On examination fusion of the eyelid margins by skin web in congenital cases and by adhesions in acquired cases is seen.

Treatment

Treatment is by excision of the skin web or adhesions. Care should be taken to keep the raw surfaces apart during the healing process.

MADAROSIS*

Definition

Loss or decrease in the number of cilia of eyelashes and/or eyebrows is called madarosis (Fig. 2.3.9).

Etiology

Ocular causes: Blepharitis, trachoma, local trauma (mechanical, thermal following radiotherapy or cryotherapy) of the eyelids, tumors of the eyelids.

Dermatological causes: Atopic dermatitis, seborrheic dermatitis, ichthyosis, psoriasis, generalized alopecia.

Systemic diseases: Hypothyroidism, hyperthyroidism, hypoparathyroidism, hyperparathyroidism, hypopituitarism.

Autoimmune diseases: Vogt-Koyanagi-Harada syndrome, scleroderma, lupus erythematosus.

Nutritional diseases: Marasmus, iron deficiency, hypoproteinemia.

Infective diseases: Leprosy, syphilis, human immunodeficiency virus (HIV).

Drugs: Miotics, antithyroid drugs, anticoagulants.

Inherited Diseases Associated with Madarosis

- Treacher Collins syndrome (mandibulofacial dysostosis).
- Xeroderma pigmentosum.
- Oculodentodigital dysplasia.
- Tietze syndrome (albinism, deafness).

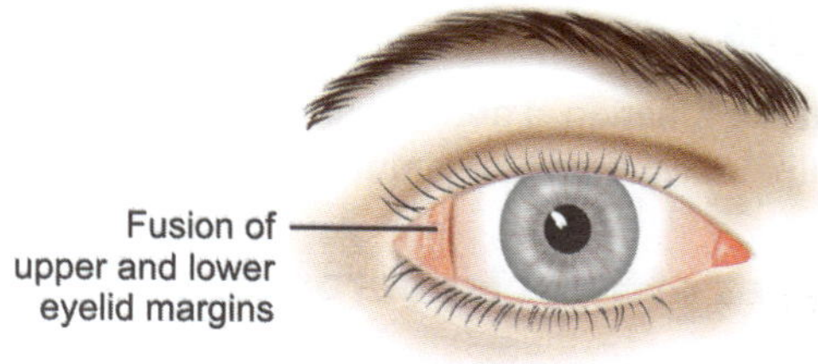

FIG. 2.3.8: Ankyloblepharon

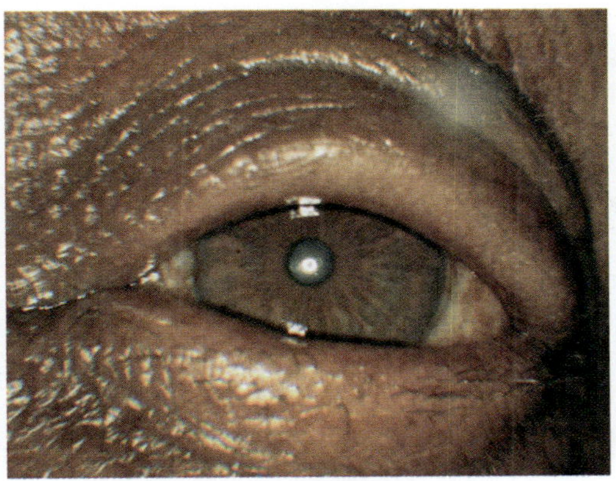

FIG. 2.3.9: Madarosis (*Note:* Decreased number of eyelashes).

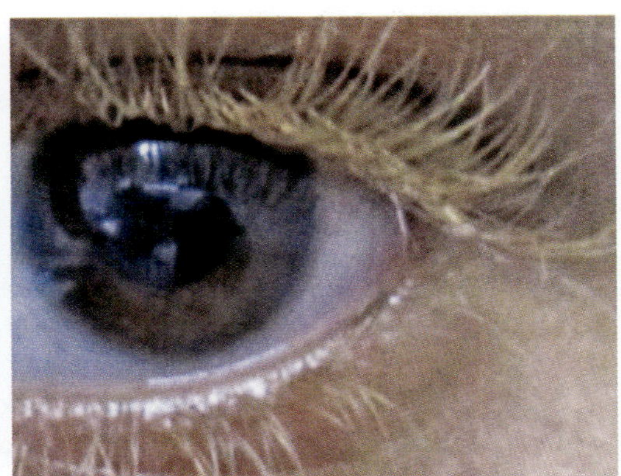

FIG. 2.3.10: Poliosis (*Note:* Presence of hypopigmented eyelashes).

Treatment

1. Treatment is done by identifying the underlying disease and treatment of the primary cause for madarosis. In non-scarring causes, regrowth of the eyelashes/follicles of eyebrows occurs after treatment of the primary disease.
2. For madarosis involving eyelashes: In cases involving scarring eyelash grafting is required. Topical prostaglandin analogs, e.g. bimatoprost, are used to stimulate the growth of eyelashes in non-scarring causes of madarosis of eyelashes.
3. For madarosis involving eyebrows: In cases involving scarring, eyebrow reconstruction is required and it is done by follicular unit transplantation. Topical minoxidil is used in the treatment of madarosis of eyebrows caused due to alopecia.

HYPERTRICHOSIS AND TRICHOMEGALY*

Hypertrichosis is defined as presence of increased number of eyelashes.

Trichomegaly is defined as presence of abnormally long and thick eyelashes.

Causes for Hypertrichosis and Trichomegaly

1. Congenital causes include familial hypertrichosis, oculocutaneous albinism.
2. Acquired causes include:
   a. Infections (e.g. HIV type 1).
   b. Systemic diseases such as dermatomyositis, systemic lupus erythematosus.
   c. Side effect of topically applied ocular drugs such as latanoprost, bimatoprost (antiglaucoma drugs), topical cyclosporine (immunosuppressor).
   d. Side effect of systemic drugs such as interferon alpha (IFN-α) cyclosporine.

POLIOSIS*

Poliosis is defined as presence of localized hypopigmented hair follicles involving eyelashes and/or eyebrows (Fig. 2.3.10).

Causes for Poliosis

Sarcoidosis, Vogt-Koyanagi-Harada syndrome, sympathetic ophthalmitis, blepharitis, vitiligo and side effect of topically administered prostaglandins.

GIST BOX 2.3

- *Trichiasis:* Misdirection of eyelashes toward the globe with normal position of eyelid margin.
- *Entropion:* Inward turning of the eyelid margin.
- *Ectropion:* Outward turning of the eyelid margin.
- *Symblepharon:* Adhesion between palpebral and bulbar conjunctiva resulting in adherence of the eyelid to the globe.
- *Ankyloblepharon*: Fusion of the upper and lower eyelid margins.
- *Madarosis:* Loss or decrease in the number of cilia of eyelashes and/or eyebrows.
- *Hypertrichosis:* Presence of increased number of eyelashes.
- *Trichomegaly:* Presence of abnormally long and thick eyelashes.
- *Poliosis:* Presence of localized hypopigmented hair follicles involving eyelashes and/or eyebrows.

CHAPTER

2.4 Inflammations and Infections of Eyelids

STYE (HORDEOLUM EXTERNUM)**

Definition

Acute suppurative inflammation of eyelash follicle and associated gland of Zeis or Moll (Figs 2.4.1A and B, Table 2.4.1).

Etiopathogenesis

Stye is more common in children and adolescents. Poor personal hygiene, habitual rubbing of eyes, refractive errors, exposure to dusty weather, decreased immunity are predisposing factors. *Staphylococcus aureus (S. aureus)* is the most common causative agent.

Symptoms

Symptoms are painful swelling of the eyelid margin pointing toward the skin side involving the eyelash.

Signs

On examination:

1. Swelling shows tenderness and other inflammatory signs such as redness and edema of the affected area.
2. Located at the lid margin and pointing toward the skin side involving the eyelash as it arises from the gland of Zeis or Moll.

A

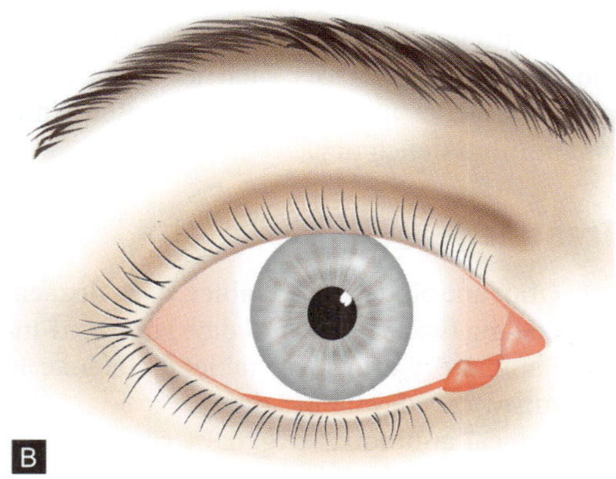

FIGS 2.4.1A and B: Stye. **A.** Photograph; **B.** Diagrammatic representation (*Note:* Swelling at the lid margin with inflammatory signs).

TABLE 2.4.1: Differences between stye, internal hordeolum and chalazion

Features	*Stye*	*Chalazion*	*Internal hordeolum*
Definition	Acute suppurative inflammation of gland of Zeis or Moll	Chronic non-suppurative inflammation of meibomian gland	Acute suppurative inflammation of meibomian gland
Etiology	*Staphylococcus aureus (S. aureus)*	Blockage of the ducts of the meibomian gland	*S. aureus*
Clinical features	Painful swelling involving the eyelid margin pointing toward the skin side	Painless swelling away from the eyelid margin pointing toward the conjunctival side	Painful swelling away from the eyelid margin pointing toward the conjunctival side
Treatment	Medical management by antibiotics	Intralesional injection of steroids or incision and curettage is required	Medical management by antibiotics

Complications

Stye may progress to cellulitis, generalized infection of the eyelid mainly in patients with decreased immunity or when the virulence of the organism causing infection is high.

Differential Diagnosis

Stye should be differentiated from internal hordeolum and chalazion.

Investigations

They should be done in patients with repeated stye. Investigations should be aimed to find out the predisposing factors such as uncorrected refractive errors, uncontrolled diabetes mellitus and immunodeficiency.

Treatment

1. Oral antibiotics (e.g. tablet ciprofloxacin 500 mg twice a day for 5 days) and anti-inflammatory drugs (e.g. tablet diclofenac 50 mg twice a day for 3–5 days).
2. Topical antibiotics (e.g. 0.3% ciprofloxacin in the form of eyedrops or ointment).
3. Hot compress.
4. Removal of the affected eyelash by epilation.

CHALAZION**

Definition

Subacute or chronic non-suppurative inflammation of meibomian gland (Figs 2.4.2A to C) (refer Table 2.4.1).

Etiopathogenesis

Chalazion is more common in patients with poor hygiene of the eyelids and in those with blepharitis or meibomianitis.

Histopathologically, chalazion is lipogranulomatous inflammation with histological picture (Fig. 2.4.3) showing inflammatory cells surrounding the areas of lipid indicated by clear spaces.

Symptoms

Painless swelling involving either upper or lower eyelid.

Signs

On examination:

1. Swelling is non-tender and inflammatory signs are absent.
2. Swelling is located away from the lid margin and pointing toward the conjunctival

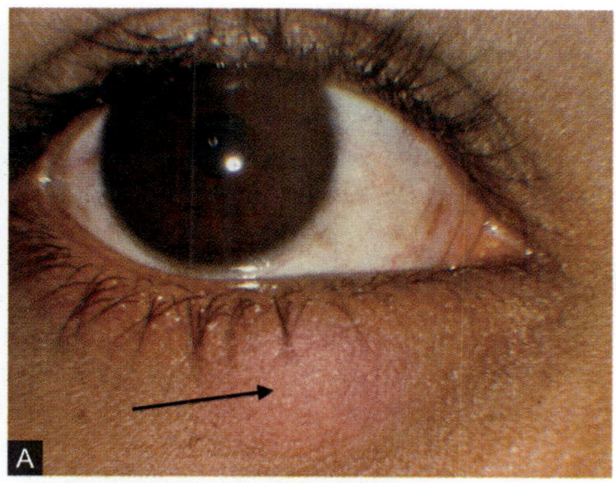

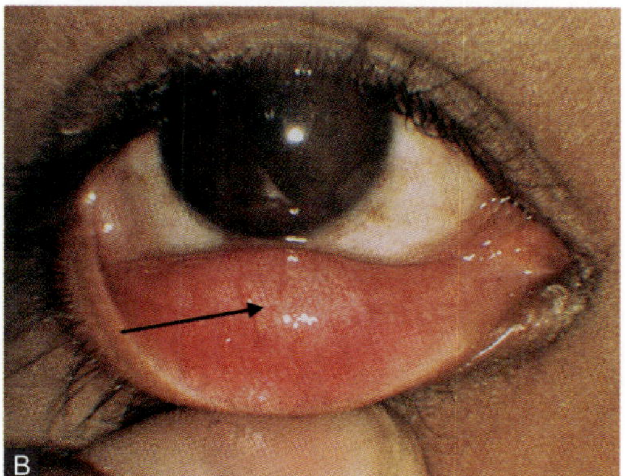

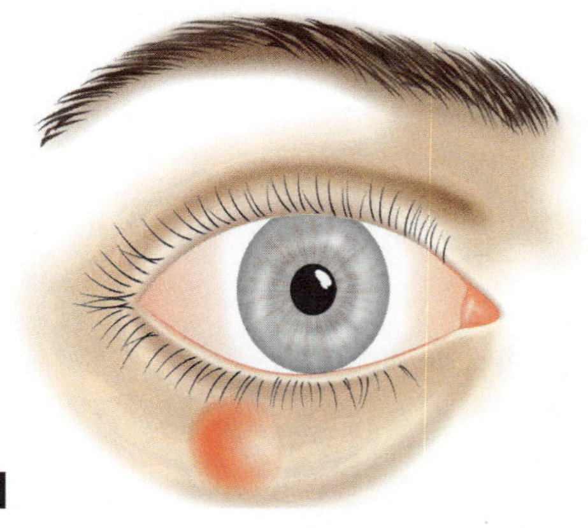

FIGS 2.4.2A to C: Chalazion. **A and B.** Photograph; **C.** Diagrammatic representation (*Note:* Swelling away from the lid margin with absence of inflammatory signs, which is pointing toward the conjunctival side).

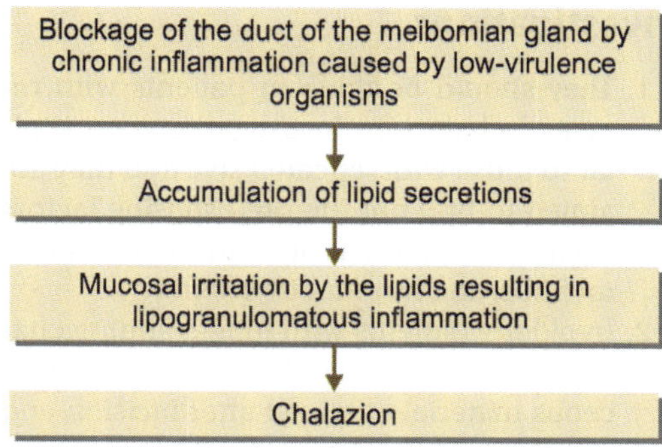

FIG. 2.4.3: Lipogranulomatous inflammation

side as it involves the meibomian gland present in the tarsal plate.

Complications*

1. Cosmetic disfigurement.
2. Secondary infection leading to formation of internal hordeolum and progression to preseptal orbital cellulitis.
3. Mechanical ptosis by large chalazion involving upper eyelid.
4. Diminution of vision secondary to astigmatism caused by pressure over cornea by large chalazion of the upper eyelid.

Marginal chalazion: The chalazion presenting at the lid margin because of extension via the meibomian ducts.

Burst chalazion: The chalazion, which ruptures and opens on the conjunctival side mimicking conjunctival granuloma.

Differential Diagnosis

Chalazion should be differentiated from internal hordeolum and stye. In elderly age people chalazion should be differentiated from meibomian gland carcinoma (Fig. 2.4.4).

Investigations

1. They should be done in patients with repeated chalazion. Investigations are similar to those with repeated stye and they are aimed to find out the predisposing factors such as blepharitis, uncontrolled diabetes mellitus, and immunodeficiency.
2. In elderly patients with long-standing chalazion or recurrent chalazion, the sebaceous material obtained after incision and curettage of chalazion should be sent for histopathological examination to rule out sebaceous gland carcinoma.

Treatment

1. About one fourth of the chalazion cases undergo spontaneous resolution when they are small. These patients require hot compress and digital massage to the eyelid margin to open the blocked ducts of the glands.
2. Intralesional injection of long-acting steroid, e.g. triamcinolone acetate, which acts by reducing inflammation.
3. Incision and curettage of the chalazion are required for large chalazion. After local infiltration of the lignocaine vertical incision is put on the conjunctival side and the cheesy material is scooped out. The incision has to be put vertically to avoid damage to the ducts of the neighboring glands.

Recurrent Chalazion and Multiple Chalazia (Fig. 2.4.5)

- They are common in patients with posterior blepharitis or meibomianitis, or in patients with poor lid hygiene.
- In elderly patients it may be masquerade syndrome of sebaceous gland carcinoma.
- Uncontrolled diabetics and those with immunodeficiency can have recurrent chalazion or multiple chalazia.

INTERNAL HORDEOLUM**

Definition

Acute suppurative inflammation of the meibomian gland (Figs 2.4.6A and B) (refer Table 2.4.1).

Etiopathogenesis

Staphylococcus aureus is the most common causative agent. Predisposing factors are similar to external hordeolum.

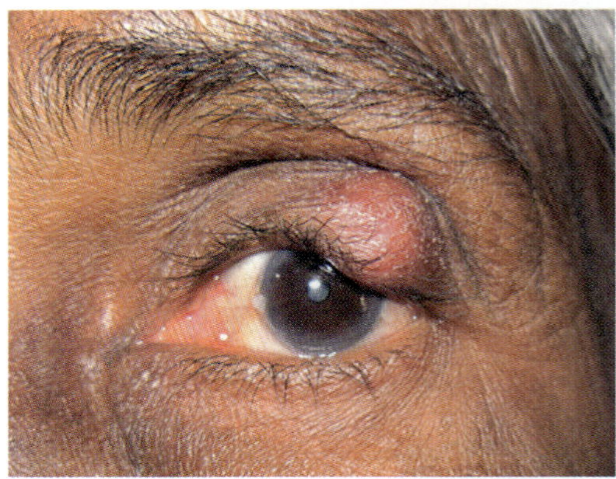

FIG. 2.4.4: Chalazion of the upper eyelid in an elderly female patient, which has to be differentiated from meibomian gland carcinoma.

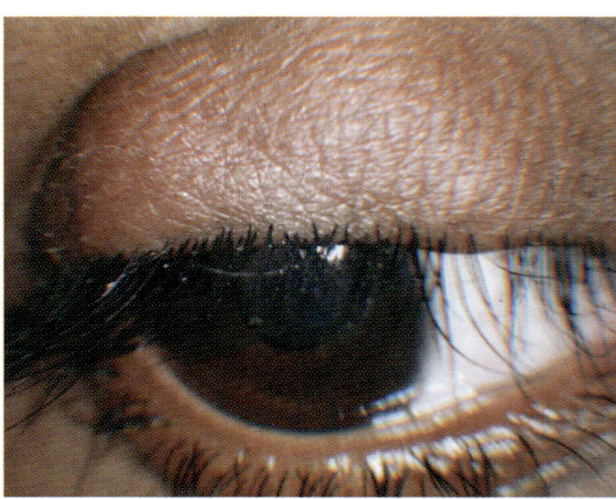

FIG. 2.4.5: Multiple chalazion involving upper eyelid

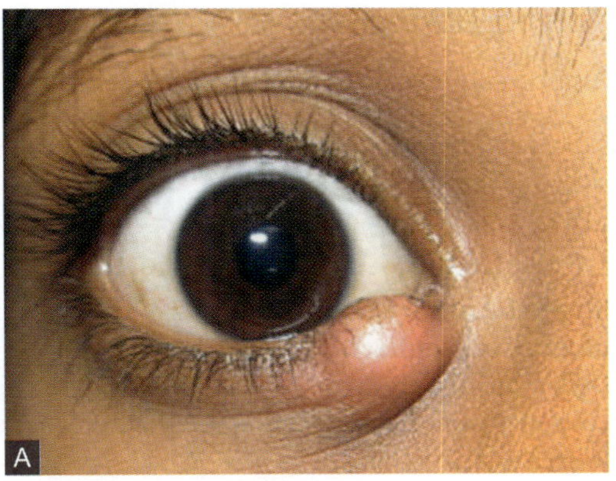

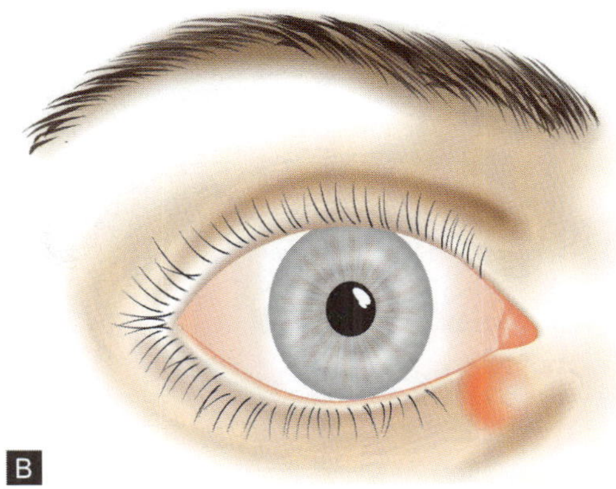

FIGS 2.4.6A and B: Internal hordeolum. **A.** Photograph; **B.** Diagrammatic representation (*Note:* Swelling away from lid margin with inflammatory signs).

Symptoms

Painful swelling of the eyelid.

Signs

On examination:

1. Swelling shows tenderness and other inflammatory signs such as redness, edema of the affected area.
2. Located away from the lid margin and pointing toward the conjunctival side as it arises from the meibomian gland.

Investigations

They are similar to those with stye. They are aimed to find out the predisposing factors, such as blepharitis, uncontrolled diabetes mellitus and immunodeficiency.

Complications

Internal hordeolum may progress to cellulitis, generalized infection of the eyelid mainly in patients with decreased immunity or when the virulence of the organism causing infection is high.

Differential Diagnosis

Internal hordeolum should be differentiated from stye and chalazion.

Treatment

Treatment is by:

1. Oral antibiotics (e.g. tablet ciprofloxacin 500 mg twice a day for 5 days) and anti-inflammatory drugs (e.g. tablet diclofenac 50 mg twice a day for 3-5 days).
2. Topical antibiotics (e.g. 0.3% ciprofloxacin in the form of eyedrops or ointment).
3. Hot compress.
4. Incision and drainage.

BLEPHARITIS**

Definition

Inflammation of the eyelid margin involving the eyelashes and glands of the eyelids (Fig. 2.4.7).

Etiology

Blepharitis is usually associated with:

1. Poor lid hygiene.
2. Bacterial infection or colonization of the eyelids.
3. Parasitic infestation.
4. Meibomian gland dysfunction resulting in the production of altered lipids.
5. Common diseases associated with blepharitis are seborrheic dermatitis and acne rosacea.

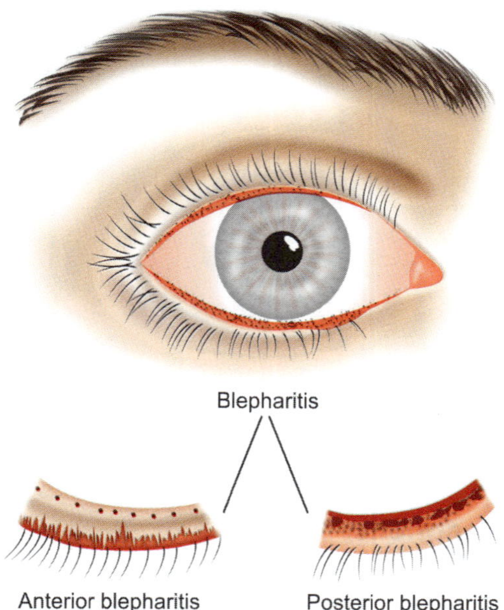

FIG. 2.4.7: Blepharitis (anterior and posterior)

Classification

Blepharitis is divided into:

- Anterior blepharitis involving eyelashes on the anterior margin of the eyelids
- Posterior blepharitis involving the meibomian glands on the posterior margin.

Anterior Blepharitis

Anterior blepharitis is further classified into:

- Staphylococcal or ulcerative blepharitis
- Squamous blepharitis or seborrheic blepharitis
- Mixed staphylococcal and seborrheic blepharitis.

Staphylococcal or ulcerative blepharitis**

Definition: It is a type of anterior blepharitis caused by bacterial colonization of the eyelids (Figs 2.4.8A and B).

Etiopathogenesis: It is due to hypersensitivity response to bacterial antigens. *S. aureus* is the most commonly isolated organism. Other organisms include *Staphylococcus epidermidis, Propionibacterium acnes* and *Corynebacterium* species.

Symptoms: Patient presents with a chronic course with acute exacerbations of symptomatic phase with symptoms of redness, itching around the eyelid margins, foreign body sensation, crusting of the eyelashes.

Signs: On examination, the anterior eyelid margin shows crusts or scales with dilated blood vessels surrounding the eyelash follicles. Removal of crusts may cause bleeding due to formation of ulcers, hence it is called ulcerative blepharitis.

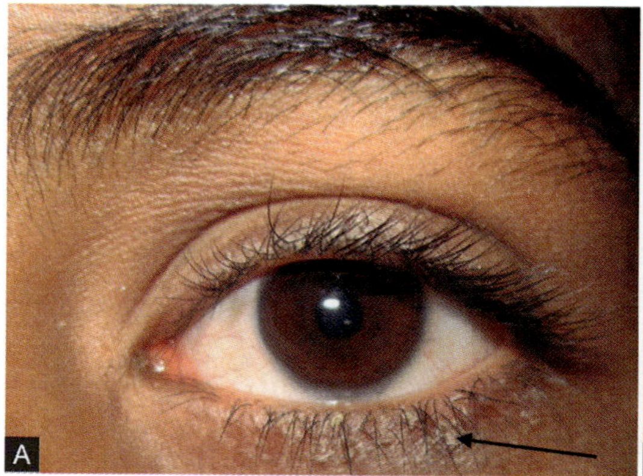

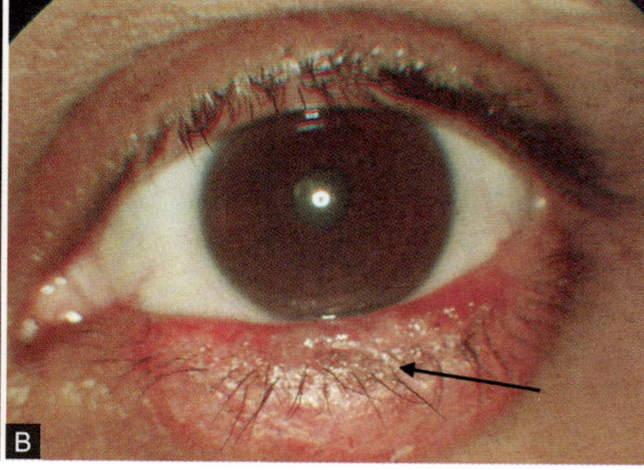

FIGS 2.4.8A and B: Anterior blepharitis (*Note:* Eyelid margin showing crusts with dilated blood vessels surrounding the eyelash follicles).

Complications: Madarosis—loss of eyelashes, chronic blepharoconjunctivitis, marginal keratitis, phlyctenular conjunctivitis and keratitis.

Treatment: Lid hygiene by using lid scrubs and warm compress, commercially available lid scrubs or baby shampoo or diluted povidone-iodine solution can be used for cleaning of the eyelid margins. Topical antibiotics such as 0.3% ciprofloxacin preferably in the form of eye ointment applied to lid margins. Systemic antibiotics such as tetracycline or doxycycline, topical steroids such as 0.1% dexamethasone are indicated in unresponsive cases and in cases with complications (e.g. marginal keratitis).

Squamous blepharitis or seborrheic blepharitis**

Definition: It is a type of anterior blepharitis associated with dandruff or seborrhea of the scalp.

Etiopathogenesis: It is due to excessive seborrheic secretions involving the hair follicles of scalp and eyelash follicles.

Symptoms: They are similar to staphylococcal blepharitis. Patient presents with a chronic course with acute exacerbations of symptomatic phase with symptoms of redness, itching around the eyelid margins, foreign body sensation, crusting of the eyelashes.

Signs: On examination, the eyelid margin shows white scales or flakes along the eyelashes. Removal of the scales will not cause bleeding as in ulcerative blepharitis. Examination of the scalp may show associated seborrhea of the scalp.

Complications: They are similar to those in ulcerative blepharitis, but they are less frequent.

Treatment: It is similar to treatment of ulcerative blepharitis and includes:

- Lid hygiene by using lid scrubs and warm compress
- Treatment of the associated seborrhea of the scalp
- Oral and topical antibiotics are usually not required as for ulcerative blepharitis.

Posterior Blepharitis

Posterior blepharitis is also called meibomianitis (Fig. 2.4.9).

Etiopathogenesis: It is due to meibomian gland dysfunction resulting in alteration of the lipids secreted by the meibomian glands. The alteration in the lipids results in increased viscosity, which results in obstruction of the orifices of the meibomian glands. The altered lipids are further broken by bacterial lipase enzyme produced by the common colonizing organisms (e.g. *S. aureus*). Epidermidis releasing free fatty acids, which cause ocular irritation and tear film dysfunction.

Symptoms: It include foreign body sensation, burning, blurring of vision because of tear film dysfunction.

Signs: On examination of eyelid margin show thickening, foamy discharge along the posterior eyelid margin, capping of the meibomian gland orifices by thickened secretions.

Complications: Keratoconjunctivitis sicca or dry eye, recurrent corneal erosions because of altered tear film.

Treatment: As follows:

1. Lid hygiene by using lid scrubs and warm compress.

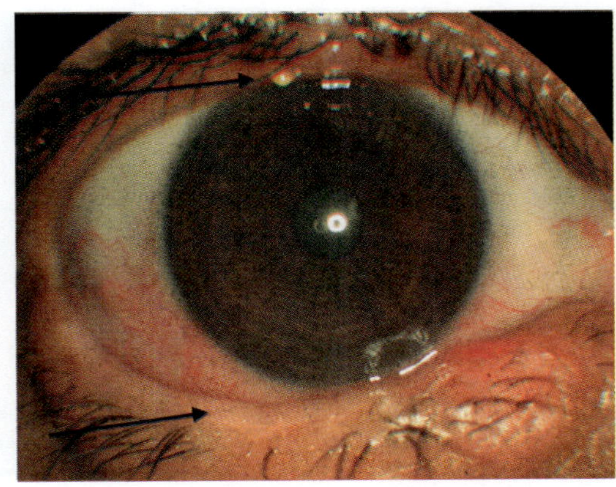

FIG. 2.4.9: Posterior blepharitis (*Note:* Thickening of the eyelid margin with capping of the meibomian gland orifices by thickened secretions).

2. Systemic tetracycline or doxycycline for 2–3 months in unresponsive cases, they act mainly by inhibiting bacterial lipase enzymes.

Parasitic Blepharitis

Definition: It is a subtype of blepharitis caused by parasites.

Etiology: Demodex folliculorum and phthiriasis palpebrarum (crab louse).

Symptoms: Symptoms are similar to other types of blepharitis and include redness, itching around the eyelid margins, foreign body sensation, crusting of the eyelashes.

Signs: On examination lice eggs or nits are seen at the lid margin.

Treatment: This is by mechanical removal of the nits at the eyelid margin by forceps and treatment of the underlying parasitic infestation by delousing.

EDEMA OF THE EYELIDS

Definition

Edema of the eyelids is a condition characterized by swelling of the eyelids due to accumulation of the fluids (Figs 2.4.10A and B).

Causes

1. Active edema is due to inflammation of the eye or its surrounding structures and the causes include inflammations of the lid (e.g. blepharitis), conjunctiva (e.g. conjunctivitis), lacrimal sac (e.g. dacryocystitis), cornea (e.g. keratitis), uvea (e.g. uveitis), orbit (e.g. orbital cellulitis), paranasal sinuses (e.g. sinusitis).
2. Allergic reaction of the eyes to drugs or pollen, angioedema, contact dermatitis.
3. Passive edema is due to circulatory disturbances. Causes include systemic diseases such as cardiac failure, renal failure and local diseases (e.g. cavernous sinus thrombosis).

Reasons for Easy Swelling of the Eyelids

- Skin of the eyelids is the thinnest in the body. It does not have a subcutaneous fatty layer.
- Layer of loose subcutaneous tissue gets distended easily by blood in case of injuries to head and by fluid in cardiac failure, which presents as puffiness of face.
- The submuscular areolar tissue of upper eyelids is in continuity with subaponeurotic space of scalp allowing easy passage of fluid and blood to the upper eyelids leading to black eye or ecchymosis of upper eyelids in cases of head injuries.

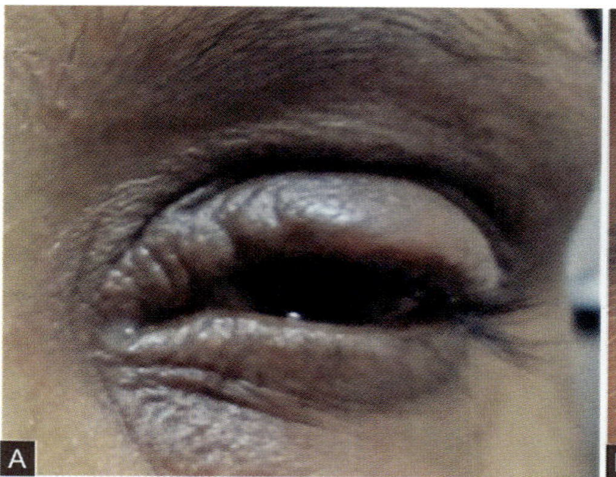

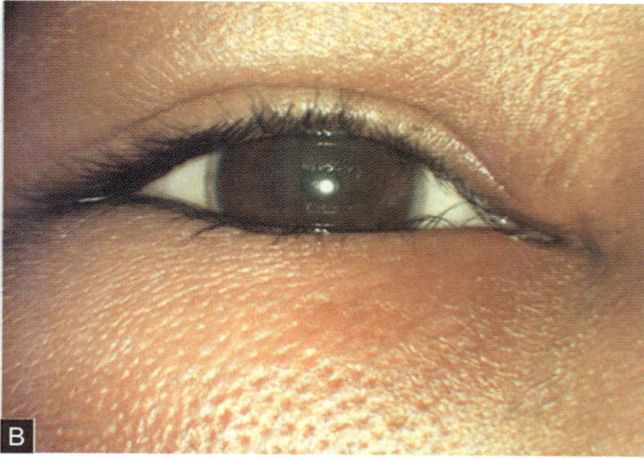

FIGS 2.4.10A and B: Edema of eyelids

Treatment

Eyelid edema is treated by the treatment of the underlying cause.

VIRAL INFECTIONS OF EYELIDS

Molluscum Contagiosum

Molluscum contagiosum is infection of the skin of the eyelids by molluscum contagiosum virus, a poxvirus.

Etiology

Molluscum contagiosum is a common viral infection seen in children and it spreads by direct contact. Being cutaneous infection it can involve skin over any part of the body, but it is more frequently seen over face, neck, trunk and extremities.

Histopathology

Molluscum contagiosum shows presence of intracytoplasmic inclusion bodies called Henderson-Patterson bodies, also called molluscum bodies.

Clinical Features

1. Molluscum contagiosum presents with pale, waxy umbilicated nodules single or multiple. Each nodule measures about 1–5 mm in diameter with an umbilicated center containing the virus.
2. Chronic follicular conjunctivitis may be seen because of shedding of virus into the conjunctival fornix mainly from the lesions involving the eyelid.
3. Larger and confluent molluscum lesions are seen in adults with human immunodeficiency virus (HIV) infection.

Treatment

Small lesions may show spontaneous resolution and treatment is indicated for non-resolving or bigger lesions. Treatment options are excision of the lesion, incision and curettage of the lesion, and destruction of the lesion by cryotherapy or laser.

Cutaneous Wart or Verruca Vulgaris

Cutaneous wart is infection of skin by human papilloma virus. It is more commonly seen in

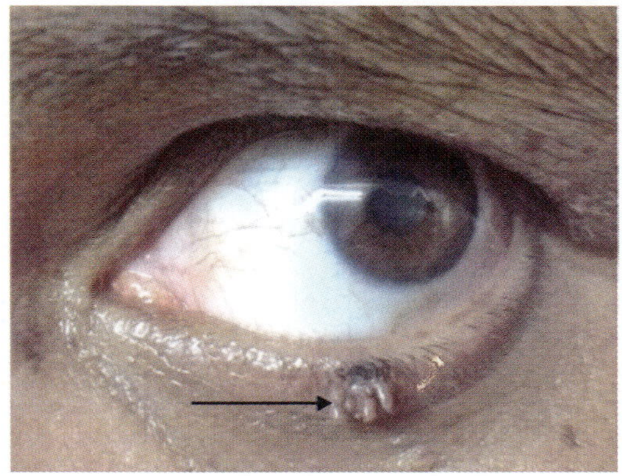

FIG. 2.4.11: Cutaneous wart

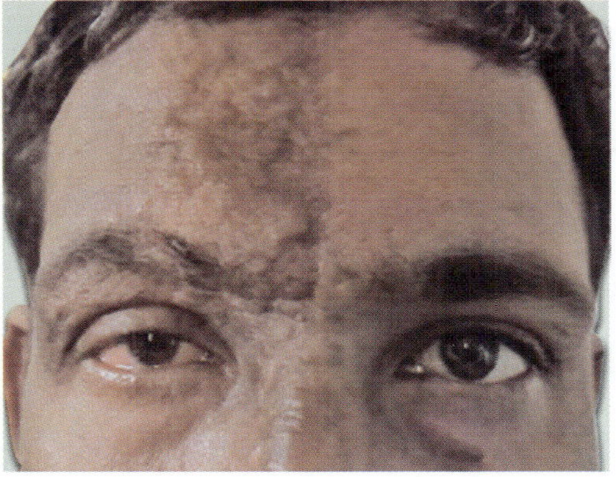

FIG. 2.4.12: Scar resulting from herpes zoster ophthalmicus (*Note:* Scar limited to midline of face along the distribution of trigeminal nerve).

children and young adults, and it spreads by close contact. Extensive warts are seen in individuals with decreased immunity as in infection with HIV (Fig. 2.4.11).

Cutaneous wart presents as irregular elevated finger-like projections resembling a cauliflower. Treatment is by surgical excision or by cryotherapy, or by laser.

Herpes Zoster Ophthalmicus and Herpes Simplex

Herpes zoster ophthalmicus and herpes simplex are common viral infections caused by varicella zoster virus, and herpes simplex virus respectively. They are described in detail under infections of cornea (Fig. 2.4.12).

GIST BOX 2.4

- *Hordeolum externum:* Acute suppurative inflammation of eyelash follicle and associated gland of Zeis or Moll.
- *Hordeolum internum:* Acute suppurative inflammation of the meibomian gland.
- *Chalazion:* Subacute or chronic non-suppurative inflammation of meibomian gland.
- *Blepharitis:* Inflammation of the eyelid margin involving the eyelashes and glands of the eyelids.

CHAPTER

2.5 Diseases of Eyelid Position and Movement

BLEPHAROPTOSIS/PTOSIS***

Definition

The word ptosis is derived from Greek and it means falling downward or drooping of any organ (Figs 2.5.1A and B).

Blepharoptosis is defined as drooping of the upper eyelid from its normal position. In ophthalmology blepharoptosis is generally referred as ptosis. Normally upper eyelid covers 2 mm of cornea. In ptosis the upper eyelid covers more than 2 mm of cornea.

Etiopathogenesis

Ptosis or drooping of the upper eyelid is because of weakness of the elevators/retractors of upper eyelid (levator palpebrae superioris and Müller's muscle). The cause for weakness may be in the muscle, aponeurosis, neuromuscular junction or in the nerves supplying the muscle.

Classification*

Ptosis can be classified into different types based on the etiology or onset and pathology, or cause:

- Based on etiology, ptosis is classified into:
  - Congenital ptosis
  - Acquired ptosis.
- Based on the pathology, ptosis is classified into:
  - Neurogenic ptosis
  - Myogenic ptosis
  - Aponeurotic ptosis
  - Mechanical ptosis.

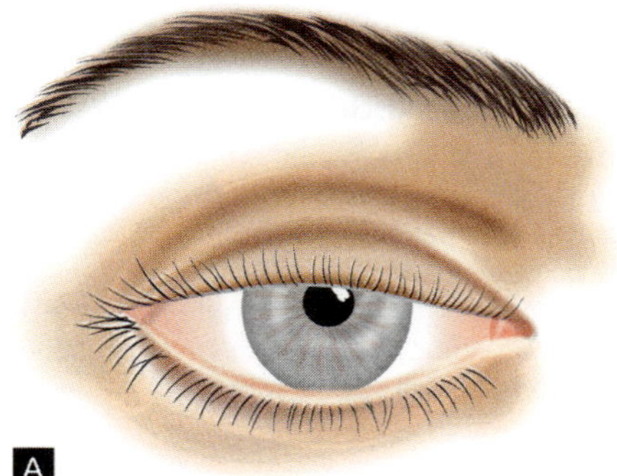

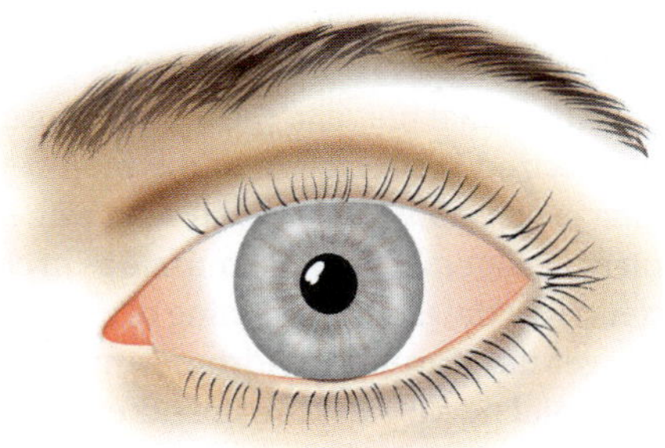

FIGS 2.5.1A and B: Ptosis. **A.** Right eye—ptosis; **B.** Left eye—normal.

CONGENITAL PTOSIS**

Congenital ptosis is usually present at birth and it may be unilateral or bilateral.

Congenital Myogenic Ptosis

Congenital myogenic ptosis is the most common type of congenital ptosis. It is due to maldevelopment of levator muscle. It is characterized by absence of upper eyelid crease, poor levator function and increased palpebral aperture width on down gaze on ptotic side because of the limitation of mobility of eyelid by the fibrotic levator muscle:

1. Simple congenital ptosis not associated with any ocular or systemic anomalies.
2. Congenital ptosis in association with other anomalies such as:
   a. Blepharophimosis syndrome (ptosis, blepharophimosis, telecanthus and epicanthus).
   b. Associated with weakness of superior rectus muscle resulting in ptosis with vertical squint or hypotropia.

Congenital Neurogenic Ptosis

Congenital neurogenic ptosis is seen in the following conditions.

*Congenital Synkinetic Ptosis (Marcus Gunn Jaw-winking Ptosis)**

Congenital synkinetic ptosis is because of misdirection of mandibular division of the V cranial nerve or III cranial nerve to the levator muscle. It is characterized by retraction of the ptotic eyelid resulting in elevation of the eyelid seen with stimulation of ipsilateral pterygoid muscle as in chewing, clenching the teeth or opening of mouth.

Congenital Horner's syndrome and congenital III cranial nerve palsy are the other causes of congenital neurogenic ptosis.

Congenital Aponeurotic Ptosis

Congenital aponeurotic ptosis is rare type of congenital ptosis. It is caused by faulty insertion or failure of insertion of levator aponeurosis on to the anterior surface of tarsus. It is usually seen in association with birth trauma.

Congenital Mechanical Ptosis

Congenital mechanical ptosis is seen in congenital malformations involving the upper eyelid such as hemangioma, plexiform neurofibroma.

Treatment of Congenital Ptosis*

1. Surgery is the treatment of choice. Timing of surgery depends on the severity of ptosis.

   Mild ptosis: Upper eyelid covers 2–4 mm of cornea (Fig. 2.5.2).

   Moderate ptosis: Upper eyelid covers 4–6 mm of cornea (Fig. 2.5.3).

   Severe ptosis: Upper eyelid covers more than 6 mm of cornea (Fig. 2.5.4).

   Mild-to-moderate ptosis: Surgery may be delayed till 4–5 years of age so that accurate measurements can be taken when the child can cooperate for ptosis measurements.

   Severe ptosis: Surgery should be performed as early as possible to prevent amblyopia.
2. The type of surgery is determined by amount of ptosis and levator muscle function.

Levator Muscle Function Measurement

It is measured by Berke's method. It is done by measuring the amount of excursion of the upper eyelid margin when a patient looks from downgaze to extreme upgaze after blocking the action of the frontalis muscle by applying direct pressure to the eyebrow. Normal levator function is 15 mm. Levator function of below 4 mm is taken as poor function.

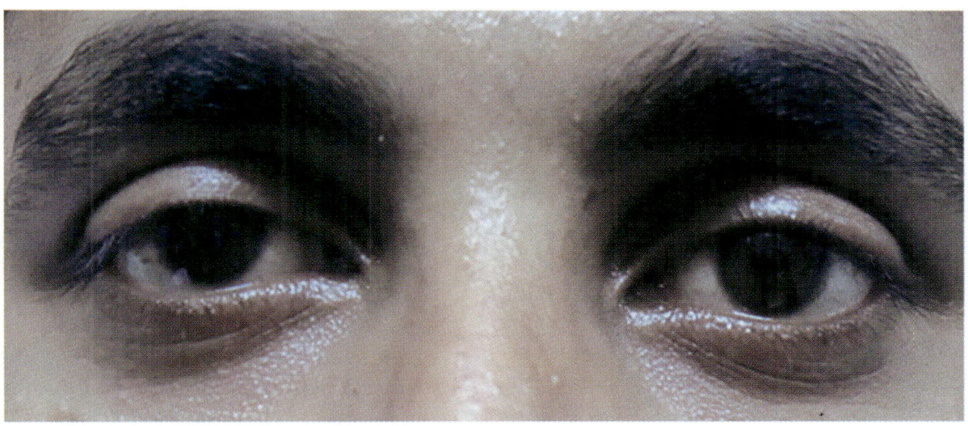

FIG. 2.5.2: Mild ptosis of right eye

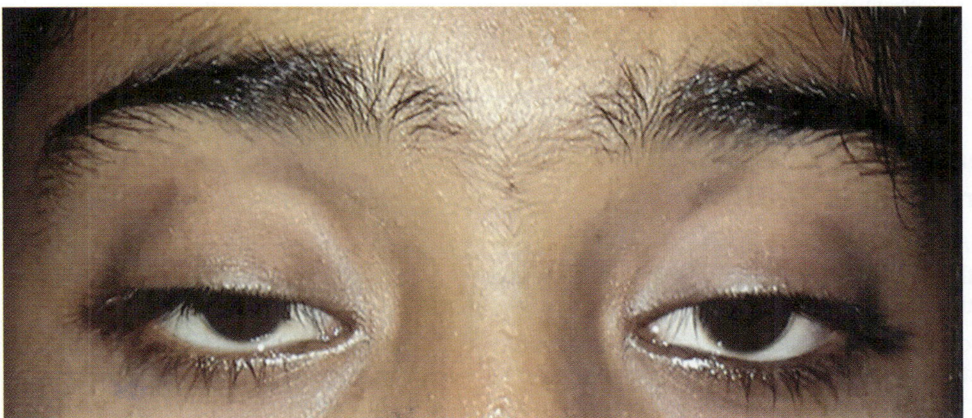

FIG. 2.5.3: Moderate ptosis of right eye

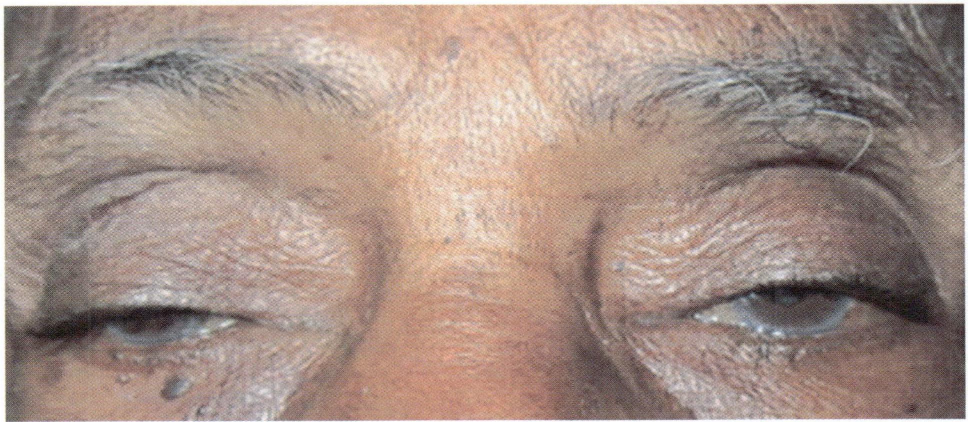

FIG. 2.5.4: Severe ptosis of both eyes

3. The principle of surgery is to strengthen the retractors of the upper eyelid.
   Fasanella-Servat operation: It is done in mild ptosis with good levator muscle function. Here a part of tarsal plate and Müller's muscle are excised (resected) to strengthen the Müller's muscle.
   Levator resection: It is done in moderate-to-severe ptosis with good-to-moderate levator function. It is the surgery of choice for most of the cases of ptosis with good levator function since levator palpebrae superioris (LPS) is the primary retractor of the upper eyelid. Here LPS is shortened (resected) to strengthen the LPS muscle.
   Frontalis sling operation: It is done in severe ptosis with poor levator muscle function. Here upper eyelid is anchored to the frontalis muscle by a sling. Synthetic sutures or autogenous fascia lata are used as sling.

Treatment of Associated Conditions in Ptosis

Blepharophimosis syndrome is treated by medial canthal tendon plication for telecanthus and epicanthus, and frontalis sling operation for ptosis.

Marcus Gunn jaw-winking syndrome is treated by levator resection in mild cases, and by levator disinsertion and frontalis sling suspension in severe cases.

Mechanical ptosis is treated by treatment of the mechanical factor causing ptosis.

ACQUIRED PTOSIS

Acquired ptosis is acquired later in adult life and depending on the causes. It is further classified as:

1. Myogenic ptosis seen in myasthenia gravis, progressive muscular dystrophy, chronic progressive external ophthalmoplegia, oculopharyngeal muscular dystrophy.
2. Neurogenic ptosis seen Horner's syndrome causing oculosympathetic paralysis and in paralysis of oculomotor nerve (Fig. 2.5.5).
3. Aponeurotic ptosis due to senile weakness of the levator aponeurosis or weakness of the aponeurosis following trauma. It is the most common type of ptosis.
4. Mechanical ptosis is due to excessive weight over the upper eyelid by large chalazion or tumors of the upper eyelid.

Symptoms

Patient presents with:

1. Cosmetic disfigurement because of drooping of the upper eyelid.
2. Diminution of vision in severe degree of ptosis when the pupillary area is covered by the upper eyelid.
3. Symptoms of the causative disease.

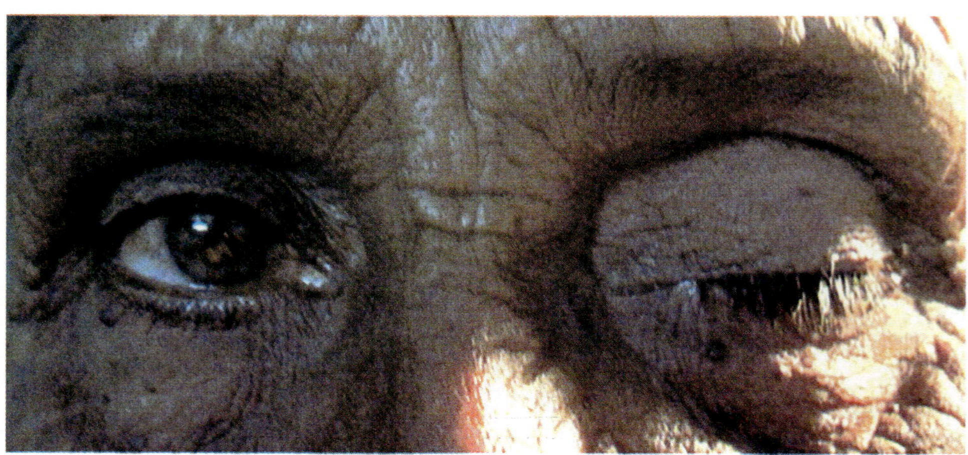

FIG. 2.5.5: Patient presenting with complete ptosis of left upper eyelid as a result of paralysis of oculomotor nerve

Signs

1. On examination drooping of the upper eyelid of varying degree is seen.
2. Signs of the primary disease causing ptosis are seen.

Investigations

Investigations are carried out to find out the primary cause of ptosis is acquired ptosis. Investigations are tailored depending on the detailed history.

Myasthenia gravis is an autoimmune disorder characterized by abnormal fatigability of the muscles because of deficiency of acetylcholine receptors as a result of destruction of acetylcholine receptors by the antibodies directed against them. Ocular myasthenia gravis presents with history of variable degree of ptosis, increasing with fatigue.

Ice test: It is applied to the eyelid for 5–10 minutes. Improvement in the amount of ptosis is seen in myasthenia gravis. It is because of the fact that cold temperature enhances neuromuscular transmission by inhibiting the action of acetylcholinesterase.

Neostigmine test: It is a reversible acetylcholinesterase inhibitor. The test is done by intramuscular injection of neostigmine 4 mg. Improvement in the amount of ptosis is seen in myasthenia gravis.

Tensilon test (edrophonium test): It is also reversible acetylcholinesterase inhibitor. The test is done by intravenous injection of 10 mg of edrophonium. Improvement in the amount of ptosis is seen in myasthenia gravis. Edrophonium is safer than neostigmine.

Serum assay for acetylcholine receptor antibodies and electromyography are the laboratory investigations required for confirmation of myasthenia gravis.

Horner's syndrome is because of oculosympathetic paresis. It is characterized by ptosis, miosis of pupil, inverse ptosis of lower eyelid, anhidrosis of ipsilateral face and enophthalmos. It is diagnosed by phenylephrine test.*

Phenylephrine test: It is done by instilling one drop of phenylephrine into the conjunctival sac of both eyes after measuring the amount of ptosis. Improvement in ptosis and dilatation of the miotic pupil more than the normal pupil because of denervation supersensitivity after 5 minutes indicates Horner's syndrome.

Chronic progressive external ophthalmoplegia (CPEO) is a type of mitochondrial myopathy characterized by slowly progressive paralysis of extraocular muscles. Electromyography and mitochondrial assay are the definitive laboratory tests for CPEO.

Oculopharyngeal muscular dystrophy is a muscular dystrophy characterized by ptosis and dysphagia, usually seen in elderly individuals. The diagnosis is made on clinical criteria and muscle biopsy is the confirmative laboratory test.

Oculomotor nerve or third nerve palsy shows other clinical features associated with ptosis such as limitation of extraocular movements involving the muscles innervated by third nerve, dilatation of the pupil and downward, and outward displacement of the eyeball. Third nerve palsy has to be evaluated for medical and surgical causes.

Aponeurotic ptosis is the most common type of all the types of ptosis. It is characterized by the absence of eyelid crease or presence of high eyelid crease because of loss of insertion, or upward insertion of levator fibers.

Treatment

Treatment of acquired ptosis is done by identifying the underlying cause of ptosis and treatment of the causative disease. Surgery is done only after the primary disease causing ptosis is treated. Surgery, if required is chosen as for the congenital ptosis.

Evaluation of a Patient with Ptosis

Kindly refer Chapter 4 'Case Presentation' in Author's textbook 'Clinical Methods in Ophthalmology'.

PSEUDOPTOSIS

Pseudoptosis involves conditions, which appear apparently (e.g. ptosis) because of decrease in vertical palpebral aperture width (Fig. 2.5.6). These are differentiated from ptosis by the presence of normal action of the retractors of the upper eyelid. The causes include:

1. Anophthalmos, enophthalmos, microphthalmos, phthisis bulbi because of lack of support to the upper eyelid from behind by the eyeball.
2. Dermatochalasis and blepharochalasis because of excessive laxity of skin of upper eyelid.
3. Contralateral lid retraction.
4. Ipsilateral hypotropia.

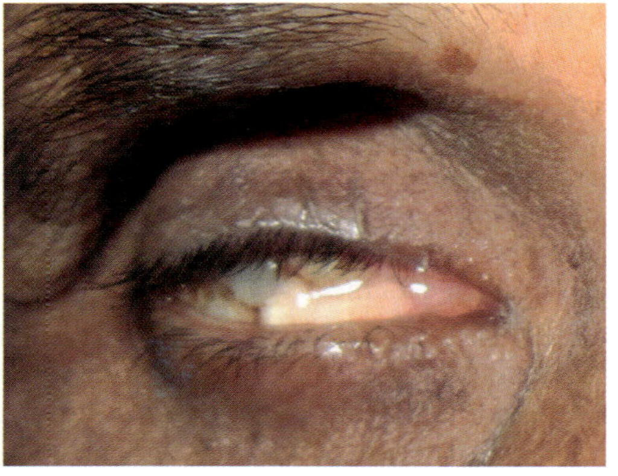

FIG. 2.5.6: Pseudoptosis (*Note:* Pseudoptosis in a patient with phthisis bulbi)

Inverse Ptosis

- Elevation of the lower eyelid from its normal position, covering cornea is called inverse ptosis.
- It is due to weakness of retractors of lower eyelid.
- It is seen in Horner's syndrome because of weakness of Müller's muscle as a result of paresis or paralysis of sympathetic supply.

LID RETRACTION*

Definition

Upward movement of the upper eyelid or downward movement of the lower eyelid with exposure of sclera between the limbus and eyelid margin is called lid retraction (Fig. 2.5.7).

Pathogenesis

The upper eyelid retraction is because of overaction of retractors of the upper eyelid and the cause for lower eyelid retraction is underaction of the retractors of the lower eyelid. The cause may be either in the muscle or in the nerve supplying the muscle.

The most common cause for both upper and lower eyelid retraction is thyroid eye disease.

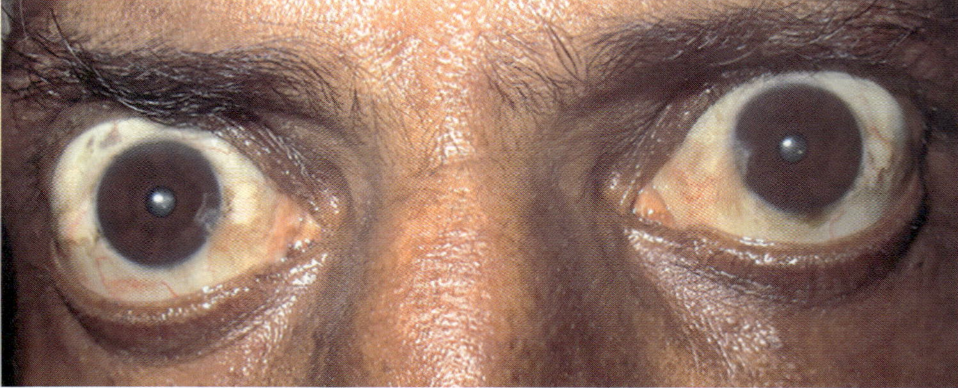

FIG. 2.5.7: Lid retraction in a patient with thyroid eye disease

Causes

Neurogenic causes: Parinaud's syndrome, hydrocephalus, Marcus Gunn jaw-winking syndrome, third nerve misdirection syndrome.

Myogenic causes: Grave's eye disease, following overcorrection in ptosis surgeries.

Mechanical causes: Proptosis, buphthalmos, pathological myopia.

Treatment

Mild cases are treated by müllerectomy. Moderate-to-severe cases require levator recession.

BLEPHAROCHALASIS

1. Idiopathic self-limiting inflammatory edema of the eyelids leading to thinning and wrinkling of the skin of the eyelids is called blepharochalasis (Fig. 2.5.8). It is seen in young girls.
2. The exact etiology is not known. It is thought to be a variant of hereditary angioneurotic edema.
3. Recurrent episodes cause redundancy of the skin of the eyelids and may lead to ptosis because the weakness of LPS.
4. Blepharochalasis has to be differentiated from dermatochalasis, which mainly occurs in elderly individuals because of prolapsed orbital fat.
5. Medical line of management in the form of systemic steroids is used during inflammatory stage.
6. Surgical management is indicated for advanced stages with redundancy of skin of eyelids and blepharoptosis. Redundancy of skin of the lids is corrected by blepharoplasty and ptosis is corrected by repair of dehiscence of levator muscle.

DERMATOCHALASIS

1. Laxity and redundancy of the skin of the upper eyelid seen in elderly people because of prolapse of orbital fat is called dermatochalasis (Figs 2.5.9A and B).
2. It is usually seen in middle-aged and elderly patients. This is because of age-related decrease in the elasticity of connective tissue of eyelids leading to prolapse of the orbital fat.
3. Symptoms are because of hanging of redundant skin of the eyelids over the edge of the lids. In severe cases it may cause diminution of visual field because of manual obstruction.
4. Symptomatic patients are treated by blepharoplasty to excise the redundant skin.

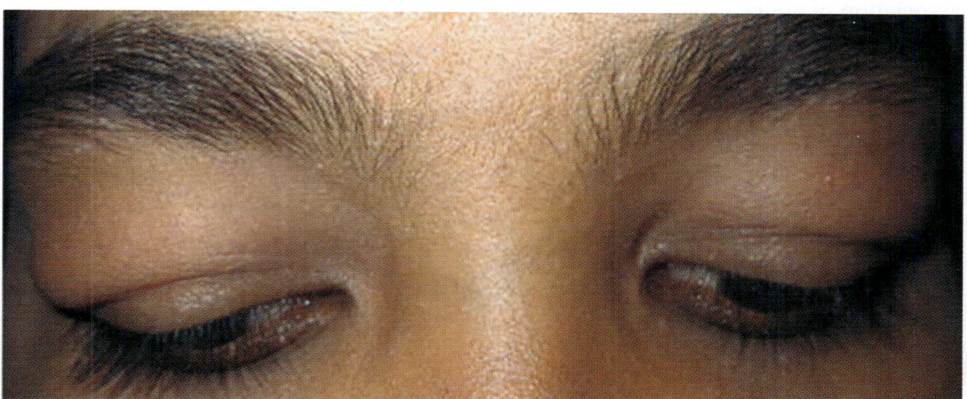

FIG. 2.5.8: Blepharochalasis

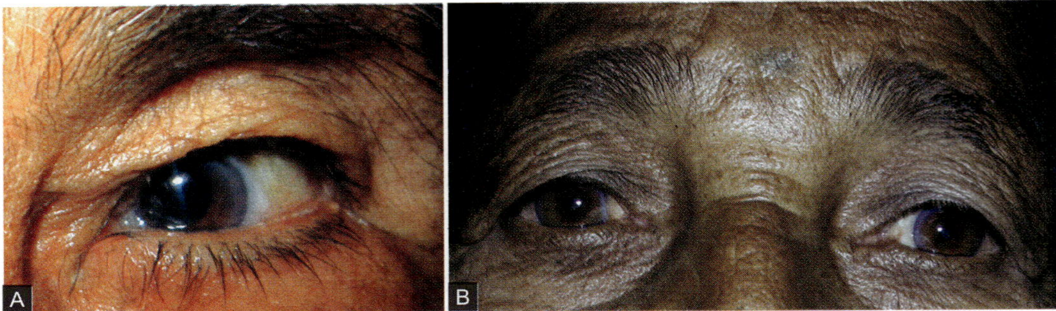

FIGS 2.5.9A and B: Dermatochalasis

FLOPPY EYELID SYNDROME

1. It is a clinical condition characterized by lax, floppy and rubbery eyelids.
2. It is usually associated with obesity and obstructive sleep apnea. Keratoconus is the common ocular association.
3. Ocular features include easily everted, rubbery and floppy upper eyelids, and chronic papillary conjunctivitis.
4. The underlying pathogenesis is because of upregulation of elastin degrading enzymes leading to lax tarsus of eyelids and mechanical factors such as eversion of the lax eyelids in people who sleep in prone position because of contact with pillow. Low nocturnal oxygen perfusion leading to ischemic damage of the tarsus may explain the association of floppy eyelid syndrome with obstructive sleep apnea. The chronic exposure of the conjunctiva leads to chronic papillary conjunctivitis.
5. Treatment of floppy eyelid syndrome is done by lubricating eyedrops to keep the ocular surface moist, eyelid taping in the night to prevent exposure of the ocular surface. Horizontal lid shortening is done in severe cases to correct horizontal lid laxity.

EYELID IMBRICATION SYNDROME

1. It is a rare disease characterized by overriding of a horizontally lengthened upper eyelid over the margin of the lower eyelid.
2. It is characterized by symptoms of chronic irritation because of chronic rubbing of the tarsal conjunctiva against the eyelashes of the lower eyelid because of the overlapping of the upper eyelid over the lower eyelid.
3. Eyelid imbrication syndrome may be associated with floppy eyelid syndrome.
4. Treatment is by tightening of the upper eyelid by full thickness of upper lid wedge resection.

Floppy eyelid syndrome and eyelid imbrication syndrome are rare clinical entities and should be suspected in patients presenting with chronic red eye presenting as chronic papillary conjunctivitis of upper tarsal conjunctiva not responding to treatment.

BLEPHAROSPASM

Definition

Involuntary closure of the eyelids caused by spasm or contraction of orbicularis oculi is called blepharospasm (Fig. 2.5.10).

Blepharospasm is of two types:

- Essential blepharospasm
- Reflex blepharospasm.

*Essential Blepharospasm**

Essential blepharospasm is a rare condition characterized by increased blinking because

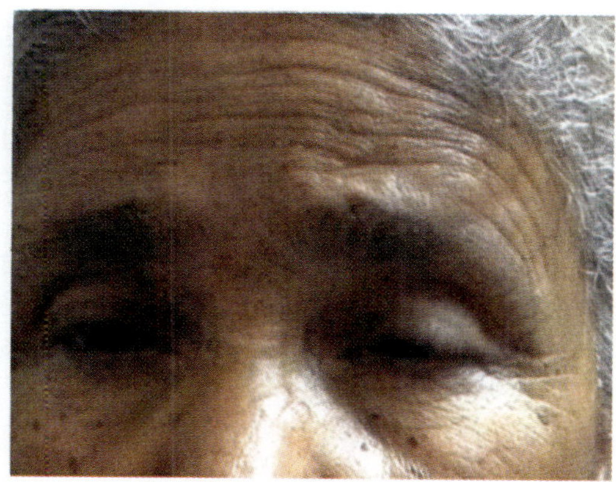

FIG. 2.5.10: Blepharospasm

of involuntary spasms of orbicularis oculi. It is usually seen in elderly individuals more common in females.

It is characterized by mild spasms of orbicularis oculi resulting in increased blinking rate in the early stages and sustained contraction of the orbicularis oculi in later stages leading to forceful contractions of the eyelids thereby affecting the patient's daily activities. This may lead to development of spastic entropion in elderly people.

Treatment is done by:

- Botulinum toxin injection is the most commonly employed treatment initially
- Surgical myectomy of orbicularis oculi muscle and surgical ablation of facial nerve are the less commonly employed surgical techniques in non-responsive patients.

Botulinum Toxin

Botulinum toxin is a neurotoxin derived from *Clostridium botulinum.* It acts by preventing the release of acetylcholine from presynaptic junction. It causes localized muscle paralysis on local intramuscular injection. The action of botulinum toxin lasts for 3–4 months.

There are seven types of botulinum toxin, i.e. A, B, C, D, E, F and G. Type A is commonly used in ophthalmology. Botulinum toxin is used in ophthalmology in the treatment of:

- Strabismus by injection into extraocular muscles.
- Essential blepharospasm by injection into orbicularis oculi.
- Spastic entropion by injection into pretarsal portion of orbicularis oculi.
- Some types of acquired nystagmus by retrobulbar injection.

Reflex Blepharospasm

Reflex blepharospasm is a common condition characterized by increased blinking because of reflex between the facial nerve motor for orbicularis oculi and trigeminal nerve sensory for cornea, and conjunctiva. It is seen in conditions such as keratitis, corneal or conjunctival foreign body, iridocyclitis and conjunctivitis. Treatment of reflex blepharospasm is by treatment of the underlying cause.

LAGOPHTHALMOS**

Definition

Lagophthalmos is defined as inability to close the eyelids completely (Figs 2.5.11A and B).

The word lagophthalmos is derived from Greek word, which means hare eye. This is based on the belief that hares sleep with their eyes open. In reality this is not true as hares sleep with their eyes closed.

Etiology

Lagophthalmos is seen in:

1. Weakness of orbicularis oculi muscle as a result of paresis or paralysis of facial nerve.
2. Cicatricial conditions, which prevent complete closure of the eyelids as in symblepharon, cicatricial ectropion.
3. Diseases of eyelids and orbit preventing the closure of eyelids with function of the orbicularis oculi being normal. These conditions include diseases such as:
   - Symblepharon
   - Cicatricial ectropion
   - Proptosis.

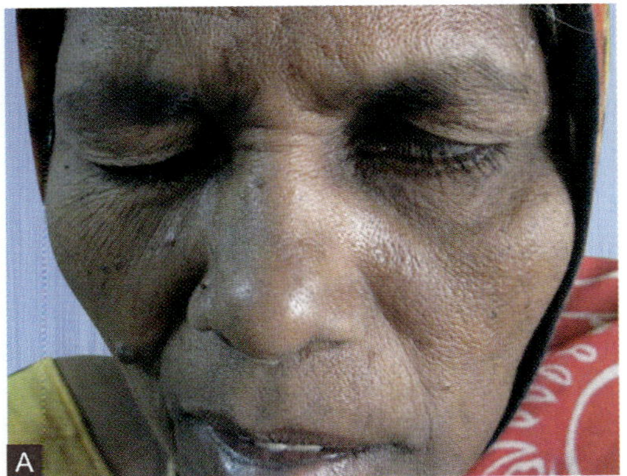

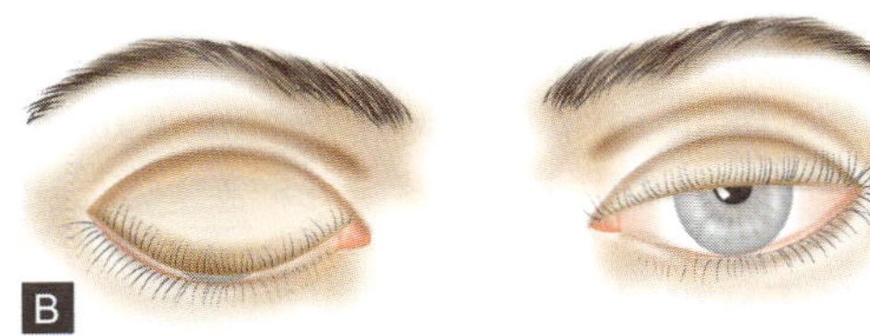

FIGS 2.5.11A and B: Lagophthalmos of left eye. **A.** Photograph; **B.** Diagrammatic representation (*Note:* Complete closure of right eye; incomplete closure of left eye).

Clinical Features

Normal blinking and closure of the eyelids are essentials for maintenance of tear film. Incomplete closure of the eyelids leads to dryness of cornea and conjunctiva resulting in exposure keratopathy.

Investigations

Investigations are aimed at finding the underlying cause of lagophthalmos.

Treatment

Self-limiting causes such as idiopathic facial nerve palsy (Bell's palsy) require temporary treatment measures to prevent development of complications (e.g. exposure keratopathy). Diseases of the eyelids and orbit need to be treated before treating lagophthalmos.

Medical treatment: It is done by using lubricating eyedrops and taping of the eyelids to prevent corneal and conjunctival xerosis, and development of exposure keratopathy. Medical line of management is employed as a temporary measure.

Surgical treatment: Tarsorrhaphy and gold weight implantation in the upper eyelid are usually done in cases of lagophthalmos causes paralytic facial palsy.

Tarsorrhaphy**

Tarsorrhaphy is a surgical procedure to reduce the palpebral aperture width to decrease the exposure of cornea by suturing the upper and lower eyelids together. It can be temporary tarsorrhaphy or permanent tarsorrhaphy.

Temporary tarsorrhaphy: It is done as a temporary measure by simple suturing of the upper and lower eyelid margins. It is done as a temporary measure in lagophthalmos associated with exposure keratopathy, while the patient is on treatment for the primary cause in which complete recovery is expected. For example, Bell's palsy, which will recover over 4–6 months.

Permanent tarsorrhaphy: It is done by overlapping of the two eyelids together and suturing them together. It is done in cases of lagophthalmos associated with exposure keratopathy in which complete recovery is not possible. For example, traumatic or paralytic facial nerve palsy with no chance of recovery.

FACIAL NERVE PARALYSIS

1. Facial nerve paralysis is of two types:
   - Upper motor neuron (UMN) palsy
   - Lower motor neuron (LMN) palsy.
2. Damage to the corticobulbar tract extending from cortex to brainstem results in UMN palsy.
3. Cerebrovascular diseases, multiple sclerosis and intracranial tumors are common causes for UMN facial palsy.

4. Damage to the facial nerve nucleus or facial nerve results in the LMN facial palsy (Fig. 2.5.12).
5. Idiopathic causes (e.g. Bell's palsy).
6. Infective causes such as herpes simplex, herpes zoster, leprosy, Lyme disease, fractures of base of skull.
7. Neoplastic causes such as parotid gland tumors, posterior fossa tumors, acoustic neuroma of cerebellopontine angle.
8. Autoimmune diseases such as Sjögren's syndrome, polyarteritis nodosa, sarcoidosis.

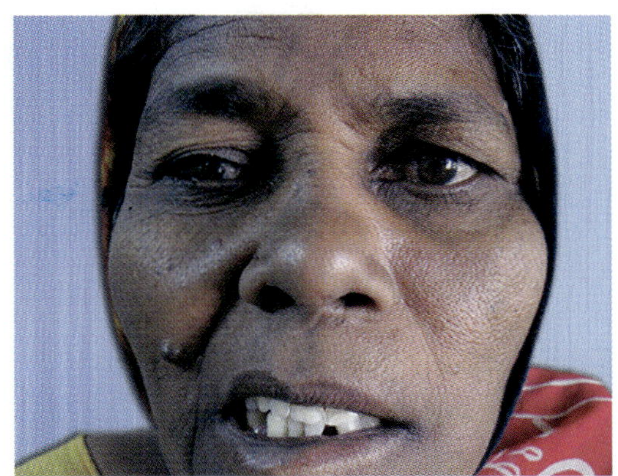

FIG. 2.5.12: Left-sided facial nerve palsy of lower motor neuron type (*Note:* Absence of wrinkling on right side of face, absence of nasolabial fold on left side of her face and deviation of angle of mouth to right side on clinching teeth).

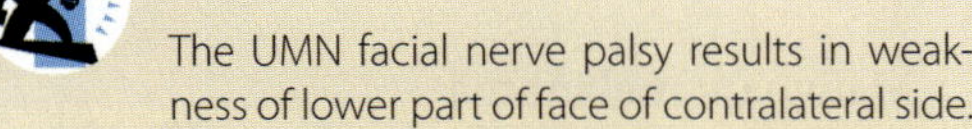

The UMN facial nerve palsy results in weakness of lower part of face of contralateral side.

The LMN facial nerve palsy result in weakness of both upper and lower part of the face of ipsilateral side.

The upper part of the face is spared in UMN palsy as upper part of face has got bilateral representation by alternative pathways. Hence lagophthalmos is not seen in UMN palsy.

Bell's Palsy

1. It is defined as idiopathic self-limiting acute peripheral facial nerve weakness.
2. It is the most common cause for acute unilateral lower motor neuron or peripheral facial nerve weakness.
3. The exact etiology is not known. It is proposed to be because of inflammation and edema of the facial nerve.
4. The diagnosis is mainly clinical. Facial weakness in Bell's palsy is acute, differentiating it from other causes such as infections, tumors in which the facial weakness progresses slowly.
5. Bell's palsy is treated by systemic steroids, which act by decreasing the inflammation and edema of the facial nerve. Ocular management is aimed at preventing exposure keratopathy by using lubricating eyedrops and eyelid taping at night.
6. About two thirds of patients with Bell's palsy show complete recovery by 6 months.

GIST BOX 2.5

- *Ptosis:* Drooping of the upper eyelid from its normal position.
- *Lid retraction:* Upward movement of the upper eyelid or downward movement of the lower eyelid, with exposure of sclera between the limbus and eyelid margin.
- *Blepharospasm:* Involuntary closure of the eyelids caused by spasm or contraction of orbicularis oculi.
- *Lagophthalmos:* Inability to close the eyelids completely.

CHAPTER

2.6 Tumors of Eyelids

Eyelids are affected by both benign and malignant tumors. The common benign tumors affecting the eyelids are:

1. Epidermal origin such as papilloma, keratoacanthoma, seborrheic keratosis, actinic keratosis, dermoid cyst.
2. Vascular origin such as hemangioma, lymphangioma, nevus flammeus, pyogenic granuloma.
3. Neural origin such as neurofibroma.
4. Xanthomatous origin such as xanthelasma, xanthogranuloma.
5. Sebaceous gland origin such as sebaceous gland adenoma, milia, cyst of Zeis.
6. Sweat gland or eccrine origin such as eccrine hidrocystoma, syringoma.
7. Modified sweat gland or gland of Moll or apocrine origin such as apocrine hidrocystoma or cyst of Moll.
8. Hair follicle origin such as pilomatrixoma, trichoepithelioma.
9. Melanocytic origin such as nevus, nevus of Ota.

The common malignant tumors of the eyelid are:

- Basal cell carcinoma (BCC)
- Squamous cell carcinoma (SCC)
- Sebaceous gland carcinoma (SGC)
- Malignant melanoma
- Kaposi's sarcoma.

Few common tumors of the eyelid are described below.

BENIGN TUMORS OF EYELID

Epidermal Origin

Squamous Papilloma

Squamous papilloma is the most common of all the benign eyelid tumors. It arises from squamous epithelium and it is usually seen in middle-aged or elderly individuals (Fig. 2.6.1).

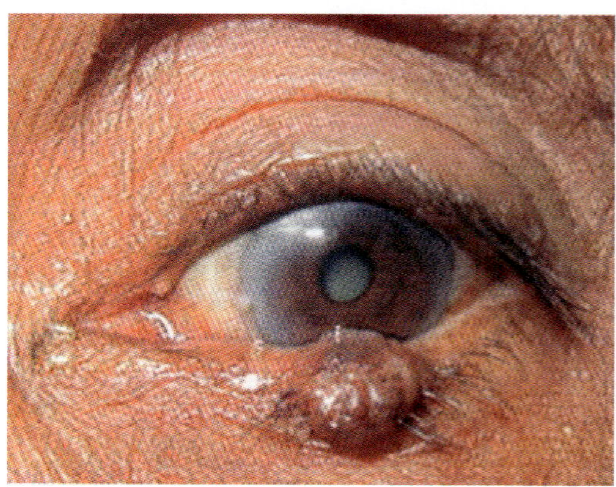

FIG. 2.6.1: Papilloma

It presents as slow growing mass usually involving the eyelid margin and it can be sessile or pedunculated. Treatment is required for cosmetic purposes and is done by surgical excision or by laser ablation.

Keratoacanthoma

Keratoacanthoma arises from epithelium and presents as rapidly growing lesion occurring in the sun exposed areas of skin. The lesion is characterized by nodular lesion with central crater having rolled up margins (Fig. 2.6.2). Keratoacanthoma can undergo malignant transformation, hence all cases should undergo complete surgical excision.

Seborrheic Keratosis

Seborrheic keratosis is a common cutaneous lesion arising from the epithelium. It is also called basal cell papilloma. It is usually seen in elderly individuals and it presents as pigmented plaque-like lesion. It has to be differentiated from other pigmented lesions such as nevus, melanoma and pigmented BCC.

Multiple or rapidly growing plaques of seborrheic keratosis are usually associated with malignant conditions such as adenocarcinoma of gastrointestinal tract called sign of Leser-Trélat.

Treatment is done by excision of the plaque along with the underlying epidermis and dermis layers of the skin.

Actinic Keratosis

Actinic keratosis is also known as solar keratosis as it is commonly seen in sun exposed areas of the body in fair-skinned individuals. It presents as flat-topped keratotic plaque, commonly seen in face, hands, scalp and eyelids.

It is the most common premalignant skin lesion and may undergo malignant transformation into SCC. It is treated by surgical excision. The cases in which complete excision cannot be done cryotherapy and local chemotherapy may be used as alternative mode of treatment.

Dermoid Cyst

Dermoid cyst is a common congenital cystic lesion seen in childhood. They are the most common epibulbar and orbital tumors in children (Fig. 2.6.3).

Etiopathogenesis: Dermoid cysts arise because of entrapment or sequestration of ectoderm at the sites of bony fusion along the sutural lines. Histologically they are called choristomas, which are defined as the presence of histologically normal tissue in abnormal location.

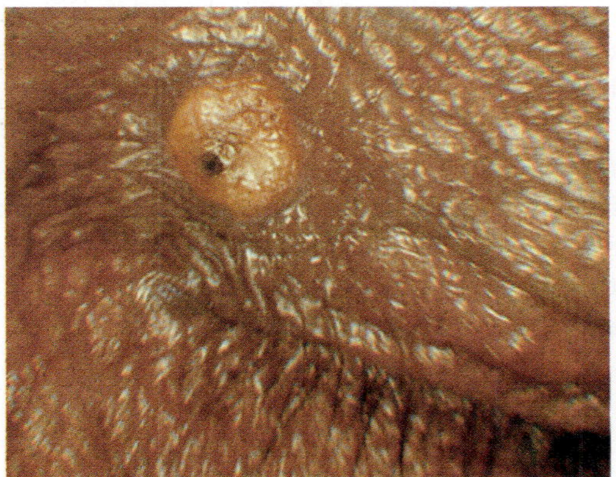

FIG. 2.6.2: Keratoacanthoma

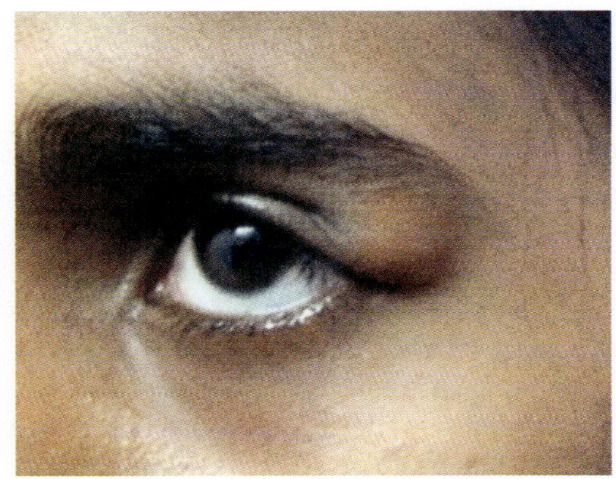

FIG. 2.6.3: Dermoid cyst

They are commonly seen on the surface of the eye, orbit and eyelids. The dermoids on the surface of the eye are seen in cornea, limbus or subconjunctival space and are called epibulbar choristomas. Epibulbar choristomas are described under congenital anomalies of conjunctiva.

Histology: The histology of dermoid cyst shows keratinized epithelium lining the cyst and the presence of hair follicles, sweat glands, and sebaceous glands in the wall of the cyst.

Clinical features: The dermoids involving bones of the orbit are called orbital choristomas. Orbital dermoids are most commonly seen in the superotemporal part of the orbit at the site of frontozygomatic suture. Dermoid cyst of the eyelids usually present as subcutaneous mass most commonly in the superotemporal part of the orbit. They are usually superficial without deeper extension. However, radiological tests such as computed tomography, should be carried out to rule out deeper orbital extension.

Treatment: This is by surgical excision. The cyst should be removed completely as rupture of the cyst may initiate inflammatory reaction and incomplete removal is usually followed by recurrence.

Vascular Origin

*Capillary Hemangioma**

Capillary hemangioma is also called strawberry nevus. It is a common congenital vascular lesion seen in children (Fig. 2.6.4). It is most often seen in females; the male to female ratio is 1:3. Though it is congenital, two thirds of the lesions manifest by 6 months of age.

Superficial lesions involving the skin of eyelids present as reddish raised patches, which typically blanch on pressure and the lesion may increase or swell on crying. Subcutaneous lesions may present as bluish or purple mass.

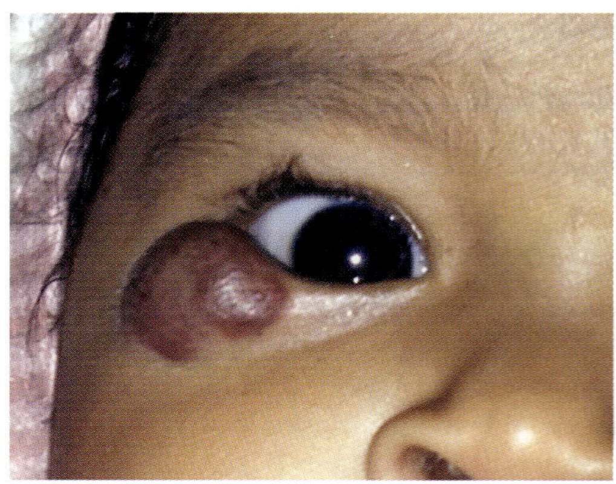

FIG. 2.6.4: Capillary hemangioma

It can occur as a superficial variety involving eyelids and a deeper variety involving orbit. The superficial variety can have deeper extensions involving the orbit.

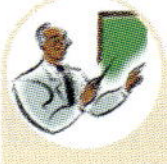

Capillary hemangioma is the most common primary orbital tumor in children.

The lesion usually shows progressive enlargement for first 6 months, later majority of the lesions undergo spontaneous regression. About two thirds of capillary hemangiomas show spontaneous regression by the age of 7 years.

Capillary hemangioma may cause amblyopia by obstruction of the visual axis because of mechanical ptosis or by induced astigmatism because of pressure of the mass over cornea.

Management is mainly by observation and follow-up. Treatment is indicated in lesions causing amblyopia. Intralesional steroids or systemic steroids are the mainstay of treatment. Radiotherapy, laser therapy and surgery are considered for lesions not responding to steroids.

Kasabach-Merritt syndrome: It is a consumptive coagulopathy seen in enlarging hemangioma or extensive visceral hemangiomas resulting in bleeding diathesis because of thrombocytopenia.

Cavernous Hemangioma

Cavernous hemangioma involves eyelids less frequently compared to capillary hemangioma. It does not undergo spontaneous resolution as in capillary hemangioma. The age of onset is in middle age in fourth decade. It also usually affects females more than males as in capillary hemangioma. It presents as deep blue patches. Treatment is by surgical excision.

Cavernous hemangioma is the most common primary benign orbital tumor in adults.

Nevus Flammeus

Nevus flammeus is also called port-wine stain. It is a congenital vascular lesion seen often in association with Sturge-Weber syndrome.

It presents as a flat reddish pink lesion involving the skin over face along the distribution of branches of trigeminal nerve. Unlike capillary hemangioma, nevus flammeus does not undergo spontaneous regression. The lesion becomes darker as the age advances and it appears reddish purple in color. Treatment is done for cosmetic purposes and it is done by ablation of the lesion to prevent scarring by pulsed dye laser.

Sturge-Weber syndrome: It is a phakomatosis involving the facial vessels and the cerebellar vessels. It is characterized by port-wine stain and ipsilateral leptomeningeal hemangioma.

The ocular features are glaucoma, choroidal hemangioma, heterochromia of iris, tortuous retinal vessels and conjunctival angiomas.

Pyogenic Granuloma

Pyogenic granuloma is a common acquired vascular lesion, which follows trauma (Fig. 2.6.5). It presents as fast growing fleshy mass. It is because of proliferation of granulation tissue following mechanical trauma or surgical trauma. Treatment is by surgical excision.

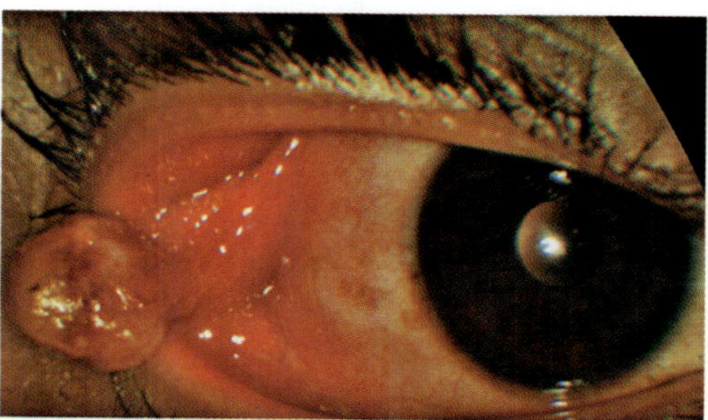

FIG. 2.6.5: Pyogenic granuloma

Neural Origin

Neurofibroma

Neurofibroma is a neural tumor consisting of neurons and fibroblasts. Plexiform neurofibroma is usually found in association with type 1 neurofibromatosis. It affects the upper eyelid resulting in ptosis and S-shaped deformity. The lesion is soft in consistency and gives bag of worms feeling on palpation. Treatment is by surgical debulking as complete excision of the lesion is usually not possible.

Xanthomatous Origin

*Xanthelasma**

Xanthelasma of the eyelids called xanthelasma palpebrarum is the most common type of xanthoma (Fig. 2.6.6). It is characterized by accumulation of fat laden macrophages in the subcutaneous layer of eyelids appearing as yellow, slightly raised plaque.

It involves upper eyelid more commonly than lower eyelid and it is usually present near the medial canthus. Xanthelasma is more common in women in fourth or fifth decade.

Around 50% of patients with xanthelasma are known to be associated with hyperlipidemia. Its presence suggests an increased risk for atherosclerosis and hence increased risk of ischemic heart disease.

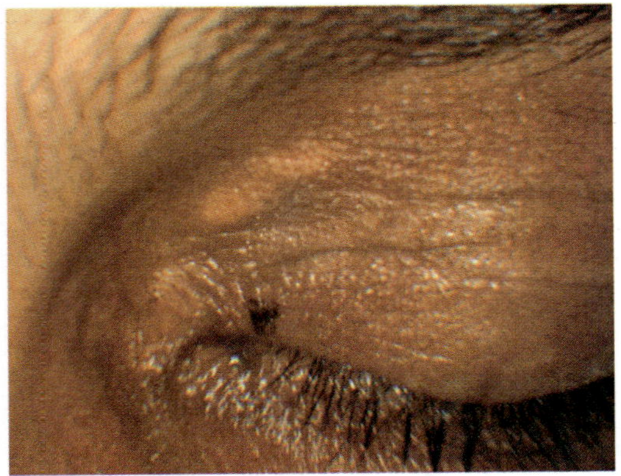

FIG. 2.6.6: Xanthelasma

Patients with xanthelasma should be investigated for hyperlipidemia. Treatment is usually required for cosmetic reasons and it is done by surgical excision or by vaporizing the lesion by carbon dioxide laser or yttrium-aluminum-garnet (YAG) laser or by topical application of trichloroacetic acid.

Sebaceous Gland Origin

Milia

Milia are multiple tiny white lesions caused by occlusion of pilosebaceous glands commonly involving the eyelids and skin over the nose. Treatment is by incision and expression of the contents.

Cyst of Zeis

Cyst of Zeis is small opaque cyst occurring at the eyelid margin because of obstruction of sebaceous gland or gland of Zeis associated with eyelash hair follicle (Fig. 2.6.7).

It is opaque because of accumulation of oily secretions and these oily secretions give it yellow color. Treatment is required for cosmetic reason and is done by simple excision.

Sweat Gland or Eccrine Origin

Eccrine Hidrocystoma

Eccrine hidrocystoma presents as single or multiple translucent fluid-filled cyst as a result of occlusion of the sweat glands. It is translucent because of accumulation of clear sweat gland secretions.

Modified Sweat Gland or Apocrine Origin

Apocrine Hidrocystoma or Cyst of Moll

Apocrine hidrocystoma presents as translucent fluid-filled cyst occurring at the eyelid margin as a result of occlusion of modified sweat glands or glands of Moll present at the eyelid margin. It is translucent because of accumulation of clear sweat gland secretions. It is similar to eccrine hidrocystoma except for the location.

Hair Follicle Origin

Pilomatrixoma

Pilomatrixoma is a benign tumor arising from matrix of the hair follicle. It presents as firm nodule with most of the lesions showing calcification. Treatment is by surgical excision.

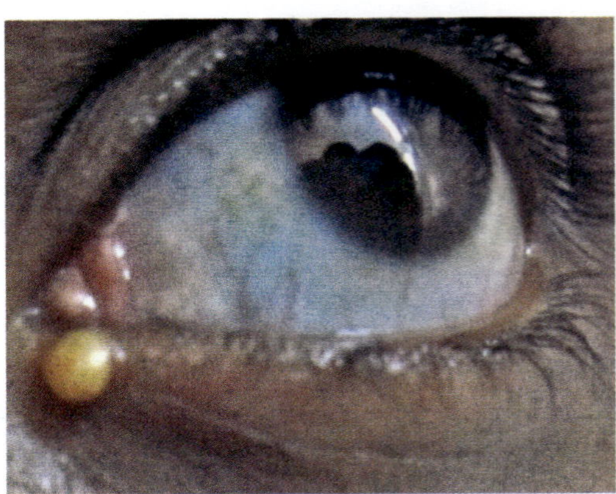

FIG. 2.6.7: Cyst of Zeis

Melanocytic Origin

Melanocytic Nevus

Melanocytic nevus is a common benign tumor of melanocytic origin consisting of melanocytes derived from neural crest. It can be congenital or acquired.

Congenital nevus is present at birth and it may present as kissing nevus in which melanocytes are present in both upper and lower eyelids at symmetrical position.

Acquired nevus usually begins in childhood and it may be:

- Junctional nevus involves epidermis
- Intradermal nevus involves dermis
- Compound nevus involves both epidermis and dermis.

Clinically nevus presents as flat (junctional nevus) or dome-shaped (intradermal nevus) (Fig. 2.6.8), or pedunculated lesion (compound nevus). Intradermal nevus is most commonly seen in adults and it may less pigmented or amelanotic.

Malignant transformation is possible with nevus, hence they have to be followed up and lesions showing features of malignancy such as rapid growth, change in pigment pattern and vascularity should be excised.

Nevus of Ota

Nevus of Ota is a congenital condition characterized by oculodermal melanocytosis. It presents as brown hyperpigmentation of face within the distribution of first and second branches of trigeminal nerve, and ocular involvement in the form of pigmentation of skin of eyelids, conjunctiva, episclera, sclera and uveal tissue.

Malignant transformation to malignant melanoma is known to occur from nevus of Ota. Hence, regular follow-up of patients are required. Treatment is by laser ablation by using Q-switched neodymium-doped yttrium aluminum garnet (Nd-YAG) laser.

MALIGNANT TUMORS OF EYELID

Basal Cell Carcinoma**

Basal cell carcinoma is slow growing, non-metastasizing malignant tumor of skin. It is the most common malignant tumor of the eyelid accounting for 90% of the malignant tumors of the eyelid (Fig. 2.6.9).

> The BCC is most common malignancy of skin. Head and neck is the most common site of occurrence accounting for 90%. BCC of eyelid accounts for 90% of the malignant tumors of eyelid.

Etiopathogenesis

Cells of origin: It arises from the basal cells found in the basal layer of the epidermis.

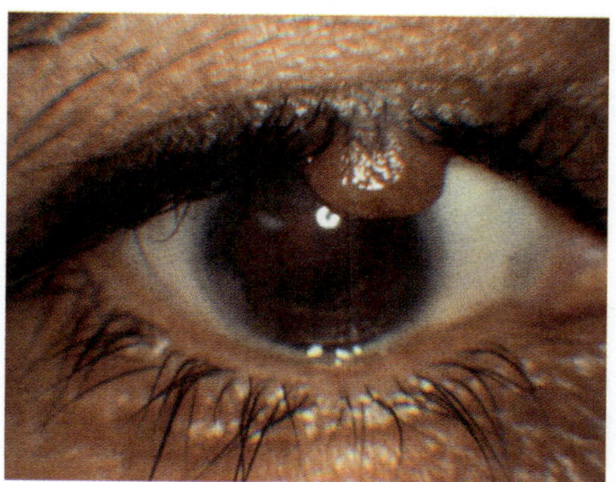

FIG. 2.6.8: Dome-shaped intradermal nevus

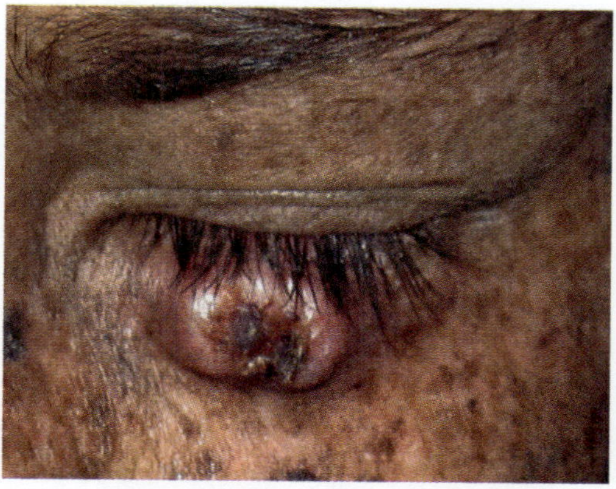

FIG. 2.6.9: Basal cell carcinoma

Risk factors: Fair skin or light-skinned people and chronic exposure to ultraviolet rays of sunlight.

Location: Lower eyelid is the most common site accounting for 50%, followed by medial canthus (25%), upper eyelid (15%) and lateral canthus (5%).

Clinical Features

The clinical features depend on the clinical type of BCC. The clinical types of BCC are:

- Nodular BCC
- Noduloulcerative BCC
- Sclerosing BCC.

Basal cell carcinoma presents as nodule (nodular BCC), or ulcer (noduloulcerative BCC) or plaque (sclerosing BCC) involving the eyelid with features suggestive of malignancy such as rolled border, or irregular border and destruction of lid margin.

Rodent Ulcer

Noduloulcerative BCC presenting with rolled edges and central ulceration is called rodent ulcer.

Treatment

Diagnosis is confirmed by incision biopsy. Surgical excision is the treatment of choice for BCC. Excision biopsy with frozen section or Mohs' micrographic surgery is the most commonly employed surgical techniques. Radiotherapy and cryotherapy are less commonly employed.

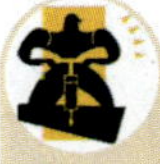

Mohs' Micrographic Surgery

It is a surgical technique for complete removal of the tumor tissue and preservation of normal healthy tissue. It is done by using horizontal frozen section histopathological slides to obtain precise microscopic tumor margin. This technique is used in the treatment of skin carcinomas.

Squamous Cell Carcinoma

Squamous cell carcinoma is the second most common malignant tumor of the eyelid accounting for 5% of all malignant lid tumors. Though it is less common than BCC, it is more aggressive tumor as it can undergo metastasis to regional lymph nodes.

Etiopathogenesis

Cells of origin: It arises from squamous cells of the epidermis.

Risk factors: Fair skin or light-skinned people and chronic exposure to ultraviolet rays of sunlight.

Location: Lower eyelid and medial canthus are most commonly involved.

Clinical Features

The clinical features depend on the clinical type of SCC. The clinical types of SCC are:

- Nodular SCC
- Ulcerative SCC.

Squamous cell carcinoma presents as indurated nodule or ulcer with everted margins.

Treatment

1. It is on similar lines as for BCC.
2. Diagnosis is confirmed by incision biopsy.
3. Treatment options are surgical excision either by excision biopsy with frozen section or Mohs' micrographic surgery. Since, SCC is more aggressive than BCC more aggressive surgery is required for SCC. Local involved lymph nodes need treatment. Radiotherapy and chemotherapy are the other treatment options available.

Sebaceous Gland Carcinoma**

Sebaceous gland carcinoma (SGC) is the third most common malignant tumor of the eyelid accounting for 1–5% of all malignant lid tumors.

Etiopathogenesis

Cells of origin: It commonly arises from meibomian glands. Rarely, it can arise from glands of Zeis or Moll or from sebaceous glands of caruncle.

Risk factors: It is a highly aggressive tumor seen in elderly females and it is characterized by high rate of local recurrence, regional, and distant metastases. More incidences are seen in individuals with prior radiation therapy.

Location: Upper eyelid is most commonly involved because of presence of more number of meibomian glands in upper eyelid.

Multifocal origin of the tumor and superficial spreading of the tumor called pagetoid spread are the two unique features of SGC, differentiating it from other tumors of eyelid.

Clinical Features

Clinical features depend on the clinical type of SGC. SGC presents in two clinical types.

Nodular SGC: It presents as firm yellow nodule resembling chalazion. It shows features of malignancy such as thickening of the tarsal plate with destruction of meibomian gland orifices and madarosis because of tumor invading eyelash follicles.

Superficial spreading SGC: It presents as plaque lesion with diffuse thickening of the lid margin and loss of eyelashes.

Diagnosis

A high index of suspicion is required for diagnosis of SGC. Full thickness biopsy of the eyelid is required for confirmation of diagnosis.

Masquerade Syndrome

The diagnosis of SGC is usually missed in the initial stages as it simulates chalazion or chronic blepharitis.

The SGC should be suspected in elderly patients diagnosed with chalazion, when chalazion is associated with features such as madarosis and destruction of meibomian gland orifices; and recurrence after incision and curettage for more than three times.

The SGC should also be suspected in elderly individuals presenting with chronic blepharitis not responding to treatment and associated with features such as diffuse thickening of the lid margin, and loss of eyelashes.

Treatment

1. Wide surgical excision is the treatment of choice. Patients presenting late with the intraocular and orbital spread may require exenteration.
2. Involvement of the lymph nodes is treated by lymph node dissection or radical neck dissection.
3. Metastasis occurs by regional spread to lymph nodes and distant spread by hematogenous route.

Prognosis

1. Prognosis for SGC is poor because of difficulties in diagnosis.
2. The SGC without distant metastasis has got mortality rate of 10%.
3. The SGC with distant metastasis is associated with mortality rate of 25–40%.
4. Poor prognostic factors are tumor size more than 10 mm, duration more than 6 months, hematogenous spread and orbital extension.
5. Tumors arising from glands of Zeis and tumors less than 6 mm are associated with good prognosis.

Malignant Melanoma

Malignant melanoma of the eyelids is rare accounting for 1% of all eyelid malignancies.

Etiopathogenesis

Cells of origin: It arises from melanocytes.

Risk factors: Chronic sun exposure, white race, congenital nevi.

Clinical Features

Clinical features depend on the clinical type. Malignant melanoma of eyelids presents in three clinical types.

Superficial spreading characterized by a pigmented plaque-like lesion and nodular characterized by pigmented nodular lesion.

Lentigo maligna melanoma occurring in Hutchinson's freckle (a premalignant lesion occurring in sun exposed skin of elderly individuals), presents as pigmented macule.

Acral lentiginous melanoma, one more variant of malignant melanoma usually affects the palms and soles, and it does not affect the eyelids.

> Though pigmentation is supposed to be the characteristic feature of melanomas, 50% of melanomas involving eyelids are amelanotic.

Treatment

It is done by wide surgical excision. Involved lymph nodes are treated by lymph node dissection. Prognosis depends on the presence or absence of metastasis. Tumors invading the subcutaneous tissues are prone for metastasis and are usually associated with poor prognosis.

PREDISPOSING CONDITIONS FOR MALIGNANT TUMORS OF EYELID

Xeroderma Pigmentosum*

1. Xeroderma pigmentosum (XP) is a rare hereditary precancerous condition of the skin characterized by hyperpigmented spots on skin all over the body and malignant growths (Fig. 2.6.10).
2. The XP is transmitted as an autosomal recessive trait and it is characterized by defective repair of deoxyribonucleic acid (DNA) following exposure to normal sunlight.
3. The disease manifests early in childhood. The initial manifestations are areas of erythema freckles, which progress to hyperpigmented spots developing on the areas of skin exposed to sunlight. Multiple BCCs and other skin malignancies such as SCCs, malignant melanomas develop later. The disease is fatal and death is because of metastatic SCCs, and malignant melanoma.

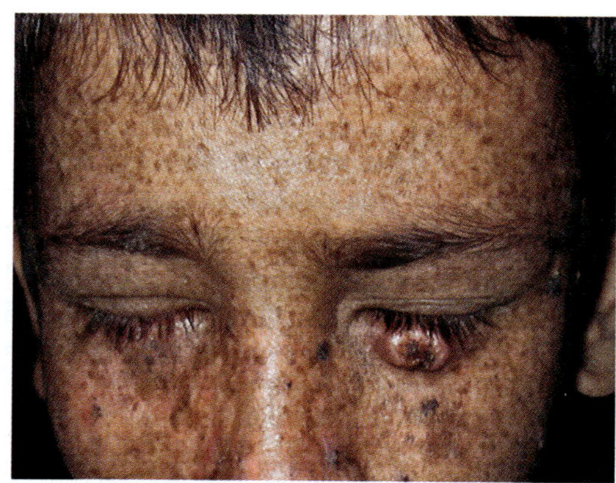

FIG. 2.6.10: Xeroderma pigmentosum

4. Ocular manifestations are seen up to 80% of cases of XP. The ocular features are destruction of the eyelids, symblepharon and carcinomas of the eyelids.
5. The prognosis of the disease is poor because of development of multiple skin malignancies. Treatment is mainly preventive by preventing exposure to sunlight. The affected children are advised to work in night and sleep during day time. Treatment of the malignant growths is done by surgical excision.

Gorlin-Goltz Syndrome

Gorlin-Goltz syndrome is a rare autosomal dominant syndrome characterized by increased predisposition to develop BCC with clinical manifestations involving multiple organs such as:

- Dental anomalies in the form of odontogenic keratocysts, mandibular prognathism
- Skeletal system anomalies, e.g. bifurcated ribs, kyphoscoliosis
- Ophthalmic anomalies, e.g. hypertelorism, strabismus
- Central nervous system anomalies, e.g. hydrocephalus, mental retardation.

GIST BOX 2.6

- Squamous papilloma is the most common of all the benign eyelid tumors.
- Actinic keratosis or solar keratosis is the most common premalignant skin lesion and may undergo malignant transformation into squamous cell carcinoma.
- Basal cell carcinoma is the most common malignant tumor of the eyelid accounting for 90% of the malignant tumors of the eyelid.
- Squamous cell carcinoma is the second most common malignant tumor of the eyelid accounting for 5% of all malignant lid tumors. Though, it is less common than basal cell carcinoma (BCC), it is more aggressive tumor as it can undergo metastasis to regional lymph nodes.

FREQUENTLY ASKED QUESTIONS (FAQs)

*Short Answers

1. Mention the layers of the eyelid.
2. Draw a diagram of the cross section of the upper eyelid.
3. Draw a diagram of the cross section of the lower eyelid.
4. Glands of the eyelids.
5. Muscles of the eyelids.
6. Cryptophthalmos.
7. Distichiasis.
8. Pseudotrichiasis.
9. Senile entropion.
10. Mention the clinical types of entropion.
11. Treatment of entropion.
12. Mention the clinical types of ectropion.
13. Madarosis.
14. Hypertrichosis and trichomegaly.
15. Poliosis.
16. Complications of chalazion.
17. Classify ptosis.
18. Congenital synkinetic ptosis.
19. Treatment of congenital ptosis.
20. Horner's syndrome.
21. Lid retraction.
22. Essential blepharospasm.
23. Xeroderma pigmentosum.
24. Xanthelasma.
25. Capillary hemangioma.

**Short Essays

1. Trichiasis.
2. Define entropion. Mention the different types and treatment of entropion.
3. Define ectropion. Mention the different types and treatment of ectropion.
4. Symblepharon.
5. Hordeolum externum.
6. Chalazion.
7. Internal hordeolum.
8. Classify blepharitis. Add a note on clinical features and treatment of blepharitis.
9. Ulcerative blepharitis.
10. Squamous blepharitis.
11. Congenital ptosis.
12. Lagophthalmos.
13. Tarsorraphy.
14. Basal cell carcinoma of eyelids.
15. Sebaceous gland carcinoma of eyelids.

***Long Essays

1. Define ptosis. Classify ptosis. Describe the different types of ptosis and management of ptosis.

BIBLIOGRAPHY

1. Bartley GB. The differential diagnosis and classification of eyelid retraction. Trans Am Ophthalmol Soc. 1995;93:371-87.
2. Bergman R. The pathogenesis and clinical significance of xanthelasma palpebrarum. J Am Acad Dermatol. 1994;30(2 Pt 1):236-42.
3. Braiteh F, Kurzrock R, Johnson FM. Trichomegaly of the eyelashes after lung cancer treatment with the epidermal growth factor receptor inhibitor. J Clin Oncol. 2008;26(20):3460-2.
4. Dubey AK, Nagar M, Gupta A, et al. Xeroderma pigmentosum (case report). Indian J Ophthalmol. 1990;38(2):94-6.
5. Gulati GC, Ahluwalia BK. Ocular involvement in xeroderma pigmentosum. J All India Ophthalmol Soc. 1967;15(6):233-5.
6. Hamada S, Kersey T, Thaller VT. Eyelid basal cell carcinoma: non-Mohs excision, repair, and outcome. Br J Ophthalmol. 2005;89(8):992-4.

7. Jawa DS, Sircar K, Somani R, et al. Gorlin-Goltz syndrome. J Oral Maxillofac Pathol. 2009;13(2):89-92.
8. Kanski JJ. Clinical Ophthalmology Systematic Approach, 5th edition. Philadelphia: Butterworth-Heinemann; 2003.
9. Kay KM, Kim JH, Lee TS. Poliosis of eyelashes as an unusual sign of a halo nevus. Korean J Ophthalmol. 2010;24(4):237-9.
10. Kumar A, Karthikeyan K. Madarosis: a marker of many maladies. Int J Trichology. 2012;4(1):3-18.
11. Malhotra C, Waris A, Nagpal RC. Ocular uses of Botulinum toxin: an overview. JK science: Journal of Medical Education and Research. 2008;10(2).
12. Miller NR, Newman NJ, Walsh FB. Walsh & Hoyt's Clinical Neuro-Ophthalmology. Philadelphia: Lippincott Williams & Wilkins; 1998.
13. Misra MC. Xeroderma pigmentosum with eye affection. J All India Ophthalmol Soc. 1963;11:62-7.
14. Murthy JM, Saxena AB. Bell's palsy: Treatment guidelines. Ann Indian Acad Neurol. 2011;14(Suppl 1):S70-2.
15. Nambi GI, Beck B, Gupta AK. An unusual cause of lagophthalmos. Oman J Ophthalmol. 2010;3(1):32-3.
16. Pandeshwar P, Jayanthi K, Mahesh D. Gorlin-Goltz syndrome. Case Rep Dent. 2012;2012:247239.
17. Paul LJ, Cohen PR, Kurzrock R. Eyelash trichomegaly: review of congenital, acquired, and drug-associated etiologies for elongation of the eyelashes. Int J Dermatol. 2012;51(6):631-46.
18. Pham TT, Perry JD. Floppy eyelid syndrome. Curr Opin Ophthalmol. 2007;18(5):430-3.
19. Sharma G, Nagpal A. Nevus of ota with rare palatal involvement: a case report with emphasis on differential diagnosis. Case Rep Dent. 2011;2011:670-679.
20. Shields JA, Carol LS. Eyelid, Conjunctival, and Orbital Tumors: An atlas and Textbook, 2nd edition, Philadelphia: Lippincott Williams & Wilkins; 2007.
21. Shukla Y, Ratnawat PS. Tuberous xanthoma of upper eye lids (a case report). Indian J Ophthalmol. 1982;30(3):161-2.
22. Tanenbaum M. A rational approach to the patient with floppy/lax eyelids. Br J Ophthalmol. 1994;78(9):663-4.
23. Verma L, Kumar A, Garg SP, et al. Iris neovascularization in Sturge–Weber syndrome. Indian J Ophthalmol. 1991;39(2):82-3.
24. Wali UK, Al-Mujaini A. Sebaceous gland carcinoma of the eyelid. Oman J Ophthalmol. 2010;3(3):117-21.
25. Wiafe B. Herpes Zoster Ophthalmicus in HIV/AIDS. Community Eye Health. 2003;16(47):35-6.
26. Yanoff M, Duker JS. Ophthalmology, 3rd edition. China: Mosby Elsevier; 2008.

SECTION 3

Conjunctiva

CHAPTER

3.1 Anatomy of Conjunctiva

INTRODUCTION

Conjunctiva is a transparent, thin mucous membrane, which lines the anterior surface of globe up to limbus and posterior surface of eyelids. The word conjunctiva means a membrane, which conjoins eyeball with eyelids.

FUNCTIONS OF CONJUNCTIVA

1. Provides lubrication by production of mucin from goblet cells, an essential component of tear film.
2. Provides protection to globe as it lines the anterior surface of eyeball.
3. Takes part in immune function and defensive mechanisms of eye against microbial organisms by secretion of antibacterial proteins.

GROSS ANATOMY

Conjunctiva is subdivided into:

1. *Palpebral conjunctiva or tarsal conjunctiva:* It lines the posterior surface of eyelids.
2. *Bulbar conjunctiva:* It lines the anterior surface of sclera.
3. *Forniceal conjunctiva:* It is the junction between the palpebral conjunctiva and bulbar conjunctiva. It is divided into superior, inferior, nasal and temporal fornices.
4. Plica semilunaris is a fold of bulbar conjunctiva present in the medial canthus. It is the vestigial remnant of nictitating membrane or third eyelid present in animals such as reptiles and birds.

Caruncle is modified skin tissue situated in the medial canthus, medial to plica semilunaris. It contains sweat glands, sebaceous glands, accessory lacrimal glands and hair follicles (Fig. 3.1.1).

HISTOLOGY*

The histology of conjunctiva shows:

1. *Epithelium:* It is non-keratinizing stratified squamous epithelium. Its thickness varies according to the part of conjunctiva. It is about five cells thick at limbus, 3–4 cells thick at fornices and 2–3 cells thick over palpebral conjunctiva. The basal cells are cuboidal, whereas the superficial cells are flat polyhedral cells.
2. *Stromal layer:* It consists of a superficial adenoid layer consisting of lymphocytes and

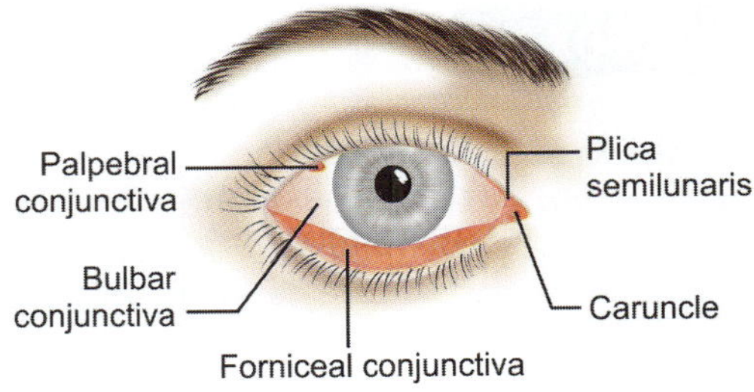

FIG. 3.1.1: Gross anatomy of conjunctiva

connective tissue, and deeper fibrous layer consisting of connective tissue, nerves and blood vessels supplying conjunctiva.

The adenoid layer, which consists of lymphocytes is not present at birth; it develops at about 3 months after birth. Hence, follicular reaction is not seen in conjunctiva of newborn (conjunctival follicles are usually seen in viral infections of conjunctiva).

GLANDS OF CONJUNCTIVA*

Mucin-secreting Glands (Goblet Cells, Crypts of Henle and Glands of Manz)

Mucin-secreting glands are present in the innermost layer of the tear film and they secrete mucin. Goblet cells are located in the epithelium of conjunctiva, and they are most numerous in the nasal bulbar conjunctiva and in inferior fornix. Crypts of Henle and glands of Manz are not true glands; they are folds of mucous membrane. Crypts of Henle are present in tarsal conjunctiva and glands of Manz are present in limbal conjunctiva.

Accessory Lacrimal Glands of Krause and Wolfring

Accessory lacrimal glands of Krause and Wolfring are located deep in the stroma of conjunctiva and they secrete aqueous layer of tear film along with the main lacrimal gland (Fig. 3.1.2).

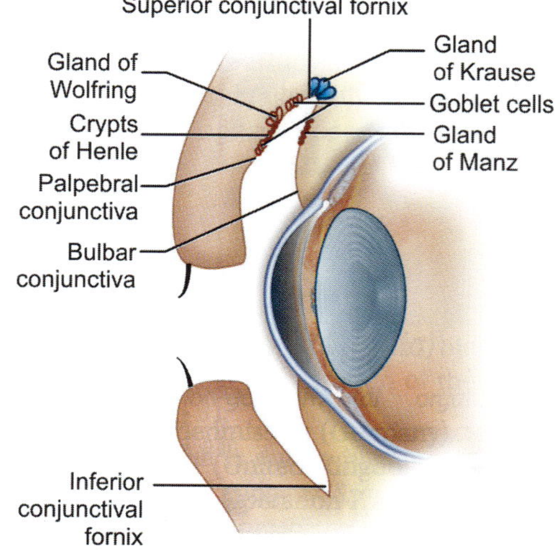

FIG. 3.1.2: Glands of conjunctiva

Blood Supply of Conjunctiva

Conjunctiva is supplied by palpebral branches of lacrimal artery and anterior ciliary artery. Venous drainage is by superior and inferior ophthalmic veins.

Nerve Supply of Conjunctiva

Conjunctiva is supplied by nasal, frontal and nasociliary branches of trigeminal nerve.

Lymphatic Drainage

Submandibular lymph nodes drain the medial half of conjunctiva and lateral half drains into preauricular lymph nodes.

GIST BOX 3.1

- Conjunctiva is a transparent, thin mucous membrane, which lines the anterior surface of globe up to limbus and posterior surface of eyelids.
- Conjunctiva is subdivided into palpebral conjunctiva, bulbar conjunctiva and forniceal conjunctiva.
- Glands of conjunctiva include mucin-secreting glands such as goblet cells, crypts of Henle, glands of Manz, and accessory lacrimal glands of Krause and Wolfring.

CHAPTER

3.2 Symptomatology of Conjunctiva

HYPEREMIA

Definition

Redness of conjunctiva due to congestion of the conjunctival vessels is called hyperemia of conjunctiva (Fig. 3.2.1).

Causes for Hyperemia of Conjunctiva*

1. Hyperemia of conjunctiva is seen in all varieties of conjunctivitis, i.e. infective, allergic, toxic, traumatic, etc.
2. Transient hyperemia is seen in conditions such as on exposure to dust, fumes, wind, on rubbing of eyes, after head bath, lack of sleep, etc.
3. Reflex hyperemia is seen in inflammations of the surrounding structures of the eyes such as rhinitis, sinusitis, etc. and in systemic febrile conditions.

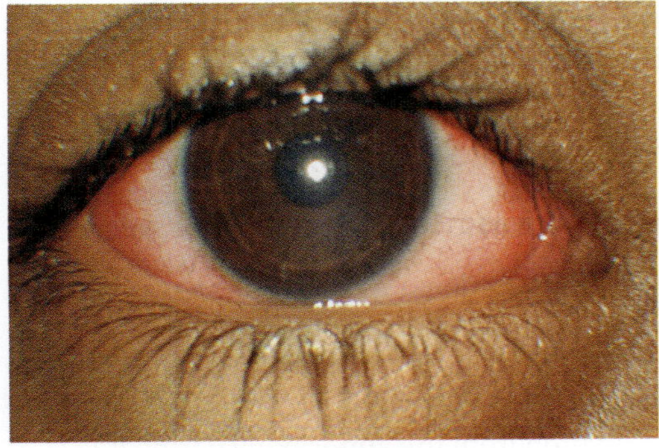

FIG. 3.2.1: Hyperemia of conjunctiva

Clinical Features

On examination, congestion is seen prominently in the conjunctival fornices, bulbar conjunctiva and fading toward the limbus. Congested vessels are bright red in color, move with conjunctiva on moving the conjunctiva and blanch on applying topical vasoconstrictor.

Treatment

Treatment of hyperemia is done by treating the underlying condition. Symptomatic treatment is done by topical vasoconstrictor eyedrops such as phenylephrine.

ECCHYMOSIS (SUBCONJUNCTIVAL HEMORRHAGE)**

Definition

Collection of blood under the bulbar conjunctiva is called ecchymosis (Figs 3.2.2A to D).

Causes

1. Trauma is the commonest cause for subconjunctival hemorrhage. It may be because

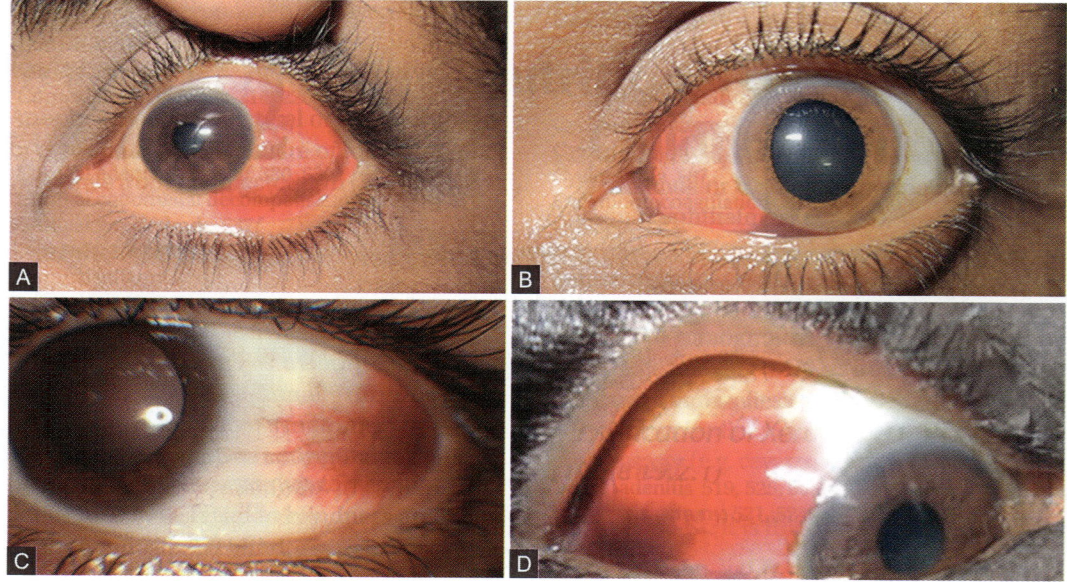

FIGS 3.2.2A to D: Ecchymosis of conjunctiva or subconjunctival hemorrhage

of direct trauma to conjunctiva resulting in rupture of conjunctival capillaries or because of seepage of blood along the floor of the orbit as in fractures of base of skull and head injuries.

2. Hemorrhagic conjunctivitis caused by enteroviruses, pneumococci, etc.
3. Vascular diseases such as diabetes, hypertension and arteriosclerosis because of spontaneous rupture of the capillaries.
4. Bleeding diseases: Hemophilia and blood dyscrasias such as leukemia, anemia, etc.

Clinical Features

Subconjunctival hemorrhage is usually painless condition with only symptom being redness of the eye. Pain may be seen in cases of subconjunctival hemorrhage caused by trauma.

Evaluation of Patient with Subconjunctival Hemorrhage

Look for the posterior limit of the subconjunctival hemorrhage. If posterior limit cannot be made out, retrobulbar hemorrhage has to be ruled out particularly in patients with history of moderate-to-severe eye trauma or head injury.

Evaluate for other causes of subconjunctival hemorrhage in patients with no history of trauma.

Treatment

Subconjunctival hemorrhage does not require treatment; it will be absorbed completely over a period of 4–6 weeks. Hence, reassurance and placebo eyedrops are sufficient. Treatment of the underlying cause and associated causes is required.

CHEMOSIS**

Definition

Swelling or edema of the conjunctiva is called chemosis (Figs 3.2.3A and B). Chemosis is because of collection of fluid under the loosely attached bulbar conjunctiva arising because of exudation from the abnormally permeable conjunctival capillaries.

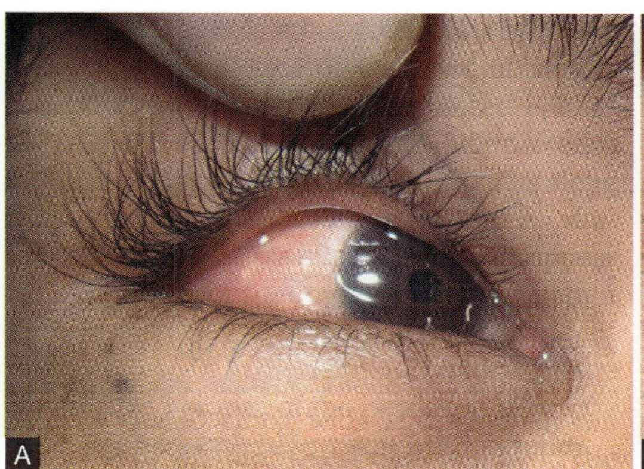

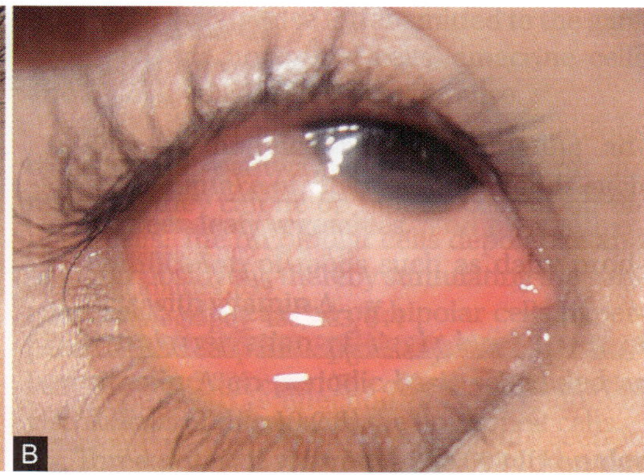

FIGS 3.2.3A and B: Chemosis of conjunctiva

Causes

1. Ocular inflammatory conditions such as conjunctivitis, keratitis, iridocyclitis, endophthalmitis, panophthalmitis, etc. and allergic conditions of eye—allergic conjunctivitis.
2. Systemic conditions such as congestive cardiac failure, anemia, hypoproteinemia, nephritic syndrome, angioneurotic syndrome, etc.
3. Passive congestion due to mechanical obstruction to venous outflow as in exophthalmos, orbital tumors, cavernous sinus thrombosis, etc.

Clinical Features

Discoloration of Conjunctiva

Normal conjunctiva is transparent mucous membrane. It may show discoloration in various ocular and systemic conditions (Fig. 3.2.4 and Table 3.2.1).

Conjunctival Discharge

Abnormal excess production of secretions from the conjunctiva in response to inflammation consisting of tears, mucus, inflammatory cells with or without microbial organisms is called conjunctival discharge. It varies according to the type of conjunctivitis (Table 3.2.2).

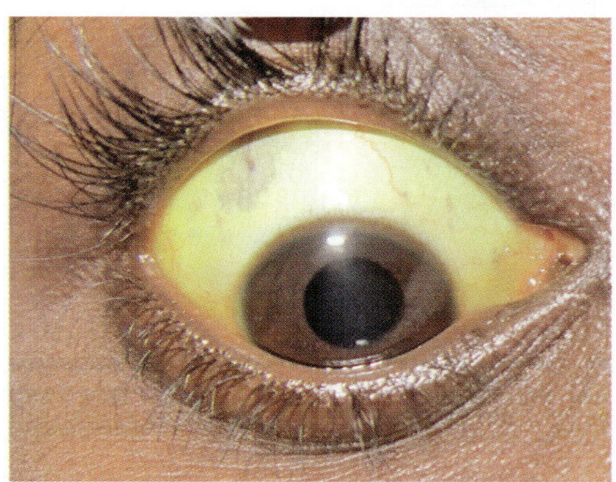

FIG. 3.2.4: Yellowish discoloration of conjunctiva in jaundice

Treatment

Milder cases are treated with topical vasoconstrictor eyedrops—phenylephrine. Chemosis because of allergic conditions is treated by topical and systemic steroids. Along with this, the underlying causes such as inflammatory conditions of the eye or systemic conditions causing chemosis must be treated.

TABLE 3.2.1: Types of conjunctival discoloration

Discoloration	*Features*
Yellow discoloration	Jaundice (due to the presence of bile pigments)
Red discoloration	Subconjunctival hemorrhage
Brownish discoloration	• Argyrosis (due to long-term application of silver nitrate and other drugs such as adrenaline) • Conjunctival melanosis, benign nevus, precancerous melanosis, malignant melanoma

TABLE 3.2.2: Different types of conjunctival discharges in response to different kinds of conjunctivitis

Discharge	*Conjunctivitis*
Watery discharge (transparent)	Viral conjunctivitis
Mucopurulent or purulent discharge (yellowish green)	Bacterial conjunctivitis
Mucoid serous discharge (white)	Allergic conjunctivitis

GIST BOX 3.2

- *Hyperemia of conjunctiva:* Redness of conjunctiva due to congestion of the conjunctival vessels.
- *Ecchymosis of conjunctiva or subconjunctival hemorrhage:* Collection of blood under the bulbar conjunctiva.
- *Chemosis of conjunctiva:* Swelling or edema of the conjunctiva.

CHAPTER

3.3 Congenital Anomalies of Conjunctiva

EMBRYOLOGY

Surface ectoderm gives rise to epithelium of conjunctiva and stroma of conjunctiva develops from mesoderm.

CONGENITAL ANOMALIES

Epitarsus

Epitarsus is a rare congenital anomaly of conjunctiva characterized by the presence of a fold of conjunctiva attached to the tarsal plate. It is usually due to persistence of hypertrophic fold of plica semilunaris.

Treatment: It is usually not required. It is required either for cosmetic reasons or when it covers cornea. Treatment when required is done by excision of the epitarsus.

Choristomas of Conjunctiva

Choristomas are defined as the presence of histologically normal tissue in abnormal location. They are the commonest epibulbar and orbital tumors in children. Choristomas involving the surface of the eye either cornea, limbus or subconjunctival space are called epibulbar choristomas and those involving bones of the orbit are called orbital choristomas. Epibulbar choristomas may be dermoid or dermolipoma.

Dermoid

Etiopathogenesis

Dermoid is usually sporadic and non-hereditary inheritance may be associated with Goldenhar syndrome. Dermoid contains ectodermal structures such as hair, sebaceous glands, sweat glands and mesodermal structures such as blood vessels, cartilage (Figs 3.3.1A and B).

Clinical features

1. Dermoid presents as flat or elevated growth, commonest site is inferotemporal part of limbus.
2. Smaller dermoid is asymptomatic, larger ones produce symptoms such as irritation, blurring of vision either because of astigmatism or because of manual encroachment of the pupillary area.

Treatment

Treatment is indicated for symptomatic lesions and for cosmetic growth. Treatment when required is done by surgical excision. Deeper extension into the iris and ciliary body must be ruled out before attempting surgery. Lesions with corneal involvement may require lamellar or full thickness keratoplasty following excision of the dermoid.

Dermolipoma

Etiopathogenesis

Dermolipoma is usually less common compared to dermoid and it contains fat. It may be associated with Goldenhar syndrome such as dermoid.

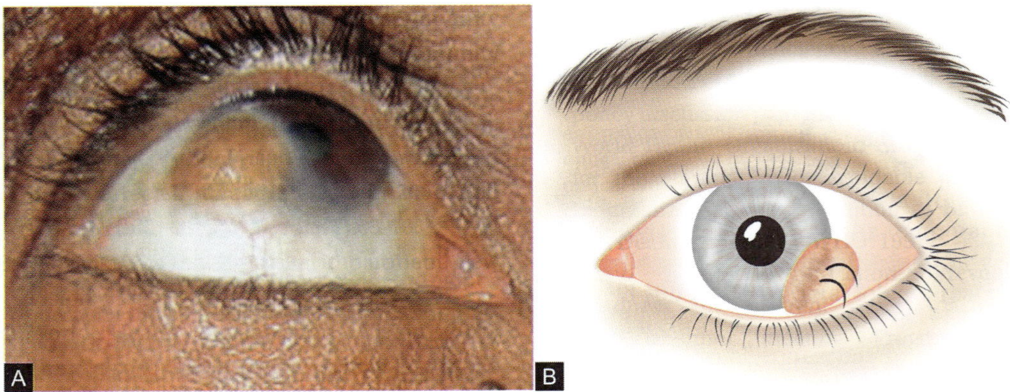

FIGS 3.3.1A and B: Limbal dermoid. **A.** Photograph; **B.** Diagrammatic representation (*Note:* Solid mass lesion in the inferotemporal part of limbus showing hair shafts).

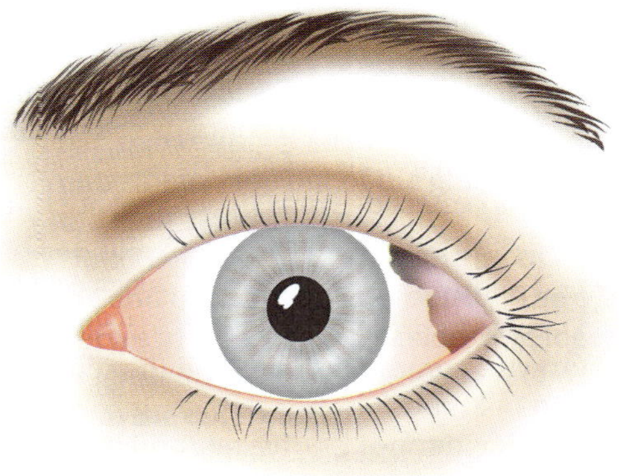

FIG. 3.3.2: Dermolipoma (*Note:* Growth in the superotemporal fornix)

Clinical features

1. Dermolipoma presents as soft yellow growth usually away from limbus and most common site being superotemporal fornix.
2. Since it is away from cornea, visual symptoms are not seen.
3. Usually, dermolipoma has orbital extension.
4. It has to be differentiated from prolapsed orbital fat and palpebral lobe of lacrimal gland.

Treatment

Treatment is not indicated for smaller lesions. Larger lesions need surgical excision. Orbitotomy is required for complete excision of lesions with orbital extension (Fig. 3.3.2).

Goldenhar syndrome (oculoauriculovertebral dysplasia): It is a rare syndrome characterized by ocular epibulbar dermoid, auricular-preauricular skin tags and vertebral-vertebral hypoplasia. Other defects seen are hypoplasia of face, cleft lip, cleft palate, etc.

GIST BOX 3.3

- Epibulbar choristomas are the commonest epibulbar and orbital tumors in children. Choristomas involving the surface of the eye either cornea, limbus or subconjunctival space are called epibulbar choristomas and those involving bones of the orbit are called orbital choristomas.
- Epibulbar choristomas may be dermoid or dermolipoma.

CHAPTER

3.4 Inflammatory Diseases of Conjunctiva

CONJUNCTIVITIS

Definition

Inflammation of conjunctiva is called conjunctivitis. It is characterized by:

- Hyperemia or redness of conjunctiva
- Cellular infiltration
- Exudation or discharge, which can be watery, mucoid, mucopurulent or purulent.

Classification

Conjunctivitis is broadly classified as:

- Infectious conjunctivitis
- Non-infectious conjunctivitis.

Infectious conjunctivitis is further classified into:

- Bacterial conjunctivitis
- Viral conjunctivitis
- Chlamydial conjunctivitis
- Fungal conjunctivitis
- Protozoal conjunctivitis
- Spirochaetal conjunctivitis
- Microsporidal conjunctivitis.

Non-infectious conjunctivitis is further classified into:

- Allergic conjunctivitis
- Toxic conjunctivitis
- Traumatic conjunctivitis.

Conjunctivitis associated with diseases of skin and mucous membrane such as Steven-Johnson syndrome, ocular cicatricial pemphigoid, etc.

BACTERIAL CONJUNCTIVITIS

Bacterial conjunctivitis is the most common ocular infection worldwide.

ETIOPATHOGENESIS

Normally, conjunctiva has got natural defense mechanisms against any microbial invasion in the form of:

1. Presence of normal conjunctival flora resisting the invasion by pathogenic microbes.
2. Protective action of the eyelids.
3. Antimicrobial activity of tear film due to presence of lysozymes and immunoglobulins.

Disruption of these normal defense mechanisms predisposes to infection of the ocular surface as occurring in the following conditions:

1. Replacement of normal conjunctival flora by pathogenic flora as in diseases affecting local ocular or systemic immune mechanism such as in patients with diabetes mellitus, human immunodeficiency virus (HIV) infection, patients on immunosuppressive therapy, etc.
2. Diseases of eyelids such as entropion, ectropion, lagophthalmos.
3. Diseases affecting tear film such as dry eye, obstructions in the lacrimal drainage system (chronic dacryocystitis).

Conjunctivitis is seen all over the world with increased incidence and epidemics of conjunctivitis being seen in people in dry climate, unhygienic sanitation as in underdeveloped countries.

Mode of Spread

Exogenous route is the commonest mode of spread of conjunctivitis. Discharge from infected persons is the source of infection. Infection usually spreads by fingers, flies, fomites, towels, etc. Other routes of infection are from surrounding structures (e.g. from sinusitis) and endogenous route (usually rare).

CLASSIFICATION**

The classification of bacterial conjunctivitis is based on the etiological agent and clinical features as detailed in Table 3.4.1.

Acute Mucopurulent Conjunctivitis

Acute mucopurulent conjunctivitis is the most common type of conjunctivitis. It is characterized by hyperemia of conjunctiva and mucopurulent discharge (Figs 3.4.1A and B).

Etiology

Acute mucopurulent conjunctivitis is caused by bacteria such as *Staphylococcus aureus (S. aureus), Streptococcus pneumoniae (S. pneumoniae), Haemophilus influenzae.* Mode of spread is by discharge of infected persons from exogenous route.

Clinical Features

Symptoms

1. Acute or sudden onset of redness, grittiness, foreign body sensation and discharge—initially watery, later mucopurulent.
2. Symptoms will be unilateral initially; other eye will be invariably involved in 1–2 days (source of infection being the affected eye, hence both the eyes should be treated).

Signs

1. Lid edema seen in severe cases.
2. Conjunctiva shows features of conjunctival congestion.
3. Stickiness of eyelashes due to mucopurulent discharge.

TABLE 3.4.1: Classification of bacterial conjunctivitis

Types	*Causative agents*	*Clinical features*
Acute mucopurulent conjunctivitis	*Staphylococcus aureus, Streptococcus pneumoniae (S. pneumoniae), Haemophilus influenzae*	Conjunctival congestion, mucopurulent discharge
Hyperacute purulent conjunctivitis	*Neisseria gonorrhoeae, Neisseria meningitidis*	Lid edema, conjunctival congestion, purulent discharge
Acute membranous conjunctivitis	*Corynebacterium diphtheriae*	Lid edema, conjunctival discharge, true membrane formation
Acute pseudomembranous conjunctivitis	Virulent bacterial strains of *S. pneumoniae* and *Streptococcus haemolyticus*	Lid edema, conjunctival discharge, pseudomembrane formation
Angular conjunctivitis	*Moraxella lacunata*	Congestion at the medial and lateral canthus
Chronic conjunctivitis	*Staphylococcus aureus*	Chronic symptoms of more than 3 weeks duration
Granulomatous conjunctivitis	*Mycobacterium tuberculosis, Mycobacterium leprae, Treponema pallidum*	Conjunctival granuloma

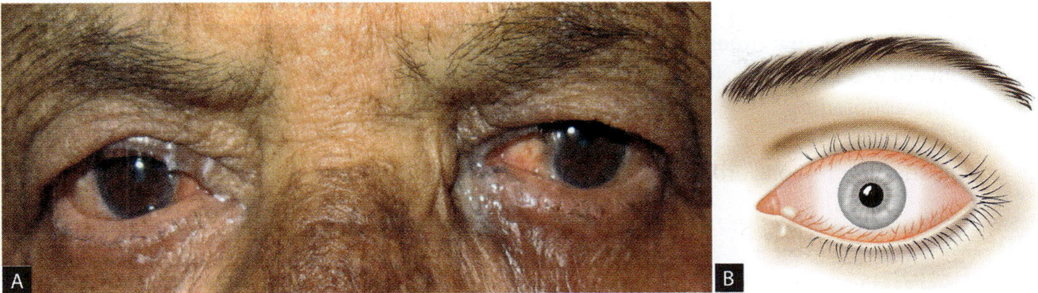

FIGS 3.4.1A and B: Acute mucopurulent conjunctivitis. **A.** Photograph; **B.** Diagrammatic representation (*Note*: Conjunctival congestion, lid edema, mucopurulent discharge).

Clinical Course and Complications

Usually acute mucopurulent conjunctivitis is self-limiting condition. Complications are rare. Complications seen are corneal involvement in the form of corneal ulceration and spread of infection to surrounding structures resulting in preseptal or postseptal orbital cellulitis.

Investigations

Investigations are not required routinely in all cases. These are required in severe non-responsive cases:

1. Investigations carried out in severe conjunctivitis are gram staining of conjunctival discharge, conjunctival swab for culture and sensitivity.
2. In non-responsive cases, polymerase chain reaction (PCR) is done to rule out chlamydial and viral conjunctivitis.

Differential Diagnosis

Acute conjunctivitis has to be differentiated from other causes of acute red eye, other types of bacterial conjunctivitis, viral conjunctivitis and allergic conjunctivitis.

Treatment

Acute mucopurulent conjunctivitis is treated by broad-spectrum antibiotic eyedrops and eye ointment.

Eye ointments are more effective than eyedrops as they are retained in the conjunctival sac for longer time as compared to eyedrops, which are drained by lacrimal drainage system. Eye ointments usually cause stickiness of eyelids; hence, they are used in nighttimes.

1. Broad-spectrum antibiotics: Quinolones such as ciprofloxacin (0.3%), moxifloxacin (0.3%), ofloxacin (0.3%) or levofloxacin (0.3%) are commonly used. Aminoglycosides such as gentamicin or tobramycin, chloramphenicol, polymyxin are the other drugs commonly used. Initially, eyedrops are advised as frequently as hourly, later may be tapered to two times a day. Eye ointments are used preferably at night.

Don'ts in All Types of Bacterial Conjunctivitis

No steroids: Though steroids decrease inflammation and prevent scarring especially in membranous conjunctivitis, use of steroids is not advised as it may result in corneal ulceration.

No contact lenses: Contact lenses should not be worn till 2 days after complete resolution of symptoms as use of contact lenses may cause corneal abrasion, which may be infected resulting in corneal ulceration.

No eye patch: The eye patch should not be applied as this converts and this increase the temperature of the conjunctival sac increasing the multiplication of the bacteria.

2. Oral anti-inflammatory drugs: Tablet diclofenac (50 mg), two times a day are used initially for 2–3 days.
3. Systemic antibiotics: These are not required in all the cases; they are required in complications such as preseptal orbital cellulitis, etc.

Hyperacute Purulent Conjunctivitis**

Definition

Acute severe inflammation of the conjunctiva characterized by purulent conjunctival discharge is called hyperacute purulent conjunctivitis (Figs 3.4.2A and B).

Etiopathogenesis

The causative organism is usually *Neisseria gonorrhoeae (N. gonorrhoeae)* and less frequently *Neisseria meningitidis*. Gonococcal infection usually spreads from genitals to eye by direct contact.

Acute severe purulent conjunctivitis caused by virulent strains of *S. aureus* and *S. pneumoniae* is referred sometimes as hyperacute conjunctivitis.

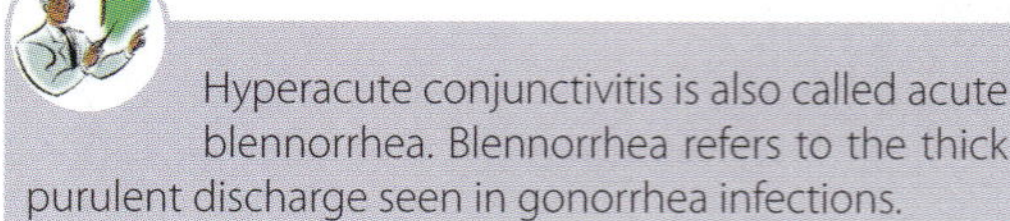

Hyperacute conjunctivitis is also called acute blennorrhea. Blennorrhea refers to the thick purulent discharge seen in gonorrhea infections.

Depending on the age of onset, it is of two types:

1. Hyperacute purulent conjunctivitis of adults.
2. Hyperacute purulent conjunctivitis of neonates called ophthalmia neonatorum (it is described in detail in next page).

Hyperacute purulent conjunctivitis of adults

Clinical features

1. The disease is characterized by acute onset of redness of the eyes associated with thick green purulent discharge.
2. Ocular pain, chemosis, lid edema and preauricular lymphadenopathy are commonly seen as associated features.
3. The disease usually starts as unilateral, but rapidly progresses to become bilateral.

Hyperacute purulent conjunctivitis caused by gonorrhea is usually seen in neonates and in sexually active young adults. The mode of infection is usually from direct contact from the genital infection. The infection may rarely spread as metastatic infection from gonococcal urethritis.

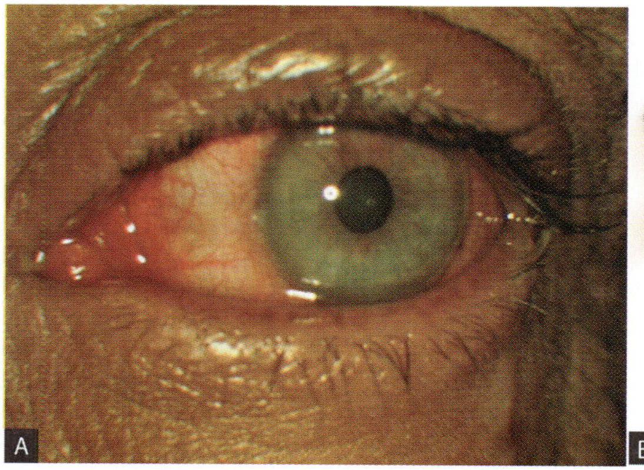

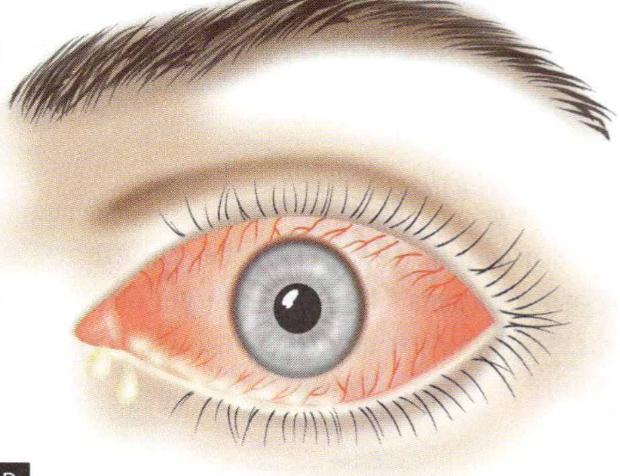

FIGS 3.4.2A and B: Hyperacute purulent conjunctivitis. **A.** Photograph; **B.** Diagrammatic representation (*Note:* Severe conjunctival congestion, lid edema, purulent discharge).

Complications

1. Corneal involvement in the form of corneal ulceration and corneal perforation.

> Corneal ulceration is more frequent in gonococcal infection as *N. gonorrhoeae* can penetrate intact corneal epithelium. Organisms, which can penetrate intact corneal epithelium are:
> - *Neisseria gonorrhoeae.*
> - *Listeria monocytogenes.*
> - *Corynebacterium diphtheriae (C. diphtheriae).*
> - *Haemophilus influenzae.*

2. Symblepharon formation because of virulent infection leading to membrane formation.
3. Spread of infection to surrounding structures leading to orbital cellulitis.
4. Systemic complications such as septicemia can occur rarely.

Laboratory diagnosis

Laboratory diagnosis is done by:

1. Gram staining, which shows gram-negative diplococci.
2. Culture by using enriched agar or selective medium such as Thayer-Martin medium.

> Laboratory diagnosis is essential to diagnose hyperacute conjunctivitis caused by *Neisseria* as its treatment is different from all other types of bacterial conjunctivitis.
>
> Systemic treatment is compulsory for all neisseria conjunctivitis and treatment by topical antibiotics as done for all other bacterial conjunctivitis is not effective.

Treatment

Systemic treatment is indicated in hyperacute conjunctivitis caused by *Neisseria*. In other cases, systemic treatment is not compulsory:

1. Systemic treatment is the most important aspect in treating neisseria conjunctivitis.
2. This is done by a single intramuscular injection of ceftriaxone (1 g) in cases of neisseria conjunctivitis. The cases with corneal involvement require intravenous injection of ceftriaxone (1 g) two times a day for 3–5 days.

Topical treatment is done by moxifloxacin (0.5%) eyedrops and tobramycin (0.3%) eyedrops used as frequently as one drop every half-an-hour depending on the severity of infection. Other treatment is similar to the treatment of acute mucopurulent conjunctivitis.

> All patients with neisseria conjunctivitis should be evaluated for other sexually transmitted diseases including HIV infection.
>
> About one third of patients with neisseria conjunctivitis are known to have coexisting chlamydial infection; concurrent treatment for chlamydial infection with tetracycline or azithromycin is indicated.

Ophthalmia neonatorum***

Definition

Inflammation of the conjunctiva occurring in a neonate within first 28 days of life is called ophthalmia neonatorum. It is also called neonatal conjunctivitis (Figs 3.4.3A and B).

Epidemiology

It was one of the commonest causes of childhood blindness in past. Its incidence has come down significantly with the improvement in socioeconomic status and healthcare system. The prevalence of ophthalmia neonatorum varies worldwide depending on the socioeconomic status. The prevalence in worldwide varies between 0.9 and 21%, in India it varies between 0.5 and 33%.

Etiopathogenesis

Transmission from mother during birth from infected birth canal is the commonest mode of infection of neonatal conjunctivitis (Table 3.4.2).

Clinical features

1. Redness of eyes due to the conjunctival hyperemia.
2. Watering and discharge from eyes either unilateral or bilateral. Purulent discharge is seen in gonococcal ophthalmia neonatorum and mucopurulent discharge is seen in other microbial causes. Serous discharge is seen in herpes simplex ophthalmia neonatorum.
3. Chemosis of conjunctiva and lid edema may be seen depending on the severity of inflammation (Table 3.4.3).

Complications

If not treated properly, neonatal conjunctivitis may involve cornea resulting in:

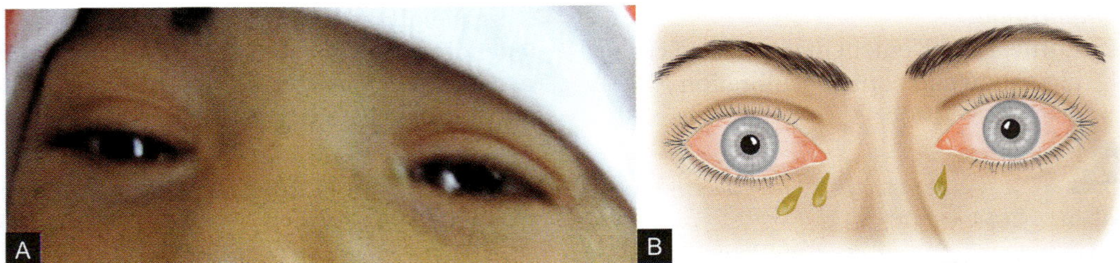

FIGS 3.4.3A and B: Ophthalmia neonatorum. **A.** Photograph; **B.** Diagrammatic representation (*Note:* Bilateral conjunctival congestion and purulent discharge).

TABLE 3.4.2: Causes of ophthalmia neonatorum

Cause	*Causative agent*	*Onset*		*Source*
Chemical cause	Silver nitrate	< 24 hour		Prophylactic agent
Microbial				
Common bacteria	*Neisseria gonorrhoeae* *Staphylococcus aureus, Streptococcus pneumoniae, Haemophilus, Escherichia coli*	2–5 day 5–7 day	Most dangerous	Birth canal Acquired from external source
Chlamydia	*Chlamydia trachomatis*	5–14 day	Most common	Birth canal
Virus	Herpes simplex	5–30 day	Rare cause	Birth canal

TABLE 3.4.3: Different types of ophthalmia neonatorum

Causative agents	*Clinical features*
Chemical conjunctivitis	Self-limiting inflammation caused by silver nitrate used as prophylaxis against infectious neonatal conjunctivitis.
Gonococcal conjunctivitis	It is usually bilateral presenting as hyperacute blennorrhea with purulent discharge usually associated with lid edema and chemosis of conjunctiva. Delay in treatment may lead to corneal ulceration with rapid progression to perforation of corneal ulcer. Hence, it is the most dangerous type of neonatal conjunctivitis.
Neonatal conjunctivitis due to other bacteria	It is less severe than gonococcal conjunctivitis either unilateral or bilateral and presents with mucopurulent discharge.
Chlamydial neonatal conjunctivitis	It is the commonest cause for neonatal conjunctivitis. It presents as unilateral or bilateral conjunctivitis with clinical features similar to neonatal conjunctivitis due to other bacteria. Follicular response, which is seen in adult chlamydial conjunctivitis is not seen in neonatal conjunctivitis as lymphoid follicles are absent in neonatal conjunctiva (lymphoid follicles develop in conjunctiva by 2 months).
Herpes simplex neonatal conjunctivitis	It is a rare cause of neonatal conjunctivitis. It may be associated with skin lesions; dendritic keratitis seen with primary herpes.

- Keratitis
- Corneal ulcer
- Corneal opacity
- Anterior staphyloma.

*Differential diagnosis**

Ophthalmia neonatorum should be differentiated from:

- Congenital dacryocystitis (congenital nasolacrimal duct obstruction)
- Congenital glaucoma.

Tears are produced from eyes after 7 days. Hence, congenital dacryocystitis should be suspected in neonates with watering and discharge after 7 days. It can be differentiated from ophthalmia neonatorum by the presence of positive regurgitation test and onset of watering and discharge after 7 days.

Congenital glaucoma can be differentiated from ophthalmia neonatorum by the presence of other signs such as corneal edema, buphthalmos and raised intraocular pressure.

Investigations

- Gram staining and Giemsa staining of the conjunctival scrapings
- Culture on blood agar for bacteria
- Polymerase chain reaction for other bacteria and *Chlamydia*
- Direct fluorescent antibody test for herpes simplex virus and for detecting *Chlamydia.*

*Treatment***

Treatment depends on the type of ophthalmia neonatorum:

1. Chemical ophthalmia neonatorum does not require specific treatment as it is self-resolving condition.
2. Gonococcal ophthalmia neonatorum is treated by single intramuscular injection of ceftriaxone 50 mg/kg to a maximum of 125 mg. Single intramuscular injection of kanamycin 100 mg can be used as an alternative to ceftriaxone. Alternatively, cefotaxime may be used 25 mg/kg twice daily either intramuscularly or intravenously for 7 days. Topical antibiotic eyedrops alone are inadequate in the treatment of gonococcal ophthalmia neonatorum and they are indicated in corneal involvement.
3. Ophthalmia neonatorum due to other bacteria is treated by topical antibiotics such as erythromycin (0.5%) or tetracycline (1%) for gram-positive organisms and tobramycin (0.3%) or gentamicin (0.3%) for gram-negative organisms.
4. Chlamydial ophthalmia neonatorum is treated by erythromycin oral suspension 50 mg/kg/day in four divided doses for 2 weeks and topical treatment by erythromycin (0.5%) eye ointment applied four times a day for 2 weeks. Alternatively, instead of erythromycin, azithromycin 20 mg/kg orally may be used once daily for 3 days. Topical treatment alone is inadequate; hence, it should always be combined with systemic therapy.
5. Ophthalmia neonatorum due to herpes simplex virus is treated by systemic acyclovir 30 mg/kg for 14 days and topical acyclovir eye ointment.

Prophylaxis

1. It is done by antenatal screening of pregnant women for genital infections and treatment of infections to prevent transmission of infection to newborn.
2. Silver nitrate (1%), erythromycin (0.5%), tetracycline (1%) or povidone-iodine (2.5%) for single application is effective in prophylaxis for high risk or suspected cases.

In 1881, Carl Crede, a German obstetrician used silver nitrate (2%) for prophylaxis against ophthalmia neonatorum, which was the leading cause of childhood blindness in 19th century. This was called Crede's prophylaxis method. Later, the concentration was reduced to 1%, but since it was found to be toxic to conjunctiva causing chemical conjunctivitis; Crede's method of prophylaxis has been replaced by other agents such as erythromycin (0.5%), tetracycline (1%) or povidone-iodine (2.5%).

Since, the incidence of ophthalmia neonatorum has come down drastically, and as it is no longer considered as leading cause for childhood blindness particularly in developed and developing countries where prophylaxis for all newborns is no longer followed. It is advised in only high-risk cases or suspected cases.

Acute Membranous Conjunctivitis**

Definition

Acute membranous conjunctivitis is a type of acute conjunctivitis characterized by formation of true membrane on the conjunctiva (Fig. 3.4.4).

Etiopathogenesis

Membranous conjunctivitis is caused by *C. diphtheriae*. The rare causes include virulent bacterial strains of *S. pneumoniae* and *Streptococcus haemolyticus* (*S. haemolyticus*), viral infections such as herpes simplex virus, adenovirus, and alkali injuries.

> Conventionally, membranous conjunctivitis caused by *C. diphtheriae* is referred as true membranous conjunctivitis and all other remaining causes are grouped as pseudomembranous conjunctivitis.
>
> Because of the effective universal immunization against diphtheria, the incidence of membranous conjunctivitis caused by *Corynebacterium* has decreased drastically and it has become a rare entity.

The pathogenesis of membranous conjunctivitis is characterized by violent inflammation of conjunctiva resulting in coagulative necrosis of inflamed conjunctiva. The coagulative necrosis results in the formation of membrane consisting of fibrin within the substance of conjunctiva. Since, the membrane occurs within the stroma of conjunctiva, it cannot be removed without causing bleeding.

Clinical Features

The disease is usually seen in children in the age group of 2–10 years living in crowded conditions and from low socioeconomic strata. The mode of spread is from airborne droplets or secretions from respiratory tract in case of respiratory diphtheria, or from secretions from skin lesions in case of cutaneous diphtheria.

Stage of infiltration

The first stage of the disease and it is characterized by moderate-to-severe inflammation of conjunctiva with congestion, chemosis, mucopurulent conjunctival discharge and lid edema. The characteristic feature of the disease is the presence of grayish yellow membrane covering the palpebral conjunctiva. Preauricular lymphadenopathy is usually present. Systemic features such as fever and additional features in the form of sore throat, and membrane over the tonsils and pharynx are usually seen in associated respiratory diphtheria.

Stage of suppuration

Follows the stage of infiltration and it is characterized by suppurative necrosis of the conjunctiva resulting in sloughing of the exudative membrane formed in the stage of infiltration. The sloughing of the membrane results in the formation of raw surfaces over the palpebral conjunctiva.

Stage of cicatrization

Stage of cicatrization is seen as last stage and it is characterized by healing of the raw conjunctival surfaces by cicatrization leading to cicatricial entropion, trichiasis and symblepharon. Symblepharon results due to healing of the raw surfaces over palpebral conjunctiva.

Complications

1. Corneal involvement in the form of corneal ulceration and corneal perforation. Corneal involvement is more frequent similar to hyperacute conjunctivitis caused by gonococci as *C. diphtheriae* can also penetrate intact corneal epithelium.

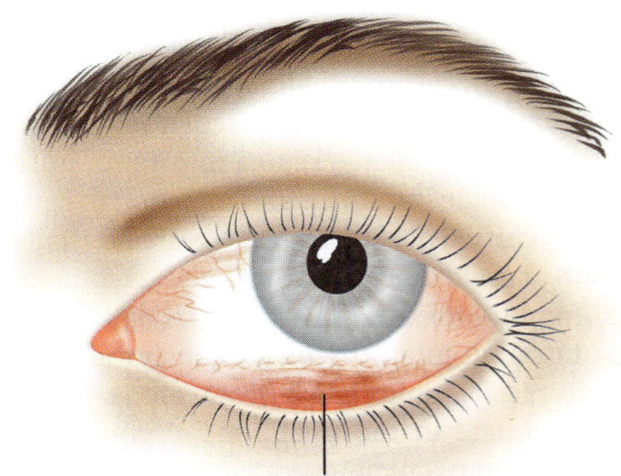

FIG. 3.4.4: Membranous conjunctivitis

2. Symblepharon, cicatricial entropion, trichiasis because of cicatrization.

Investigations

Clinical diagnosis is confirmed from Gram staining of the conjunctival secretions.

Treatment

Local treatment

Local treatment is done by topical application of antibiotics and antidiphtheric serum:

1. Penicillin eyedrops in 1:10,000 dilution instilled hourly and erythromycin eye ointment at bedtime are the preferred antibiotics.
2. Antidiphtheric serum instillation into conjunctival sac hourly.

Systemic treatment

Systemic treatment is done by antibiotics and antidiphtheric serum:

1. Benzylpenicillin and erythromycin are the preferred antibiotics. Benzylpenicillin is administered in a dosage of 50,000 U/kg intramuscular injection two times a day for children below 10 years of age. In adults, 1.2 million units per day intramuscular injection in two divided doses. Erythromycin is administered in patients who are allergic to penicillin. It is administered in a dosage of 50 mg/kg. Antibiotics are administered for 10–14 days.
2. Antidiphtheric serum is administered in a dose of 40,000–60,000 U by intravenous injection.

Prevention of Complications

Complications such as symblepharon can be avoided by prevention of healing of conjunctival surfaces together by application of contact shell or by repeated sweeping of the conjunctival fornices by glass rod.

Prophylaxis

Prophylaxis is done by immunization against diphtheria by diphtheria, pertussis and tetanus (DPT) vaccine.

Diphtheria is an infectious disease caused by gram-negative bacillus *C. diphtheriae*. The disease is characterized by formation of a membrane especially in the respiratory tract. The name diphtheria is derived from the word diphtheria, a Greek word, which means leather indicating the tough membrane produced in the disease. The systemic effects of diphtheria are because of production of an exotoxin, which causes potential cardiovascular system and central nervous system effects.

Pseudomembranous Conjunctivitis**

Pseudomembranous conjunctivitis is a type of acute conjunctivitis characterized by the formation of pseudomembrane over the conjunctiva.

Etiopathogenesis

Pseudomembranous conjunctivitis is caused by virulent bacterial strains of *S. pneumoniae* and *S. haemolyticus*, viral infections such as herpes simplex virus, adenovirus and alkali injuries.

The pathogenesis of pseudomembranous conjunctivitis is characterized by violent inflammation of conjunctiva resulting in necrosis of inflamed conjunctiva that results in the formation of membrane consisting of fibrin over the surface of conjunctiva. Since, the membrane occurs on the surface of conjunctiva, it can be removed easily leaving behind intact conjunctival epithelium.

In membranous conjunctivitis, membrane occurs in the stroma of conjunctiva; hence, it cannot be removed easily, whereas in pseudomembranous conjunctivitis, membrane formation occurs on the surface of conjunctiva that can be removed easily leaving behind intact conjunctival epithelium.

Clinical Features

1. Pseudomembranous conjunctivitis is characterized by formation of a pseudomembrane, which can be removed easily.
2. Other clinical features are similar to acute mucopurulent conjunctivitis and characterized by conjunctival congestion, chemosis, lid edema and mucopurulent discharge.

Treatment

It is similar to treatment of acute mucopurulent conjunctivitis and is done by antibiotic eyedrops and anti-inflammatory drugs.

Ligneous Conjunctivitis*

Ligneous conjunctivitis is relatively rare type of chronic conjunctivitis characterized by formation of recurrent pseudomembranes over the conjunctiva.

The membrane is because of fibrin deposits. It is regarded as an ocular manifestation of systemic plasminogen deficiency. Plasminogen is essential for breaking of fibrin, the deficiency of plasminogen results in the formation of fibrin membrane.

Ligneous conjunctivitis is characterized by the formation of yellowish white membrane over the conjunctiva of woody consistency. The importance of this condition is that it has to be differentiated from membranous and pseudomembranous conjunctivitis.

Treatment is usually unsatisfactory. Use of corticosteroids and topical immunosuppressive drugs such as cyclosporine has not given good results. Surgical excision of the membrane is also associated with recurrence. Use of topical plasminogen has yielded better results.

Angular Conjunctivitis**

Definition

Subacute or chronic inflammation of conjunctiva mainly involving the conjunctiva and the skin of the lid margins at the angles of the eye at medial, and lateral canthus is called angular conjunctivitis (Figs 3.4.5A and B).

Etiopathogenesis

Angular conjunctivitis is caused by Morax-Axenfeld, a gram-negative diplobacillus. Rarely, it can be caused by staphylococci. Morax-Axenfeld is named after Morax and Axenfeld who separately published reports regarding the gram-negative diplobacillus. It is normal saprophyte of nasal mucosa. It is associated with angular conjunctivitis and dacryoadenitis.

Morax-Axenfeld bacillus produces proteolytic enzyme, which collects in the angles of the eye and this causes maceration of the epithelium of the conjunctiva, and the surrounding eyelids. It is associated with deficiency of vitamin A and riboflavin.

Clinical Features

Symptoms: Redness, mucopurulent discharge, irritation of eyes, itching and excoriation of skin at the medial and lateral canthus.

Signs: On examination, the eye shows congestion of the bulbar conjunctiva near the angles and excoriation of skin at the medial, and lateral canthus.

Complications

Blepharitis and marginal corneal ulcer are the most common complications associated with chronic angular conjunctivitis.

Treatment

1. Angular conjunctivitis is treated by tetracycline eye ointment three times a day. It is continued for 3 weeks to eliminate the infection.
2. The mainstay of treatment is by zinc. Zinc acts here by inhibiting the proteolytic enzyme produced by the Morax-Axenfeld bacillus. Zinc oxide eyedrops three to four times per day and zinc ointment for the skin at the medial and lateral canthus.
3. Vitamin A and riboflavin supplementation in patients showing other features of the deficiency to hasten the treatment process.

Riboflavin is an essential nutrient required for cellular respiration along with protein compounds together forming flavoprotein enzymes. Morax-Axenfeld bacillus destroys the protein component leading to deficiency of flavoprotein enzymes. This explains similar mucocutaneous lesions seen in riboflavin deficiency such as angular stomatitis. Morax-Axenfeld infection manifests mainly as angular conjunctivitis because of local deficiency of flavoprotein enzymes.

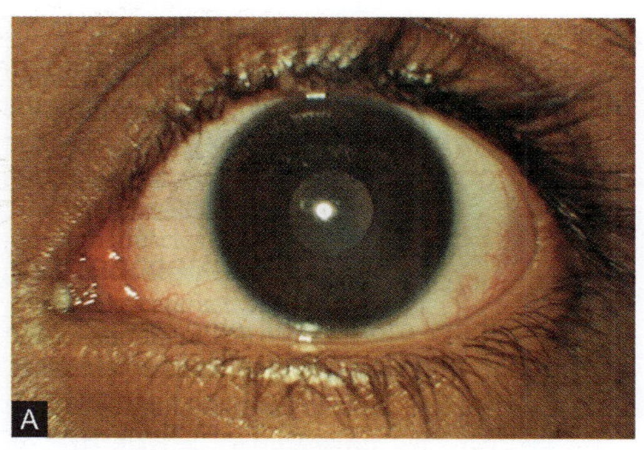

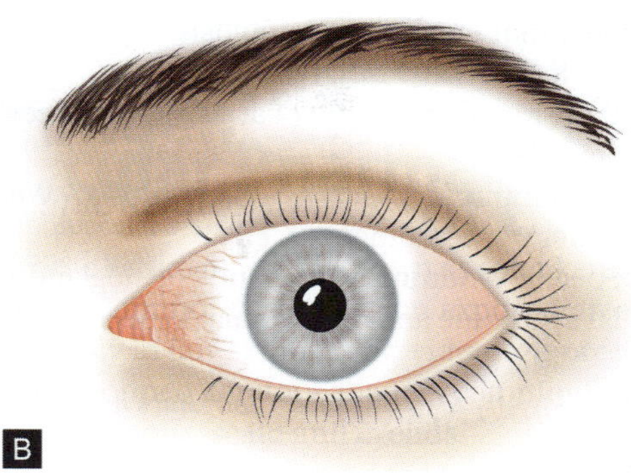

FIGS 3.4.5A and B: Angular conjunctivitis. **A.** Photograph; **B.** Diagrammatic representation.

Vitamin A is responsible for maintenance of normal epithelium and blepharitis of the lid margin associated with the angular conjunctivitis shows improvement with administration of vitamin A.

Chronic Bacterial Conjunctivitis

Definition

Chronic inflammation of the conjunctiva of more than 3 weeks' duration is called chronic bacterial conjunctivitis.

Etiopathogenesis

Staphylococcus aureus is the most common cause for chronic bacterial conjunctivitis. Other causes are *Escherichia coli, Klebsiella pneumoniae, Proteus* and *Moraxella lacunata* (Morax-Axenfeld bacillus). The commonest causative agent, *S. aureus,* colonizes the skin of the eyelids and it causes chronic conjunctivitis either by direct infection or indirectly because of the liberated exotoxins.

Clinical Features

Symptoms: Chronic redness, foreign body sensation and minimal mucopurulent discharge are the symptoms of chronic conjunctivitis.

Signs: On examination, conjunctiva shows signs such as hyperemia of conjunctiva and papillary hypertrophy or follicular reaction. Eyelids may show features such as thickening, redness, madarosis and recurrent stye.

Differential Diagnosis

Chronic bacterial conjunctivitis has to be differentiated from other causes of chronic conjunctivitis, which include viral conjunctivitis, allergic conjunctivitis, conjunctivitis seen in eyelid abnormalities such as floppy eyelid syndrome and conjunctivitis caused by *Chlamydia,* drugs, toxins, etc.

Treatment

Chronic bacterial conjunctivitis is treated by antibiotic therapy along with lid hygiene to eliminate the colonization of the bacteria. Broad-spectrum antibiotics are used as eyedrops and eye ointments for 2–3 weeks.

Granulomatous Conjunctivitis

Definition

Granulomatous conjunctivitis is a chronic inflammation of conjunctiva characterized by formation of granuloma of conjunctiva.

Causes

Common causes of granulomatous conjunctivitis are:*

1. Bacterial causes: Tuberculosis, leptospirosis, leprosy, syphilis, etc.
2. Parasitic causes: Toxocariasis, onchocerciasis, etc.
3. Autoimmune diseases: Sarcoidosis, Wegener's granulomatosis, etc.
4. Specific syndromes: Parinaud's oculoglandular syndrome and ophthalmia nodosa.

*Ophthalmia Nodosa**

Definition

Chronic granulomatous inflammatory reaction of the conjunctiva to hairs of certain insects and vegetables is called ophthalmia nodosa.

Initially, it was described as pseudotuberculosis because of its resemblance to granulomas associated with tuberculosis. It is now called ophthalmia nodosa because of the characteristic nodular reaction.

Etiopathogenesis

Opthalmia nodosa is also called caterpillar hair conjunctivitis, since it commonly occurs in response to retained hair of caterpillar. It is because of chronic inflammation initiated by retained hair. The inflammatory cells are mainly lymphocytes and giant cells.

Clinical features

In India, ophthalmia nodosa is more common in winter season as the caterpillars are abundant during winter.

Usually, there is a symptomless period following the entry of caterpillar hair into conjunctiva. The symptoms are chronic irritation and foreign body sensation. On examination, characteristic nodule is present on the conjunctiva.

Treatment

Treatment is mainly by surgical removal of the caterpillar hair. Topical steroids are indicated for control of associated inflammation.

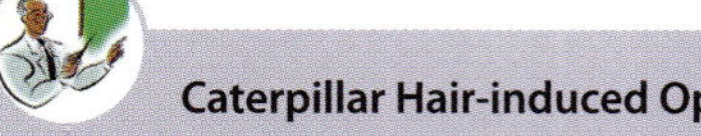

Caterpillar Hair-induced Ophthalmitis

It is defined as inflammatory reaction of eye induced by intraocular penetration of the caterpillar hair.

Very few patients are known to have intraocular penetration of the caterpillar hair leading to caterpillar hair-induced ophthalmitis. Direct toxicity, mechanical effects and inflammatory reaction induced by the caterpillar hair are responsible for ocular damage. Granulomatous iridocyclitis because of anterior segment penetration and posterior segment involvement in the form of vitritis, and chorioretinitis because of posterior segment penetration are seen in caterpillar hair-induced ophthalmitis.

Treatment is by steroids to control the inflammation and surgical removal of the caterpillar hair wherever possible. In cases where caterpillar hair removal is associated with more intraocular damage, lysis of the hair by argon laser or neodymium-doped yttrium aluminum garnet (Nd-YAG) laser has given good results.

*Parinaud's Oculoglandular Syndrome**

Definition

Parinaud's oculoglandular is a syndrome characterized by unilateral chronic granulomatous conjunctivitis associated with ipsilateral submandibular and preauricular or postauricular lymphadenopathy.

Etiology

Cat scratch disease caused by *Bartonella henselae* is the commonest cause for Parinaud's oculoglandular syndrome. The other common causes are:

1. Bacterial infections: Tularemia, tuberculosis, treponema pallidum.
2. Fungal infections: Sporotrichosis, blastomycosis and coccidioidomycosis.
3. Viral infections: Mumps and infectious mononucleosis.
4. Chlamydia infections: Lymphogranuloma venereum.
5. Rickettsial causes: Rickettsiosis or Mediterranean spotted fever.

Clinical features

The clinical features are characterized by chronic granulomatous inflammatory conjunctivitis and involvement of the ipsilateral lymph nodes.

Investigations

Patients have to be evaluated based on history and other constitutional symptoms for the various etiological agents mentioned above. The usual investigations done are:

1. Microbiological tests of the conjunctival secretions by Gram staining, Giemsa staining and culture of the conjunctival secretions to find out the etiological agent.
2. Serological tests tailored depending on the history such as Veneral Disease Research Laboratory (VDRL) to rule out syphilis, indirect immunofluorescence test to rule out cat scratch disease, etc.

Treatment

Treatment depends on the underlying cause.

VIRAL CONJUNCTIVITIS

Viral conjunctivitis is one of the commonest types of conjunctivitis. The salient features of viral conjunctivitis are:

1. Most of the times it is self-limiting and it may or may not require treatment.
2. Frequently associated with infection of corneal epithelium leading to keratitis.
3. Commonest cause of follicular conjunctivitis.

ETIOLOGY

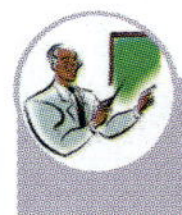

Adenovirus is the most common virus causing viral conjunctivitis.

Other viruses include:

- Herpes simplex virus
- Herpes zoster virus
- Enterovirus
- Coxsackievirus
- Rubeola (measles) virus
- Mumps virus
- Cytomegalovirus
- Epstein-Barr virus
- Newcastle virus.

CLASSIFICATION

Adenoviral Conjunctivitis**

Adenoviral conjunctivitis is the most common type of viral conjunctivitis.

Etiopathogenesis

Adenovirus is a non-enveloped double-stranded deoxyribonucleic acid (DNA) virus. It is called adenovirus as it was first isolated from human adenoid glands. There are 57 different serotypes of adenovirus of which 19 are known to cause conjunctivitis. They are usually associated with respiratory infection and gastrointestinal infection also. The infection spreads by direct contact with the infected secretions such as discharge from the eyes or from respiratory droplets.

Clinical Features

The common types of presentation are:

- Acute follicular conjunctivitis
- Pharyngoconjunctival fever
- Epidemic keratoconjunctivitis
- Chronic papillary or follicular conjunctivitis.

Acute follicular conjunctivitis

1. It is the most common type of clinical presentation of adenoviral conjunctivitis. It is characterized by the formation of follicles due to aggregation of lymphocytes in the adenoid layer of conjunctiva usually in the inferior fornix of conjunctival sac (Fig. 3.4.6).
2. Ocular involvement and ocular symptoms are milder and often self-limiting in acute follicular conjunctivitis. Acute follicular conjunctivitis due to other causes is described below.

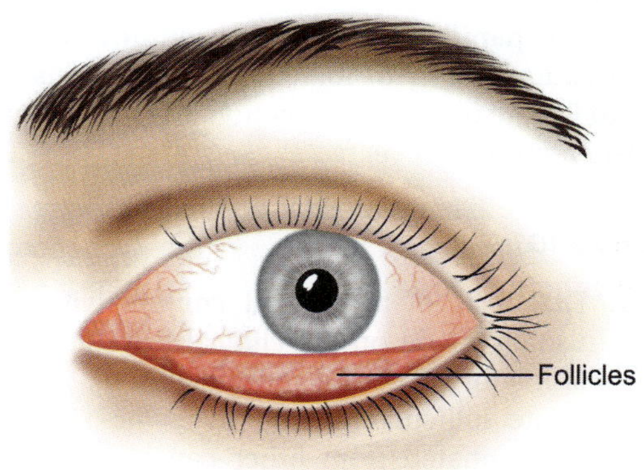

FIG. 3.4.6: Follicular conjunctivitis

Pharyngoconjunctival fever

1. Pharyngoconjunctival fever is most commonly caused by serotypes 3, 4 and 7.
2. The clinical features are characterized by acute follicular conjunctivitis associated with pharyngitis, fever and preauricular lymphadenopathy.
3. Corneal involvement is usually mild in the form of punctuate keratitis.

Epidemic keratoconjunctivitis

1. It is most commonly caused by serotypes 8 and 19.
2. The clinical features are characterized by significant involvement of cornea along with conjunctival involvement presenting as keratoconjunctivitis. The typical clinical features involve initial presentation as uniocular follicular conjunctivitis, which usually becomes bilateral.
3. Conjunctival hyperemia, chemosis of conjunctiva, lid edema and petechial hemorrhages are usually associated features.
4. Pseudomembrane formation is seen in severe varieties.
5. Corneal involvement is seen in the form of punctuate epithelial keratitis because of active multiplication of adenovirus within the corneal epithelium. Subepithelial and anterior stromal infiltrates develop in the cornea later usually as a result of immunological response to virus present in the epithelium of cornea.

Chronic papillary or follicular conjunctivitis

Chronic papillary or follicular conjunctivitis is usually rare type of presentation, but it can persist for months or years.

Diagnosis

1. Diagnosis of adenoviral conjunctivitis is usually made on the clinical features and laboratory diagnosis is not required.
2. Acute follicular conjunctivitis has to be differentiated from other causes such as trachoma, adult inclusion conjunctivitis, Newcastle conjunctivitis, herpetic conjunctivitis, etc.
3. Giemsa staining of the conjunctival secretions shows predominance of mononuclear cells. Isolation of the virus can be done from viral culture, but not done routinely as it is expensive and time consuming procedure.

Treatment

1. At present, no effective antiviral drug is available against adenovirus. Hence, treatment is mainly supportive.
2. Mild cases of follicular conjunctivitis are treated by symptomatic treatment in the form of cold compress, topical vasoconstrictor drugs and antibiotic eyedrops to prevent secondary bacterial infection.
3. Topical steroids are used in severe cases. The indications for the use of steroids are presence of pseudomembranous conjunctivitis and subepithelial corneal infiltrates. Steroids should not be used in presence of active epithelial keratitis and when used should be tapered slowly to prevent recurrence of the infiltrates.
4. Proper prophylactic measures should be taken to prevent the spread of the disease as it is very contagious. Prophylactic measures include avoiding contact with infected persons and personal hygiene measures.

Herpes Simplex Conjunctivitis

Herpes simplex conjunctivitis is usually seen in primary ocular herpes lesions.

Etiopathogenesis

Herpes simplex type 1 is responsible for majority of ocular infections. It spreads by close contact and by kissing. Herpes simplex type 2 rarely causes ocular lesions and the mode of spread is by orogenital contact.

Clinical Features

1. The typical presentation is in the form of follicular conjunctivitis with vesicular skin

lesions involving the face and eyelids. Preauricular lymphadenopathy is usually seen.

2. Corneal involvement is rare, if seen, it is usually in the form of punctuate keratitis and dendritic keratitis is rare. Stromal involvement of the cornea is not seen in primary ocular herpes.

Diagnosis

Diagnosis is usually done by clinical features and associated herpetic skin lesions. Laboratory diagnosis is made by examination of the conjunctival secretions, which shows intranuclear inclusion bodies and multinucleated giant cells. Serological tests such as enzyme-linked immunosorbent assay (ELISA) and immunofluorescence can be used for serological diagnosis.

Treatment

1. Treatment is not required as primary ocular herpes infection is self-limiting. It usually resolves within 1–2 weeks.
2. Topical antiviral drugs such as acyclovir eyedrops and eye ointment are used in patients with corneal involvement.
3. Steroid drugs should be avoided as they increase the severity of corneal epithelial keratitis.

Acute Hemorrhagic Conjunctivitis*

Definition

Acute hemorrhagic conjunctivitis is a type of acute conjunctivitis characterized by multiple hemorrhages of conjunctiva.

Etiology

Enterovirus 70 and coxsackievirus A24 belonging to picornavirus family are the etiological agents responsible for acute hemorrhagic conjunctivitis. It is highly contagious disease and spreads through close contact.

Apollo Conjunctivitis

Acute hemorrhagic conjunctivitis was first recognized in West Africa as an epidemic conjunctivitis. It is also called Apollo conjunctivitis as it was recognized first in the year 1969, the year Apollo 11 landed on the moon.

Clinical Features

1. The disease is self-limiting and runs a short, but severe course lasting for 1 week.
2. Acute hemorrhagic conjunctivitis presents with all the features of conjunctivitis such as redness, watering, discharge, lid edema and ocular pain.
3. The characteristic feature is the presence of multiple conjunctival petechial hemorrhages, which coalesce to form multiple subconjunctival hemorrhages.
4. Conjunctival follicles and preauricular lymphadenopathy are usually seen in majority of viral conjunctivitis.
5. Corneal involvement is rare, if seen, it is usually in the form of punctate keratitis.

Diagnosis

The diagnosis is mainly clinical. Since, specific antiviral drugs are not available and the disease is usually self-limiting; laboratory diagnosis is not required.

Treatment

Treatment is usually symptomatic and supportive in the form of topical vasoconstrictor drugs; topical antibiotic eyedrops to prevent secondary bacterial infection and oral analgesic drugs for pain relief.

CHLAMYDIAL CONJUNCTIVITIS

CHLAMYDIA

1. *Chlamydia* exhibits the properties of viruses, bacteria and parasites.

2. Chlamydiae are obligate intracellular parasite; initially, they were included under viruses because of the features such as failure to grow in cell-free media and filterability.
3. Now, they are considered under bacteria because of many features resembling bacteria—presence of both deoxyribonucleic acid (DNA) and ribonucleic acid (RNA), cell wall, and susceptibility to antibiotic drugs.
4. They are called parasites since they lack enzymes required for energy synthesis and depend upon host cell for energy requirements.
5. *Chlamydia trachomatis (C. trachomatis), Chlamydophila psittaci (C. psittaci)* and *Chlamydophila pneumoniae (C. pneumoniae)* are the species of *Chlamydia* causing disease in human beings.
6. *Chlamydia trachomatis* causes trachoma, adult inclusion conjunctivitis, genital infections such as urethritis in males and cervicitis in females, lymphogranuloma venereum and pneumonia. *C. psittaci* causes psittacosis and *C. pneumoniae* causes pneumonia.

Chlamydia exhibits the properties of viruses, bacteria and parasites. Chlamydia infections are one of the most common sexually transmitted infections worldwide. Trachoma caused by *C. trachomatis* was one of the most common causes of blindness in the last century.

Chlamydia trachomatis is called trachoma inclusion conjunctivitis (TRIC) agent as it can cause trachoma and inclusion conjunctivitis.

CLASSIFICATION

Inclusion Conjunctivitis

Inflammation of the conjunctiva characterized by the presence of inclusion bodies in the conjunctival epithelial cells is called inclusion conjunctivitis. It is caused by *C. trachomatis*. Inclusion conjunctivitis is of two types:

1. Adult inclusion conjunctivitis.
2. Neonatal inclusion conjunctivitis.

*Adult Inclusion Conjunctivitis***

Definition

Inclusion conjunctivitis seen in adults caused by *C. trachomatis* is called adult inclusion conjunctivitis.

Etiopathogenesis

Chlamydia trachomatis serotypes D to K are the causative agents for adult inclusion conjunctivitis. It is more commonly seen in sexually active young adults. The source of infection is from genital infection in the form of urethritis in males and cervicitis in females. The mode of transfer from genitals to eye is either from direct transfer or indirect transfer through contaminated fingers.

Swimming Pool Conjunctivitis

Adult inclusion conjunctivitis is also called swimming pool conjunctivitis as the disease used to spread through swimming pools contaminated with genital secretions of infected persons. With the use of chlorination to treat the water of the swimming pools, this mode of spread has come down drastically.

The incubation period is 5–12 days. The infection begins as follicular conjunctivitis. Inclusion conjunctivitis is usually less severe compared to trachoma.

Clinical features

1. Symptoms are similar to bacterial conjunctivitis such as redness, grittiness, foreign body sensation and mucopurulent discharge.
2. Examination of the eye shows acute or chronic follicular conjunctivitis and preauricular lymphadenopathy.
3. Corneal involvement if seen, it will be in the form of superficial punctate keratitis and pannus involving the superior part of the cornea.

Differential diagnosis

Adult inclusion conjunctivitis has to be differentiated from other causes of follicular conjunctivitis.

Investigations

Giemsa staining of conjunctival scraping shows basophilic inclusion bodies in the conjunctival epithelial cells. ELISA and PCR of the conjunctival scrapings are available for faster diagnosis.

Investigations have to be done to rule out other associated sexually transmitted infections such as gonorrhea, syphilis, HIV, etc.

Treatment

1. Adult inclusion conjunctivitis requires topical treatment for conjunctivitis and systemic treatment is compulsory to treat the associated genital infection.
2. Topical treatment is in the form of tetracycline (1%) or erythromycin eye ointment four times a day for 4–6 weeks.
3. Systemic treatment is done by tetracycline 250 mg four times a day or doxycycline 100 mg two times a day or erythromycin 500 mg four times a day for 4–6 weeks. Tetracycline is avoided in children less than 7 year old, in pregnant and in lactating women.
4. Treatment of the sexual partner is also important to prevent reinfection.

Neonatal Inclusion Conjunctivitis

Neonatal inclusion conjunctivitis is the commonest type of neonatal conjunctivitis. It is described under ophthalmia neonatorum.

Trachoma***

Definition

Trachoma is defined as chronic inflammation of conjunctiva caused by *C. trachomatis* characterized by chronic follicular reaction and papillary hypertrophy of the conjunctiva.

The word 'trachoma' is derived from Greek word, which means 'rough' describing the characteristic rough appearance of palpebral conjunctiva due to the presence of follicles and papillae in trachoma.

Trachoma History

It is one of the oldest known infectious diseases with the earliest references of the disease dating back to 16th century BC from Egypt. Hence, it is also known as Egyptian ophthalmia.

It might have affected great scholars such as Galileo, St Paul, etc.

It affected thousands of soldiers of Napoleon's army when Napoleon fought against Egypt army. Because of the campaign of Napoleon, trachoma spread rapidly across Europe and Africa. Trachoma spread rapidly among the soldiers because of close contact and when the soldiers who went back to their homes they were spreading the disease to the civilian society. Hence, it is also known as military ophthalmia.

Etiopathogenesis

Trachoma is caused by *C. trachomatis* serotypes A, B, Ba and C.

Chlamydia is present in two forms, one is infective form called elementary body present extracellularly and other is intracellular variety called initial body or reticulate body. Elementary body is the infective form and the infection begins by attachment of the elementary body to the epithelial cell, which is endocytosed into the epithelial cell. Within the epithelial cell, elementary body is converted into initial body. The initial body divides rapidly by binary fission and when initial body is mature it contains about 100–500 elementary bodies, and this is called inclusion body. The inclusion body is called Halberstaedter-Prowazek body. The inclusion body swells up and bursts to release the elementary bodies, which again infect the neighboring epithelial cells:

1. Elementary body attaches to epithelial cell.
2. Endocytosed by epithelial cell, converted into initial body.
3. Initial body is converted into inclusion body containing 100–500 elementary bodies.
4. Inclusion body bursts to release elementary bodies, which again infect the neighboring epithelial cells.

Trachoma is more common in people from low socioeconomic strata living in overcrowded conditions with poor personal hygiene and presence of abundant flies. Usually in endemic areas the disease is acquired in infancy or childhood. The disease is more common in females compared to males.

The source of infection is usually the conjunctival discharge from infected person. The mode of spread is by close contact resulting in direct eye-to-eye transmission, through flies and by materials such as contaminated towels, handkerchiefs and sticks used to apply eye cosmetics (surma).

Trachoma is one of the world's leading causes of preventable blindness. It is the leading cause of infectious blindness worldwide. Though, trachoma is eradicated from the developed countries, it continues to be an important cause of blindness basically in the underdeveloped countries of Asia and Africa. Trachoma still affects about 41 million people in 56 different countries. It has caused complete blindness in about 8 million people worldwide. As per the reports, though trachoma is eradicated from India, still many more cases continue to be present in India, particularly the cases with sequelae of trachoma.

The incubation period is 5–12 days. The disease in the absence of secondary bacterial infection is usually mild and has spontaneous resolution even without treatment. The sequelae of the disease responsible for blindness occur 15–20 years later and include trichiasis, entropion and corneal opacity.

Clinical Features

Symptoms

The symptoms depend on the presence or absence of secondary bacterial infection:

1. In the absence of secondary bacterial infection, the symptoms are mild and include mild irritation, redness and discharge.
2. In the presence of secondary bacterial infection, typical symptoms of acute mucopurulent conjunctivitis such as redness, grittiness, foreign body sensation and mucopurulent discharge are seen.

Signs

The signs of trachoma are seen in the epithelium of both conjunctiva and cornea as *C. trachomatis* usually causes keratoconjunctivitis.

Conjunctiva

Conjunctiva shows congestion, follicular reaction and diffuse papillary hypertrophy.

Follicles: It is because of aggregation of lymphocytes and in trachoma they are seen commonly on the upper palpebral conjunctiva. Follicles can be seen on lower palpebral conjunctiva and rarely on the bulbar conjunctiva. Follicles seen on the bulbar conjunctiva and rarely near the limbus are pathognomonic of trachoma are called Herbert's follicle. Once the Herbert's follicles heal, they leave behind scar called Herbert's pit (Figs 3.4.7 and 3.4.8).

Papillary hypertrophy: It is because of vascular hyperplasia and seen in both upper and lower palpebral conjunctiva.

Conjunctival scarring: It is seen later after moderate-to-severe inflammation of conjunctiva. Small linear or stellate scars are seen in moderate inflammation and bigger confluent scars are seen in severe inflammation. Horizontal linear conjunctival scar seen in the sulcus subtarsalis is called Arlt's line. Severe conjunctival scarring and cicatrization may lead to potential blinding complications such as trichiasis, entropion, etc.

Cornea

Cornea shows punctate keratitis and pannus.

Keratitis: It is usually in the form of superficial punctate keratitis and it more commonly involves the upper part of the cornea.

Pannus: It is the fibrovascular membrane arising from limbus and extending over the cornea. Pannus is because of infiltration by inflammatory cells associated with vascularization. Pannus can be progressive pannus (Fig. 3.4.9) in which the cellular infiltration is ahead of vascularization or regressive pannus (Fig. 3.4.10) in which cellular infiltration is behind vascularization.*

Corneal scarring: It is seen in the end stages because of healing of pannus and corneal ulcers caused by lid abnormalities—trichiasis, entropion, etc.

Classification (Tables 3.4.4 to 3.4.6)**

Mac Callan's classification is based on the conjunctival signs and describes the evolution of the disease.

Clinical diagnosis of trachoma is made by the presence of at least two of the following signs:

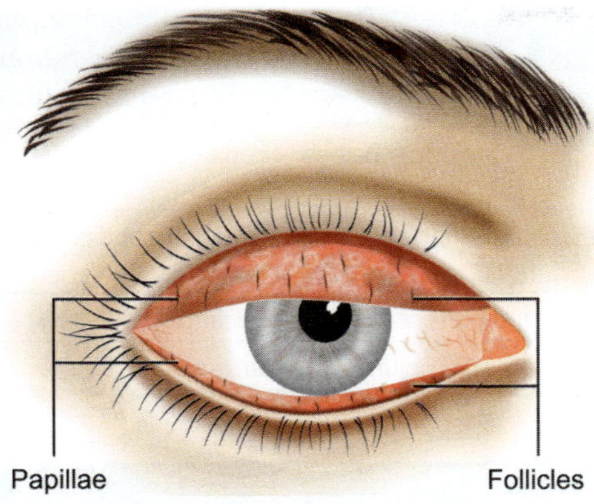

FIG. 3.4.7: Follicles and papillae of palpebral conjunctiva

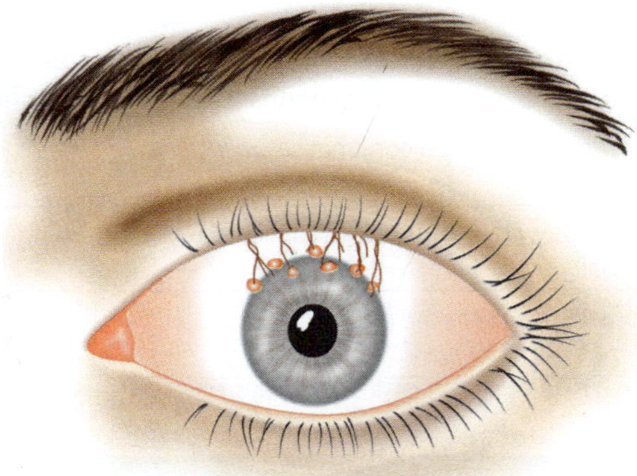

FIG. 3.4.8: Herbert's limbal follicles and pits

1. Presence of follicles in the upper tarsal conjunctiva.
2. Presence of conjunctival scarring.
3. Presence of Herbert's limbal follicles or pits.
4. Presence of pannus of cornea.

*Complications and Sequelae of Trachoma**

1. Cicatrization of conjunctiva leads to complications such as entropion and trichiasis.
2. Inflammation of conjunctiva and lids leads to complications such as concretions, ptosis, ectropion, tylosis, pseudopterygium and symblepharon.

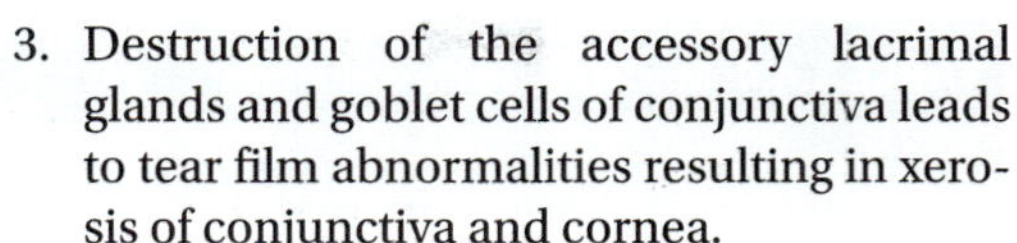

3. Destruction of the accessory lacrimal glands and goblet cells of conjunctiva leads to tear film abnormalities resulting in xerosis of conjunctiva and cornea.

The complications of trachoma can be summarized depending on the location as:

1. Lids: Entropion, trichiasis, madarosis, tylosis, ectropion and ptosis.
2. Conjunctiva: Conjunctival xerosis, symblepharon, concretions, pseudopterygium.
3. Cornea: Corneal xerosis, corneal vascularization, corneal ulcerations, corneal opacity and keratectasia.
4. Lacrimal apparatus: Dacryocystitis and dacryoadenitis.

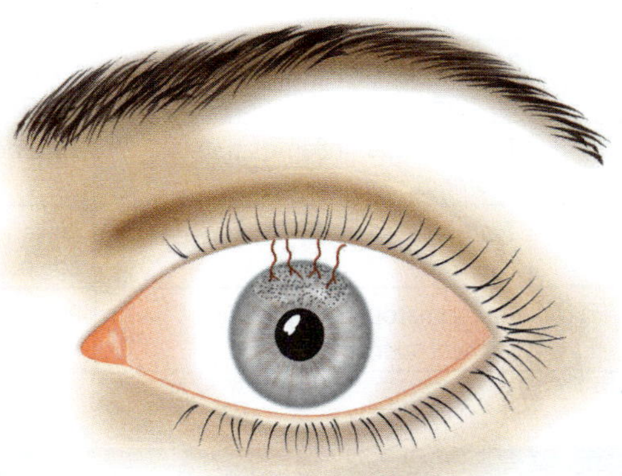

FIG. 3.4.9: Progressive pannus

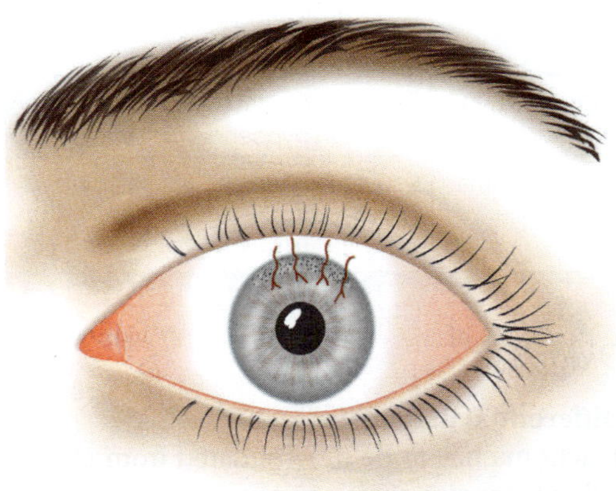

FIG. 3.4.10: Regressive pannus

TABLE 3.4.4: Mac Callan's classification

Stage	*Type*	*Features*
Stage I	Incipient trachoma	Presence of immature follicles on the upper palpebral conjunctiva and punctate keratitis
Stage II	Established trachoma	Presence of mature follicles, papillae in the palpebral conjunctiva and corneal pannus
Stage III	Cicatrizing trachoma	Resolution of papillae, follicles and presence of signs of cicatrization
Stage IV	Healed trachoma	Presence of complications because of conjunctival cicatrization

TABLE 3.4.5: World Health Organization classification

Index	*Type*	*Features*
TF	Trachomatous inflammation *(follicular)*	Presence of five or more follicles on the upper palpebral conjunctiva
TI	Trachomatous inflammation *(intense)*	Presence of inflammatory thickening of the tarsal conjunctiva obscuring the view of more than half of normal deep tarsal vessels
TS	Trachomatous inflammation *(scarring)*	Presence of scarring in the tarsal conjunctiva
TT	Trachomatous inflammation *(trichiasis)*	Presence of trichiasis with at least one misdirected eyelash rubbing against the eyeball
TO	Trachomatous inflammation *(corneal opacity)*	Presence of corneal opacity in the pupillary area

TABLE 3.4.6: Jones classification

Type	*Pathogen*	*Features*
Blinding trachoma	Caused by *Chlamydia trachomatis* (C. *trachomatis)* serotypes A, B, Ba, C in hyperendemic areas	Associated with secondary bacterial infection and spreads from eye to eye
Non-blinding trachoma	Caused by *C. trachomatis* serotypes A, B, Ba, C in hypoendemic areas	Not associated with secondary bacterial infection and transmission from eye to eye is limited
Paratrachoma	Caused by *C. trachomatis* serotypes D to K	Manifests as inclusion conjunctivitis in adults and ophthalmia neonatorum in neonates; mode of transmission is by genital infection

Diagnosis

Differential diagnosis

Trachoma has to be differentiated from chronic follicular conjunctivitis and vernal conjunctivitis.

Trachoma can be differentiated from chronic follicular conjunctivitis by the presence of associated features caused by the causative agent of chronic follicular conjunctivitis and the absence of papillae, and pannus in chronic follicular conjunctivitis. The follicles in chronic follicular conjunctivitis are typically found in lower palpebral conjunctiva, whereas in trachoma they are more commonly seen in upper tarsal conjunctiva.

Trachoma can be differentiated from vernal conjunctivitis by the presence of symptoms such as itching and ropy discharge. Signs such as cobblestone appearance of papillae and absence of follicles in vernal conjunctivitis.

Laboratory diagnosis

1. Conjunctival smears stained by Giemsa stain show plasma cells, neutrophils, macrophages and lymphocytes. This mixed cellular morphology is typical of chlamydia infection.
2. Detection of inclusion bodies (Halberstaedter-Prowazek bodies) by Giemsa stain, iodine stain and immunofluorescent stains in conjunctival smears.
3. Isolation of the *Chlamydia* by inoculation of conjunctival scrapings into tissue culture or yolk sac of embryonated eggs. The cell lines used are McCoy cells and HeLa cells.
4. Detection of specific antibodies by using complement fixation, microimmunofluorescence, ELISA and PCR.

*Treatment**

Treatment of trachoma is based on the SAFE strategy as advised by WHO. SAFE stands for:

- S—surgical care
- A—antibiotics
- F—facial cleanliness
- E—environmental improvement.

Surgical care (S)

Surgical care in trachoma is mainly aimed at correction of entropion and trichiasis.

Antibiotics (A)

Chlamydia is sensitive to sulfonamides, tetracycline, erythromycin, azithromycin and rifampicin. World Health Organization (WHO) has recommended oral azithromycin and local tetracycline for treatment of trachoma.

Local antibiotics

Tetracycline (1%) eye ointment four times a day or sulfacetamide (20%) eyedrops three times a day and tetracycline (1%) eye ointment at night for 6 weeks.

Systemic antibiotics

1. Tetracycline 250 mg or erythromycin 250 mg orally four times a day for 4 weeks.
2. Azithromycin 20 mg/kg single dose in children and 1.5 g in adults is the drug of choice now to avoid long schedule of treatment with tetracycline or erythromycin.

Facial cleanliness (F)

Facial cleanliness in the form of washing of face and maintaining facial cleanliness.

Environmental improvement (E)

Environment improvement in the form of improving sanitation facilities to reduce the flies, which spread the infection. Facial cleanliness and environmental improvement are important for preventing the spread of trachoma and to prevent reinfection. Treatment of sequelae of trachoma is based on its site:

1. Trachoma sequelae in the eyelids: Trichiasis and entropion are treated by corrective surgeries.
2. Sequelae in the conjunctiva: Xerosis are treated by artificial tears; symblepharon and pseudopterygium are treated by surgery.
3. Sequelae in cornea: Vascularization are treated by peritomy and corneal opacity is treated depending on the grade, and the site of the opacity.

Prophylaxis for Trachoma

Prophylaxis of trachoma is done by improvement of personal hygiene, environmental sanitation and health education.

Intermittent treatment: The WHO has recommended intermittent treatment or blanket treatment in endemic areas. Intermittent treatment consists of antibiotic eye ointment usually tetracycline (1%) in children twice daily for 5 consecutive days in a month for 6 months in a year.

FOLLICULAR CONJUNCTIVITIS**

Definition

Follicular conjunctivitis includes a group of diseases characterized by inflammation of conjunctiva associated with formation of follicles in the conjunctiva.

Follicles*

Follicles are formed as a result of lymphoid hyperplasia resulting in aggregation of lymphocytes within the adenoid layer of conjunctiva. They appear as small, round swellings usually involving the palpebral conjunctiva and conjunctival fornices. Follicular reaction is not seen in conjunctiva of newborn as lymphoid layer is absent in conjunctiva of newborn. They should be differentiated from papillae, which represent vascular hypertrophy and are usually seen in allergic conjunctivitis.

Etiology

Follicular conjunctivitis is caused by a wide range of causes, which can be infectious or non-infectious. Follicular conjunctivitis may present as acute follicular conjunctivitis (duration < 3 week) and chronic follicular conjunctivitis (duration > 3 week).

The causes for acute follicular conjunctivitis are as follows:

1. Viral conjunctivitis: Adenoviral conjunctivitis (acute follicular conjunctivitis, epidemic keratoconjunctivitis, pharyngoconjunctival fever), herpes simplex conjunctivitis, Newcastle virus conjunctivitis, etc.
2. Chlamydial conjunctivitis: Adult inclusion conjunctivitis.

The causes for chronic follicular conjunctivitis are:

1. Viral conjunctivitis: Chronic follicular conjunctivitis caused by adenovirus, Epstein-Barr viral conjunctivitis, conjunctivitis caused by mumps and measles, etc.
2. Chlamydial conjunctivitis: Trachoma caused by *C. trachomatis.*
3. Bacterial conjunctivitis: Angular conjunctivitis caused by Morax-Axenfeld bacillus.
4. Parinaud's oculoglandular syndrome.
5. Drugs: Pilocarpine, atropine, idoxuridine, eserine, epinephrine, brimonidine.
6. Toxic causes follicular conjunctivitis as a response to shedding of viral toxins from molluscum contagiosum of the eyelids.

Benign Lymphoid Folliculosis or School Folliculosis

It is bilateral condition characterized by the presence of non-inflammatory follicular hypertrophy of the conjunctiva. It is a benign condition seen in children usually along with lymphoid hyperplasia. It is also called school folliculosis as it is commonly seen in children of school age group. It is differentiated from other causes by the absence of inflammatory features.

Clinical Features

The clinical features depend on the causative agent causing follicular conjunctivitis. The common feature involving all the varieties is the presence of follicles commonly involving the palpebral (tarsal) conjunctiva and less commonly involving the bulbar conjunctiva.

Treatment

Treatment depends on the cause.

ALLERGIC CONJUNCTIVITIS

Allergic conjunctivitis is defined as inflammation of conjunctiva as a response to immunological response elicited by allergens.

ETIOPATHOGENESIS

Conjunctiva is the most commonly involved site in allergic diseases affecting the eye because of high vascularity and direct exposure of conjunctiva to the exogenous allergens. The overall incidence of allergic conjunctivitis worldwide is about 20%.

Allergic conjunctivitis is because of hypersensitivity reaction as a result of immunological response initiated by allergens or antigens. Immediate hypersensitivity and delayed cell-mediated immune responses play a crucial role in the development of allergic conjunctivitis. The important mediators of inflammation are histamine, prostaglandins and eosinophil major basic protein.

CLASSIFICATION

Allergic conjunctivitis is classified into:

- Seasonal allergic conjunctivitis
- Perennial allergic conjunctivitis
- Vernal conjunctivitis or keratoconjunctivitis
- Atopic conjunctivitis
- Phlyctenular conjunctivitis or keratoconjunctivitis
- Giant papillary conjunctivitis
- Contact dermatoconjunctivitis.

Seasonal Allergic Conjunctivitis

Definition

Seasonal allergic conjunctivitis is the most common type of allergic conjunctivitis characterized by seasonal occurrence caused by pollens.

Etiopathogenesis

Seasonal allergic conjunctivitis is caused by seasonal airborne allergens such as grass pollen. The exposure to these grass pollen leads to immunoglobulin E-mediated hypersensitivity reaction resulting in allergic conjunctivitis.

Since pollens are seen in specific period of the year, it is seen in the pollen bearing season, which is usually after summer season. It is also called hay fever conjunctivitis as it is caused by grass pollens.

Hay means grass, which is dried and used for feeding animals. Hay fever indicates allergic inflammation caused by hay.

Clinical Features

Symptoms

Redness and itching of the eyes showing characteristic seasonal incidence are the main complaints.

Signs

On examination, edema of the eyelids, chemosis and hyperemia of the conjunctiva are the usual signs (Figs 3.4.11A and B).

Differential diagnosis

Seasonal allergic conjunctivitis has to be differentiated from other types of allergic conjunctivitis. Diagnosis is made from the history and characteristic seasonal incidence.

Treatment

Identification of the allergen and avoiding it or carrying out desensitization is the ideal treatment, but it is not possible in majority of the cases. Treatment is done depending on the severity of inflammation by using one or more of the following drugs:

1. Topical vasoconstrictors: Epinephrine, naphazoline, etc.
2. Topical antihistaminic drugs: Azelastine.
3. Topical mast cell stabilizers: Sodium cromoglycate.
4. Topical antihistaminic and mast cell stabilizers: Olopatadine, ketotifen, etc.
5. Topical non-steroidal anti-inflammatory drugs: Ketorolac.
6. Topical steroid drugs: Fluorometholone, loteprednol, dexamethasone, prednisolone, etc.
7. Systemic antihistaminic drugs: Chlorpheniramine maleate, cetirizine, etc.

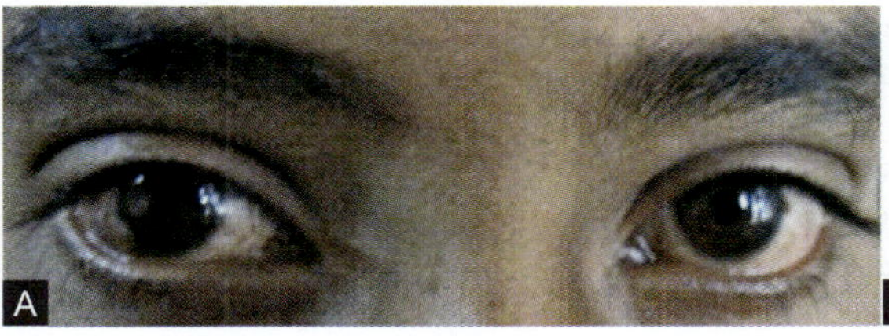

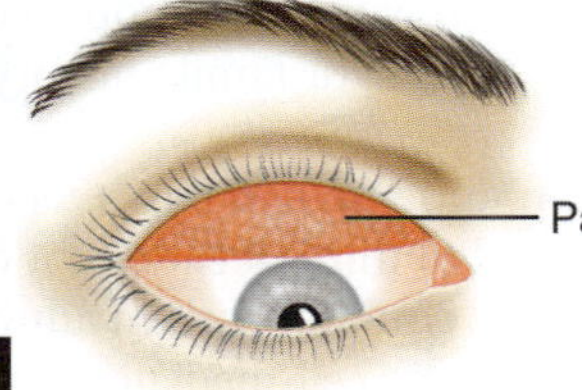

FIGS 3.4.11A and B: Allergic conjunctivitis. **A.** Dusky red congestion seen in allergic conjunctivitis; **B.** Conjunctival papillae.

Perennial Allergic Conjunctivitis

Perennial allergic conjunctivitis is a type of allergic conjunctivitis characterized by its persistence throughout the year. It is usually caused by allergens, which exist throughout the year across all the seasons such as house dust mites.

Etiopathogenesis, clinical features and treatment of perennial allergic conjunctivitis are similar to seasonal allergic conjunctivitis with only difference being presence of perennial symptoms in case of perennial allergic conjunctivitis.

Vernal Conjunctivitis**

Definition

Vernal conjunctivitis is an allergic conjunctivitis typically seen in children characteristically presenting as bilateral may be asymmetrical, recurrent inflammation of conjunctiva with seasonal incidence, which peaks in summer or late spring season.

It is called vernal because of its peak incidence in the spring season. The word vernal means spring season.

Etiopathogenesis

1. It is usually seen in the first and second decade, more commonly affecting boys in first decade of life.
2. It is more commonly seen in hot and dry climate, hence more commonly seen in tropical countries in summer season.
3. The disease usually becomes more symptomatic during late spring or summer season, but mild symptoms can persist throughout the year.
4. It can be associated with other atopic conditions such as asthma or family history of atopy.
5. The disease can undergo spontaneous resolution by second to third decade or it can continue as atopic conjunctivitis in adults.
6. Immunoglobulin E and cell-mediated hypersensitivity reactions play an important role in the pathogenesis of vernal conjunctivitis.

Pathology

Pathology is characterized by:

1. Infiltration by eosinophils.
2. Proliferation of conjunctival epithelium.
3. Hyaline degeneration of fibrous layer of conjunctiva.
4. Hypertrophy of vessels of conjunctiva resulting in the formation of papillae.

Clinical Features

Symptoms

Itching, watering, photophobia, ocular discomfort, foreign body sensation, ropy mucoid discharge, etc.

Signs

The signs depend on the type of vernal conjunctivitis and are described below in the classification (Figs 3.4.12 and 3.4.13).

Classification

Depending on the clinical signs vernal conjunctivitis is classified into (Table 3.4.7):

- Palpebral vernal conjunctivitis
- Limbal or bulbar vernal conjunctivitis
- Mixed vernal conjunctivitis.

Vernal Keratopathy**

Cornea is frequently involved in both palpebral and limbal varieties of vernal conjunctivitis; hence, the disease is frequently called vernal keratoconjunctivitis.

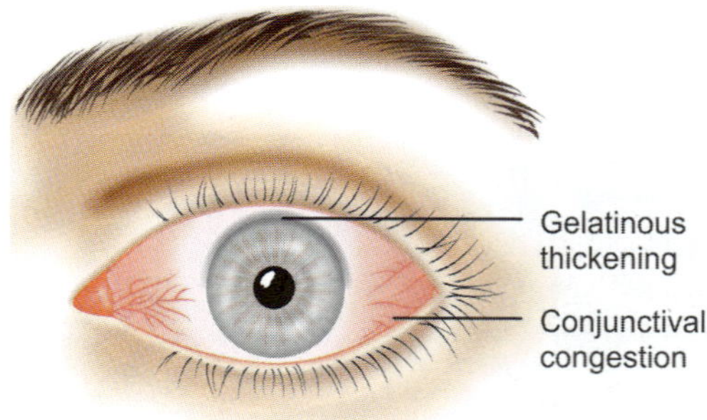

FIG. 3.4.12: Gelatinous thickening around limbus

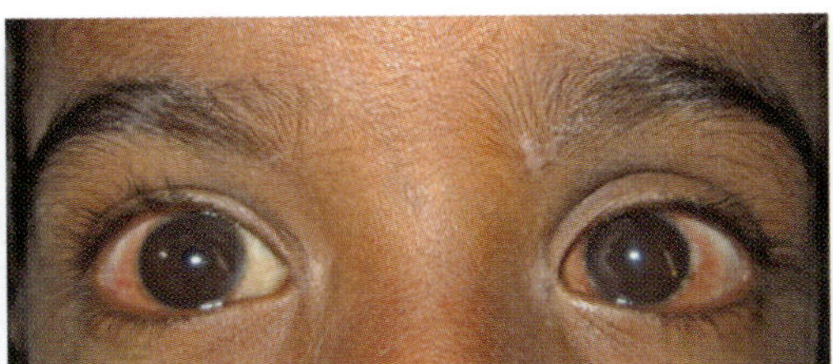

FIG. 3.4.13: Dusky red congestion in vernal conjunctivitis

Clinical Features

Vernal keratopathy can present as follows.

Superficial punctate corneal erosions and superficial punctate epithelial keratitis: These are the commonest lesions seen in vernal keratopathy and these are because of the toxic effect of the inflammatory mediators released as a result of inflammation of conjunctiva.

Ulcerative keratitis or shield ulcer: The punctate corneal erosions can coalesce together resulting in formation of macroerosion called shield ulcer.

Corneal plaques: A shield ulcer when coated by exudates results in the formation of corneal plaque. Corneal plaques prevent re-epithelialization; hence, prevent healing of the shield ulcer.

Subepithelial scars: Healing of shield ulcer will lead to subepithelial scars.

Pseudogerontoxon: It resembles senilis arcus and it is because of lipid deposition in the superficial stroma in the periphery of the cornea (Fig. 3.4.14).

> Keratoconus is seen more frequently in patients with vernal keratoconjunctivitis and other allergic diseases. Chronic repeated rubbing of the eyes is proposed as one of the causative factors for keratoconus.

Vernal conjunctivitis by itself will not cause diminution of vision; however, it may be caused by vernal keratopathy including shield ulcer, corneal plaques, corneal scarring or because of adverse effects of steroids used for the treatment of vernal conjunctivitis (Figs 3.4.15A and B).

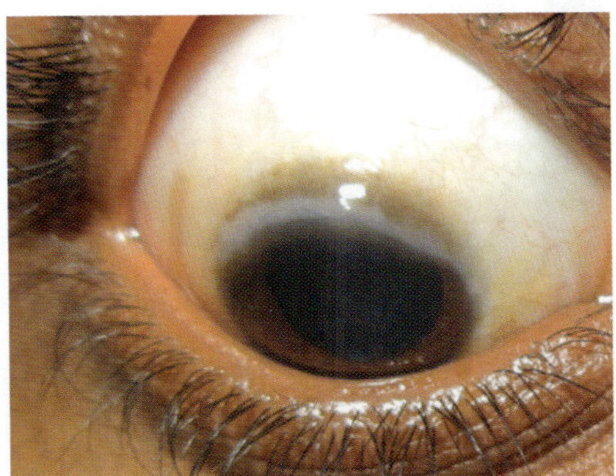

FIG. 3.4.14: Pseudogerontoxon

TABLE 3.4.7: Classification of vernal conjunctivitis on the basis of clinical signs

Palpebral vernal conjunctivitis	*Limbal or bulbar vernal conjunctivitis*	*Mixed vernal conjunctivitis*
Typically affects the upper palpebral conjunctiva characterized by papillary hyperplasia	Marked hyperemia around the limbus	Presents with the features of both palpebral and bulbar types
The papillary hyperplasia gives raise to flat topped hexagonal appearance resembling cobblestone appearance	Gelatinous thickening around the limbus	
Giant papillae result later because of fusion of papillae with individual papillae measuring more than 1 mm	Aggregates of eosinophils and degenerated epithelial cells along the limbus presenting as white dots usually along the superior limbus called Horner-Trantas dots	

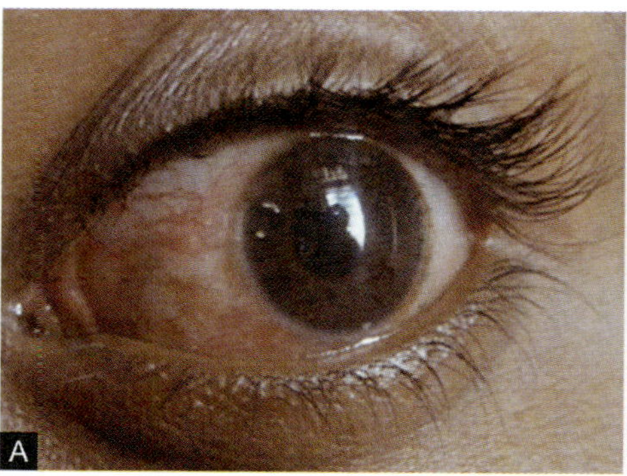

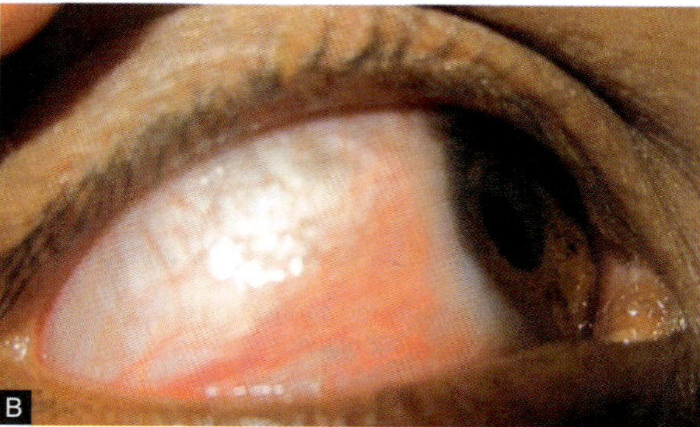

FIGS 3.4.15A and B: Vernal conjunctivitis

Shield Ulcer*

A typical shield ulcer will be superficial, horizontally oval shallow corneal ulcer with irregular borders.

A shield ulcer is produced by combined effect of the toxins released from the inflammatory mediators and by the mechanical effect of the giant papillae on the cornea.

Shield ulcer is classified into three types:
- Grade I: Shield ulcer with clear base.
- Grade II: Shield ulcer with inflammatory debris at the base.
- Grade III: Shield ulcer with elevated plaques.

The treatment of shield ulcer is by cycloplegic drugs such as atropine or homatropine, antibiotic eyedrops. Steroid eyedrops should be used carefully in case of epithelial defect.

Shield ulcer needs aggressive management to prevent complications such as secondary infection resulting in infective corneal ulcer, corneal perforation and corneal blindness.

Grade I ulcers respond favorably to treatment. Grade II ulcers require scraping of the ulcer to remove the inflammatory debris. Grade III ulcers respond poorly to treatment, and may require surgical treatment in the form of amniotic membrane transplantation and superficial keratectomy.

Differential Diagnosis

Vernal conjunctivitis has to be differentiated from other types of allergic conjunctivitis. This is done based on the clinical features and clinical presentation.

Vernal conjunctivitis can be differentiated from trachoma by the presence of symptoms such as itching and ropy discharge; and signs such as cobblestone appearance of papillae, and absence of follicles in vernal conjunctivitis.

Treatment

Local treatment

1. Topical antihistaminic drugs: Azelastine.
2. Topical mast cell stabilizers: Sodium cromoglycate.
3. Topical antihistaminic and mast cell stabilizers: Olopatadine, ketotifen, etc.
4. Topical non-steroidal anti-inflammatory drugs: Ketorolac.
5. Topical steroid drugs: Fluorometholone, loteprednol, dexamethasone, prednisolone, etc.
6. Topical immunomodulatory drugs: Cyclosporine (0.05%) and tacrolimus (0.005%), etc.
7. Topical mucolytic agents: Acetylcysteine.
8. Large papillae are treated by intralesional injection of long-acting steroids such as triamcinolone acetate.

Systemic treatment

Systemic treatment is indicated for short duration in severe cases and drugs used are:

1. Systemic antihistaminic drugs.
2. Oral steroids.

Surgical treatment

Surgical treatment is usually required for treatment of non-responding shield ulcers in the form of amniotic membrane transplantation and superficial keratectomy.

Atopic Conjunctivitis

Definition

Atopic conjunctivitis is a type of allergic conjunctivitis seen in the middle-aged adults and associated with atopic conditions such as atopic dermatitis or eczema.

Etiopathogenesis

Allergic diseases with family history of hypersensitivity are called atopic diseases. The common atopic diseases associated with atopic conjunctivitis are atopic dermatitis and asthma. The mechanism of allergy is similar to that of vernal conjunctivitis and differentiated from vernal conjunctivitis on the basis of clinical features.

Clinical Features

Symptoms

Atopic conjunctivitis tend to be more severe than vernal conjunctivitis and present as itching, watering and stringy mucus discharge. The disease is usually bilateral and seen in middle-aged adults.

Signs

The disease runs more chronic course than vernal conjunctivitis and the characteristic associated features are presence of periorbital eczema. Severe cases present as cicatrizing conjunctivitis leading to complications such as symblepharon, shortening of fornices of conjunctiva, etc. which can lead to blindness.

Papillary hypertrophy, gelatinous thickening of limbus and Horner-Trantas dots are seen similar to vernal conjunctivitis.

Differential Diagnosis

Atopic conjunctivitis has to be differentiated from vernal conjunctivitis (Table 3.4.8).

Treatment

Treatment is on similar guidelines as for vernal conjunctivitis and it is done by antihistaminic drugs, mast cell stabilizers, steroids and antimetabolites drugs such as cyclosporine.

Phlyctenular Keratoconjunctivitis***

Definition

Phlyctenular keratoconjunctivitis is a delayed type hypersensitivity reaction of conjunctival and/or corneal epithelium to endogenous allergens characterized by formation of nodules in the conjunctiva, limbus or cornea.

The word phlycten is derived from a Greek word meaning 'blister' or 'bleb' indicating the presence of characteristic nodules.

TABLE 3.4.8: Differences between vernal conjunctivitis and atopic conjunctivitis

Vernal conjunctivitis	*Atopic conjunctivitis*
Usually seen in children	Usually seen in middle-aged adults
More common disease and the disease tends to be seasonal with the disease being more common in summer	Disease is perennial
Periorbital changes involving the eyelids are absent	Periorbital changes involving the skin around the eyelids are characteristically seen
Cicatricial changes in conjunctiva are absent	Cicatricial changes resulting in loss of vision are seen in severe form of the disease

Etiopathogenesis

1. The disease is more common in undernourished people living in unhygienic conditions where the infections are common, hence more common in underdeveloped and developing countries.
2. It is more commonly affects people in younger age of first and second decade with incidence being more common in girls as girls tend to involve in indoor activities with more incidences of bacterial, and other infections because of overcrowded and unhygienic conditions.
3. Hypersensitivity to *Mycobacterium tuberculosis* remains the most common cause in underdeveloped countries.
4. Hypersensitivity to *S. aureus, Propionibacterium acnes, Chlamydia, Candida* and parasitic infections caused by roundworm are the other common organisms associated with phlyctenular keratoconjunctivitis.

Histologically, phlyctens are composed of plasma cells, histiocytes and lymphocytes.

> Vernal conjunctivitis is more common in boys probably because of the fact that boys tend to involve more in outdoor activities and more exposed to exogenous allergens, which are implicated as a cause for vernal conjunctivitis.
>
> Phlyctenular conjunctivitis is more common in girls probably because of the fact that girls tend to involve more in indoor activities and in conditions such as overcrowded seen in low socioeconomic strata, so there are more chances of acquiring microbial infections, and hence more chances of endogenous allergy to the acquired microbes.

Clinical Features

Based on the involvement of conjunctiva or cornea or both conjunctiva and cornea, it can be phlyctenular conjunctivitis, phlyctenular keratitis or phlyctenular keratoconjunctivitis respectively.

Phlyctenular conjunctivitis

Phlyctenular conjunctivitis presents as a unilateral condition with symptoms of ocular irritation and watering. On examination, characteristic raised nodule with pink to gray or white in color measuring about 1 mm in diameter surrounded by conjunctival hyperemia is observed. The nodule is usually situated on the bulbar conjunctiva near the limbus (Fig. 3.4.16).

The nodule gets liquefied and becomes ulcer in a period of 1 week. The ulcer heals slowly over 1–2 weeks with re-epithelialization. Rarely, the phlycten undergoes necrosis resulting in necrotizing phlyctenular conjunctivitis.

Necrotizing phlyctenular conjunctivitis: It is a rare complication of phlyctenular conjunctivitis characterized by necrosis of the phlyctenular nodule.

Miliary phlyctenular conjunctivitis: It is a rare type of phlyctenular conjunctivitis characterized by the presence of multiple phlyctens commonly distributed around the limbus.

Phlyctenular keratitis**

Phlyctenular keratitis usually begins as phlycten beginning at the limbus and extending toward the center of the cornea surrounded by vessels extending in a straight course from limbus to the nodule. It presents with clinical features of ocular pain, lacrimation and photophobia because of involvement of cornea.

The clinical course of phlyctenular keratitis resembles the phlyctenular conjunctivitis. The corneal phlycten gets liquefied and it becomes ulcer, which heals with or without opacity by re-epithelialization.

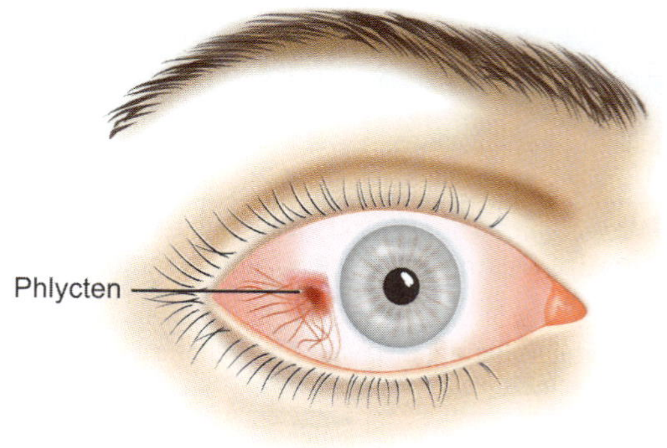

FIG. 3.4.16: Phlyctenular conjunctivitis

Phlyctenular keratitis can present as ulcerative keratitis characterized by the formation of corneal ulcer or infiltrative keratitis characterized by corneal infiltration. The corneal ulcer caused by phlyctenular keratitis can be of two types.

Fascicular ulcer: It is caused by extension of phlycten from margin of cornea or limbus toward the center of the cornea with presence of superficial blood vessels along the path of extension of the phlycten. It rarely perforates and usually heals leaving behind a corneal opacity.*

Scrofulous ulcer: It is caused by ulceration of limbal phlycten and presents at the margin of cornea resembling marginal ulcer. It can be differentiated from marginal ulcer by the absence of clear area between the ulcer and the limbus, which is present in a true marginal ulcer. It usually heals quickly without causing any residual corneal opacity.

Phlyctenular keratoconjunctivitis

Phlyctenular keratoconjunctivitis is because of extension of phlyctenular conjunctivitis; the clinical features by extension of conjunctival phlycten to involve the cornea. It presents with the clinical features of both phlyctenular conjunctivitis and phlyctenular keratitis.

Differential Diagnosis

Phlyctenular conjunctivitis should be differentiated from other inflammatory conditions such as:

- Inflamed pterygium
- Inflamed pinguecula
- Episcleritis
- Scleritis.

Phlyctenular keratitis should be differentiated from infective keratitis and marginal keratitis.

Investigations

Investigations are required in presence of multiple phlycten or in case of recurrent phlyctens. The investigations done are to rule out any present or recent past microbial infection:

1. Chest X-ray and Mantoux test to rule out tuberculosis.
2. Stool examination to rule out any parasitic infestations.
3. Systemic examination, ear, nose and throat (ENT) examination in particular to rule out any infection such as tonsillitis commonly seen in younger age.

Treatment

1. Local treatment is by topical steroid eyedrops or eye ointments. Commonly used steroid eyedrops are prednisolone, dexamethasone, betamethasone, fluorometholone, etc.
2. Topical antibiotic eyedrops are used along with steroid eyedrops to prevent secondary bacterial infection.
3. Cycloplegic drugs such as atropine or homatropine are indicated in case of corneal involvement.
4. Treatment of the underlying cause such as tuberculosis, parasitic infestations and other infections should be carried out along with local treatment to prevent recurrences.

Giant Papillary Conjunctivitis**

Definition

Giant papillary conjunctivitis is a type of allergic conjunctivitis involving the upper palpebral conjunctiva caused by repeated exposure of conjunctiva to an irritating agent (Fig. 3.4.17).

It is most commonly associated with the use of contact lenses. Hence, it is also called contact lens-associated papillary conjunctivitis.

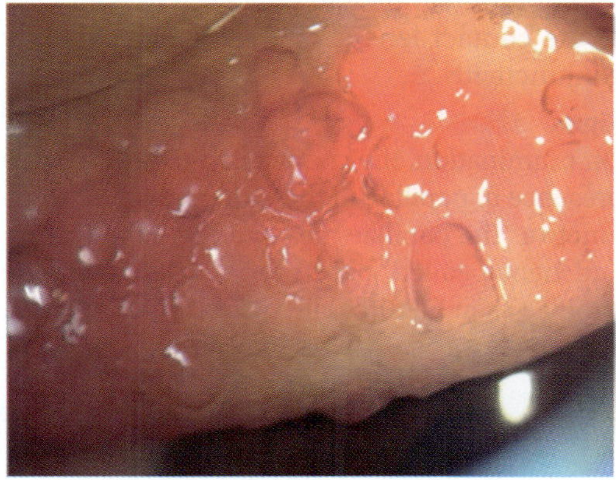

FIG. 3.4.17: Giant papillae

Etiology

The commonly involved etiological agents in the development of giant papillary conjunctivitis are:

1. The use of contact lenses is the most common etiological agent associated with the disease. It is more frequently seen with the use of soft contact lenses compared to rigid gas permeable or hard contact lenses.
2. Exposed corneal or conjunctival sutures following surgeries such as keratoplasty, trabeculectomy, pterygium surgery with suturing of the graft and ocular prosthesis are the etiological factors associated with the development of giant papillary conjunctivitis.

Pathogenesis

The pathogenesis of giant papillary conjunctivitis is explained as a combined result of:

1. Repeated irritation to conjunctiva caused by chronic exposure of conjunctiva to foreign particles such as contact lenses, sutures, prosthesis, etc.
2. Immunological reaction of the conjunctiva caused by antigens in the form of deposits on the contact lenses, sutures, prosthesis, etc.

Clinical Features

Symptoms

It presents with the symptoms of itching, irritation and intolerance to contact lenses in case of the contact lens-associated giant papillary conjunctivitis.

Signs

On examination, the characteristic feature is the presence of papillae in the upper palpebral conjunctiva. The papillae measure more than 1 mm and hence called giant papillae differentiating papillae seen in other allergic conditions, which are usually measure 0.3–1 mm in diameter.

Differential Diagnosis

It has to be differentiated from other allergic conjunctivitis such as vernal conjunctivitis.

Treatment

1. The main treatment is by discontinuing or removing the causative agent such as stopping the contact lenses, removal of exposed sutures and by preventing the deposits on contact lenses, and prosthesis by proper cleaning.
2. Antihistaminic drugs and mast cell stabilizers are the usual drugs used for treatment. Resistant cases are treated by steroid eyedrops.

Contact Dermatoconjunctivitis

Definition

Contact dermatoconjunctivitis is defined as a type of allergic conjunctivitis involving the skin of the eyelids and conjunctiva following exposure to various drugs or other toxic products.

Etiopathogenesis

The common agents known to cause contact dermatoconjunctivitis are:

1. Cosmetics applied to the eye or to the face.
2. Ophthalmic medications such as atropine, neomycin, brimonidine, bimatoprost, etc.

Conjunctivitis medicamentosa: Conjunctivitis seen secondary to use of drugs such as atropine, neomycin, brimonidine, bimatoprost and other drugs, which can also cause contact dermatoconjunctivitis is called conjunctivitis medicamentosa.

Clinical Features

Eczematous reaction of skin of eyelids associated with redness of conjunctiva following exposure to cosmetics or drugs are the typical clinical features.

Treatment

1. Diagnosis can be confirmed by patch test.
2. Treatment is by discontinuing the causative agent, and by treating with antihistaminic drugs and steroid drugs.

GIST BOX 3.4

- Inflammation of conjunctiva is called as conjunctivitis. It is characterized by hyperemia or redness of conjunctiva, cellular infiltration and exudation or discharge, which can be watery, mucoid, mucopurulent or purulent.
- Conjunctivitis can be because of infective, allergic, toxic, traumatic causes, etc.
- Bacterial conjunctivitis is the most common ocular infection.
- Hyperacute purulent conjunctivitis caused by gonorrhea is usually seen in sexually active young adults and neonates.
- Inflammation of conjunctiva occurring in a neonate within first 28 days of life is called ophthalmia neonatorum.
- Acute membranous conjunctivitis is caused by *Corynebacterium diphtheriae.*
- Angular conjunctivitis is caused by Morax-Axenfeld gram-negative diplobacillus.
- Ophthalmia nodosa is chronic granulomatous inflammatory reaction of the conjunctiva to hairs of certain insects and vegetables.
- Adenovirus is the most common virus causing viral conjunctivitis.
- Trachoma is the chronic inflammation of conjunctiva caused by *Chlamydia trachomatis* and it is characterized by chronic follicular reaction and papillary hypertrophy of the conjunctiva.
- Vernal conjunctivitis is an allergic conjunctivitis typically seen in children characteristically presenting as bilateral may be asymmetrical, recurrent inflammation of conjunctiva with seasonal incidence, which peaks in summer or late spring season.
- Atopic conjunctivitis is type of allergic conjunctivitis seen in the middle-aged adults and associated with atopic conditions such as atopic dermatitis or eczema.
- Phlyctenular keratoconjunctivitis is a delayed type hypersensitivity reaction of conjunctival and/or corneal epithelium to endogenous allergens characterized by formation of nodules in the conjunctiva, limbus or cornea.
- Giant papillary conjunctivitis is a type of allergic conjunctivitis involving the upper palpebral conjunctiva caused by repeated exposure of conjunctiva to an irritating agent.

CHAPTER

3.5 Degenerative Diseases of Conjunctiva

PTERYGIUM***

The word pterygium is derived from Greek word 'pterygos' meaning 'wing'.

Definition

Pterygium is a degenerative condition of the conjunctiva characterized by proliferation of subconjunctival tissue as a triangular fleshy mass to invade the cornea involving the Bowman's membrane and the superficial stroma (Fig. 3.5.1).

Etiology

Definite etiology is not known. Pterygium is known to be because of damage to limbal stem cells because of cumulative effect and exposure to:

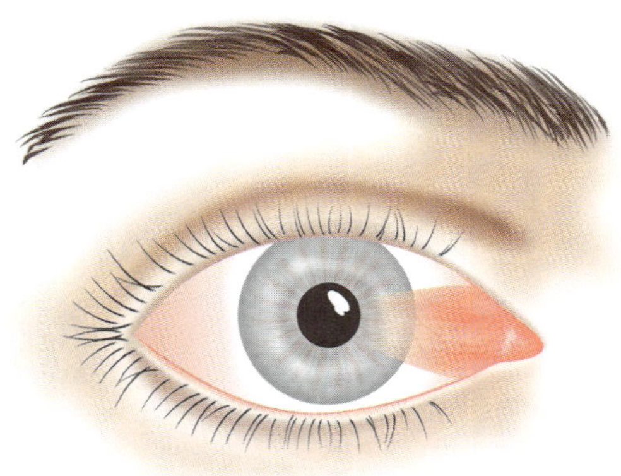

FIG. 3.5.1: Pterygium

- Ultraviolet radiation
- Dry, dusty and sandy weather.

Pathogenesis (Fig. 3.5.2)

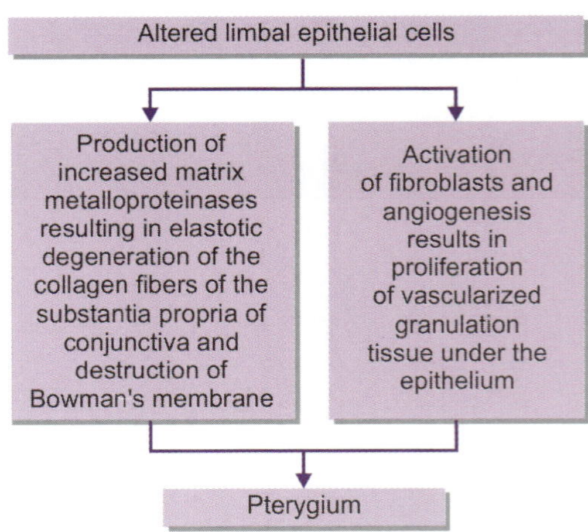

FIG. 3.5.2: Pathogenesis of pterygium

Pathology

Elastotic degeneration of the collagen fibers of the substantia propria of conjunctiva.

Clinical Features

Symptoms

1. Asymptomatic in the initial stages.
2. Irritation, foreign body sensation and cosmetic disfigurement.

3. Diminution of vision due to corneal astigmatism or manual encroachment of the visual axis by pterygium.
4. Pain, redness and other inflammatory symptoms because of recurrent inflammation of pterygium.
5. Rarely diplopia due to limitation of extraocular movements.

Signs

1. Pterygium presents as triangular fibrovascular fold in the nasal or temporal bulbar conjunctiva encroaching cornea (Fig. 3.5.3).
2. Atrophic pterygium presents as thin, attenuated fold with little vascularization and infiltrations in front of the head of the pterygium (cap) are absent (Fig. 3.5.4).
3. Progressive pterygium presents as thick fleshy vascular with infiltrations in front of the head of the pterygium (cap of the pterygium) (Figs 3.5.5 and 3.5.6).

Parts of Pterygium

1. Apex or head: Apical part present on the cornea.
2. Neck: Limbal part.
3. Body: Scleral part.
4. Cap: Infiltrates in front of the apex (seen in progressive pterygium).

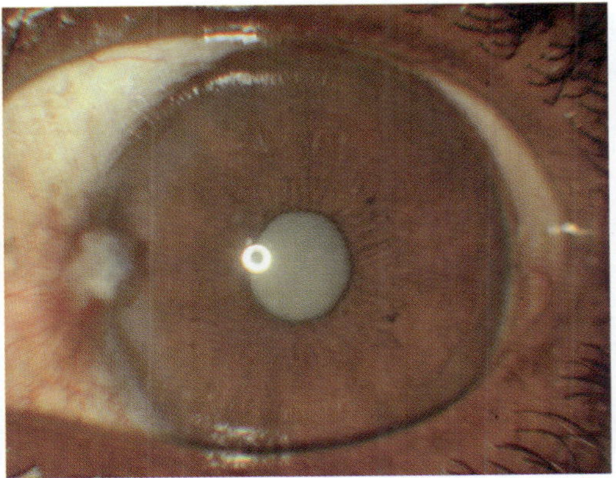

FIG. 3.5.3: Early pterygium

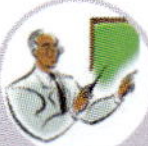

Pseudopterygium*

Adhesion of a fold of scarred conjunctiva to part of peripheral cornea or sclera following inflammation.

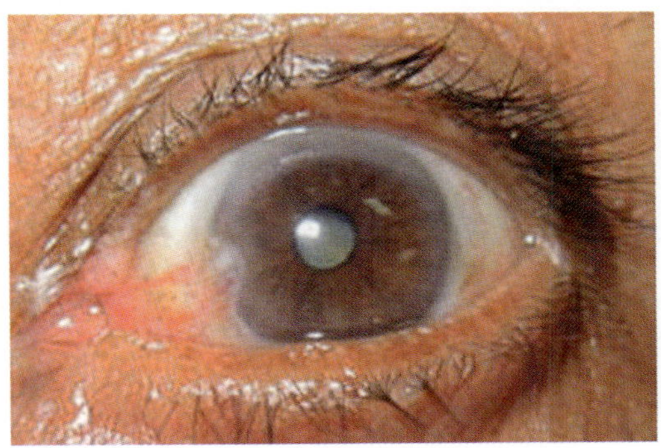

FIG. 3.5.4: Atrophic pterygium

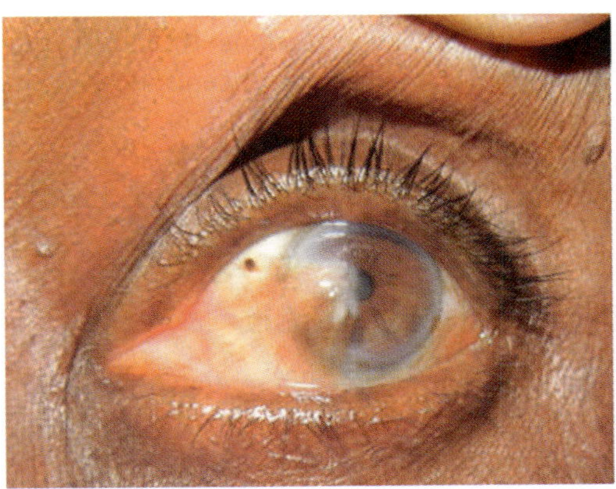

FIG. 3.5.5: Progressive pterygium

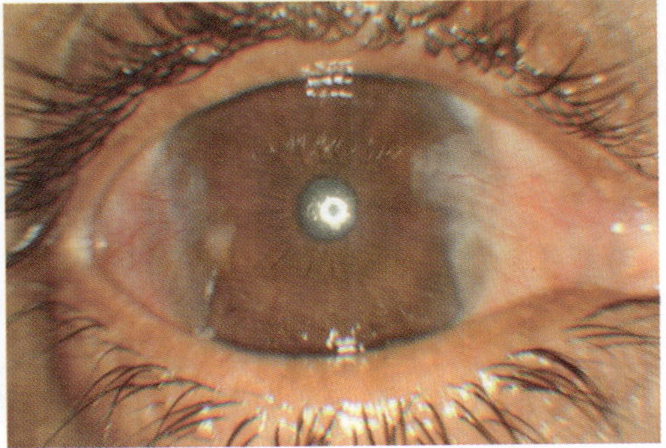

FIG. 3.5.6: Nasal and temporal progressive pterygium

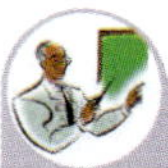

Deposition of Iron in Cornea

Fleischer's ring: Iron deposition seen at the base of the keratoconus.

Hudson-Stahli line: Iron deposition seen as horizontal line in cornea at the junction of meeting of upper and lower eyelids.

Ferry's line: Iron deposition seen in front of filtering bleb.

Coat's ring: Iron deposition seen in rust ring left after removing corneal foreign body.

Stocker Busaca's Line: Deposition of iron in front of the apex of the pterygium.

Complications

1. Recurrent inflammations (inflamed pterygium) causing recurrent episodes of pain, redness, etc.
2. Cystic degeneration.
3. Neoplastic change to epithelioma and fibrosarcoma (very rare complication).

Differential Diagnosis

Pterygium has to be differentiated from pinguecula, pseudopterygium, papilloma and ocular surface squamous neoplasia (OSSN).

Pinguecula appears as a yellowish nodule near the limbus with apex away from the cornea. Papilloma and OSSN have lobulated appearance with sentinel vessel.

Inflamed pterygium has to be differentiated from episcleritis, scleritis and phlyctenular conjunctivitis. All three present as nodular inflammation, whereas pterygium will have characteristic wing-shaped or triangular appearance (Table 3.5.1).

Treatment*

1. Atrophic pterygium is managed symptomatically by topical vasoconstrictor eyedrops and lubricant eyedrops.
2. Surgical excision is the only treatment available for progressive pterygium.
3. Inflamed pterygium is managed by topical steroid eyedrops and oral anti-inflammatory drugs.

Indications for Excision of Pterygium

1. Optical: Pterygium causing diminution of vision either due to corneal astigmatism or due to obstruction of the visual axis.
2. Cosmetic: For cosmetic reasons.
3. Therapeutic: Recurrent inflammation of pterygium.

Surgical excision is the treatment of choice for pterygium. The various methods of pterygium excision are:

TABLE 3.5.1: Differences between pterygium and pseudopterygium*

Features	*Pterygium*	*Pseudopterygium*
Definition	Degenerative condition	Inflammatory condition
Etiology	Ultraviolet radiation, dry, dusty and sandy weather	Chemical burns and trauma
Age	Middle age and elderly people	Seen at any age
Clinical course	Progressive or stationary	Stationary
Site	Nasal or temporal bulbar conjunctiva in the horizontal meridian	Seen at any meridian
Probe test	Probe cannot be passed under the neck of the pterygium	Probe can be passed under the neck of the pterygium as it is attached only at the apex
Treatment	Treatment is by surgical excision; recurrence following surgery is seen and the incidence varies according to the method of surgical excision	Treatment is by surgical excision and recurrence is not seen

1. Simple pterygium excision:
   a. Simple pterygium excision with primary closure of the conjunctiva.
   b. Pterygium excision with bare sclera technique.
2. Pterygium excision with grafting:
   a. Pterygium excision with free conjunctival graft.
   b. Pterygium excision with amniotic membrane graft.
   c. Pterygium excision with mucous membrane graft.
   d. Pterygium excision with limbal conjunctival graft.
   e. Pterygium excision with rotational conjunctival graft.
   f. Pterygium PERFECT—Pterygium Extensive Resection Followed by Extended Conjunctival Graft.
3. Surgeries to prevent recurrence of pterygium: The pterygium recurrence is attributed to the fact that pterygium is due to altered limbal stem cells, which continue to proliferate resulting in recurrence.

   The recurrence rate is in the range of 30–50%. It is highest with simple pterygium excision by bare sclera technique and least with limbal conjunctival grafting as in the latter method altered stem cells are replaced by normal ones:
   a. McReynolds operation: Transplantation of the head of the pterygium under bulbar conjunctiva. This will change the direction of pterygium in which it grows, thereby prevents corneal encroachment, but cosmetically it may not be acceptable.
   b. Pterygium excision with adjunct antimetabolites:
      - Thiotepa eyedrops four times daily for 6 weeks
      - Mitomycin C (0.02%) applied topically to the bare sclera during surgery.
   c. Pterygium excision by β-irradiation.

Mitomycin C is also used in trabeculectomy for topical application over sclera to prevent its recurrence other than its use in pterygium excision.

4. Treatment of pterygium encroaching the pupillary area of cornea: Surgical excision of pterygium is followed by treatment of the residual opacity. Residual corneal opacity is treated by phototherapeutic keratectomy or lamellar keratoplasty.

Pterygium Surgery

Anesthesia for pterygium surgery:
1. Topical anesthesia with lignocaine (4%) and infiltration of lignocaine (2%) into the pterygium.
2. Sub-Tenon's anesthesia or peribulbar anesthesia is required when conjunctival graft is planned.

Procedure of pterygium excision
1. Eye is painted and draped.
2. Head of the pterygium is dissected from the cornea.
3. Separation of the body of the pterygium from the surrounding conjunctiva, Tenon's capsule.
4. Excision of the pterygium with precautions not to injure horizontal rectus muscle.
5. The next step depends on the type of surgery planned such as in pterygium excision with conjunctival graft. Conjunctival graft taken from the superotemporal bulbar conjunctiva is sutured to the cut ends of pterygium, in pterygium excision with adjunctive use of antimetabolites, antimetabolite drugs in required concentration are applied locally to the bare sclera after pterygium excision (Fig. 3.5.7).

Complications of pterygium surgery
1. Recurrence of pterygium is the most common complication. Recurrence rate is highest in simple pterygium excision.
2. Residual corneal opacity: Pterygium cannot be removed without leaving behind a corneal opacity as it invades deeper to Bowman's membrane.
3. Injury to underlying horizontal rectus muscle, if pterygium is not dissected carefully, is one of the rare intraoperative complications.
4. Scleral thinning and sclera melting are seen following deeper dissection of the pterygium and most commonly in intraoperative use of topical antimetabolite drugs.

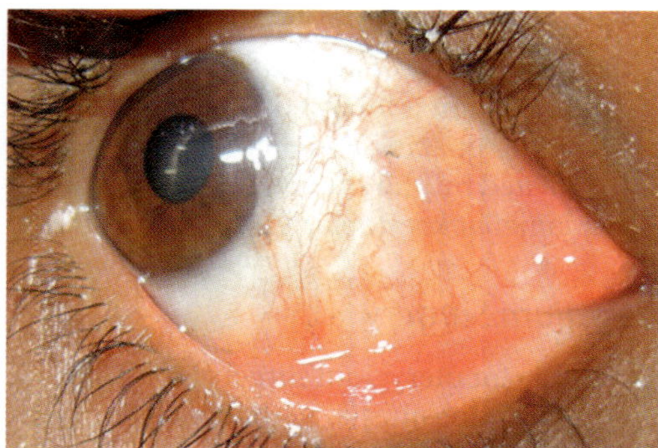

FIG. 3.5.7: Postpterygium surgery with conjunctival grafting

PINGUECULA*

The word pinguecula is derived from Latin word 'pinguis' meaning 'fat'.

Definition

Pinguecula is a degenerative condition of the conjunctiva characterized by yellowish white deposit in the conjunctiva near the limbus (Figs 3.5.8A and B).

It is a misnomer; it is called so because of its appearance similar to fat (yellowish white-colored deposit). It is due to deposition of hyaline material in the conjunctiva.

Etiology

It is similar to etiology of pterygium. It is seen in middle-aged and elderly people, and it is more common in people who are exposed to ultraviolet radiation, dry and dusty weather.

Pathology

Pathology of pinguecula is characterized by elastotic degeneration of the substantia propria of conjunctiva and infiltration of hyaline material.

Clinical Features

Symptoms

1. Asymptomatic in most of the cases.
2. Irritation, foreign body sensation and cosmetic disfigurement.
3. Pain, redness and other inflammatory symptoms because of recurrent inflammation of pinguecula (pingueculitis).

Signs

1. Pinguecula presents as triangular yellowish white deposit in the nasal or temporal bulbar conjunctiva near the limbus with apex of the triangle directed away from the limbus.
2. It is usually stationary condition and will not cause visual symptoms such as pterygium (Table 3.5.2).

Treatment

Treatment is indicated for cosmetic disfigurement and for therapeutic purpose in case of

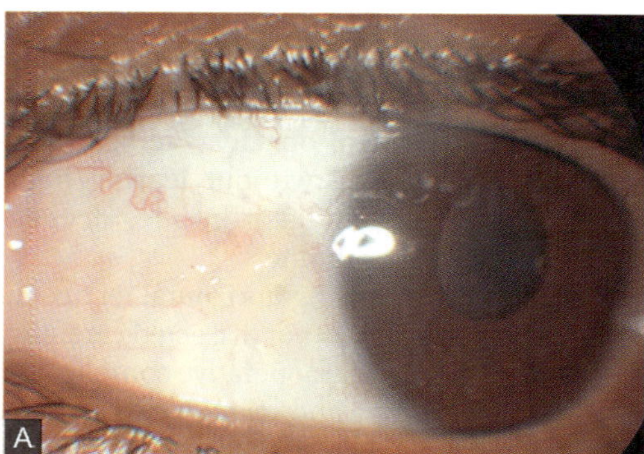

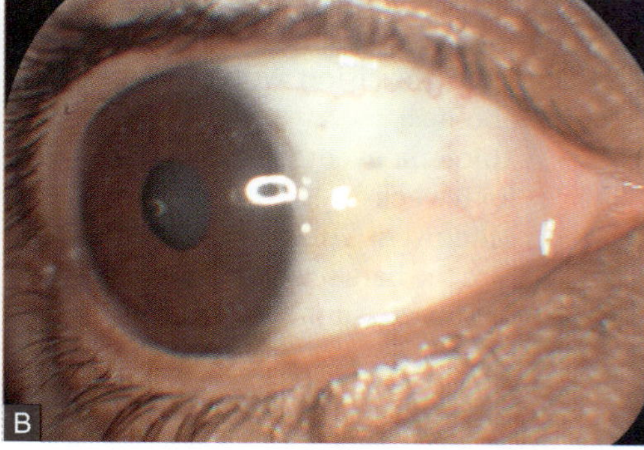

FIGS 3.5.8A and B: Pinguecula

TABLE 3.5.2: Differences between pinguecula and pterygium

Features	*Pterygium*	*Pinguecula*
Definition	Degenerative condition characterized by fibrovascular proliferation	Degenerative condition characterized by hyaline deposition
Pathology	Elastotic degeneration of substantia propria of conjunctiva and fibrovascular proliferation	Elastotic degeneration of substantia propria of conjunctiva and hyaline degeneration
Clinical features	Triangular fibrovascular proliferation of bulbar conjunctiva encroaching the cornea with apex of the triangle toward the cornea	Triangular yellowish white deposition in the bulbar conjunctiva near the limbus with apex of the triangle away from cornea Encroachment of cornea is not seen
Clinical course	Progressive or stationary	Stationary

recurrent episodes of pingueculitis. Treatment is done by excision of the pinguecula.

Both pterygium and pinguecula are more common in nasal bulbar conjunctiva compared to temporal side as:
- Nasal bulbar conjunctiva is exposed more to sunlight because of reflection of light rays from nasal bones onto nasal conjunctiva.
- As tears are collected in medial canthus in lacus lacrimalis before they are drained, nasal bulbar conjunctiva is exposed more to toxic waste products, which are carried from the tears.

CONCRETIONS

The word 'concretion' means calcified deposits. It is a misnomer as deposits are due to accumulation of dead and degenerated epithelial cells in the depressions (Henle's loops) of conjunctiva (Fig. 3.5.9).

Definition

Concretion is a common degenerative condition of conjunctiva characterized by deposition of yellowish deposits in the palpebral and forniceal conjunctiva.

Etiopathogenesis

Concretions, seen in elderly individuals, are due to accumulation of dead and degenerated epithelial cells in depressions (Henle's loops) of conjunctiva.

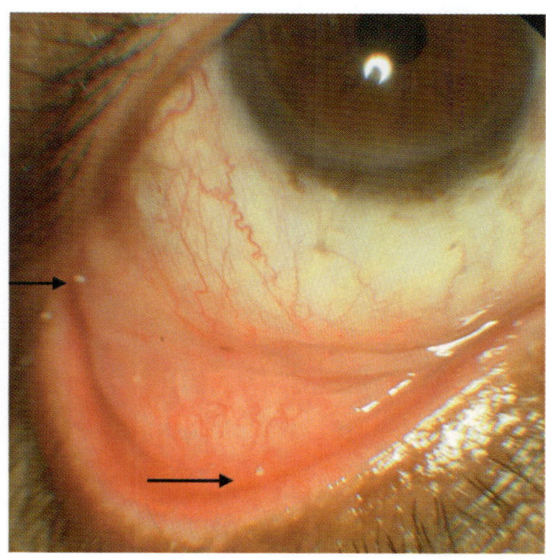

FIG. 3.5.9: Concretions

Clinical Features

- Asymptomatic in most of the cases
- Irritation, foreign body sensation.

Treatment

Concretions are treated by simple removal with a hypodermic needle when they are causing irritation and foreign body sensation.

GIST BOX 3.5

- Pterygium and pinguecula are the most common degenerative conditions of the conjunctiva.
- Pterygium is a degenerative condition of the conjunctiva characterized by proliferation of subconjunctival tissue as a triangular fleshy mass to invade the cornea involving the Bowman's membrane and the superficial stroma.
- Pinguecula is a degenerative condition of the conjunctiva characterized by yellowish white deposit in the conjunctiva near the limbus.

CHAPTER

3.6 Tumors of Conjunctiva

Tumors of conjunctiva include cysts of conjunctiva, benign tumors of conjunctiva and malignant tumors of conjunctiva.

CYSTS OF CONJUNCTIVA

The common cysts of conjunctiva include:

1. Congenital choristomas such as dermoid and dermolipoma: They are described under congenital anomalies of conjunctiva.
2. The other cystic lesions of conjunctiva include retention cysts, lymphatic cysts and cysts of infective origin such as hydatid cyst and cysticercus cyst.

BENIGN TUMORS OF CONJUNCTIVA

The common benign tumors of conjunctiva are papilloma, nevus, fibroma and angiomas of conjunctiva such as lymphangioma and hemangioma.

Papilloma of Conjunctiva

Conjunctival papilloma can be squamous papilloma or viral papilloma. Conjunctival papilloma presents as finger like or cauliflower appearance. Viral papilloma is caused by human papilloma virus. The treatment of the condition is by surgical excision.

Capillary Hemangioma

Capillary hemangioma may be seen alone or along with capillary hemangioma of eyelids or orbit. It is described under tumors of eyelids.

Pyogenic Granuloma

Pyogenic granuloma is described under tumors of eyelids.

Nevus of Conjunctiva

1. Conjunctival nevus is a common benign condition commonly seen in the bulbar conjunctiva. Few nevi may involve the caruncle or palpebral conjunctiva. It presents as a flat or raised pigmented lesion varying from dark brown to light brown or yellow in color. It is usually seen in children (Fig. 3.6.1).
2. Rarely nevus is known to undergo malignant transformation, the risk being less than 1%.
3. Nevi of conjunctiva are managed by observation to look for any increase in the size or pigmentation suggestive of malignant transformation.
4. Treatment is indicated for those nevi showing increase in size and for cosmetic reasons. Treatment is by complete surgical excision.

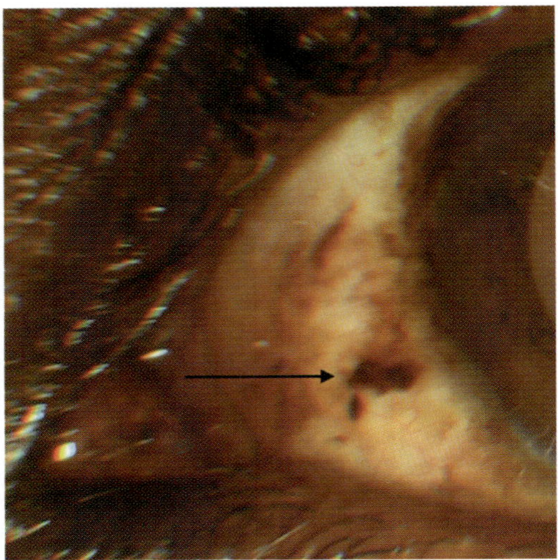

FIG. 3.6.1: Nevus of conjunctiva

Primary Acquired Melanosis

1. It is a benign slow growing tumor usually seen in middle age and elderly age people more commonly seen in fair-skinned people.
2. It is considered as premalignant condition as up to 50% chances of malignant transformation are present.
3. It presents as flat lesion with ill-defined margins and the histopathological picture showing presence of abnormal melanocytes.
4. Treatment is by complete surgical excision followed by with or without cryotherapy or topical chemotherapy.

MALIGNANT TUMORS OF CONJUNCTIVA

The common malignant tumors of conjunctiva are squamous cell carcinoma, malignant melanoma, basal cell carcinoma and Kaposi's sarcoma.

Malignant Melanoma of Conjunctiva

1. It is a rare malignant tumor of conjunctiva seen commonly in elderly individuals. Exposure to the ultraviolet radiations is considered as risk factor. 50–75% of the melanomas arise from pre-existing primary acquired melanosis (PAM).
2. Bulbar conjunctiva is the most common site and rarely seen in palpebral or forniceal conjunctiva.
3. It presents as a raised or flat pigmented lesion with variable amount of pigmentation and amelanotic lesions are also seen rarely (Fig. 3.6.2).
4. Rapid growth, absence of mobility in relation to underlying sclera, presence of feeder sentinel vessels and encroachment of cornea are the clinical features suggestive of malignancy.
5. Treatment is by wide surgical excision followed by either chemotherapy or cryotherapy or radiotherapy. Sentinel lymph node biopsy is indicated in cases of regional lymph node metastasis. Orbital exenteration is done for cases with orbital invasion. Cases presenting with distant metastasis to lung, brain, etc. are treated by palliative therapy.

Kaposi's Sarcoma

- Kaposi's sarcoma is a malignant vascular tumor
- It is the most common tumor seen in acquired immunodeficiency syndrome (AIDS) patients and it is rarely seen in others
- It presents as reddish flat or elevated lesion resembling subconjunctival hemorrhage
- The treatment options available are surgical excision, radiotherapy or cryotherapy.

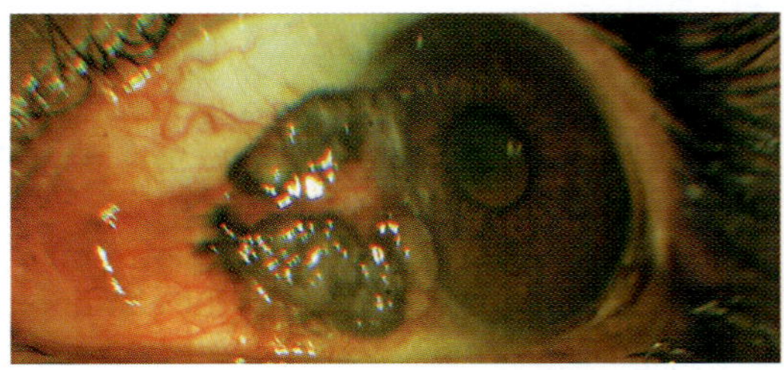

FIG. 3.6.2: Melanoma of conjunctiva

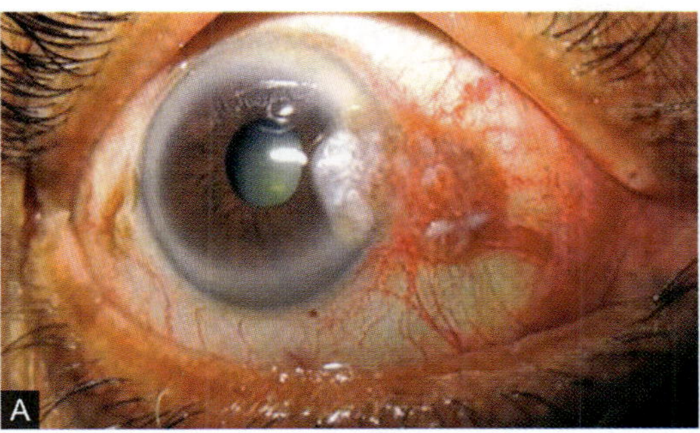

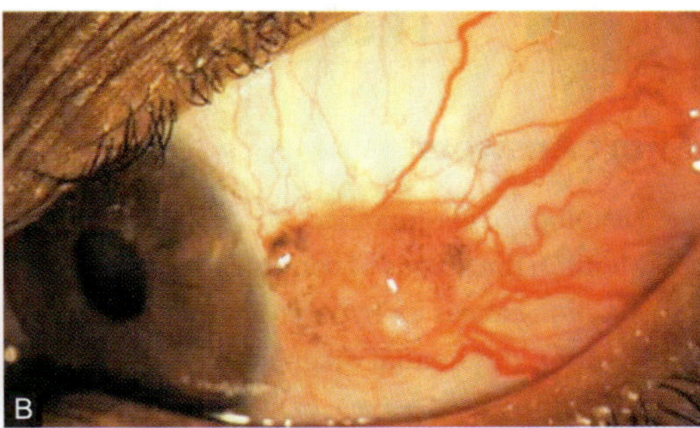

FIGS 3.6.3A and B: Ocular surface squamous neoplasia

Ocular Surface Squamous Neoplasia

1. Ocular surface squamous neoplasia (OSSN) includes a group of neoplastic conditions affecting the epithelium of cornea and conjunctiva such as dysplastic conditions, carcinoma in situ, and squamous cell carcinoma (Figs 3.6.3A and B, Fig. 3.6.4).
2. It is usually seen in elderly people, more common in males. However, in patients with HIV infection, it is known to occur in younger age.
3. Exposure to ultraviolet light and infection by human papilloma virus are the proposed etiological factors responsible for OSSN.
4. It presents as lobulated lesion with prominent vessel called sentinel vessels involving the bulbar conjunctiva more commonly.
5. It has to be differentiated from benign conditions such as papilloma, pterygium and pyogenic granuloma.

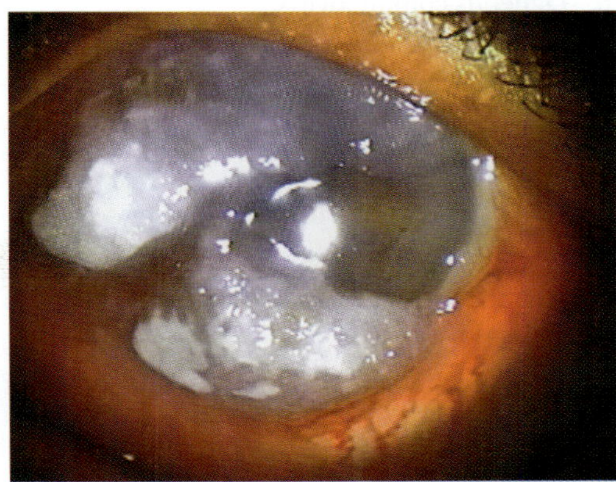

FIG. 3.6.4: Ocular surface squamous neoplasia involving cornea

6. The diagnosis of the condition is by cytology or by excisional biopsy.
7. The treatment of the condition is by surgical excision combined with or without use of either cryotherapy or radiotherapy, or local chemotherapy.

GIST BOX 3.6

- The common benign tumors of conjunctiva are papilloma, nevus, fibroma and angiomas of conjunctiva such as lymphangioma and hemangioma.
- The common malignant tumors of conjunctiva are squamous cell carcinoma, malignant melanoma, basal cell carcinoma and Kaposi's sarcoma.
- Ocular surface squamous neoplasia includes a group of neoplastic conditions affecting the epithelium of cornea and conjunctiva such as dysplastic conditions, carcinoma in situ and squamous cell carcinoma. It is usually seen in elderly people more common in males. However, in patients with HIV infection, it is known to occur in younger age.

FREQUENTLY ASKED QUESTIONS (FAQs)

*Short Answers

1. Histology of conjunctiva.
2. Mention the glands of conjunctiva.
3. Mention causes for hyperemia of conjunctiva.
4. Mention differential diagnosis of ophthalmia neonatorum.
5. What are the causes for granulomatous conjunctivitis?
6. Ligneous conjunctivitis.
7. Ophthalmia nodosa.
8. Parinaud's oculoglandular syndrome.
9. Pannus.
10. Treatment of trachoma.
11. WHO classification of trachoma.
12. Conjunctival follicles.
13. Mention the causes for acute hemorrhagic conjunctivitis.
14. Mention the complications and sequelae of trachoma.
15. Shield ulcer.
16. Fascicular ulcer.
17. Mention the differences between pterygium and pseudopterygium.
18. Pseudopterygium.
19. Describe the treatment of pterygium.
20. Pinguecula.

**Short Essays

1. Ecchymosis (subconjunctival hemorrhage).
2. Chemosis.
3. Classify bacterial conjunctivitis.
4. Hyperacute purulent conjunctivitis.
5. Treatment for ophthalmia neonatorum.
6. Acute membranous conjunctivitis.
7. Pseudomembranous conjunctivitis.
8. Angular conjunctivitis.
9. Adult inclusion conjunctivitis.
10. Classify trachoma.
11. WHO classification of trachoma.
12. Follicular conjunctivitis.
13. Adenoviral conjunctivitis.
14. Vernal conjunctivitis.
15. Phlyctenular keratitis.
16. Vernal keratopathy.
17. Giant papillary conjunctivitis.

***Long Essays

1. Mention the differential diagnosis of acute red eye. Describe clinical features and treatment of bacterial conjunctivitis.
2. Define ophthalmia neonatorum. Describe etiology, clinical features and treatment of ophthalmia neonatorum.
3. Describe etiology, pathogenesis, clinical features and management of trachoma.
4. Classify allergic conjunctivitis. Describe etiology, clinical features and management of vernal conjunctivitis.
5. Describe etiology, clinical features and management of phlyctenular conjunctivitis.
6. Define pterygium. Describe the etiology, clinical features and management of pterygium.

BIBLIOGRAPHY

1. Agarwal A. Handbook of Ophthalmology, 1st edition. Slack Incorporated; 2006. p. 204.
2. Basak SK. Essentials of Ophthalmology. Current Books International, 2nd edition. pp. 106-8.
3. Bonnet JM, Begg NT. Control of diphtheria: guidance for consultants in communicable disease control. World Health Organization. Commun Dis Public Health. 1999;2(4):242-9.

4. Cameron JA. Shield ulcers and plaques of the cornea in vernal keratoconjunctivitis. Ophthalmology. 1995;102(6):985-93.
5. Chatterjee S. Neonatal Conjunctivitis Modern Ophthalmology, 3rd edition. Jaypee Brothers Medical Publishers (P) Ltd.
6. Dawson CR, Daghfous T, Whitcher J, et al. Intermittent trachoma chemotherapy: a controlled trial of topical tetracycline or erythromycin. Bull World Health Organ. 1981;59(1):91-7.
7. Dawson CR, Whitcher JP, Schmidt NJ. Editorial: Acute hemorrhagic conjunctivitis. JAMA. 1974;230(5):727-8.
8. Dushku N, John MK, Schultz GS, et al. Pterygia pathogenesis: corneal invasion by matrix metalloproteinase expressing altered limbal epithelial basal cells. Arch Ophthalmol. 2001;119(5):695-706.
9. Fraser SG, Dowd TC, Bosanquet RC, et al. Argon and YAG lasers in the treatment of ophthalmia nodosa. Eye (Lond). 1995;9(Pt 5):638-40.
10. Gupta S, Sinha R, Sharma N, et al. Ocular surface squamous neoplasia. Del Ophthalmol. 2012;23(2):89-96.
11. Haase DA, Nash RA, Nsanze H, et al. Single-dose ceftriaxone therapy of gonococcal ophthalmia neonatorum. Sex Transm Dis. 1986;13(1):53-5.
12. International Trachoma Initiative 10th Anniversary Report.
13. Latif A, Mason P, Marowa E, et al. Management of gonococcal ophthalmia neonatorum with single-dose kanamycin and ocular irrigation with saline. Sex Transm Dis. 1988;15(2):108-9.
14. Leonardi A, Hall A. Mechanisms of corneal allergic reaction: New options for treatment. Expert Rev Ophthalmol. 2010;5(4):545-56.
15. Maia S, Gomes M, Oliveira L, et al. Isolated Bulbar Conjunctival Kaposi's Sarcoma as a Primary Presentation of AIDS: A Case Report. Case Rep Ophthalmol Med. 2013;2013:469195.
16. Majmudar PA. Atopic and vernal keratoconjunctivitis. Advanced Ocular Care; March 2010.
17. Mansour AM, Barber JC, Reinecke RD, et al. Ocular choristomas. Surv Ophthalmol. 1989;33(5):339-58.
18. Mukherjee PK. Pediatric Ophthalmology. New Age International (P) Limited; 2005.
19. Narsani AK, Jatoi SM, Khanzada MA, et al. Recurrence of pterygium with conjunctival autograft versus mitomycin C. Pak J Ophthalmol. 2008;24(1):29-33.
20. Palafox SKV, Jasper S, Tauber, et al. Ophthalmia neonatorum. J Clinic Experiment Ophthalmol. 2011;2:119.
21. Sathe SM. Angular conjunctivitis with associated dermatitis. Indian J Ophthalmol. 1955;3(1):1-9.
22. Schlosser K. Trachoma through history. International Trachoma Initiative.
23. Schneider G. Silver nitrate prophylaxis. Can Med Assoc J. 1984;131(3):193-6.
24. Schott D, Dempfle CE, Beck P, et al. Therapy with a purified plasminogen concentrate in an infant with ligneous conjunctivitis and homozygous plasminogen deficiency. N Engl J Med. 1998;339(23):1679-86.
25. Sengupta S, Reddy PR, Gyatsho J, et al. Risk factors for intraocular penetration of caterpillar hair in Ophthalmia Nodosa: a retrospective analysis. Indian J Ophthalmol. 2010;58(6):540-3.
26. Sethi PK, Dwivedi N. Ophthalmia nodosa. Indian J Ophthalmol. 1982;30(1):11-4.
27. Sharma V, Varma P, Vaidya S. Bilateral lipoderma in adult: a rare case. Int J Ophthalmol Vis Sci. 2006;4(1).
28. Shields CL, Shields JA. Conjunctival tumors in children. Curr Opin Ophthalmol. 2007;18(5):351-60.
29. Shields JA, Shields CL. Eyelid, Conjunctival, and Orbital Tumors: An Atlas and Textbook, 2nd edition. Lippincott Williams & Wilkins; 2007.
30. Smolin and Thoft. In: Foster CS, Azar DT, Dohlman CH (Eds). The Cornea: Scientific Foundations and Clinical Practice, 4th edition. Philadelphia: Lippincott Williams & Wilkins; 2005.

31. Strategies for Prevention of Blindness in National Programs, 2nd edition. Geneva: WHO; 1997.
32. Takamura E, Uchio E, Ebihara N, et al. Japanese guideline for allergic conjunctival diseases. Allergol Int. 2011;60(2):191-203.
33. Tasman W, Jaeger EA. The Wills Eye Hospital: Atlas of Clinical Ophthalmology, 2nd edition. Philadelphia: Lippincott Williams & Wilkins; 2001.
34. Varma BM, Ga BK. Congenital epitarsus. J All India Ophthalmol Soc. 1969;17(4):163-5.
35. Venkataswamy G. Angular conjunctivitis and riboflavine deficiency. Indian J Ophthalmol. 1960;8(2):33-41.
36. Wadhwani M, D'souza P, Jain R, et al. Conjunctivitis in the newborn-a comparative study. Indian J Pathol Microbiol. 2011;54(2):254-7.
37. Williams DC, Edney G, Maiden B, et al. Recognition of allergic conjunctivitis in patients with allergic rhinitis. World Allergy Organ J. 2013;6(1):4.
38. World Health Organization. Conjunctivitis of the newborn: prevention and treatment at the primary health care level. Geneva; 1986.
39. Zaka-ur-Rab Z, Mittal S. Optic Nerve Head Drusen in Goldenhar Syndrome. JK Science. 2007;9(1):33-4.
40. Zembowicz A, Mandal RV, Choopong P. Melanocytic lesions of the conjunctiva. Arch Pathol Lab Med. 2010;134(12):1785-92.

SECTION 4

Optics and Refraction

CHAPTER 4.1 Optics of Human Eye

OPTICS

Optics is a branch of physics and involves the study of light.

Light/Visible light is the portion of the electromagnetic spectrum, which is visible to the human eye. It ranges from 390 to 750 nm. Visible light includes seven spectrums of colors ranging from violet to red situated between 390 and 750 nm wavelengths. The portion of the electromagnetic spectrum below violet is called ultraviolet (UV) light and the portion above is called infrared light.

Ultraviolet light is the portion of the electromagnetic spectrum with wavelength shorter than visible light ranging from 10 to 390 nm. The UV light is invisible to the human eye. Most of the UV light is blocked by the ozone layer of the atmosphere. The UV light is necessary for production of vitamin D. Long-term exposure to the UV light is implicated in many conditions of the eyes such as cataract, pterygium, skin cancers, etc.

Infrared light is the portion of the electromagnetic spectrum with wavelength longer than visible light with wavelength more than 750 nm.

Reflection of Light

Reflection of light is the phenomenon of turning back of light into the same medium after striking the boundary of other medium.

The boundary between the two media is called reflective surface, the light rays falling on the reflective surface are called incident rays and the rays reflected back from the reflective surface are called reflected rays.

Laws of Reflection (Fig. 4.1.1)

1. The incident rays, reflected rays and normal (a line drawn perpendicular to the reflecting surface between incident rays and reflected rays) all lie in same plane.
2. The angle of incidence (angle between the incident ray and normal) is equal to the angle of reflection (angle between the reflected ray and normal).

Types of Reflection

Reflection is of two types:

1. Regular reflection: It occurs when light rays fall on smooth surfaces (e.g. mirror). Here, the parallel light rays falling on the smooth

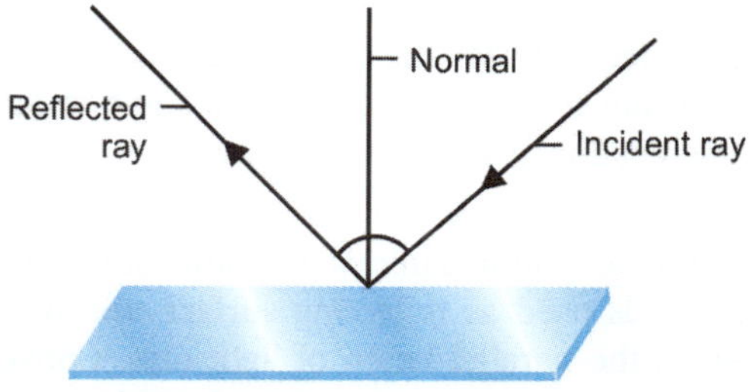

FIG. 4.1.1: Laws of reflection

reflective surface will lead to parallel reflected rays leading to the formation of image.

2. Irregular reflection: It occurs when light rays fall on rough surfaces (e.g. stone). Here, the parallel light rays falling on the smooth reflective surface will lead to divergent reflected rays and thus image is not formed.

Mirror: It is a reflective surface and the light rays falling on it undergo regular reflection. It can be plane mirror or spherical mirror.

Plane mirror

A mirror with plane reflective surface is called plane mirror. The image formed by a plane mirror is virtual, erect, laterally inverted and lies as far behind the mirror as the object is in front of it.

Spherical mirror

A mirror with spherical reflective surface is called spherical mirror. It can be concave spherical mirror or convex spherical mirror depending on the reflecting surface.

Concave spherical mirror

In concave spherical mirror, the inner side of the sphere is used as reflecting surface and it converges the parallel beam of light rays. The image formed by a concave mirror depends on the position of the object:

- Object at infinity forms real, minified, inverted image at principal focus of the mirror
- Object at the center of curvature of the mirror forms inverted and same size image at the center of curvature
- Object at the principal focus of the mirror forms real, magnified and inverted image at the infinity
- Object between the principal focus and pole of the mirror forms virtual, magnified and erect image behind the mirror.

Convex spherical mirror

In convex spherical mirror, the outer side of the sphere is used as reflecting surface and it diverges the parallel beam of light rays. Convex mirror forms virtual, erect and minified image.

Refraction of Light

Refraction of light is the phenomenon of change in the direction of light due to change in the density of transmission medium, when light travels from one medium to another medium.

When light passes from a medium with higher density to a medium with lower density, the light moves away from the midline and when light moves from a medium with lower density to a medium of high density, the light moves toward the midline.

Laws of Refraction (Fig. 4.1.2)

- The incident rays and refracted rays lie on either side of the normal and all lie in the same plane
- The ratio of sine of the angle of incidence and sine of angle of refraction is constant.

This constant is called refractive index, when the light travels from air or vacuum. Refractive index is the ratio of speed of light in vacuum or air to the speed of light in the medium.

LENS

Lens is a transparent refractive medium with two surfaces. Lenses are of two types, spherical lenses and cylindrical lenses.

Spherical lenses are bounded by two surfaces, which form part of a sphere. A spherical lens can be convex spherical lens or concave spherical lens.

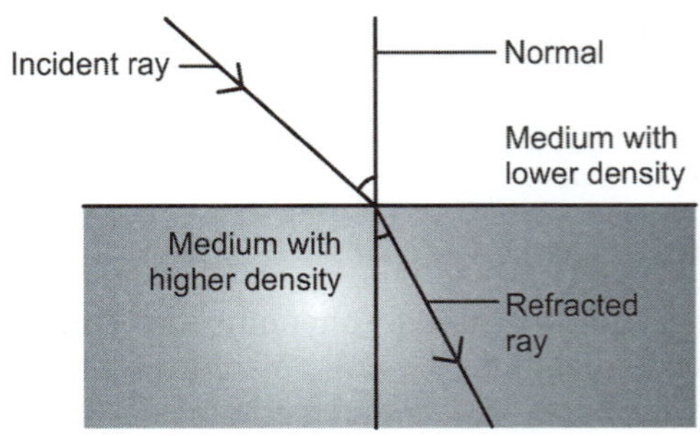

FIG. 4.1.2: Laws of refraction

Cylindrical lenses are bounded by two surfaces, which form part of a cylinder. A cylindrical lens can be convex cylindrical lens or concave cylindrical lens.

The image formation in convex lens depends on the position of the object and it is similar to the image formation in concave mirror. The image formation in concave lens is always virtual, erect and minified, similar to the image formation in convex mirror.

For Ophthalmic lenses refer Author's textbook *'Clinical Methods in Ophthalmology',* Chapter 7, 'Ophthalmic Lenses'.

Sturm's Conoid (Fig. 4.1.3)*

The Sturm's conoid indicates the path of the light through a toric lens. In toric lens, the two principal meridians are unequal with one median being more curved than the other; hence, the light does not come to a point focus, but forms a line focus with two lines being perpendicular to each other. The best focusing occurs in between these two lines of focus and it is called circle of least confusion. The distance between the two lines of focus is called focal interval of Sturm.

The circle of least confusion indicates that spherical equivalent of the cylindrical lens. This corresponds to a point where the horizontal and vertical dimensions of the image are equal and the goal of a spherical refractive correction is to choose a lens that produces circle of least confusion.

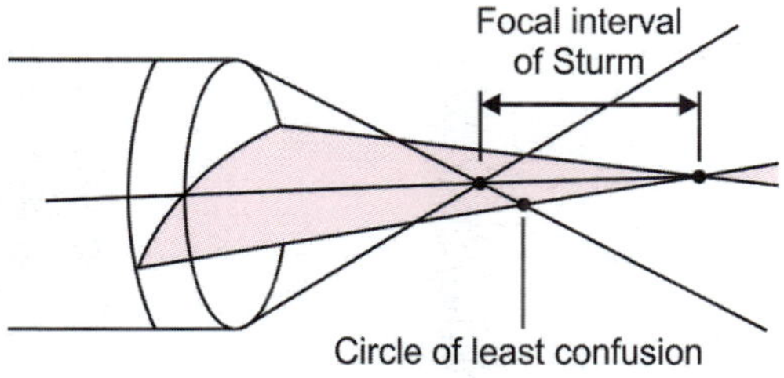

FIG. 4.1.3: Sturm's conoid

OPTICS OF HUMAN EYE

Eye has a compound optical system with two refractive mediums, cornea and lens, which focus the light rays onto the retina.

Schematic Eye*

Allvar Gullstrand has described the schematic eye with two nodal points, two principal points and two principal foci.

Gullstrand's Schematic Eye

- The total refractive power of the eye is +58 D with cornea +43 D and lens +15 D
- The two principal points are situated 1.35 mm (P_1) and 1.60 mm (P_2) behind the anterior surface of cornea respectively
- The two nodal points are situated 7.08 mm (N_1) and 7.33 mm (N_2) behind the anterior surface of cornea respectively
- The two principal foci are situated 15.70 mm (F_1) in front of and 24.38 mm (F_2) behind the cornea, respectively.

Allvar Gullstrand, a Swedish ophthalmologist was awarded Nobel Prize for description of schematic eye. He was the one who invented slit lamp.

Reduced Eye*

The reduced eye model was described to simplify the complex optical system of the eye by considering a single refractive surface.

Listing's Reduced Eye

- The total refractive power of the eye is +60 D
- The principal point is situated 1.5 mm (P) behind the anterior surface of cornea
- The two nodal points are situated 7.2 mm (N) behind the anterior surface of cornea
- The two principal foci are situated 15.70 mm (F_1) in front of and 24.38 mm (F_2) behind the cornea respectively

- The anterior focal length of the eye measuring 17.2 mm and posterior focal length of the eye measuring 22.9 mm.

Donders' Reduced Eye

- The total refractive power of the eye is +60 D
- The principal point is situated 2 mm (P) behind the anterior surface of cornea
- The nodal point is situated 7 mm (N) behind the anterior surface of cornea
- The anterior focal length of the eye is 15 mm and posterior focal length of the eye is 20 mm.

The schematic eye model of the human eye with two principal points and two nodal points is simplified by the reduced eye model with one principal point and one nodal point to simplify the calculations of the size and positions of the images produced by the human eye.

GIST BOX 4.1

- Eye has a compound optical system with two refractive mediums, cornea and lens, which focus the light rays onto the retina.
- The total refractive power of the eye is +60 D.
- The principal point is situated 1.5 mm (P) behind the anterior surface of cornea.
- The two nodal points are situated 7.2 mm (N) behind the anterior surface of cornea.
- The two principal foci are situated 15.70 mm (F_1) in front of and 24.38 mm (F_2) behind the cornea, respectively.
- The anterior focal length of the eye measuring 17.2 mm and posterior focal length of the eye measuring 22.9 mm.

CHAPTER

4.2 Techniques of Refraction

Refraction in eye is defined as a process by which the light rays are focused onto the light-sensitive layer of the retina. Refraction occurs in the eye at the:

1. Cornea, which is the first and the most important refractive surface with refractive power of 44 D accounting for two thirds of the refractive power of the eye.
2. Lens with refractive power of 16 D accounting for rest of the power of the eye.

The refractive power is determined by the curvature of cornea and lens, and index of lens. In emmetropia, the refractive power and axial length are in proportion to each other; hence, the light rays are focused onto the retina.

Emmetropia is determined by:
- Curvature of cornea.
- Curvature, position and index of lens.
- Axial length.

Any abnormality in any one of the above factors will lead to emmetropia.

The techniques of determining the refractive status of the eye and correcting the refractive errors are included under refraction. The techniques of refraction are broadly classified into two types.

TYPES OF REFRACTION

1. Objective refraction: It is done without active participation of the patient.
2. Subjective refraction: It is done by participation of the subject or the patient.

TECHNIQUES OF OBJECTIVE REFRACTION*

The different techniques of objective refraction are as follows:
- Retinoscopy
- Automated refractometry
- Keratometry.

Retinoscopy**

Retinoscopy is an objective method of finding the refractive error based on the principle of neutralization.

Principle

Retinoscopy is based on the principle that when light is reflected into eye, the direction in which light will travel in the pupillary area depends on the refractive status of the eye.

Types

1. Dry retinoscopy: Retinoscopy without the use of cycloplegic drugs is called dry retinoscopy.
2. Wet retinoscopy: Retinoscopy with the use of cycloplegic drugs is called wet retinoscopy.
3. Static retinoscopy: Retinoscopy done by relaxing the accommodation by cycloplegic

drugs or by asking the subject to fix at a distant target is called static retinoscopy.

4. Dynamic retinoscopy: Retinoscopy done by use of active accommodation by asking the subject to look at a near target.

Dry and static retinoscopy is done in elderly individuals, in whom the amplitude of accommodation is decreased. Wet and static retinoscopy is done in children and young adults in whom the accommodation is active. Dynamic retinoscopy is rarely done in clinical practice.

Mydriatics and Cycloplegic Agents in Retinoscopy

Cycloplegic drugs are used in retinoscopy in children and young adults in whom the accommodation is active. In children aged less than 7 years, atropine is used. In children between 7 and 12 years, homatropine is used and in children between the age group of 12 and 20 years, cyclopentolate is used. In the age group of 20–35 years with hypermetropia, homatropine or cyclopentolate is used.

In elderly individuals, only mydriatic drugs such as phenylephrine or tropicamide are used to enhance the visibility of pupillary reflex or to overcome the opacities of the media.

Procedure

Retinoscopy is done in a darkroom. The instruments required are retinoscope, trail set, trial frame and vision charts.

The examiner (ophthalmologist or optometrist) sits at a distance of 1 m from the subject/patient. Light is thrown into the subject's eye and the examiner observes the movement of red reflex in the pupillary area in both horizontal and vertical meridians by moving the retinoscope. The results are interpreted as:

1. Movement of red reflex with the movement of the retinoscope: Emmetropia, myopia of < 1 D, hypermetropia.
2. Movement of red reflex opposite to the movement of the retinoscope—myopia > 1 D.
3. No movement of red reflex: Myopia of 1 D.

The refractive error is estimated by neutralizing the movement of red reflex in both the vertical and horizontal meridian:

1. Red reflex, when moving opposite to the movement of the retinoscope is neutralized by concave lens (image moves with the movement in case of concave lens).
2. Red reflex, when moving with the movement of the retinoscope is neutralized by convex lens (image moves against the movement in case of convex lens).

In case of myopia or hypermetropia, the red reflex comes to neutralization in both the meridian by a single lens either concave or convex. In case of refractive errors associated with astigmatism, the neutralization of red reflex requires two different lenses of different refractive powers.

Postmydriatic test

When retinoscopy is done under mydriatics and cycloplegics, postmydriatic test (PMT) is done to check for the subjective acceptance of the objective refraction values, once the action of the mydriatic and cycloplegic drugs has completely disappeared. The PMT is done after 3 weeks in cases where atropine is used, after 3 days for homatropine, 1 day for cyclopentolate and after 4–6 hours where phenylephrine or tropicamide is used.

The refractive error is estimated by subtracting the deductions for the cycloplegic use and for the distance from the retinoscopy readings.

Deductions for mydriatics and cycloplegics: Atropine 1 D, homatropine 0.5 D, cyclopentolate 0.75 D, phenylephrine nil and tropicamide nil.

Deductions for distance: 1 for 1 m distance and 1.5 for 2/3 m.

The final values obtained after the deductions are checked for subjective acceptance before prescribing the glasses. Few examples are given below:

1. Calculate the refractive power in a patient with the retinoscopic readings of +2 in both the axes with retinoscopy done from 1 m distance using atropine as cycloplegic agent.

Ans: The refractive power is obtained by,

Refractive power = +2–1–1 = 0

where,

+2 : Retinoscopic reading
1 : Deduction for distance
1 : Deduction for cycloplegic

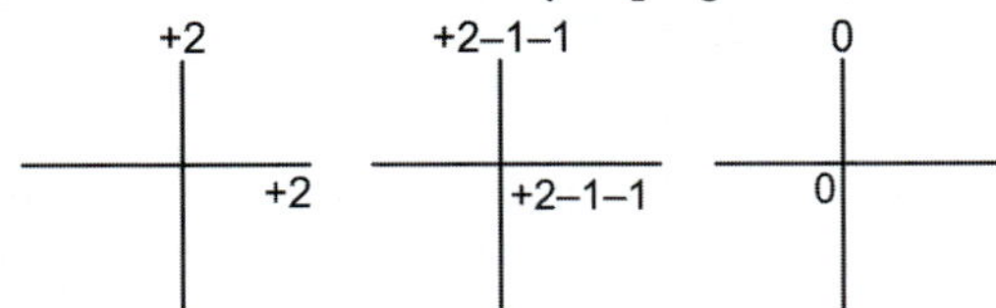

The refractive power correction required is 0 D, patient is emmetropic.

2. Calculate the refractive power in a patient with the retinoscopic readings of -2 in both the axes with retinoscopy done from 1 m distance using atropine as cycloplegic agent.

Ans: The refractive power is obtained by,

Refractive power = -2–1–1 = –4

where,

–2 : Retinoscopic reading
1 : Deduction for distance
1 : Deduction for cycloplegic

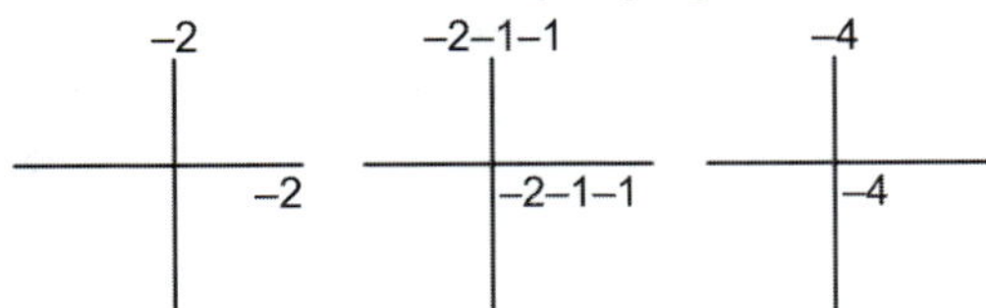

The refractive power correction required is –4 D, patient is myopic.

3. Calculate the refractive power in a patient with the retinoscopic readings of +3 in vertical axis and +4 in horizontal axis, both the axes with retinoscopy done from 1 m distance using atropine as cycloplegic agent.

Ans: The refractive power is calculated in axis separately.

Refractive power in vertical axis
= +3–1–1 = +1

Refractive power in horizontal axis
= +4–1–1 = +2

+3
+4
+3–1–1
+4–1–1
+1
+2

The refractive power correction required is +1 D in vertical axis and +2 D in horizontal axis. The correction is given as a combination of spherical and cylindrical lens. +1 D sphere and +1 D cylindrical at 90°. Cylindrical lens is always given at 90° from the desired axis as cylindrical lens acts at 90° to its axis. In the example described here, +1 D more power is required in horizontal axis, hence it is given in vertical axis at 90°.

Retinoscope

Retinoscope is an instrument used to do retinoscopy. There are two types of retinoscopes:

1. Mirror retinoscope, which reflects light into the eye. Priestley-Smith retinoscope is an example for mirror retinoscope.
2. Self-illuminated retinoscope consisting of source of light in the instrument itself.

Automated Refractometry (Fig. 4.2.1)

Automated refractometry is done by computerized autorefractometer. It is the most popular method of objective refraction. It is used as an alternative to the retinoscopy as it is less time consuming and provides the refractive power readings rapidly.

Keratometer

Keratometer is an instrument, which measures the curvature of the cornea. It is used for measurement of corneal astigmatism.

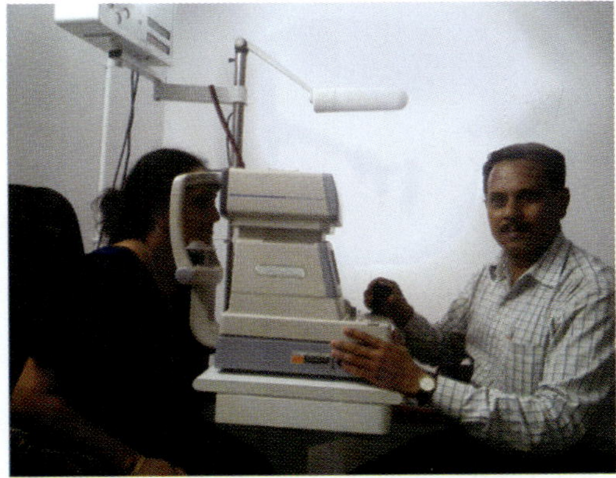

FIG. 4.2.1: Automated refractometry

TECHNIQUES OF SUBJECTIVE REFRACTION

Subjective refraction is done after objective refraction to find out the refractive power of the lenses to be prescribed depending on the subjective acceptance.

Subjective refraction is done in all patients, who can cooperate for subjective refraction by telling through which lenses they are subjectively better. Hence, subjective refraction cannot be done in children below the age of 1 year and mentally retarded patients. In them, the glasses are given based on the objective refraction findings.

Trial and Error Method

Trial and error method is the most common method of subjective refraction. In this method, each eye is tested separately after occluding the other eye by placing the weakest concave lens in case of myopia and strongest convex lens in case of hypermetropia. The power of the lens is increased or decreased depending on the subjective response from the patient. In case of cylindrical lenses, both power and axis are varied, and the best lens is chosen from the subjective response. The similar trial and error method is repeated in the other eye.

After subjective refraction, subjective verification of the refractive power is done. The spherical power is verified by duochrome test or FRIEND test. The cylindrical power is verified by Jacksons cross cylinder or astigmatic fan test.

Correction for near vision, if required is done and added to the distant correction. Finally, the refractive power is prescribed for correction of the refractive error either in the form of spectacles or contact lenses.

GIST BOX 4.2

- Refraction in eye is defined as a process by which the light rays are focused onto the light sensitive layer of the retina.
- Objective refraction is done without active participation of the patient. The various techniques of objective refraction are retinoscopy, automated refractometry and keratometry.
- Subjective refraction is done by participation of the subject or the patient. Trial and error method is the most common type of subjective refraction.

CHAPTER

4.3 Refractive Errors

Eye works as a convex lens focusing the rays of light, which enter the eye into a single point called focal point. The distance between the focal point to the center of the lens is called focal length. The ability of the eye to change its focal length depending on the distance of the object from the eye in order to focus the objects makes the eye a unique optical system. This ability of the eye to adjust or vary the refractive power is because of accommodation.

EMMETROPIA*

The word emmetropia is derived from Greek word emmetros means well-proportioned indicating that refractive power and axial length of the eye are in proportion, so that parallel rays of light coming from more than 6 m or infinity are focused on the retina with lens being in a relaxed state or without exerting accommodation.

Definition

Emmetropia is a state of normal refraction of the eye in which parallel rays of light coming from more than 6 m or infinity are focused on the retina with lens being in a relaxed state or without exerting accommodation (Fig. 4.3.1).

AMETROPIA*

Ametropia is a state of abnormal refraction of eye, in which parallel rays of light coming from more than 6 m or infinity are focused either in front or behind of retina with lens being in a relaxed state or without exerting accommodation.

Ametropia or refractive error affects millions of people in worldwide and it is the most common cause for which people visit ophthalmologist or eye clinic.

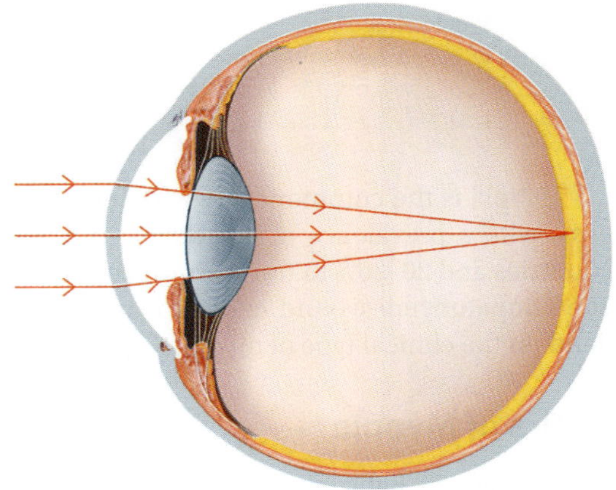

FIG. 4.3.1: Emmetropia

Ametropia includes:
- Myopia
- Hypermetropia
- Astigmatism.

At birth, the eyes show ametropia, with full-term babies showing hypermetropia. The hypermetropia is in the range from +2 to +3 diopters. The preterm babies show myopia. Emmetropia is achieved by 6–7 years of age.

The interesting fact is that the hypermetropia will come back as the age advances because of sclerosis of lens, thus making it in the normal course of hypermetropia at both extremes of ages.

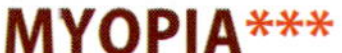

MYOPIA***

Definition

Myopia is a type of anisometropia in which parallel rays of light coming from more than 6 m or infinity are focused in front of the retina with lens being in a relaxed state or without exerting accommodation (Fig. 4.3.2).

The word myopia is derived from Greek words 'myein' and 'ops', which means 'to shut or squeeze the eyes', because of the fact that myopic individuals see by squeezing the eyes, as this improves the vision because of pinhole effect.

Myopia is called nearsightedness or shortsightedness, as myopics will be able to see only near objects clearly and distant objects are blurred.

Myopia is the commonest type of refractive error with a prevalence of up to 80% in Asian countries and 20–30% in the Western countries. The etiopathogenesis and clinical features depend on the clinical type of myopia.

Optics of Myopia

Parallel rays of light coming from infinity are focused in front of the retina with accommodation at rest.

Optical treatment of myopia is by prescription of concave lens to diverge the rays and to make them fall on the retina.

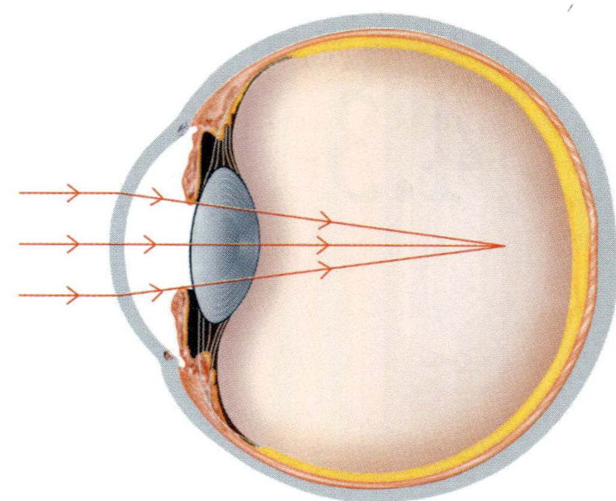

FIG. 4.3.2: Myopia

Divergent rays of light coming from near are focused on the retina without the effort of accommodation; hence, near vision is good. Since accommodation is not required for near vision in myopics, it may lead to convergence insufficiency.

Classification of Myopia

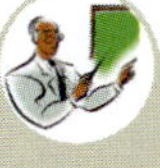

Depending on the amount of myopia, it is classified into:
- Low myopia: Myopia of less than –3.0 D
- Medium myopia: Myopia of –3.0 to –6.0 D.
- High myopia: Myopia of more than –6.0 D.

By convention, myopia of more than –6.0 D is called pathological myopia.

Clinically, myopia is classified into:
- Congenital myopia
- Simple myopia
- Pathological myopia
- Nocturnal myopia
- Pseudomyopia
- Induced myopia.

Congenital Myopia

Congenital myopia is a clinical type of myopia seen since birth. Myopia is seen more commonly in preterm babies. It can be unilateral or bilateral condition and may be associated with other congenital anomalies such as megalocornea. The refractive error is up to –10 D. It presents similar to pathological myopia with enlarged or elongated eyeball at birth and all the fundus features except that progression is absent or rare. Unilateral cases of congenital myopia may lead to amblyopia.

Simple Myopia or Developmental Myopia

Simple myopia is the most common clinical variety of myopia seen in children and in adults.

Etiopathogenesis

Etiopathogenesis is because of physiological error in the growth of the eyeball caused by one of the mechanisms mentioned below:

- Increase in the axial length of the eyeball leading to axial myopia
- Increase in the curvature of the cornea and or lens leading to curvature myopia.

> Normally, the axial length and power of the eyeball are inversely and proportionately related to each other.
>
> An increase in the axial length without proportionate increase in the refractive power of the eye or increase in the refractive power of the eye without proportionate increase in the axial length of the eye causes simple myopia.

More close work, e.g. reading, watching television (TV) from near and excessive use of computers, in childhood has been implicated as a cause for myopia. The explanation put forth is excessive near work leading to near point stress affecting the extraocular and intrinsic muscles of the eye altering the shape of the eye causing myopia. However, this theory fails to explain the occurrence of myopia in illiterates.

> Myopics have problem in seeing far objects, which make it uncomfortable for them to participate in outdoor games or activities; hence, myopics will involve more in reading, watching computer or TV. The advantage is myopic children sit in the front benches in school and has a look of being studious.

Clinical course

1. Simple myopia usually presents in children called childhood myopia, presenting at the age of 5–10 years. It usually progresses with increase in the refractive error progressing at the rate from –0.5 D to –1.0 D per year. The progression usually stops by teenage and the refractive error usually will not exceed –5.0 D.
2. Simple myopia can present in the adults in the age group of 20–40 years and late adult onset simple myopia presenting in the age group of more than 40 years. The adult onset and late adult onset simple myopia usually progresses at a slower rate and progression stop by fifth decade.

Symptoms

- Diminution of vision for distance of varying degrees depending on the amount of refractive error
- Asthenopic symptoms such as eye strain, headache seen in cases of mild refractive error.

Signs

Examination usually shows normal eye; large prominent eye is seen in cases associated with increased axial length of the eyeball. Retinoscopy shows myopic refraction and the refractive error usually will not exceed –6.0 D. Fundus examination shows normal retina; degenerative retinal changes commonly seen in pathological myopia are usually absent.

Diagnosis

Diagnosis is made by clinical features and by retinoscopy findings.

Treatment

1. Optical treatment of myopia: It is done by appropriate concave lenses to diverge the rays of light and to make them fall on the retina to form the image. Concave lenses can be prescribed in the form of spectacles and contact lenses (Fig. 4.3.3).
2. Surgical treatment of myopia: It is done by refractive surgeries. Laser-assisted in situ keratomileusis (LASIK), photorefractive keratectomy, phakic intraocular lens (IOL) implantation and radial keratotomy are the commonly performed refractive surgeries to correct myopia.

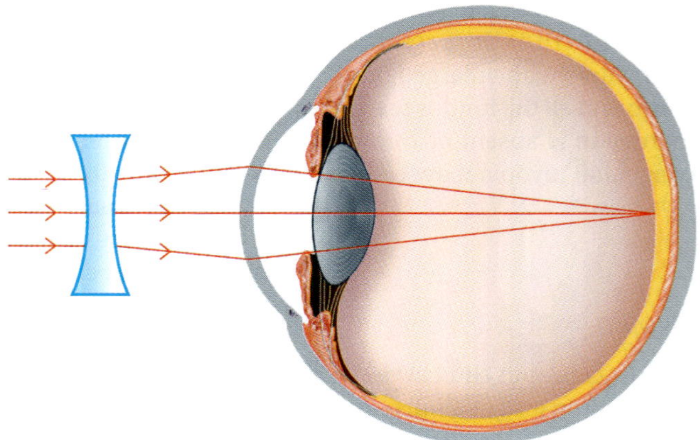

FIG. 4.3.3: Optical treatment of myopia by concave lens

Refractive surgeries for myopia are:*

- Radial keratotomy
- Photorefractive keratectomy
- LASIK
- Laser-assisted subepithelial keratectomy (LASEK)
- Epi-LASIK
- Customized LASIK
- IntraLase LASIK
- Phakic IOL
- Intrastromal corneal ring segments.

Pathological or Degenerative Myopia

Pathological myopia is a clinical type of myopia characterized by degenerative changes because of rapid increase in the axial length of the eyeball. Pathological myopia is usually more than –6.0 D with axial length of more than 25 mm.**

Etiopathogenesis

Etiopathogenesis is characterized by manifestation in early childhood by 5 years of age and increasing rapidly reaching –15 to –30 D by 25 years of age. Hereditary factors play an important role in the pathogenesis of the disease. The pathogenesis of development of pathological myopia is explained by following two theories:

1. Mechanical theory: This theory states that distension of sclera or weakening of sclera caused by prolonged elevated intraocular pressure, sustained accommodation and increased close work causes myopia by increasing the axial length.
2. Biological theory: This theory states that hereditary and growth factors play an important role in the development of myopia. Normally, two thirds of the growth in the length of the eyeball is achieved by 4 years of age; afterwards, it shows slow growth. If the growth of the eyeball continues rapidly, it leads to pathological myopia.

Pathological myopia is seen in association with systemic conditions such as Marfan's syndrome, Stickler's syndrome, Down syndrome, gyrate atrophy, albinism, etc.

Pathology

The pathological changes in pathological myopia are because of increased axial length of the eyeball as a result of hereditary and growth factors leading to degeneration of the choroid, retina and vitreous. The elongation of the eyeball is more pronounced in the posterior part of the eyeball predominantly involving the structures behind the lens.

The retina shows tessellated appearance because of atrophy of the retinal pigment epithelium and exposure of the underlying large choroidal vessels. The atrophy of the retinal pigment epithelium and choroid results in visibility of underlying white sclera visible around the optic disk called myopic crescent.

Pathological myopia is one of the leading causes of legal blindness across the world. Pathological myopia accounts for up to 30% of all cases of myopia. The causes for loss of vision are choroidal neovascularization membrane, macular degeneration and retinal detachment.

Clinical features

Symptoms

- Gross diminution of vision for distance depending on the severity of refractive error
- Floaters because of associated vitreous liquefaction and degeneration
- Delayed dark adaptation or night blindness because of chorioretinal degeneration.

Signs

- Eyeball appears prominent resembling proptosis called pseudoproptosis
- Large cornea, deep anterior chamber and sluggishly reacting large pupil
- Retinoscopy shows myopic refractive error of more than –6 D.

Examination of fundus (Fig. 4.3.4, Figs 4.3.5A to D)*

1. Optic disk: It is appears large with large physiological cup, temporal crescent or annular crescent and may show tilted appearance.
2. Macula: It shows Förster-Fuchs spot because of accumulation of pigment associated with subretinal neovascularization and choroidal hemorrhage. Myopic foveoschisis and macular hole are the other pathologies seen in the macula.
3. Background: The retina shows tessellated appearance and patches of choroidal atrophy.
4. Periphery of the retina: Cystoid degeneration, lattice degeneration and other retinal degenerations are seen commonly in the periphery of the retina.
5. Vitreous: It shows degenerations such as vitreous liquefaction, muscae volitantes or vitreous opacities and posterior vitreous detachment.
6. Choroid: It shows lacquer cracks indicating breaks in the Bruch's membrane with choroidal atrophy.
7. Sclera: Scleral thinning in the posterior part of the eyeball with ectasia of sclera in the posterior pole resulting in posterior staphyloma.

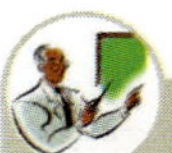

Pathological Myopia and Retinal Detachment

Pathological myopia is associated with high incidence of retinal detachment because of increased incidence of peripheral retinal degenerations, e.g. lattice degeneration, predisposing to the development of retinal tear or retinal hole. Hence, all individuals with pathological myopia should undergo indirect ophthalmoscopy with scleral indentation for examination of the periphery of the retina to look for lattice degeneration, when present should be preferably treated by prophylactic laser photocoagulation.

Treatment

Optical treatment is similar to simple myopia by concave lenses in the form of spectacles or contact lenses and refractive surgeries.

High concave lenses required for correction of pathological myopia are associated with complications such as minification of the image, spherical aberration leading to image distortion and reduced peripheral field of vision. Hence, contact lenses, which cause less image minification and less spherical aberration are better alternative to spectacles in cases with high pathological myopia.

The optical treatment will not prevent the complications associated with the pathological myopia, which are because of elongation of the eyeball. The treatment to prevent the elongation of the eyeball is not yet well-developed; however, many options have been tried, but have not yielded good results. The treatment options are:

- Scleral reinforcement surgery by using grafts to prevent elongation of sclera and scleral thinning
- Reducing the intraocular pressure by using antiglaucoma medications
- Relaxing the accommodation by using anticholinergic drugs such as atropine and homatropine as topical eyedrops, and bifocal glasses

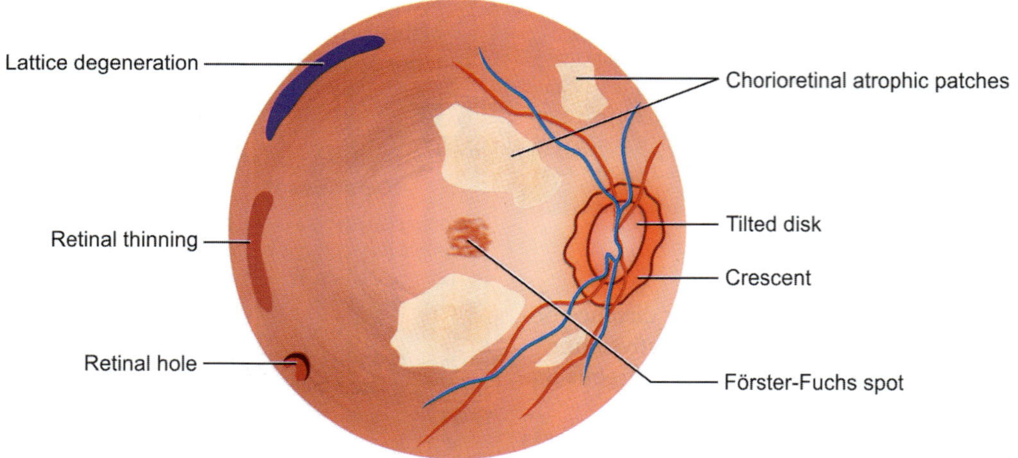

FIG. 4.3.4: Fundus picture of pathological myopia

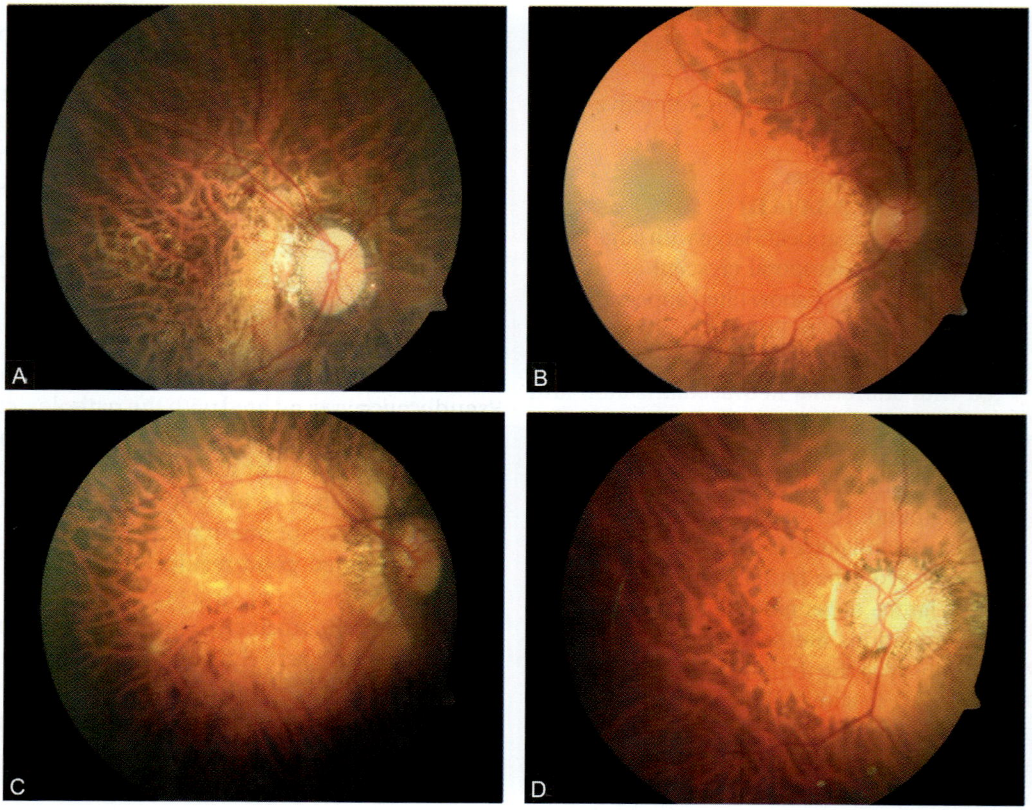

FIGS 4.3.5A to D: Fundus photographs showing changes in the retina such as tilted disk, annular crescent, temporal crescent, tessellated background, subretinal neovascularization, macular hemorrhage, etc.

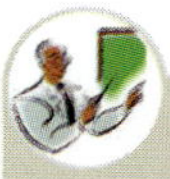

Förster-Fuchs Spot

Definition

Hyperplasia of retinal pigment epithelium associated with subretinal neovascularization and choroidal hemorrhage in the macula giving rise to the appearance of dark spot called Förster-Fuchs spot. It is named after Forster and Ernst Fuch who identified the lesion.

Clinical features

It is the common cause for loss of vision in pathological myopia. It presents as impairment of central vision in the form of metamorphopsia and impairment of color vision.

Treatment

The diagnosis is made by fundus fluorescein angiography. The treatment depends on the location of choroidal neovascularization. Treatment is by laser photocoagulation for extrafoveal lesions. Subfoveal lesions are treated by photodynamic therapy or by surgical removal of neovascularization.

Visual prognosis

The visual prognosis is usually poor in subfoveal lesions and central vision is affected because of development of macular hole or retinal detachment. Recent modalities of treatment with antivascular endothelial growth factor agents (e.g. intravitreal bevacizumab) has yielded better results compared to other modalities of treatment.

- Vitamin and nutrient supplements to improve the nutritional status.

Complications of pathological myopia*

- Retinal detachment
- Choroidal neovascularization membrane
- Posterior staphyloma
- Myopic foveoschisis and macular hole
- Ocular diseases such as posterior subcapsular cataract and open-angle glaucoma are more frequently associated with pathological myopia.

Pathological myopia is associated with increased incidence of sight-threatening retinal complications; they should be screened on a regular basis for these complications and should be educated about the symptoms of these complications.

Prevention

Since there is no effective treatment for pathological myopia, genetic counseling is necessary for the parents with pathological myopia as their child is most likely to develop pathological myopia. Children of parents with pathological myopia should be screened to detect pathological myopia and appropriate treatment to prevent development of amblyopia.

Nocturnal Myopia

Nocturnal myopia is a condition characterized by presence of nearsightedness in night or dim illumination. It is seen in people with uncorrected or undercorrected myopia. Because of increase in accommodation with decreased accommodation cues in darkness, myopia becomes more apparent in darkness.

Pseudomyopia

Pseudomyopia is a condition of artificial myopia produced by excessive accommodation or accommodative spasm. It is seen in young individuals performing excessive near work.

Pseudomyopia is treated by cycloplegic agents such as atropine, homatropine or cyclopentolate to relieve accommodative spasm.

Induced Myopia

Induced myopia is a condition of acquired myopia induced by drugs such as steroids, pilocarpine, acetylcholine, neostigmine, etc. This type of myopia is usually reversible and resolves after stopping the causative agent.

HYPERMETROPIA**

Definition

Hypermetropia/Hyperopia is a type of anisometropia in which parallel rays of light coming from more than 6 m or infinity are focused behind the retina with lens being in a relaxed state or without exerting accommodation (Fig. 4.3.6).

The word hypermetropia derived from three words 'hyper'—excess, 'met'—measuring, 'opia'—eye, meaning that light rays come to focus behind the eye, i.e. refraction in excess of the length of the eye.

Hypermetropia is also called longsightedness or farsightedness. It is called so because hypermetropics will have more difficulty in seeing objects situated at near when compared to objects situated at a distance.

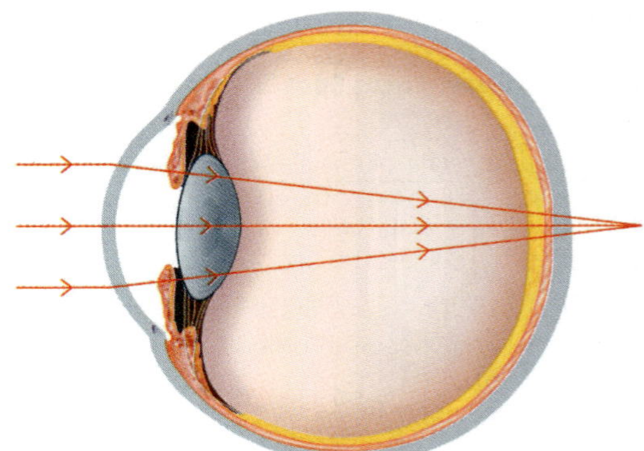

FIG. 4.3.6: Hypermetropia

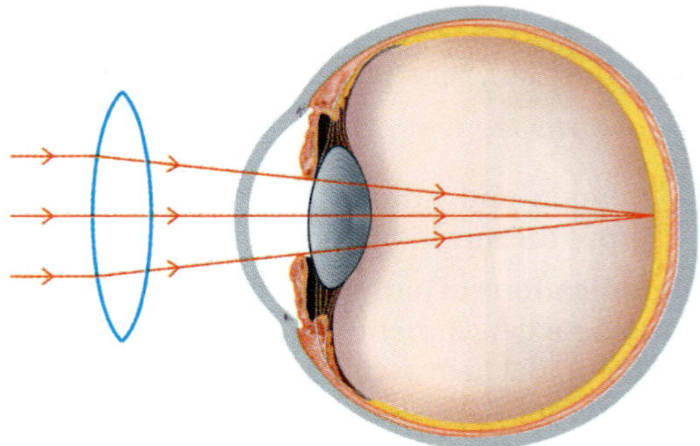

FIG. 4.3.7: Optical treatment of hypermetropia by convex lens

Optics of Hypermetropia

Parallel rays of light coming from infinity come to a focus behind the retina with accommodation at rest.

Optical treatment of hypermetropia requires prescription of convex lens to converge the rays of light onto the retina (Fig. 4.3.7).

Etiopathogenesis

1. Axial hypermetropia: Decrease in the axial length of the eyeball is the commonest cause for hypermetropia. Each millimeter of shortening in the length of the eyeball results in approximately 3 D of hypermetropia.
2. Curvature hypermetropia: Flattening of the curvature of cornea or lens or both will lead to hypermetropia. About 1 mm flattening in the curvature of cornea will result in about +6 D hypermetropia.
3. Index hypermetropia: Decrease in the refractive index of cornea or lens, or both will result in index hypermetropia.
4. Displacement or absence of lens: This type of lens following surgery or trauma will result in hypermetropia because of decrease in the total refractive power of the eye.

Accommodation plays an important role in hypermetropia. Voluntary accommodation can correct some amount of hypermetropia by increasing the curvature of the lens, thereby increasing the refractive power of the eye.

Optical Types of Hypermetropia (Fig. 4.3.8)*

Total Hypermetropia

Total hypermetropia is the amount of hypermetropia estimated after abolishing the accommodation by cycloplegic drugs. Total hypermetropia includes latent and manifest hypermetropia.

Latent hypermetropia

Latent hypermetropia is the amount of total hypermetropia, which is corrected by the tone of ciliary muscle. It is more in young children and decreases as the age advances.

Manifest hypermetropia

Manifest hypermetropia is the remaining amount of total hypermetropia, which is not corrected by the tone of ciliary muscle. It includes facultative hypermetropia and absolute hypermetropia.

Facultative hypermetropia

Facultative hypermetropia is the amount of manifest hypermetropia, which can be corrected by patient's accommodative effort over and above the normal tone of ciliary muscle.

Absolute hypermetropia

Absolute hypermetropia is the amount of manifest hypermetropia, which cannot be corrected by patient's accommodative effort.

Estimation of Hypermetropia

Total hypermetropia is calculated after using cycloplegics (e.g. atropine) to abolish the action of ciliary muscle.

Manifest hypermetropia is indicated by the power of the strongest convex lens through which hypermetropic can still have full 6/6 normal vision for distance. The strongest convex lens abolishes the accommodatory effort and gives the amount of manifest hypermetropia.

Latent hypermetropia is calculated by deducting manifest hypermetropia from total hypermetropia.

Absolute hypermetropia is indicated by the power of the weakest convex lens through which hypermetropic can have 6/6 normal vision for distance.

Facultative hypermetropia is calculated by deducting absolute hypermetropia from manifest hypermetropia.

Clinical Types of Hypermetropia

Clinically, hypermetropia is classified into three types:

- Simple hypermetropia
- Pathological hypermetropia
- Functional hypermetropia.

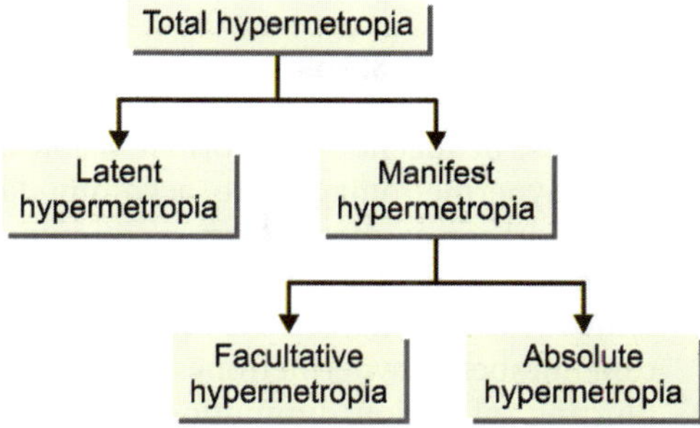

FIG. 4.3.8: Optical types of hypermetropia

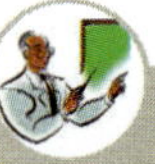

Depending on the amount of hypermetropia, it is classified into:

- Low hypermetropia: Hypermetropia of less than +2.0 D.
- Medium hypermetropia: Hypermetropia of +2.0 to +5.0 D.
- High hypermetropia: Hypermetropia of more than +5.0 D.

By convention, myopia of more than –6.0 D is called pathological hypermetropia.

Simple Hypermetropia

Simple hypermetropia is also called physiological hypermetropia occurring because of physiological errors in the growth of the eyeball. It is the commonest type of hypermetropia.

Etiopathogenesis

Etiopathogenesis is similar to simple myopia and it is because of physiological error in the growth of the eyeball caused by one of the mechanisms mentioned below.

At birth, the eyes show ametropia with full-term babies showing hypermetropia. The hypermetropia is in the range from +2 to +3 D. Emmetropia is achieved by 6–7 years of age. The infants with high hypermetropia, more than +3.5 D will remain with hypermetropia even after 7 years of age and they are more likely to develop strabismus and amblyopia:

- Decrease in the axial length of the eyeball leading to axial hypermetropia
- Decrease in the curvature of the cornea and or lens leading to curvature hypermetropia.

Clinical features

Symptoms

1. Asthenopic symptoms such as tiredness of the eyes, headache with normal vision in mild hypermetropia where accommodatory effort can correct the hypermetropia.
2. Frequent blinking, watering of the eyes, difficulty in reading, etc. are seen in significant number of hypermetropes.
3. Blurring of vision/diminution of vision more for near than for distance is seen in those in whom the accommodatory effort cannot correct the hypermetropia totally.

Signs

1. Eyeball appears small.
2. Small cornea, shallow anterior chamber.
3. Retinoscopy shows hypermetropic refractive error.
4. Apparent divergent squint because of large positive angle alpha, as the macula is situated at abnormally greater distance from the optic disk.

Examination of fundus

1. Optic disk: It appears small with ill-defined physiological cup and appearing redder in color resembling hyperemia of the optic disk as seen in papillitis, and this clinical appearance of the optic disk is called pseudopapillitis.
2. Macula: It is situated at a greater distance from the macula resulting in large positive angle alpha.
3. Blood vessels: It show undue tortuosity and abnormal branching.
4. Background: The retina gives the appearance of shot-silk retina because of presence of increased reflexes resembling shimmer of silk.

Treatment

There are two types of treatment as detailed below.

Optical treatment of hypermetropia

Optical treatment is done by appropriate convex lenses to converge the rays of light and to make them fall on the retina to form the image. Convex lenses can be prescribed in the form of spectacles and contact lenses.

Surgical treatment of hypermetropia

Surgical treatment is done by refractive surgeries:

- Hypermetropic LASIK
- Hypermetropic photorefractive keratectomy
- Automated lamellar keratoplasty

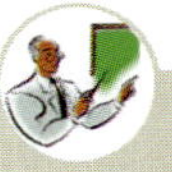

Optical Tips for Correction of Hypermetropia

Total hypermetropia should be calculated by doing retinoscopy under cycloplegia. Full cycloplegic correction for hypermetropia is given in children and in presence of accommodative squint. As the hypermetropia decreases with increasing age in children, regular follow-up once in 6 months is required to look for change in the correction. Hypermetropia in adults is treated by giving correction for manifest hypermetropia.

- Laser thermal keratoplasty
- Implantable contact lens or IOL implantation for hypermetropia caused by absence of lens or aphakia.

Complications

1. Primary angle-closure glaucoma is common in hypermetropic eyes as these eyes are smaller with shorter axial length and shallow anterior chamber.
2. Accommodative esotropia and amblyopia, especially in children.

Pathological Hypermetropia

Pathological hypermetropia is because of congenital or acquired diseases of the eye excluding the physiological errors in the growth of the eyeball.

Etiopathogenesis

Etiopathogenesis has got genetic and hereditary inheritance pattern as seen with pathological myopia. It is seen in a variety of conditions such as:

- Anomalies of the eyeball, e.g. microphthalmos and nanophthalmos
- Anomalies involving the anterior segment of the eye, e.g. cornea plana, sclerocornea, etc.
- Inherited ocular and systemic diseases, e.g. aniridia, Leber's congenital amaurosis, ocular albinism, Down syndrome, etc.

- Acquired diseases of the posterior segment, which displace the retina anteriorly, e.g. choroidal tumors, central serous retinopathy, orbital tumors, etc.

Clinical features

In addition to the clinical features seen in simple hypermetropia, other features because of the congenital or acquired ocular diseases are seen.

Treatment

Optical treatment of pathological hypermetropia is similar to that of simple hypermetropia. Along with the optical treatment, treatment of the underlying condition is required.

Visual prognosis is poor in cases of pathological hypermetropia associated with ocular anomalies.

Pathological Hypermetropia vs Pathological Myopia

Similarities

Both have got genetic and hereditary influence and both are associated with ocular and systemic diseases.

Dissimilarities

Pathological hypermetropia is relatively rare, when compared to pathological myopia. Pathological myopia by itself leads to chorioretinal degenerations causing significant loss of vision, whereas posterior segment complications seen with pathological myopia are not seen with pathological hypermetropia.

Functional Hypermetropia

Functional hypermetropia is because of paralysis of accommodation and seen in cases of internal ophthalmoplegia. It presents with symptoms similar to simple hypermetropia and treatment is by treatment of the underlying condition.

ASTIGMATISM**

Definition

Astigmatism is a type of anisometropia in which the refraction varies in the different meridian resulting in inability of the light rays to come to a point focus, but form focal lines (Fig. 4.3.9).

The word astigmatism is derived from Greek words alpha-a, meaning without and stigma, meaning point, a+ stigma meaning without point focus.

Etiopathogenesis

Astigmatism is almost present in all the eyes in mild form, which may be clinically insignificant. Clinically significant astigmatism is present in 50% of these eyes.

Astigmatism is because of different refractive powers in different meridians resulting in inability of the eye to converge the rays of light to form a point image. Based on the changes

Differences between Myopia and Hypermetropia (Table 4.3.1)

TABLE 4.3.1: Differences between myopia and hypermetropia

Myopia	*Hypermetropia*
Myopia is a type of anisometropia in which parallel rays of light coming from more than 6 m or infinity are focused in front of the retina with lens being in a relaxed state or without exerting accommodation	Hypermetropia is a type of anisometropia in which parallel rays of light coming from more than 6 m or infinity are focused behind the retina with lens being in a relaxed state or without exerting accommodation
Eyeball is of larger dimensions including larger cornea, increased axial length, larger optic disk, etc.	Eyeball is of smaller dimensions including smaller cornea, decreased axial length, smaller optic disk, etc.
Retina shows tessellated appearance and complications of the posterior segment such as retinal detachment, choroidal neovascularization, posterior staphyloma, etc.	Retina shows shot-silky appearance with optic disk showing the appearance of pseudopapillitis

Contd...

Contd...

Myopia	*Hypermetropia*
Angle alpha is negative resulting in apparent convergent squint	Angle alpha is positive resulting in apparent divergent squint
Accommodation does not seem to play an important role; in fact myopics have poor accommodation	Accommodation plays an important role in the pathogenesis of hypermetropia; hence, retinoscopy has to be evaluated by cycloplegics refraction to find out the various optical components of hypermetropia
Optical treatment is by concave lens	Optical treatment is by convex lens
Myopia predisposes to development of primary open-angle glaucoma	Hypermetropia predisposes to development of primary angle-closure glaucoma

in the refractive powers in different meridians, astigmatism is classified into:

- Regular astigmatism
- Irregular astigmatism.

Regular Astigmatism

Regular astigmatism is a type of astigmatism characterized by the presence of two principal meridians in which the refractive power changes regularly in these two principal meridians:

1. Curvature astigmatism is caused by abnormalities, involving the:
    a. Curvature of the cornea as in corneal thinning disorders such as keratoconus, cornea plana, distortion of the cornea as in encroachment of cornea by pterygium following surgeries of cornea (e.g. keratoplasty, refractive surgeries, postcataract surgery), pressure over the cornea by mass lesions of the eyelids, etc.
    b. Curvature of the lens as in lenticonus.
2. Positional astigmatism is caused by abnormalities, involving the:
    a. Position of the lens as in subluxation of the lens.
    b. Position of the macula of retina as in displacement of macula.
3. Index astigmatism is caused by abnormalities involving the refractive index of lens as in nuclear cataract.

The causes for regular astigmatism are because of abnormalities in the curvature, position and refractive index affecting the cornea, lens and retina resulting in different refractive power in the two meridians. Depending on the angle between the two principal meridians, regular astigmatism is subclassified as detailed below.

With-the-rule astigmatism

With-the-rule (WTR) astigmatism is a type of regular astigmatism characterized by presence of two principal meridians perpendicular to each other with vertical meridian being more curved than the horizontal meridian.

It is called with-the-rule astigmatism, as normally, vertical meridian is more curved than the horizontal meridian because of the pressure of the eyelids over the cornea.

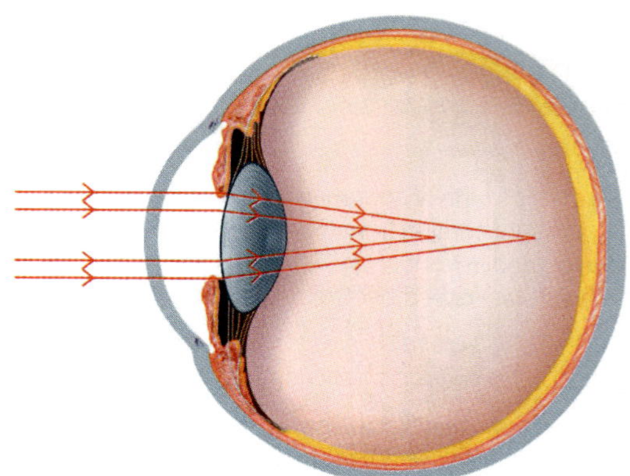

FIG. 4.3.9: Astigmatism (*Note:* Formation of focal lines)

Against-the-rule astigmatism

Against-the-rule astigmatism is a type of regular astigmatism characterized by presence of two principal meridians perpendicular to each other with horizontal meridian being more curved than the vertical meridian.

By convention, the two principal meridians in WTR astigmatism and against-the-rule astigmatism lie within 20° from 90° or 180°. If the two principal meridians lie more than 30° away from 90° or 180°, it is called oblique astigmatism. With-the-rule astigmatism is found in majority of the eyes.

Oblique astigmatism

Oblique astigmatism is a type of regular astigmatism characterized by presence of two principal meridians perpendicular to each other with horizontal meridian being found more than 30° away from 90° or 180°.

Bioblique astigmatism

Bioblique astigmatism is a type of regular astigmatism characterized by presence of two principal meridians and the principal meridians are not perpendicular to each other, but lie obliquely.

Irregular Astigmatism

Irregular astigmatism is a type of astigmatism characterized by the presence of multiple meridians with refractive power changing irregularly in these multiple meridians.

Irregular astigmatism results from abnormalities such as corneal scars following corneal tear repair, subluxation of the lens, scars involving the macula of the retina, etc.

Irregular astigmatism leads to severe visual impairment and treatment is difficult compared to regular astigmatism.

Cylindrical lenses prescribed in the form of spectacles are not effective for visual correction. Toric contact lenses are a better choice of treatment. Patients with high irregular astigmatism require refractive surgeries.

Clinical Types

Based on the formation of the two focal lines from two principal meridians to the retina regular with accommodation being relaxed, astigmatism can be of the following.

Simple myopic astigmatism: One focal line is formed in front of the retina and other focal line is formed on the retina.

Simple hypermetropic astigmatism: One focal line is formed behind the retina and other focal line is formed on the retina.

Compound myopic astigmatism: Both focal lines are formed in front of the retina.

Compound hypermetropic astigmatism: Both focal lines are formed behind the retina.

Mixed astigmatism: One focal line is formed in front of the retina and other focal line is formed behind the retina.

Clinical Features

- Distortion of vision or blurring of vision
- Asthenopic symptoms such as headache, tiredness of eyes, etc.
- Squeezing of eyes in order to get clear image of the object by avoiding distortion of the image, as squeezing of the eyes provides a stenopaic slit effect.

The image formation in patients with astigmatism is distorted with circular objects appearing elongated in any of the meridian depending on the type of astigmatism.

Diagnosis

The diagnosis of astigmatism is done by assessment of vision and visual acuity decreased because of astigmatism increases on viewing through a stenopaic slit. Retinoscopy differentiates the axis and different clinical types of astigmatism.

The other methods of diagnosis of astigmatism are by automated refractometer, keratometer and corneal topography.

Treatment

1. Optical treatment: It is done by using cylindrical lenses either concave or convex depending on the clinical type of astigmatism. Cylindrical lenses are prescribed in the form of spectacles or contact lenses.
2. Surgical treatment: It is done by surgeries such as astigmatic keratotomy, astigmatic LASIK, photoastigmatic keratotomy.

Refractive surgeries for astigmatism are:

- Astigmatic keratotomy
- Photorefractive keratectomy
- LASIK
- LASEK
- Epi-LASIK
- Customized LASIK
- IntraLase LASIK.

ANISOMETROPIA**

Definition

Anisometropia is a state of refractive condition in which the refraction of the two eyes is unequal. The word anisometropia is derived from Greek words meaning not same measurements of the two eyes.

Etiology

Anisometropia is caused by:

- Congenital causes, e.g. hereditary inheritance leading to differential growth of the eyeball
- Acquired causes, e.g. refractive errors secondary to diseases such as corneal opacity, cataract affecting one eye, or refractive errors induced by surgical trauma or mechanical trauma.

Types

Simple Anisometropia

Simple anisometropia can be simple myopic anisometropia, simple hypermetropic anisometropia, simple myopic astigmatism anisometropia and simple hypermetropic astigmatism anisometropia. In all these conditions, one eye is emmetropic and other eye is ametropic in the form of myopia, hypermetropia, myopic astigmatism and hypermetropic astigmatism respectively.

Compound Anisometropia

Compound anisometropia can be compound myopic anisometropia, compound hypermetropic anisometropia, compound myopic astigmatism anisometropia and compound hypermetropic astigmatism anisometropia.

Mixed Anisometropia

Mixed anisometropia is seen in conditions when each eye has got different types of ammetropia such as myopia, hypermetropia and so many.

Clinical Features

1. Asthenopic symptoms such as headache and tiredness of eyes because of difficulties in binocular single vision.
2. Amblyopia is seen in higher degrees of anisometropia particularly in children because of suppression of the eye with higher refractive error.
3. Alternate vision is seen in case of anisometropia with one eye being myopic, which is used for near vision and the other eye being hypermetropic or emmetropic, which is used for distance vision.

A difference of 0.25 diopter of refractive error between the two eyes results in development of 0.5% difference in the size of the retinal images. A difference of up to 2.5 D of refractive error between the two eyes or 5% difference in the size of the retinal images between the two eyes is well-tolerated. Binocular vision is present in cases of mild anisometropia and binocular vision is not possible in high degrees of anisometropia. In higher degrees of anisometropia, alternate vision or uniocular vision/amblyopia is seen.

4. Strabismus, the eye with higher refractive error develops esotropia more commonly in children and exotropia commonly in adults.
5. Diplopia is seen because of unequal size of retinal images.

Diagnosis

Diagnosis is made by retinoscopy. The state of binocular vision is assessed by Worth's 4-dot test or FRIEND test.

Treatment

Treatment is made by:

1. Spectacles: The main drawback with spectacles is prevention of fusion and development of binocular vision because of differences in the retinal image size in higher degrees of anisometropia.
2. Contact lenses: It offer better alternative as these cause less image magnification compared to spectacles.
3. Surgical treatment: It is done by refractive surgeries depending on the cause and type of refractive error.

The main problem in anisometropia in children is failure of development of binocular vision and risk of development of amblyopia. The main aspect of treatment of anisometropia is to correct anisometropia and prevent development of amblyopia.

ANISEIKONIA

Definition

Aniseikonia is a condition characterized by difference in the size of the images perceived by two eyes. The word aniseikonia is derived from Greek word meaning unequal images.

Etiopathogenesis

Aniseikonia can be produced by differences between the two eyes in the refractive apparatus or in the distribution of photoreceptors in the retina or in the cortical magnification in the visual cortex:

1. Difference in the refractive status of each eye as in different types of anisometropia.
2. Unequal distribution of the retinal elements as in retinal scar, retinal edema, epiretinal membrane, retinal folds, macular hole, etc.
3. Unequal cortical representation of the ocular images in two eyes as cortical magnification seen in dominant eye in patients with amblyopia.

Anisometropia is the commonest cause of aniseikonia. Some amount of anisometropia is almost always present and anisometropia of more than 2.5 D, which leads to an image difference of more than 5% will lead to symptoms.

Aphakia was one of the commonest causes for aniseikonia in the past as the incidence of surgical aphakia has decreased now. Aphakic glasses produce a magnification of about 30% of the image size, thereby causing significant aniseikonia in patients with unilateral aphakia.

Clinical Features

- Asthenopic symptoms such as headache, tiredness of eyes, etc.
- Diplopia
- Dizziness, nausea and vertigo
- Difficulties in depth perception.

Treatment

Aniseikonia can be measured by various methods such as space eikonometer, aniseikonia inspector, etc.

Aniseikonic glasses can be given for mild to moderate cases of aniseikonia. Aniseikonic lenses are based on the principle that magnification produced by a lens can be altered by altering the vertex distance, central thickness and the curvature of the lens. In aniseikonic glasses, magnification is adjusted between the two eyes by altering the vertex distance, central thickness and the curvature of the lens to reduce aniseikonia within the tolerable range.

Aniseikonia because of moderate to high anisometropia is corrected by contact lenses or by refractive surgeries; aniseikonia caused by retinal pathologies is treated by treatment of the underlying cause and aniseikonia because of amblyopia and magnification of the image in the cortex is managed by treatment of amblyopia.

Though aniseikonia is a more significant optical problem than anisometropia, it is less often considered, while examining the patient presenting with asthenopic symptoms. The popularity of different kinds of refractive surgeries and corneal surgeries (e.g. keratoplasty) has made increase in the incidence of anisometropia and hence increased incidence of aniseikonia. Though the evaluation and treatment of aniseikonia is difficult, the availability of high-index lenses and aspherical lenses have made optical correction possible for moderate to high aniseikonia.

GIST BOX 4.3

- Emmetropia is a state of normal refraction of the eye in which parallel rays of light coming from more than 6 m or infinity are focused on the retina with lens being in a relaxed state or without exerting accommodation.
- Ammetropia is a state of abnormal refraction of the eye in which parallel rays of light coming from more than 6 m or infinity are focused either in front or behind the retina with lens being in a relaxed state or without exerting accommodation.
- Ammetropia or refractive error affects millions of people worldwide and it is the most common cause for which people visit ophthalmologist or eye clinic.
- Myopia is a type of anisometropia in which parallel rays of light coming from more than 6 m or infinity are focused in front of the retina with lens being in a relaxed state or without exerting accommodation.
- Hypermetropia/Hyperopia is a type of anisometropia in which parallel rays of light coming from more than 6 m or infinity are focused behind the retina with lens being in a relaxed state or without exerting accommodation.
- Astigmatism is a type of anisometropia in which the refraction varies in the different meridian, resulting in inability of the light rays to come to a point focus, but form focal lines.
- Anisometropia is a state of refractive condition in which the refraction of the two eyes is unequal.
- Aniseikonia is a condition characterized by difference in the size of the images perceived by two eyes.

CHAPTER

4.4 Accommodation and Anomalies of Accommodation

ACCOMMODATION

Definition

Accommodation is defined as a process by which the divergent rays coming from a near object situated within 6 m are brought to focus on the light sensitive layer of the retina by increasing the refractive power of the lens by increasing the anterior curvature of the lens. Accommodation is brought about by accommodation reflex.

Accommodation Reflex and Mechanism of Accommodation

Afferent: Optic nerve.

Center: Edinger-Westphal nucleus.

Efferent: Oculomotor nerve.

Afferent impulses from retina induced by blurring of vision for near travel along the optic nerve, optic chiasm, optic tract, lateral geniculate body, optic radiations and striate cortex to reach the parastriate cortex.

From the parastriate cortex, the impulses reach the center, Edinger-Westphal nucleus through the occipito-mesencephalic tract.

Efferent impulses arising from the Edinger-Westphal nucleus reach the ciliary muscle, resulting in contraction of ciliary muscle, which results in relaxation of the suspensory ligaments of the lens because of forward movement of the ciliary body reducing the diameter of the circle formed by the ciliary processes. The relaxation of the suspensory ligaments of the lens results in alteration in the shape of the lens, leading to increase in the anterior curvature of the lens, thereby increasing the refractive power of the lens.

Accommodation leads to:

- Contraction of ciliary muscle and relaxation of suspensory ligaments of lens
- The radius of curvature of anterior surface of lens decreases from 10 to 6 mm equaling the radius of curvature of the posterior surface of lens, which is 6 mm.

Theories of Accommodation

Helmholtz theory is the widely accepted theory for explaining the mechanism of accommodation. It states that contraction of the ciliary muscle results in relaxation of suspensory ligaments, which reduces the tension on the capsule of the lens resulting in alteration in the shape of the lens, making it more spherical.

Range and Amplitude of Accommodation

The nearest point at which an object is seen clearly with maximum accommodation is called punctum proximum or near point. The farthest point at which an object is seen clearly without exerting any accommodation is called punctum remotum or far point. The difference between the far point and near point is called range of accommodation for that eye. The difference in the refractive power of the eye between these two points is called amplitude of accommodation (Figs 4.4.1 and 4.4.2).

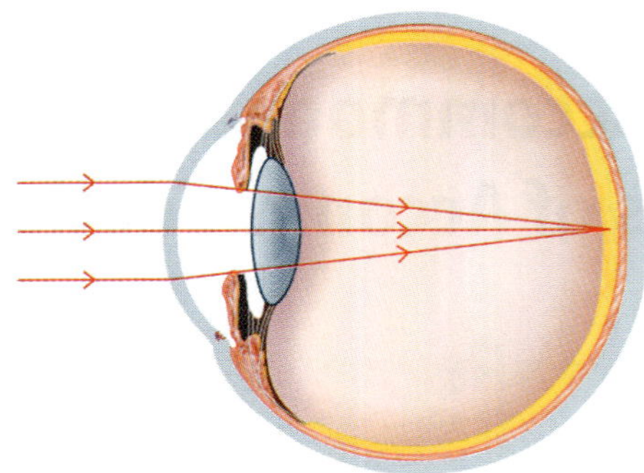

FIG. 4.4.1: Distance vision—mechanism of accommodation

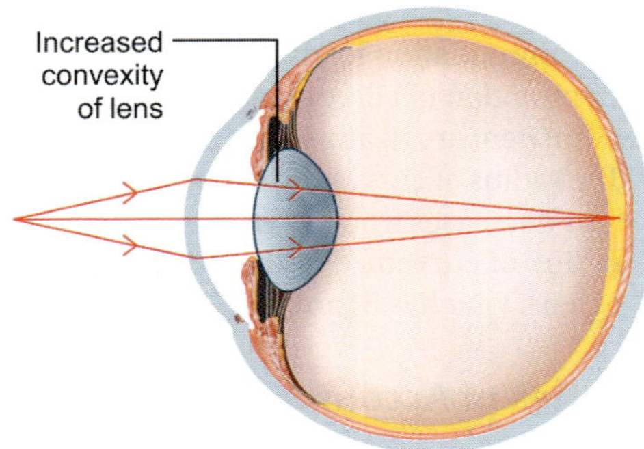

FIG. 4.4.2: Near vision—mechanism of accommodation

> The amplitude of accommodation decreases as the age increases. The accommodation is about 14 D at 10 years of age and becomes 1 D by the age of 60. This decrease in amplitude of accommodation is because of decrease in the elasticity of the lens because of age-related sclerosis of the lens, which makes the alteration in the shape of the lens not possible with increasing age.

Accommodation is accompanied by constriction of pupils and convergence. The ratio between the accommodative convergence (AC) and accommodation (A) is called AC/A ratio. The normal value varies in normal individuals from 0.5 to 4. AC/A ratio is important as high values are associated with accommodative squint.

Anomalies of Accommodation*

Anomalies of accommodation include conditions associated with:

1. Increased accommodation such as spasm of accommodation and excessive accommodation.
2. Decreased accommodation such as insufficiency of accommodation, paralysis of accommodation, ill-sustained accommodation and presbyopia.

Spasm of Accommodation

1. It indicates a condition of the excessive accommodation because of spasm of ciliary muscle.
2. It is usually seen in children because of attempt to compensate for the refractive error. It can occur following use of cholinergic drugs (e.g. pilocarpine).
3. The clinical features are asthenopic symptoms and diminution of vision for distance because of induced myopia secondary to spasm of the ciliary muscle.
4. The treatment of the condition is by using cycloplegic drugs (e.g. atropine, homatropine, cyclopentolate) to cause relaxation of the ciliary muscle, followed by treatment of the underlying predisposing condition such as treatment of refractive error or by preventing the use of cholinergic drugs.

Excessive Accommodation

1. It indicates a condition of excessive accommodation because of exertion of increased amount of accommodation than actually required.
2. It is seen in young individuals with the underlying refractive error most commonly hypermetropia.
3. The clinical features and treatment are similar to spasm of accommodation.

Insufficiency of Accommodation

1. It indicates a condition characterized by presence of decreased accommodation than the physiological lower limit for his/her age.
2. It is differentiated from presbyopia from the fact that in presbyopia accommodation is physiological and it is within the normal limit for his/her age.
3. It is seen in weakness of ciliary muscle secondary to ocular causes such as primary open-angle glaucoma as a result of constant pressure over the ciliary muscle by raised intraocular pressure or secondary to systemic causes (e.g. general debility, malnutrition, etc.).
4. The clinical features are asthenopic symptoms and diminution of vision for near.
5. The treatment is by convex lenses similar to presbyopia, treatment of the underlying cause and accommodation exercises.

Paralysis of Accommodation

1. It indicates a condition characterized by complete absence of accommodation as a result of paralysis of the ciliary muscle.
2. It is seen with cycloplegia caused by cycloplegic drugs (e.g. atropine, homatropine, etc.) following internal ophthalmoplegia because of paralysis of ciliary muscle as a result of paralysis of oculomotor nerve in conditions such as diabetes, diphtheria, etc.
3. The clinical features are similar to insufficiency of accommodation such as asthenopic symptoms and diminution of vision for near. Photophobia is seen in cases involving the sphincter pupillae as in internal ophthalmoplegia because of dilatation of the pupil.
4. The treatment is done by treating the underlying cause and by prescription of appropriate convex lenses.

Ill-sustained Accommodation

1. It is a condition characterized by episodes of insufficient accommodation in between the periods of normal accommodation.
2. It can be considered as mild variety or the beginning of insufficiency of accommodation.
3. The causes, clinical features and treatment, which are similar to insufficiency of accommodation.

PRESBYOPIA**

Definition

Presbyopia is a refractive condition of the eye characterized by decreased accommodative power of the eye as a result of physiological changes in the lens due to aging, causing progressive diminution of near vision.

The word presbyopia is derived from Greek words 'presbys'—elder and 'ops'—eye; hence, presbyopia means eyesight in elderly individuals.

Etiopathogenesis

Presbyopia is because of age-related changes such as:

- Decrease in the elasticity of the lens
- Increase in the hardness of lens as a result of sclerosis of lens
- Increase in the size of the lens
- Weakness in the power of the ciliary muscle.

Clinical Features

1. Progressively increasing difficulty in near vision and work. People with presbyopia tend to hold the books and other things away from their eyes and gradually will not be able to read small letters initially followed by progressively increasing difficulty for bigger letters.
2. Asthenopic symptoms such as headache, eyestrain following near work.

Diagnosis

Diagnosis is made based on the correlation between age and the symptoms of progressively increasing difficulty in near vision.

Treatment

Optical Treatment

Optical treatment is done by prescription of convex lenses. The weakest convex lens with which the person can read the smallest letters is prescribed. The convex lenses can be given either in the form of spectacles or contact lenses. The lenses can be prescribed in the form of unifocal, bifocal, trifocal and multifocal lenses (Table 4.4.1). Unifocal lenses are given in presence of only presbyopia without any refractive error as in myopia, hypermetropia or astigmatism. Bifocal lenses are given in presence of presbyopia associated with myopia, hypermetropia or astigmatism.

Surgical Treatment

Surgical treatment is done by:
- Scleral expansion bands
- Conductive keratoplasty
- Accommodative intraocular lenses (IOLs)
- Multifocal IOLs

TABLE 4.4.1: Types of lenses

Types	*Features*
Unifocal lenses	Correct only for fixed distance and can be used to correct either distance vision or near vision
Bifocal lenses	Correct for both distance and near vision
Trifocal lenses	Correct for distance, intermediate and near vision
Multifocal lenses	Correct for varying distances as in naturally existing accommodation

- Presbyopic laser-assisted in situ keratomileusis (LASIK).

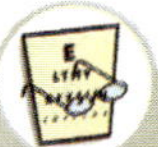

Optical Tips for Correction of Presbyopia

- In general at 40 years of age, +1.0 D convex lens is required for presbyopic correction with increase of +0.5 D for every increase of 5 years, thus making it +1.5 D, +2.0 D.....+3.0 D for 45, 50...60 years respectively. However, the power of the convex lens required has to be calculated from subjective correction.
- The required presbyopic correction is added to the refractive correction required for distance vision. The weakest convex lens with which the person can read the smallest letters at his/her usual near working distance is taken as the presbyopic correction. The required presbyopic correction is calculated in each eye separately by adding to the correction required for the distance vision. Presbyopia is better treated by undercorrection so as not to alter the normal relation between the accommodative convergence and accommodation.
- Unifocal lenses are used when only presbyopia is present without any refractive error for distance.
- Bifocal lenses are used to correct presbyopia with correction required for distance.
- Trifocal lenses are used in individuals requiring correction for distance, near and intermediate (i.e. distance between far and near) vision.
- Multifocal lenses or progressive lenses are used in individuals requiring correction for distance, near and at varying distances between distance and near.

Presbyopia usually occurs early in hypermetropes and later in myopes compared to emmetropes. Frequent change in presbyopic glasses is seen in patients of primary open-angle glaucoma because of constant pressure over the ciliary muscle resulting in the weakness of ciliary muscle.

GIST BOX 4.4

- Accommodation is defined as a process by which the divergent rays coming from a near object situated within 6 m are brought to focus on the light sensitive layer of the retina by increasing the refractive power of the lens by increasing the anterior curvature of the lens.
- Anomalies of accommodation include increased accommodation such as spasm of accommodation and excessive accommodation, and decreased accommodation such as insufficiency of accommodation, paralysis of accommodation, ill-sustained accommodation and presbyopia.
- Presbyopia is a refractive condition of the eye characterized by decreased accommodative power of the eye as a result of physiological changes in the lens due to aging causing progressive diminution of near vision.

CHAPTER

4.5 Aphakia and Pseudophakia

APHAKIA**

Definition

The word aphakia means absence of lens from the eye. Aphakia is defined as a condition in which lens is absent from its normal position, i.e. from pupillary area or patellar fossa.

Causes of Aphakia

1. Surgical aphakia resulting as a result of extraction of lens without implantation of intraocular lens (IOL) as in intracapsular cataract extraction or extracapsular cataract extraction associated with intraoperative complications such as posterior capsular rent and vitreous loss.
2. Dislocation of the lens either spontaneously as in hypermature cataract, in syndromes such as Marfan's syndrome, homocystinuria, etc. or following trauma.
3. Congenital absence of lens is a relatively rare cause for aphakia.

Optics of Aphakia*

- An emmetropic eye becomes highly hypermetropic after aphakia
- The total power of the eye is reduced from +60 D to +44 D
- The anterior focal distance becomes 23 mm from 15 mm and the posterior focal distance becomes 31 mm from 24 mm
- Accommodation is completely lost because of absence of lens (Fig. 4.5.1).

Clinical Features

Symptoms

Patients with aphakia present with gross diminution of the vision both for distance and near because of the high hypermetropia and loss of accommodation.

Signs

- Limbal scar may be present in cases of aphakia because of previous cataract surgery

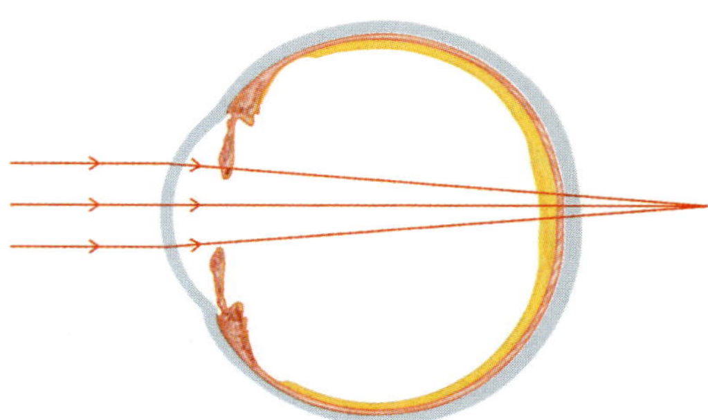

FIG. 4.5.1: Refraction in aphakic eye (*Note:* Absence of lens leading to hypermetropia)

- Anterior chamber is deep with iridodonesis or tremulousness of iris because of lack of posterior support provided by the lens
- Jet black color of the pupil
- First two Purkinje images are present with absence of third and fourth images produced by anterior and posterior capsule of lens respectively.

Diagnosis

Diagnosis is confirmed by retinoscopy, which shows high hypermetropia more than +10 D.

Treatment**

Evaluation should be made to find out the underlying cause for aphakia:

1. Aphakia because of spontaneous or traumatic dislocation of the lens into the vitreous chamber are treated by removal of the dislocated lens by posterior segment surgery in the form of three-ports pars plana vitrectomy and removal of the dislocated lens.
2. Surgical aphakia and congenital aphakia are treated by optical treatment.

   Optical treatment for aphakia is by:

- Spectacles
- Contact lenses
- Secondary IOL implantation
- Refractive surgeries.

Spectacles

- Approximately +10 D of spherical convex lens along with cylindrical lenses for correction of astigmatism in case of surgical aphakia and near addition by +3 D convex lens
- This is for previously emmetropic eyes; however, in patients with previous ametropia, the refractive power has to be calculated by retinoscopy.

Advantages	Disadvantages*
• Spectacles are the cheapest, safest and easiest method of correction of aphakia.	• Cosmetic disfigurement and discomfort to use because of heavy and thick lenses used to correct aphakia. • Spherical aberration producing pincushion distortion. • Prismatic aberration producing roving ring scotoma. • Image magnification of about 30%. • Reduced field of vision. • Anisometropia in a person in whom other eye is phakic or pseudophakic.

Ring-shaped scotoma produced by prismatic effect at the periphery of the thick convex lens is called roving ring scotoma. This scotoma shifts with the movement of the eyes resulting in appearance and disappearance of the scotoma as the eyes change their position. This is called Jack-in-the-box phenomenon.

Contact Lenses

The advantages of contact lenses are:

- Cosmetically give better appearance
- Wider field of vision
- Prismatic and spherical aberrations are absent
- Image magnification is less about 8%.

Disadvantages of contact lenses:

- Contact lens complications such as corneal abrasion, papillary conjunctivitis, infective keratitis, etc.
- Costlier than spectacles
- Requires care and maintenance of contact lenses.

Secondary Intraocular Lens Implantation

Advantages: Best method for correction of aphakia as it eliminates the disadvantages of both spectacles and contact lenses.

Disadvantages: Since it requires one more surgery, complications associated with surgery may be seen.

Secondary IOL Implantation

It is a surgical procedure for correction of aphakia by insertion of intraocular lens (IOL) by a second surgery into an eye, which is rendered aphakic by a primary surgery.

The type of IOL depends on the type of primary surgery and the status of posterior capsule.

After intracapsular cataract extraction:

- Anterior chamber IOL.
- Iris-fixated IOL.
- Scleral-fixated IOL.

After extracapsular cataract extraction:

- With intact posterior capsule:
  - Posterior chamber IOL.
- Without intact posterior capsule:
  - Anterior chamber IOL.
  - Iris-fixated IOL.
  - Scleral-fixated IOL.

Refractive Surgeries

Refractive surgeries, e.g. hypermetropic laser-assisted in situ keratomileusis (LASIK) and epikeratophakia, are the refractive surgeries for correction of aphakia.

PSEUDOPHAKIA**

Definition

Pseudophakia is defined as condition in which the natural lens is replaced by an artificial lens or IOL. The word pseudophakia means false lens, but it actually indicates artificial lens.

Optics of Pseudophakia

1. The optics of pseudophakia depends on the refractive status of the eye. The pseudophakic eye can be optically emmetropic, myopic or hypermetropic.
2. Emmetropia results when the power of the IOL is same as the power required as calculated by biometry. Myopia results when the IOL power is more than the power required and lesser IOL power than required results in hypermetropia.
3. The distance vision depends on the refractive status and the astigmatism induced by surgery.
4. Accommodation is absent in pseudophakia similar to aphakia unless accommodative IOL is implanted.
5. The near vision depends on the refractive status of the pseudophakic eye; it will be decreased in emmetropic and hypermetropic condition and remains good in myopia.

Clinical Features

Symptoms

1. Pseudophakics may not have any complaints as it is the treatment done for a disease.
2. Diminution of vision for near is present in all pseudophakics except in whom accommodative IOL, multifocal IOL is implanted or in whom there is consecutive myopia because of implantation of higher refractive power than required.
3. Diminution of vision for distance depending on the refractive status of the pseudophakic eye and astigmatism induced by surgery.

Signs

1. Limbal scar may be seen; it may be absent in cataract surgeries done by clear corneal phacoemulsification.
2. Jet black color of the pupil with the shining reflexes.
3. Presence of IOL in the eye.

Diagnosis

Diagnosis is done by history of cataract surgery and the ocular examination showing the above described signs.

Treatment

Treatment depends on the refractive condition of the pseudophakic eye. Optical treatment may or may not be required for only near vision or distance and near vision depending on the refractive status of the pseudophakic eye. Optical treatment is done by spectacles, contact lenses or refractive surgeries.

GIST BOX 4.5

- Aphakia is defined as a condition in which lens is absent from its normal position, i.e. from pupillary area or patellar fossa.
- An emmetropic eye becomes highly hypermetropic after aphakia as the power of the eye is reduced from +60 D to +44 D. Accommodation is completely lost because of absence of lens.
- Pseudophakia is defined as condition in which the natural lens is replaced by an artificial lens or intraocular lens (IOL). The optics of pseudophakia depends on the refractive status of the eye. The pseudophakic eye can be optically emmetropic, myopic or hypermetropic. Accommodation is absent in pseudophakia similar to aphakia unless accommodative IOL is implanted.

CHAPTER

4.6 Spectacles

DEFINITION

Spectacle is an optical device consisting of a pair of lenses set in a frame and worn on the eyes with sides extending onto the ears. Spectacle is also known as eyeglass.

> The earliest evidence of first use of spectacles is available from the pyramids of Egypt dating back to 500 BC. Salvino from Italy is credited with inventing the first eyeglasses in the year 1286. Benjamin Franklin from America was the first to introduce bifocal spectacles.

USES

1. Spectacles are most commonly used to correct refractive errors and spectacles are the most common mode of treatment for correction of various types of refractive errors.
2. Spectacles are used as protective glasses for safety of the eye during various occupations associated with risk of eye injury and during riding vehicles, as sunglasses to protect against ultraviolet (UV) light, etc.
3. Spectacles are also used for cosmetic purpose to improve the appearance.

PARTS OF SPECTACLES

Spectacle consists of two rims, which support and hold the lenses; the two rims are connected on the nasal side by a bridge, which is designed to rest over the nose with one nose pad on either side. Each rim is connected to an earpiece on the temporal side. Several modifications in the form of half rim or rimless spectacles with lens directly connected to bridge and earpiece are available to reduce the weight of the spectacles.

Lenses

The lenses used in spectacles are made from:

- Glass
- Plastic
- Polycarbonate.

Plastic and polycarbonate lenses are preferred because of their lesser weight resistance to impact compared to glass lenses.

Lenses are available with various coatings and properties such as:

- Antireflection coating, which decrease glare on looking at bright light
- Scratch resistance coating to reduce the scratches, particularly in plastic and polycarbonate lenses
- The UV protection coating for protection against UV rays of sun
- Photochromic lenses, which change color and become dark shaded on exposure to sunlight thus providing protection against UV light.

Depending on the type of lens used glasses can be classified (Fig. 4.6.1):*

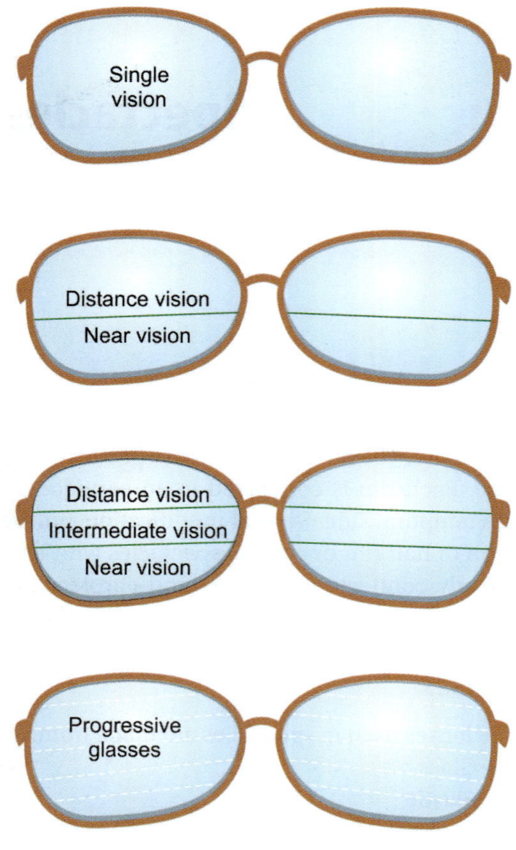

FIG. 4.6.1: Different types of spectacles

- Single vision glasses meant for correction at distance or near
- Bifocal glasses meant for correction of both distance and near vision

Progressive glasses are very popular and are used in case of myopia, hypermetropia or astigmatism associated with presbyopia. In addition to correcting for all distances from near to distance, they are cosmetically better compared to bifocal or trifocal glasses, as progressive glasses do not show line dividing the lens into different segments.

- Trifocal glasses meant for correction of distance, near and intermediate vision
- Progressive glasses meant for correction at all distances from near to distance.

DISADVANTAGES OF SPECTACLES

Though spectacles are the most accepted and common mode of correction of refractive errors, they are not devoid of disadvantages. The disadvantages are more pronounced in case of thicker lenses used to correct higher refractive errors.

The disadvantages are:

- Cosmetic blemishes particularly in case of thicker lenses used for higher refractive errors
- Discomfort because of increased weight with thicker glasses
- Difficulties to participate in outdoor sports activities because of risk of impact
- Optical aberrations such as spherical aberration, chromatic aberration, coma, image magnification, image minification, image distortion, etc.

GIST BOX 4.6

- Spectacle is an optical device consisting of a pair of lenses set in a frame and worn on the eyes with sides extending onto the ears.
- Spectacles are the most common mode of treatment for correction of various types of refractive errors.

CHAPTER

4.7 Contact Lenses

DEFINITION

Contact lens is a thin lens placed directly on the anterior surface of the cornea in contact with the cornea to correct the refractive error.

Leonardo da Vinci best known for his paintings of Mona Lisa, The Last Supper, etc. was the first one to give the idea of contact lenses in the year 1508 AD. He was the one who first noted that vision improves when a person with refractive error sees through a bowl filled with water by immersing face into the bowl.

The first contact lenses made from plastic were introduced in the year 1948. Soft contact lenses were introduced in the year 1971. Rigid gas permeable lenses were introduced by 1978. Silicone hydrogel soft contact lenses are available from 2002. It is estimated that more than 120 million people wear contact lenses worldwide.

OPTICS OF CONTACT LENS

Contact lens acts by replacing the cornea as the first refracting surface. The contact lens with radius of curvature smaller than the radius of curvature of the cornea increases the refractive power of the eye and the contact lens with radius of curvature more than that of the cornea decreases the refractive power of the eye.

Contact lens corrects the refractive error by glass/plastic lens and by fluid lens with tear film between the anterior surface of cornea and posterior surface of contact lens acting as fluid lens.

CLASSIFICATION**

Contact lenses are classified depending on the various criteria.

Depending on the Permeability of Oxygen and Materials from which the Contact Lens is Made

- Non-gas permeable rigid contact lenses made of polymethyl methacrylate (PMMA).
- Gas permeable rigid contact lenses made of silicone acrylate and fluorosilicone acrylate.
- Gas permeable soft contact lenses made of hydroxyethyl methacrylate (HEMA).

The oxygen supply to the anterior epithelium of cornea, which normally is supplied by the tear film and the atmosphere should now be able to reach the cornea through the contact lens. The oxygen permeability of a contact lens is called DK value (D is diffusion coefficient and K is solubility coefficient) and it is the most important limiting factor in the use of contact lens. Though non-gas permeable rigid contact lenses have high-optical quality, they are rarely used because of their non-gas permeability.

Depending on the Wear Time of the Contact Lens

- Daily wear: As the name itself implies, these lenses are worn during daytime for about 8–12 hours and removed during night before sleeping.
- Extended wear: They are worn throughout day and night.
- Continuous wear: They are worn continuously ranging from more than 1 day extending up to 30 days.

Rigid non-gas permeable contact lenses are also called hard contact lenses. They are made of PMMA. Though hard contact lenses offer high optical quality, they are no longer used because of poor or no oxygen permeability.

Rigid gas permeable (RGP) contact lenses called RGP contact lenses or semisoft contact lenses are made of silicone acrylate, fluorosilicone acrylate, cellulose acetate butyrate, etc. They are permeable to oxygen and have higher optical quality as in hard contact lenses.

Soft contact lenses are made of hydroxyethyl methacrylate (HEMA) and are most commonly used in clinical practice, as they are oxygen permeable and hence well tolerated.

Disposable contact lenses are meant for single use and disposed of either after 1 day or after 1 week in case of extended wear contact lenses. They are considered as safest contact lenses as they require no maintenance and chance of infection is less.

USES*

1. Optical indications include correction of refractive error. Contact lenses can be used to correct all types of refractive errors. Contact lenses are the preferred mode of treatment over spectacles for correction of aphakia, high-refractive errors.
2. Therapeutic indications include treatment of corneal perforation, corneal edema and as drug delivery system in diseases such as glaucoma.
3. Cosmetic indications include corneal scar or corneal opacities.

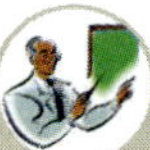

Orthokeratology

- It is a technique of correction of refractive error by altering the shape or curvature of the cornea by wearing rigid gas permeable contact lenses overnight so that patient can have good vision without spectacles in daytime.
- It is simple, non-invasive method of correction of refractive error and can be used as an alternative to refractive surgery to have freedom from spectacles during daytime.
- Since the effect is temporary and the refractive error reverses back once the patient stops wearing contact lenses during nighttime, it is not very popular.

CONTRAINDICATIONS

Contact lenses should not be used in infective and inflammatory diseases of the eye and adnexa such as conjunctivitis, dacryocystitis, blepharitis, keratitis, etc.

COMPLICATIONS*

The complications of contact lenses are related to trauma, hypersensitivity, infection, metabolic and toxic effects associated with contact lenses:

1. The conjunctival complications are because of hypersensitivity reaction to the preservatives used in contact lens solutions. The conjunctival complications are papillary conjunctivitis, giant papillary conjunctivitis and keratoconjunctivitis.
2. The corneal complications are corneal abrasion, corneal edema, infective keratitis, corneal warping, corneal neovascularization, etc.

CLINICAL PRACTICE OF CONTACT LENS (PRESCRIPTION AND FITTING)

1. Before prescription of contact lenses, history and general ocular examination is done to rule out contraindications for use of contact lenses.

2. Medical history is taken to rule out medical diseases such as:
   - Allergic diseases, as it may increase the chance of hypersensitivity-related complications of contact lenses
   - Diabetes mellitus as corneal hypoesthesia associated with diabetes may increase the risk of corneal infection
   - Psychiatric diseases as patients using contact lenses require to handle the lenses, etc.
3. Ocular examination is done to rule out infective and inflammatory diseases of the eye and adnexa such as conjunctivitis, dacryocystitis, blepharitis, keratitis, dry eye, etc.
4. Tear film evaluation as normal tear film is a prerequisite for normal functioning following wearing contact lenses.
5. Measurement of corneal diameter: Horizontal visible iris diameter is considered as corneal diameter for all practical purposes for fitting of contact lenses.
6. Estimation of the refractive error by retinoscopy and subjective correction.
7. Keratometry to measure the corneal curvature for selecting the base curve of the contact lens and usually flatter keratometer reading is taken as the base curve.
8. In case of gas permeable rigid contact lens, the usual overall diameter of the contact lens is about 9 mm and in case of soft contact lenses, the overall diameter is taken 2 mm above the horizontal visible iris diameter.
9. The contact lens fitting varies in gas permeable rigid contact lenses and soft contact lenses. In gas permeable rigid contact lenses, fluorescein is used to evaluate the fit by using trail contact lens set. Midperipheral touch and peripheral clearance indicate ideal fit in case of gas permeable rigid contact lens.

Calculation of Power

The power of the contact lenses is calculated by refraction and adjustment for the vertex distance. Vertex distance is the distance between the posterior surface of the lens either spectacle or contact lens to the anterior surface of the cornea.

Changes in the vertex distance affect the power of the lens as the focal point varies with varying vertex distance. The vertex distance in case of spectacles at which the retinoscopy is done is about 10–14 mm. Hence, the refractive power of the contact lens should be adjusted with the vertex distance. This difference becomes significant in refractive powers of 4 D or more. Hence, before prescribing contact lens power, it needs to be adjusted to the vertex distance.

Vertex distance is measured by corneal reflex pupillometer or by a simple ruler measuring the distance between the back surface of the spectacle lens to the anterior surface of cornea. The plus lens power increase on vertex distance correction for contact lens and minus lens power decrease on vertex distance correction, contact lens can be obtained by readily available vertex distance correction charts.

GIST BOX 4.7

- Contact lens is a thin lens placed directly on the anterior surface of the cornea in contact with the cornea to correct the refractive error.
- Contact lens corrects the refractive error by glass/plastic lens and by fluid lens with tear film between the anterior surface of cornea and posterior surface of contact lens acting as fluid lens.
- Classification of contact lenses depending on the permeability of oxygen and materials from which the contact lens is made—non-gas permeable rigid contact lenses made of polymethyl methacrylate (PMMA), gas permeable rigid contact lenses made of silicone acrylate and fluorosilicone acrylate and gas permeable soft contact lenses made of hydroxyethyl methacrylate (HEMA).
- Contact lenses can be used to correct all types of refractive errors. Therapeutic uses include treatment of corneal perforation, corneal edema and as drug delivery system in diseases such as glaucoma. Cosmetic uses include treatment of corneal scar or corneal opacities.

CHAPTER

4.8 Refractive Surgeries

DEFINITION

The surgical techniques for correction of refractive errors of eye such as myopia, hypermetropia, astigmatism and presbyopia are called refractive surgeries.

The refractive surgeries are becoming popular day by day because of refractive surgery being a onetime procedure and they provide the freedom from spectacles and contact lenses, which needs to be used daily.

CLASSIFICATION

The refractive surgeries are broadly classified into two categories:

1. Keratorefractive surgeries, involving the surgeries on the cornea, which correct the refractive error by altering the thickness or curvature of the cornea.
2. Intraocular refractive surgeries in which the artificial intraocular lenses are placed inside the eye.

KERATOREFRACTIVE SURGERIES

Depending on the basic mechanism involved, keratorefractive surgeries can be:*

1. Surgeries involving the addition of tissue to cornea to increase the thickness of the cornea as in epikeratophakia.
2. Surgeries involving the removal of tissue from cornea to decrease the corneal thickness such as keratomileusis and wedge resection.
3. Surgeries involving incising the cornea to alter the curvature of the cornea, e.g. radial keratotomy and astigmatic keratotomy.
4. Surgeries involving the laser ablation of the cornea, e.g. photorefractive keratectomy (PRK), laser-assisted in situ keratomileusis (LASIK), laser subepithelial keratomileusis (LASEK), Epi-LASIK, intraLase LASIK.
5. Surgeries involving coagulation to alter the curvature of the cornea, e.g. thermokeratoplasty, conductive keratoplasty.

Epikeratophakia involves addition of donor corneal lenticule by suturing to the patient's cornea to increase the corneal thickness to correct refractive errors. However, because of high incidence of complications (e.g. astigmatism induced by surgery), epikeratophakia is no longer done.

Keratomileusis also called automated lamellar keratoplasty involves removal of lamellar corneal button, reshaping it by freezing, placing it back in the cornea.

Radial keratotomy is an incisional refractive surgery done for correction of myopia. It is done by making incisions in the cornea to flatten the cornea. Because of unpredictable visual outcome and complications associated with the procedure such as weakening of the cornea, postoperative glare, etc. it is not popular now.

Lasik, which involves the laser ablation of the cornea is one of the most popular and most frequently performed refractive corneal surgeries.

Laser Refractive Surgeries

Photorefractive keratectomy and LASIK are the most commonly performed laser refractive surgeries.

Excimer laser is used in laser refractive surgeries. Excimer laser uses argon and fluorine, which emit laser energy at a wavelength of 193 nm.

Mechanism of Action

The excimer laser acts by photoablation of cornea to remove the tissue from cornea to alter the curvature of the cornea according to the type of correction for the refractive error by disrupting the chemical bonds in the cornea.

Indications

To correct refractive errors in patients older than 18 years with stable refraction.

Contraindications

Systemic contraindications

1. Autoimmune collagen vascular diseases such as rheumatoid arthritis, systemic lupus erythematosus, etc. and immunodeficiency conditions because of problems with wound healing.
2. Pregnant and nursing women because of instability of refraction.
3. Diabetes mellitus because of instability of refraction and problems in wound healing.

Ocular contraindications

1. Absolute contraindications:
   - Corneal ecstatic conditions such as keratoconus, pellucid marginal degeneration, etc.
   - Ocular surface diseases such as severe dry eye, ocular cicatricial pemphigoid, Steven-Johnson syndrome, etc.
2. Relative contraindications:
   - History of herpes zoster ophthalmicus or herpes simplex keratitis because of risk of reactivation of the infection
   - Mild dry eye.

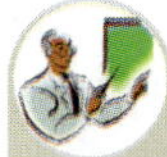

Evaluation of a Patient Posted for Laser Refractive Surgery

Patients posted for refractive laser surgery should undergo complete ocular examination involving:
- Visual acuity.
- Refraction.
- Corneal topography.
- Fundoscopy to rule out progressive retinal diseases affecting vision.
- Slit-lamp examination to rule out dry eye, corneal diseases and inflammation of eye.
- Measurement of corneal thickness of pachymetry.

Photorefractive Keratectomy

Photorefractive keratectomy is a type of refractive surgery, which involves reshaping the curvature of the cornea to correct refractive error by using excimer laser applied to cornea after removal of corneal epithelium. It is most commonly used to correct myopia. It corrects up to –10 D of myopia. It can also correct mild to moderate hypermetropia and astigmatism.

Procedure

Photorefractive keratectomy is performed under topical anesthesia under microscope. Preparation of the eye to be operated is done by painting with povidone iodine and draping. A lid speculum is used to separate the eyelids and centration is done. The corneal epithelium is removed after loosening it with 20% ethanol. The laser ablation is done by asking the patient to look at the fixation light. A bandage soft contact lens is inserted to prevent postoperative pain.

Topical antibiotic, steroid, non-steroidal anti-inflammatory eyedrops and artificial tear eyedrops are used in the postoperative period. Steroid eyedrops are tapered over 2–3 months. Bandage soft contact lens is removed by the end of the first postoperative week.

Complications

1. The main complications in the early postoperative period are postoperative pain and infectious keratitis.

2. Undercorrection or overcorrection of the refractive error, corneal haze and irregular astigmatism because of decentration during laser ablation are some of the common late postoperative complications.

Laser-assisted In Situ Keratomileusis**

Definition

The LASIK is a type of refractive surgery, which involves the use of a keratome to lift a flap of cornea and application of excimer laser to stromal bed to alter the curvature of the cornea and to correct the refractive error.

It has become the most popular refractive surgery because of quick visual rehabilitation and relatively less pain in the postoperative period. The LASIK corrects up to –12 D of myopia, 4 D of hypermetropia and 8 D of astigmatism.

Procedure

The LASIK is performed under topical anesthesia under microscope. Preparation of the eye to be operated is done by painting with povidone iodine and draping. A lid speculum is used to separate the eyelids and centration is done. Corneal flap is raised by keratome after applying the pneumatic suction ring. The laser ablation is done by lifting the corneal flap. The corneal flap is repositioned back.

Topical antibiotic, steroid, non-steroidal anti-inflammatory eyedrops and artificial tear eyedrops are used in the postoperative period. Steroid eyedrops are tapered over 1-2 months.

Central corneal thickness is very important deciding factor for deciding the amount of cornea available for laser ablation in LASIK. Normally, a corneal flap of 150–160 μm is required in LASIK to prevent flap-associated complications. A thickness of 250 μm of residual stromal bed is required to prevent postoperative ectasia of cornea.

The amount of cornea available for ablation = Total corneal thickness as measured from pachymetry – [thickness of the corneal flap (160 μm) + residual stromal bed thickness (250 μm)].

Complications

1. The intraoperative complications are usually related to raising the corneal flap and are in the form of incomplete flap, free flap, irregular flap, button holing of the flap, corneal perforation, etc.
2. The postoperative complications are overcorrection or undercorrection of refractive error, infectious keratitis, surgically induced keratectasia, irregular astigmatism because of decentration during laser ablation, diffuse lamellar keratitis and islands of uncorrected areas between the areas of corrected areas because of unequal laser ablation.

Laser Subepithelial Keratomileusis

The LASIK is a type of refractive surgery, which involves lifting of corneal epithelium and application of excimer laser and replacing the corneal epithelial flap back.

Procedure

The surgical procedure and postoperative management is similar to PRK, except for instead of removing epithelium, the epithelium is rolled as flap after treatment with 20% alcohol by using a hockey spatula and replaced back after laser ablation.

Laser subepithelial keratomileusis is similar to photorefractive keratectomy (PRK) by the fact that here also laser is applied to subepithelial cornea, but differs from the fact that corneal epithelium is not removed here, but it is folded and raised, and replaced back, which decreases postoperative pain seen with PRK.

It is similar to LASIK from the fact that LASEK also involves lifting corneal flap, but it is limited to corneal

Contd...

Contd...

epithelium, unlike in LASIK where corneal flap involves epithelium and superficial stroma of cornea, which makes the cornea week and has significant flap-associated complications. Thus, LASEK combines the advantages of both PRK and LASIK.

However, because of postoperative pain and epithelial healing problems, LASEK is performed for few indications, e.g. in patients with refractive error who have thin corneas as shown on pachymetry, and in patients who had LASIK flap-related complications.

Epi-LASIK

Epi-LASIK is almost similar to LASEK differing only by the fact that here instead of folding the epithelium, epithelial flap is made by an epikeratome, thus decreasing the postoperative pain further and decreases the epithelial healing problems.

Customized LASIK

Customized LASIK is the recent advance in conventional LASIK. It involves the correction of higher-order aberrations to improve the quality of vision. Conventional LASIK does not correct higher-order aberrations; in customized LASIK, laser ablation is done under the guidance of corneal topography or wavefront analysis guidance. Customized LASIK is available commercially as Zyoptix.

IntraLase LASIK

IntraLase LASIK is the most recent advance in the LASIK procedure. It involves the use of a femtosecond laser to raise the corneal flap. Thus, intraLase LASIK is free from microkeratome-related corneal flap complications. In intraLase LASIK, surgeon-dependent step of raising the corneal flap is replaced by raising the corneal flap by using femtosecond laser, which provides a uniform clear cut, thus reducing the microkeratome-related complications.

Small-incision Lenticule Extraction

Small-incision lenticule extraction (SMILE) is the most recent laser refractive surgery. It is done by using femtosecond laser.

Laser Thermokeratoplasty

Laser thermokeratoplasty is a surgical procedure, which involves the use of laser energy to increase temperature in the periphery of the cornea, causing coagulation of the collagen and shrinkage of the peripheral cornea resulting in flattening of the peripheral cornea and steepening of the central cornea.

The holmium-yttrium-aluminum-garnet (Ho-YAG) laser is used in laser thermokeratoplasty. Laser thermokeratoplasty is indicated to correct hypermetropia and presbyopia.

Conductive Keratoplasty

The mechanism of conductive keratoplasty is similar to laser thermokeratoplasty; it differs from it by the fact that conductive keratoplasty uses high-frequency radio waves instead of laser energy to heat the cornea. The indications are similar to conductive keratoplasty such as hypermetropia and presbyopia.

INTRAOCULAR REFRACTIVE SURGERIES

Intraocular refractive surgeries involve implantation of artificial intraocular lenses or rings into the corneal stroma, into the anterior chamber or posterior chamber of the eye to correct the refractive error.

Intrastromal Corneal Ring Segments

Intrastromal corneal ring segments are also called INTACS or intrastromal corneal ring

(ICR) and the procedure involves the implantation of ring segments into the corneal stroma.

INTACS are now commonly used in the treatment of keratoconus and other ectasias of cornea including the iatrogenic ectasia of cornea induced by LASIK.

Procedure

The procedure is done under topical anesthesia. It is done by implantation of ring segments in the periphery of the cornea after performing corneal tunnel. They act by steepening the periphery of the cornea resulting in flattening of the central cornea.

Indications

Intrastromal corneal ring are indicated in correction of myopia.

Phakic Intraocular Lenses

Definition

Intraocular lenses inserted into the anterior chamber or posterior chamber of phakic patients to correct high-refractive error without removing the naturally existing lens are called phakic intraocular lenses. They are called phakic as they are inserted in patients with presence of natural lens. They are also called implantable contact lens (ICL).

Phakic IOLs are less preferred in patients with high hypermetropia as anterior chamber tends to be shallower in hypermetropes.

Procedure

The procedure is similar to cataract surgery, except for the fact that natural lens is not removed. Depending on the site of insertion of intraocular lens (IOL), phakic IOL can be an anterior chamber IOL, iris-fixated IOL and posterior chamber IOL.

Indications

Intrastromal corneal ring segments are indicated in patients with high-refractive errors, which cannot be corrected by laser refractive surgeries.

Contraindications

They are avoided in patients with decreased corneal endothelial count and shallow anterior chamber (< 3 mm).

Complications

The major complications are damage to corneal endothelium, formation of cataract because of surgical trauma, pupillary block glaucoma and postoperative inflammation similar to cataract surgery.

Refractive Surgeries for Myopia*

- Radial keratotomy.
- Photorefractive keratectomy.
- LASIK.
- LASEK.
- Epi-LASIK.
- Customized LASIK.
- IntraLase LASIK.
- Phakic IOL.
- Intrastromal corneal ring segments.

Refractive Surgeries for Presbyopia*

- Scleral expansion bands.
- Conductive keratoplasty.
- Accommodative intraocular lenses.
- Multifocal intraocular lenses.
- Presbyopic LASIK.

Refractive Surgeries for Hypermetropia*

- Photorefractive keratectomy.
- LASIK.
- LASEK.
- Epi-LASIK.
- Customized LASIK.
- IntraLase LASIK.
- Laser thermokeratoplasty.
- Conductive keratoplasty.

Refractive Surgeries for Astigmatism

- Astigmatic keratotomy.
- Photorefractive keratectomy.
- LASIK.
- LASEK.
- Epi-LASIK.
- Customized LASIK.
- IntraLase LASIK.

GIST BOX 4.8

- The surgical techniques for correction of refractive errors of eye such as myopia, hypermetropia, astigmatism and presbyopia are called refractive surgeries.
- Keratorefractive surgeries involving the surgeries on the cornea, which correct the refractive error by altering the thickness or curvature of the cornea.
- Photorefractive keratectomy and laser-assisted in situ keratomileusis (LASIK) are the most commonly performed laser keratorefractive surgeries.
- Excimer laser is used in laser refractive surgeries. Excimer laser uses argon and fluorine, which emit laser energy at a wavelength of 193 nm.
- Intraocular refractive surgeries involve implantation of artificial intraocular lenses or rings into the corneal stroma, into the anterior chamber or posterior chamber of the eye to correct the refractive error.

FREQUENTLY ASKED QUESTIONS (FAQs)

*Short Answers

1. Schematic eye.
2. Reduced eye.
3. Sturm's conoid.
4. Mention the techniques of objective refraction.
5. FRIEND test (refer Author's textbook *'Clinical Methods in Ophthalmology'*).
6. Duochrome test (refer Author's textbook *'Clinical Methods in Ophthalmology'*).
7. Worth's 4-dot test (refer Author's textbook *'Clinical Methods in Ophthalmology'*).
8. Define Emmetropia and ametropia.
9. Mention the optical types of hypermetropia.
10. Fundus picture in pathological myopia.
11. Mention the complications of pathological myopia.
12. Define and classify astigmatism.
13. Mention the anomalies of accommodations.
14. Mention the disadvantages of aphakic glasses.
15. Optics of aphakia.
16. Mention the different types of glasses.
17. Mention the uses of contact lenses.
18. Mention the complication of contact lenses.
19. Mention the refractive surgeries for myopia.
20. Mention the refractive surgeries for hypermetropia.
21. Mention the refractive surgeries for presbyopia.
22. Classify keratorefractive surgeries.

**Short Essays

1. Retinoscopy.
2. Pathological myopia.
3. Anisometropia.
4. Astigmatism.
5. Presbyopia.
6. Define hypermetropia. Describe the clinical types and treatment of hypermetropia.
7. Aphakia.
8. Treatment of aphakia.
9. Pseudophakia.
10. Contact lenses.
11. Classify contact lenses.
12. LASIK.

***Long Essays

1. Define and classification myopia. Describe the etiology, pathogenesis, clinical features and treatment of pathological myopia.

BIBLIOGRAPHY

1. Abraham D. Duke-Elder's Practice of Refraction, 10th edition. Elsevier; 1993.
2. Achiron LR, Witkin N, Primo S, et al. Contemporary management of aniseikonia. Surv Ophthalmol. 1997;41(4):321-30.
3. American Optometric Association. Optometric Clinical Practice Guideline: Care of the Patient with Hypermetropia. St. Louis, MO; 1997.
4. American Optometric Association. Optometric Clinical Practice Guideline: Care of the Patient with Myopia. St. Louis, MO; 1997.
5. Azar DT. Part 3: Refractive surgery. In: Myron Yanoff, Jay S Duker (Eds). Ophthalmology, 2nd edition. China: Mosby; 2004.
6. Fredrick DR. Myopia. BMJ. 2002;324(7347): 1195-9.

7. Holzer MP, Sandoval HP, Solomon KD. Surgery for presbyopia. Refractive management. Am Acad Ophthalmol. 1(3).
8. Keay L, Friedman DS. Correcting refractive error in low income countries. BMJ. 2011;343:d4793.
9. Lai TYY. Retinal complications of high myopia. Medical Bulletin. 2007;12(9).
10. Manche EE, Carr JD, Haw WW, et al. Excimer laser refractive surgery. West J Med. 1998;169(1):30-8.
11. Sen DK, Malik SR. Accommodative-convergence over accommodation (AC-A) ratio (in normal Indian subjects). Indian J Ophthalmol. 1972;20(4):153-7.
12. Ursekar TN. Classification, etiology and pathology of myopia. Indian J Ophthalmol. 1983;31(6):709-11.

SECTION 5

Cornea

CHAPTER

5.1 Anatomy and Physiology of Cornea

ANATOMY OF CORNEA

Cornea is the transparent portion of the outer fibrous coat. It accounts for anterior one sixth of the outermost fibrous layer.

Dimensions (Table 5.1.1)

TABLE 5.1.1: Dimensions of cornea

Dimension	*Measurement*
Diameters of anterior surface	
Horizontal diameter	11.7–12 mm
Vertical diameter	10.5–11 mm
Diameters of posterior surface	
Horizontal diameter	11.5 mm
Vertical diameter	11.5 mm
Thickness of cornea	
Center	0.5–0.6 mm
Periphery	0.6–0.7 mm
Radius of curvature	
Anterior	7.8 mm
Posterior	6.5 mm

Functions (Table 5.1.2)

- Cornea accounts for two thirds of refractive power of the eye and acts as the refractive medium of the eye
- Along with sclera, cornea forms the outer most fibrous layer, thus protecting the intraocular structures.

Histology*

Histologically, cornea is made up of five layers; recently, a new layer is added to it making it six layers (Fig. 5.1.1):

1. *Epithelium of cornea:* It is 5–7 layers thick and it is of stratified squamous subtype. It is in continuity with epithelium of the bulbar conjunctiva. It is about 50 μ thick.

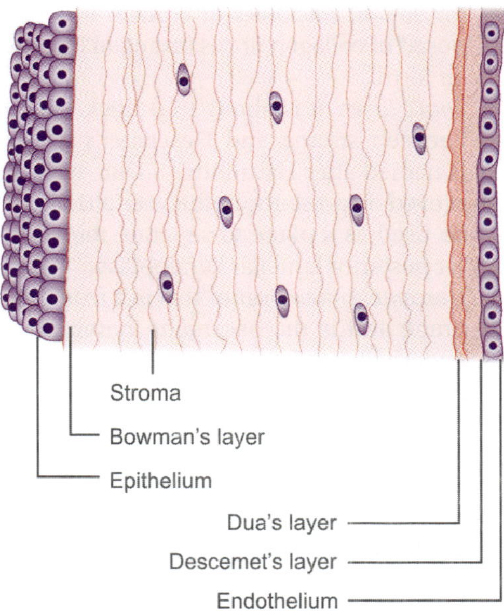

FIG. 5.1.1: Histology of cornea

TABLE 5.1.2: Functions of different layers of cornea

Layers	*Functions*
Epithelium	It provides smooth refractive surface and it heals without leading to scar formation
Bowman's layer	It is a tough layer and it provides resistance against penetration by infective microbes It cannot regenerate once damaged and any pathological process extending deeper to this layer leads to scar formation
Stroma	The collagen fibrils are arranged in lamellar fashion and this is responsible for transparency of cornea
Dua's layer	It is used as a plane to separate the cornea for posterior lamellar keratoplasty
Descemet's membrane	It is a tough layer of cornea and offers resistance to perforation of cornea
Endothelium	It is the most vital layer of cornea and is responsible for maintaining the cornea in dehydrated state by the presence of metabolic pump

The superficial layer is composed of flat cells, middle layer is composed of polygonal cells and deep layer is composed of columnar cells.

2. *Bowman's membrane*: It is not a true membrane, but is the condensation of collagen of superficial stroma. It is about 12–14 μ thick and it is a tough layer.
3. *Stroma*: It is about 500 μ thick accounting for 90% of thickness of cornea. It is composed of collagen fibrils arranged in lamellar form.
4. *Dua's layer*: It is about 15 μ thick, present between stroma and Descemet's layer. It is named after Harminder S Dua, who first proved its presence in the year 2013. It can be used as a plane to separate the cornea for posterior lamellar keratoplasty.
5. *Descemet's membrane*: This is a true membrane and is the basement membrane of endothelial cells. It is about 12 μ in thickness and is a tough layer.
6. *Endothelium*: It is the innermost layer of the cornea consisting of single layer of cells. The endothelial cells cannot regenerate and the number of endothelial cells decreases as the age increases. The endothelial cell count in children is about 4,000 cells/mm^2 and it will decrease to 2,500 cells/mm^2 by 70 years of age.

Nerve Supply*

Cornea is supplied by sensory and autonomic nerves. Sensory supply of cornea is from ophthalmic division of trigeminal nerve. The autonomic nerve supply comes from sympathetic fibers arising from ciliary ganglion.

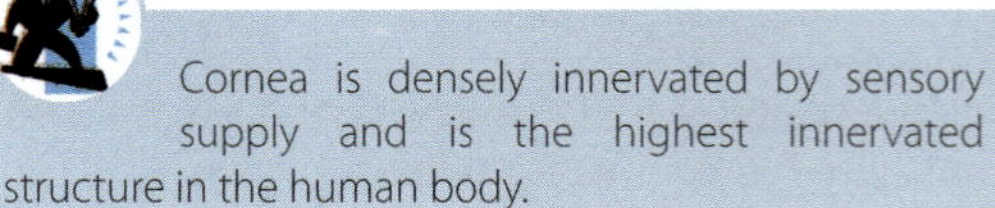

Cornea is densely innervated by sensory supply and is the highest innervated structure in the human body.

Blood Supply

Cornea has got neither blood vessels nor lymphatic supply. This uniqueness is to keep cornea transparent. However, the periphery of the cornea near the limbus is supplied by anterior ciliary vessels.

Cornea receives nutrition and oxygen by tear film and aqueous humor.

Both aerobic and anaerobic pathways are involved in metabolism of cornea. The aerobic metabolism is by Krebs (tricarboxylic acid) cycle and hexose monophosphate shunt, and anaerobic metabolism is by glycolysis.*

PHYSIOLOGY OF CORNEA

Cornea should remain transparent to act as a refractive medium, while retaining the tough fibrous properties to provide protection to the vital intraocular contents. The reasons for corneal transparency are:*

1. *Avascularity of cornea*: The cornea is avascular in nature except for periphery of cornea and this helps to keep cornea transparent.
2. *State of relative dehydration*: The hydration of cornea is about 80%, thus making it relatively dehydrated compared to tear film, which lies anterior to cornea, and aqueous humor, which lies posterior to cornea. Cornea is kept in this relatively dehydrated state by epithelium, which acts as a barrier anteriorly and by endothelium with its metabolic pump mechanism.
3. *Absence of myelinated nerve fibers*: Though cornea is densely innervated by nerve supply, the nerves in the cornea are not myelinated, which help to keep cornea transparent.
4. *Arrangement of the collagen fibrils in corneal stroma*: It contributes significantly to the transparency of cornea as explained by the following theories:
   a. *Lattice theory of Maurice*: This was proposed by David Maurice. It states that cornea is transparent because of regular lattice arrangement of the collagen fibrils, which lead to destruction of scattered light by destructive interference or mutual interference.
   b. *Goldman theory of minimal separation of collagen fibrils*: This was proposed by Goldman and Benedek. It states that cornea is transparent because of presence of small diameter collagen fibrils with small separation, which will not cause scattering of light. The collagen fibrils are separated by less than one third of wavelength of light and to cause scattering of light because of interference with transmission of light, the separation has to be more than one third of wavelength of light.

GIST BOX 5.1

- Cornea is the transparent portion of the outer fibrous coat. It accounts for anterior one sixth of the outermost fibrous layer.
- Cornea contributes to two third of refractive power of the eye.
- Histologically, cornea is made up of five layers; recently, a new layer is added to it making it six layers. The layers of cornea include epithelium, Bowman's layer, stroma, Dua's layer, Descemet's membrane and endothelium.
- Cornea is transparent to act as a refractive medium and the transparency of cornea is because of avascularity of cornea, state of relative dehydration, absence of myelinated nerve fibers and arrangement of the collagen fibrils in corneal stroma.

CHAPTER

5.2 Congenital Anomalies of Cornea

EMBRYOLOGY OF CORNEA

Cornea develops from surface ectoderm and mesoderm, with surface ectoderm giving rise to epithelium, and rest of the layers of cornea being derived from mesoderm.

Surface ectoderm gives rise to epithelium of cornea by 5–6 weeks of gestation. As the lens vesicle gets separated from surface ectoderm, the mesoderm derived from mesenchymal neural crest cells form the anterior chamber. The migration of the mesenchymal cells leads to formation of rest of the layers of cornea.

> The defective migration of the mesenchymal neural crest cells give rise to congenital anomalies of the anterior segment involving cornea, anterior chamber, iris and lens.

CONGENITAL ANOMALIES OF CORNEA

Absence of Cornea

Absence of cornea as an isolated condition will not occur, as the development of cornea is related to the other structures in the anterior segment. Hence, it can be seen in association with other anomalies such as anophthalmos and cryptophthalmos.

Microcornea (Fig. 5.2.1)*

1. Cornea with horizontal diameter of less than 10 mm is called microcornea (Table 5.2.1). It can occur as an isolated condition or associated with microphthalmos or nanophthalmos.
2. It shows either autosomal dominant or autosomal recessive or sporadic inheritance. It can be unilateral or bilateral condition. Isolated microcornea is associated with shallow anterior chamber.
3. It can be associated with other ocular anomalies such as cataract, glaucoma, aniridia, etc. The systemic associations are Ehlers-Danlos syndrome, Weill-Marchesani syndrome and Nance-Horan syndrome (a syndrome characterized by cataract, microcornea, dental anomalies and mental retardation), Turner's syndrome, etc.
4. The treatment of the condition is by correction of hypermetropia in isolated cases and by treatment of the associated conditions such as cataract and glaucoma in cases with associated ocular anomalies.

Macrocornea or Megalocornea*

1. Cornea with horizontal diameter of more than 12 mm at birth or more than 13 mm at 2 years of age is called macrocornea (refer Table 5.2.1).

TABLE 5.2.1: Comparison between microcornea and macrocornea

Microcornea	*Macrocornea*
Corneal horizontal diameter < 10 mm	Corneal horizontal diameter > 12 mm at birth or > 13 mm at 2 years
Autosomal dominant, recessive or sporadic inheritance	X-linked recessive, hence affected ones are males with females being carriers Rarely autosomal dominant, recessive or sporadic inheritance
Unilateral or bilateral	Bilateral
Can be associated with microphthalmos or nanophthalmos	Can be associated with megalophthalmos
Associated refractive error is hypermetropia	Associated refractive error is myopia

2. It usually presents as X-linked recessive condition with more than 90% of the affected people being males.
3. It can present as simple megalocornea not associated with any ocular anomaly or megalocornea in association with anterior megalophthalmos, characterized by structural enlargement of the anterior segment of eye.
4. It presents as a bilateral condition and it is because of defective growth of the optic cup.
5. It has to be differentiated from buphthalmos—a condition characterized by marked enlargement of the eyeball seen in congenital or infantile glaucoma; and keratoglobus—a condition characterized by thinning and protrusion of the cornea (Table 5.2.2).
6. The ocular conditions associated with megalocornea are high myopia, iridodonesis, phacodonesis, ectopia lentis, etc. The systemic associations are Marfan's syndrome, Ehlers-Danlos syndrome, osteogenesis imperfecta, Down syndrome, etc.
7. The treatment of the condition is by correction of associated myopia in isolated cases and by treatment of the associated conditions in cases with associated ocular anomalies.

Sclerocornea

- Scleralization of the cornea characterized by opacification and vascularization of the cornea is called sclerocornea
- It can involve only periphery of the cornea or rarely total cornea
- It can be seen in association with cornea plana.

Cornea Plana

1. Cornea plana is a congenital anomaly of the cornea characterized by flat corneal

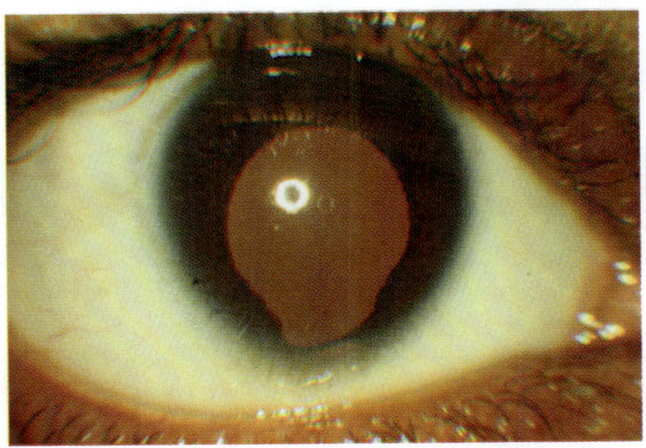

FIG. 5.2.1: Microcornea associated with coloboma iris

curvature. The corneal curvature is usually below 37 D in severe cases leading to hypermetropia.
2. The ocular conditions associated with cornea plana are sclerocornea, microphthalmos, microcornea and they are predisposed to develop angle closure glaucoma because of shallow anterior chamber.

Congenital Corneal Opacity**

The conditions are a group of diseases presenting as opacification of cornea in a newborn or in the neonatal period. Congenital and hereditary diseases, trauma, infective diseases, metabolic diseases and tumors can result in congenital corneal opacity (Table 5.2.3).

Causes

The causes for congenital corneal opacity are usually remembered by the mnemonic 'STUMPED' (Box 5.2.1), which is explained below:

1. *Sclerocornea*: It is characterized by scleralization of the cornea resulting in opacification and vascularization of the cornea.
2. *Trauma*: As the cornea in neonates is elastic in nature, it is prone to injury caused by raised intraocular pressure due to trauma resulting in breaks or tears in the Descemet's membrane. Because of tears in the Descemet's membrane, aqueous enters the stroma of cornea resulting in corneal edema and corneal opacity. Congenital glaucoma also leads to tears in Descemet's membrane and also corneal edema occurs by the same mechanism.
3. *Ulcer*: Viral keratitis such as herpetic keratitis, bacterial keratitis, etc. are the commonest causes for ulcers in neonates.
4. *Metabolic*: These causes occur because of malfunction of the lysosomal enzymes leading to accumulation of metabolic end products such as glycosaminoglycans in mucopolysaccharidoses, glycosphingolipid in sphingolipidoses resulting in corneal opacity. Corneal opacity is commonly seen

TABLE 5.2.2: Differential diagnosis of megalocornea*

Megalocornea	*Buphthalmos*	*Keratoglobus*
Cornea is enlarged in diameter with normal transparency, normal curvature with normal intraocular pressure (IOP)	Cornea is enlarged with enlargement of the whole eyeball and the enlarged cornea is hazy because of corneal edema and associated with increased IOP	Corneal diameter is normal, but thinning and protrusion of cornea resembles the appearance of megalocornea

TABLE 5.2.3: Etiology of corneal opacity

Causes	*Description*
Congenital and hereditary diseases	Sclerocornea, posterior keratoconus, Peter's anomaly, endothelial dystrophies
Trauma	Trauma leading to corneal edema caused by tears in Descemet's membrane as a result of birth trauma
Infective diseases	Corneal ulcer caused by bacteria and viruses
Metabolic diseases	Mucopolysaccharidoses, sphingolipidoses, mucolipidoses
Tumors	Limbal dermoid

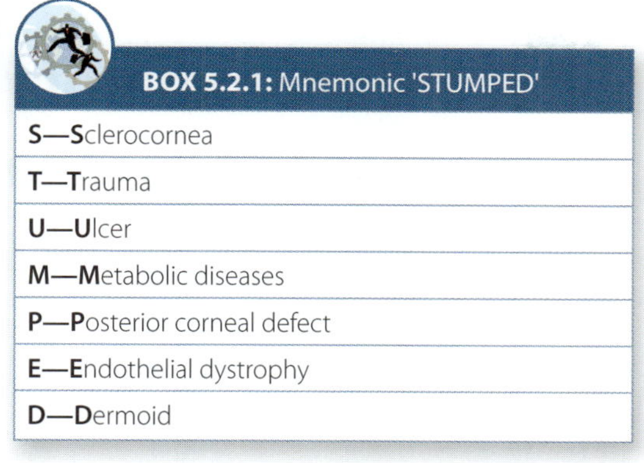

BOX 5.2.1: Mnemonic 'STUMPED'
S—Sclerocornea
T—Trauma
U—Ulcer
M—Metabolic diseases
P—Posterior corneal defect
E—Endothelial dystrophy
D—Dermoid

in types I (Hurler's syndrome), IV and VI mucopolysaccharidoses; Fabry's disease, a type of sphingolipidoses, and type III and type IV mucolipidoses. Corneal opacity is rare in types II (Hunter's syndrome) and III mucopolysaccharidoses.

5. *Posterior corneal defect*: It is seen in posterior keratoconus and Peter's anomaly. Peter's anomaly is a part of anterior segment dysgenesis or anterior chamber cleavage syndrome.
6. *Endothelial dystrophy*: Congenital hereditary endothelial dystrophy is described under corneal dystrophies.
7. *Dermoid*: Limbal dermoids usually involving the cornea or corneal dermoids result in corneal opacity.

A newborn or neonate presenting with congenital corneal opacity should be evaluated to find out the underlying disease responsible for corneal opacity, which include:

- Appropriate treatment should be done immediately to prevent the development of amblyopia and corneal blindness
- The systemic manifestations should be treated wherever possible
- The corneal opacity is treated by keratoplasty.

Posterior Keratoconus

Posterior keratoconus is a rare congenital anomaly of the cornea characterized by localized and sometimes generalized thinning of the posterior surface of cornea with anterior curvature of cornea being normal. It presents as a unilateral and non-progressive condition. It is usually identified as a localized thinning with associated corneal opacity on slit-lamp examination.

Anterior Chamber Cleavage Syndrome

The syndrome includes a spectrum of congenital diseases involving the cornea, anterior chamber, iris and lens caused by defective migration of the mesenchymal neural crest cells. The spectrum of diseases include:

1. *Posterior embryotoxon*: Prominent anteriorly displaced Schwalbe's line.
2. *Axenfeld's anomaly*: It is characterized by posterior embryotoxon with attachment of peripheral iris strands to it.
3. *Rieger's anomaly*: It is characterized by Axenfeld's anomaly plus hypoplasia of iris and corectopia of pupil.
4. *Peter's anomaly*: It is characterized by central leukomatous corneal opacity with underlying defect in the posterior cornea with iridocorneal or lenticulocorneal adhesions.

GIST BOX 5.2

- Cornea with horizontal diameter of less than 10 mm is called microcornea.
- Cornea with horizontal diameter of more than 12 mm at birth or more than 13 mm at 2 years of age is called macrocornea.
- The causes for congenital corneal opacity are sclerocornea, trauma, ulcer, metabolic diseases, posterior corneal defect, endothelial dystrophies and dermoid.

CHAPTER

5.3

Inflammatory Diseases of Cornea

KERATITIS***

Inflammatory diseases of cornea are called keratitis. It is characterized by all the signs of inflammation (Table 5.3.1).

TABLE 5.3.1: Signs of corneal inflammation

Signs	*Features*
Rubor	Redness in the form of circumcorneal congestion
Tumor	Edema in the form of corneal edema
Dolor	Pain
Functio laesa	Loss of function in the form of diminution of visual acuity

Classification of Keratitis

Etiological Classification

Based on the causative agent, keratitis is classified as discussed in Table 5.3.2.

TABLE 5.3.2: Etiological classification of keratitis

Types	*Examples*
Infective keratitis	Bacterial, viral, fungal, parasitic, spirochetal
Allergic keratitis	Vernal keratitis, phlyctenular keratitis
Traumatic keratitis	Mechanical trauma, chemical trauma
Trophic keratitis	Neurotrophic keratitis
Idiopathic keratitis	Mooren's ulcer
Keratitis associated with systemic diseases	Keratitis associated with collagen vascular diseases such as rheumatoid arthritis, systemic lupus erythematosus, etc.
Keratitis associated with diseases of skin	Rosacea keratitis

Pathological Classification

Based on the pathological features, keratitis is classified as:

- Suppurative keratitis
- Non-suppurative keratitis.

Morphological Classification

Based on the morphological features, keratitis is classified as:

- Ulcerative keratitis (Table 5.3.3)
- Non-ulcerative keratitis.

ULCERATIVE KERATITIS

Definition

Ulcerative keratitis is defined as inflammation of cornea characterized by discontinuity in the continuity of the overlying epithelium associated with necrosis of surrounding tissue. It is commonly called corneal ulcer (Fig. 5.3.1).

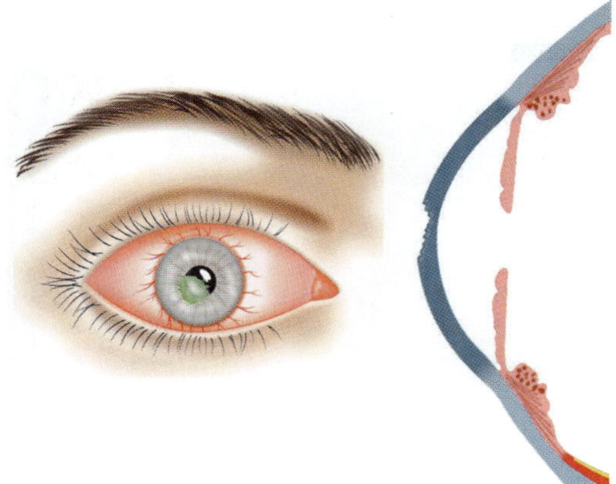

FIG. 5.3.1: Corneal ulcer or ulcerative keratitis

TABLE 5.3.3: Classification of ulcerative keratitis or corneal ulcer

Types	*Depending on*
Site	Central corneal ulcer Peripheral or marginal corneal ulcer Total corneal ulcer (Figs 5.3.2A and B)
Depth	Superficial corneal ulcer Deep corneal ulcer
Presence of hypopyon	Corneal ulcer with hypopyon Corneal ulcer without hypopyon Hypopyon corneal ulcer
Etiological agent	Infective Allergic Traumatic Trophic Idiopathic Corneal ulcer associated with systemic diseases

INFECTIVE KERATITIS OR CORNEAL ULCER

Inflammation of cornea caused by microbial infection is called infective keratitis. It can be caused by bacteria, fungi, viruses, protozoa, spirochetes, chlamydia, etc.

Infective keratitis is one of the major causes of corneal blindness across the world.

Bacterial and fungal corneal ulcers are most commonly seen in developing and underdeveloped countries, whereas viral corneal ulcers are commonly seen in developed countries.

Bacterial Corneal Ulcer***

Bacterial corneal ulcer is the most common type of infective keratitis.

Etiology

The common bacteria causing corneal ulcer are:

- Gram-positive cocci such as *Staphylococcus aureus* (*S. aureus*), *Staphylococcus epidermidis* (*S. epidermidis*), *Streptococcus pyogenes* (*S. pyogenes*), *Streptococcus pneumoniae* (*S. pneumoniae*), pneumococci
- Gram-negative cocci such as *Neisseria gonorrhoeae* (*N. gonorrhoeae*) and *Neisseria meningitidis* (*N. meningitidis*), etc.
- Gram-positive bacilli such as *Corynebacterium diphtheriae* (*C. diphtheriae*), *Bacillus cereus* (*B. cereus*), *Clostridium, Listeria monocytogenes* (*L. monocytogenes*), etc.
- Gram-negative bacilli such as *Pseudomonas aeruginosa* (*P. aeruginosa*), *Escherichia coli* (*E. coli*), *Proteus, Moraxella, Haemophilus aegyptius* (*H. aegyptius*), etc.

Pathogenesis

Since cornea along with conjunctiva is the exposed portion of the eyeball, it is at risk of getting infected by exogenous microbial agents. Like conjunctiva, cornea has got defense mechanisms to prevent infections. The defense mechanisms in cornea are:

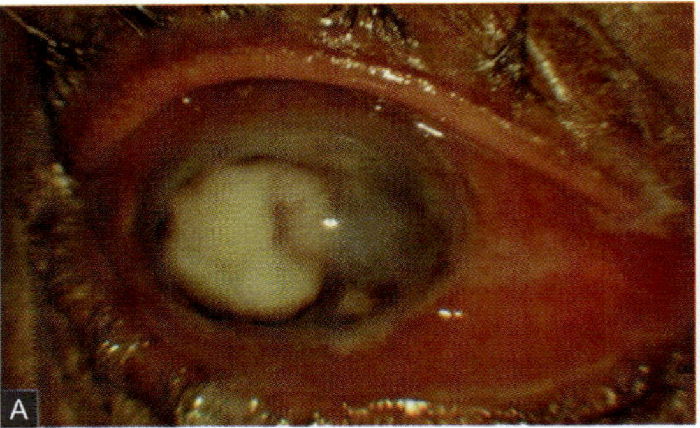
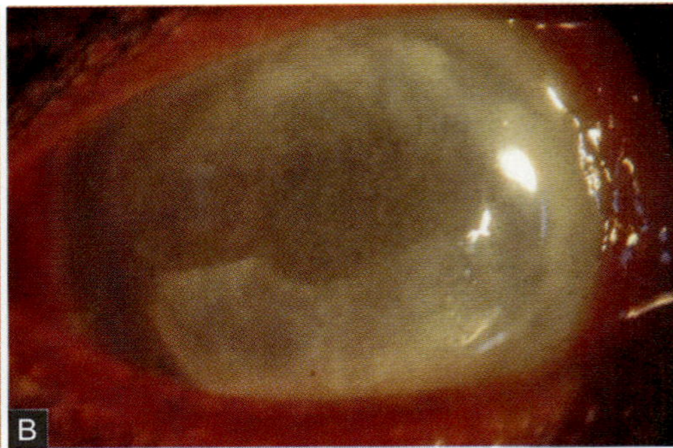

FIGS 5.3.2A and B: Total corneal ulcer

- Protective action of the eyelids
- Antimicrobial activity of tear film due to presence of lysozymes, immunoglobulins, etc.
- Presence of intact corneal epithelium.

Predisposing Risk Factors

Disruption of these normal defense mechanisms predisposes to infection of cornea as occurring in the following conditions:

- Damage to corneal epithelium as caused by vitamin A deficiency, corneal edema, exposure keratopathy, loss of corneal sensation, use of topical steroids, etc.
- Corneal abrasions caused by injury to cornea, contact lens-associated trauma, etc.
- Diseases of eyelids such as entropion leading to repeated corneal erosions, ectropion and lagophthalmos leading to exposure keratopathy
- Diseases affecting tear film, e.g. dry eyes.

Mode of Spread

1. Exogenous route is the commonest mode of infection. The infection may be acquired from external injuries with infected vegetative matter or foreign bodies.
2. The infection may be acquired by contiguous spread from the neighboring structures such as conjunctiva, sclera, uveal tract, etc.
3. Endogenous route is rarely seen because of avascularity of cornea.

Most of the bacteria cannot penetrate intact corneal epithelium except for:

- *Neisseria gonorrhoeae* and *Neisseria meningitidis*
- *Listeria monocytogenes*
- *Corynebacterium diphtheriae*
- *Haemophilus aegyptius*
- Hence, the above mentioned bacteria would not require pre-existing corneal abrasion or damage to corneal epithelium to cause corneal ulcer.

Pathology

The pathology of the disease is explained under four headings:

1. *Stage of infiltration*: This stage is characterized by infiltration of the corneal epithelium from polymorphonuclear cells, as a result of chemokines produced as a response to invasion by the microbial organism. The reaction between the inflammatory cells and the toxins produced by the microbes lead to necrosis of the corneal tissue (Figs 5.3.3A and E).
2. *Stage of ulceration*: This stage is characterized by desquamation of the necrotic and edematous epithelium resulting in the formation of ulcer. If the invading microbial organism is virulent or if the host defense mechanism is weak, the ulcer enlarges and may lead to descemetocele and perforation of corneal ulcer (Figs 5.3.3B and F).

3. *Stage of regression*: This stage is characterized by regression of the infiltration as a result of defense mechanisms of the host. This stage shows appearance of line of demarcation surrounding the ulcer; polymorphonuclear cells are replaced by mononuclear cells, which phagocytose the necrotic debris resulting in healing of the ulcer (Figs 5.3.3C and G).
4. *Stage of healing*: This stage is characterized by formation of granulation tissue resulting in cicatrization and healing of the ulcer. Depending on the depth of involvement of the inflammation, it leads to opacity and superficial lesions not penetrating Bowman's membrane heal without leaving any opacity (Figs 5.3.3D and H).

Clinical Features

Symptoms

Ocular pain, redness, watering, photophobia, diminution of vision, etc. Ocular pain and photophobia are because of stimulation of sensory nerve endings of cornea, watering is because of reflex hyperlacrimation, redness is because of congestion of circumcorneal vessels and diminution of vision is because of corneal edema, corneal infiltration, etc.

Signs

On examination

1. Eyelids show the edema because of the inflammation.
2. Conjunctiva shows chemosis and circumcorneal congestion because of the inflammation.
3. Cornea shows grayish white infiltration in the initial stages and corneal ulcer with necrosis in the later stages. The typical characteristic features of the ulcer depend on the causative organism.
4. Anterior chamber may show hypopyon.
5. Iris may show features suggestive of iritis, i.e. muddy colored iris.

Clinical Course

The clinical course of corneal ulcer depends on the virulence of the organism causing corneal ulcer, resistance offered by host immune system and the effect of treatment (Table 5.3.4).

Complications**

1. *Ectatic cicatrix*: It results because of spreading of the infection resulting in sloughing and thinning of the cornea, which bulges out because of influence of intraocular pressure (IOP).
2. *Descemetocele*: It is the herniation of Descemet's membrane as a transparent vesicle through the floor of the corneal ulcer. It is because of deeper penetration of the corneal ulcer and the resistance offered from Descemet's membrane. It may rupture leading to perforated corneal ulcer.
3. *Perforated corneal ulcer* (Figs 5.3.4A and B, Fig. 5.3.5): It is because of penetration of the corneal ulcer involving the full thickness of cornea. It results because of rupture of descemetocele due to minimal trauma or sudden exertion leading to increase in IOP.
4. *Anterior staphyloma*: It is the abnormal protrusion of uveal tissue, through weak outer coat of the eyeball. It occurs secondary to localized or diffuse thinning of the outer coat of the eyeball, cornea or sclera.

TABLE 5.3.4: Clinical course of corneal ulcer

Healed corneal ulcer	*Ectatic cicatrix*	*Perforated corneal ulcer*
This occurs when the host immune system and treatment overcome the virulence of the causative organism	This occurs when the virulence of the causative organism is high and host immune system is not able to control the infection leading to sloughing, thinning and bulging of the cornea	This occurs when thinned and sloughed cornea gives away the stroma resulting in perforation of cornea

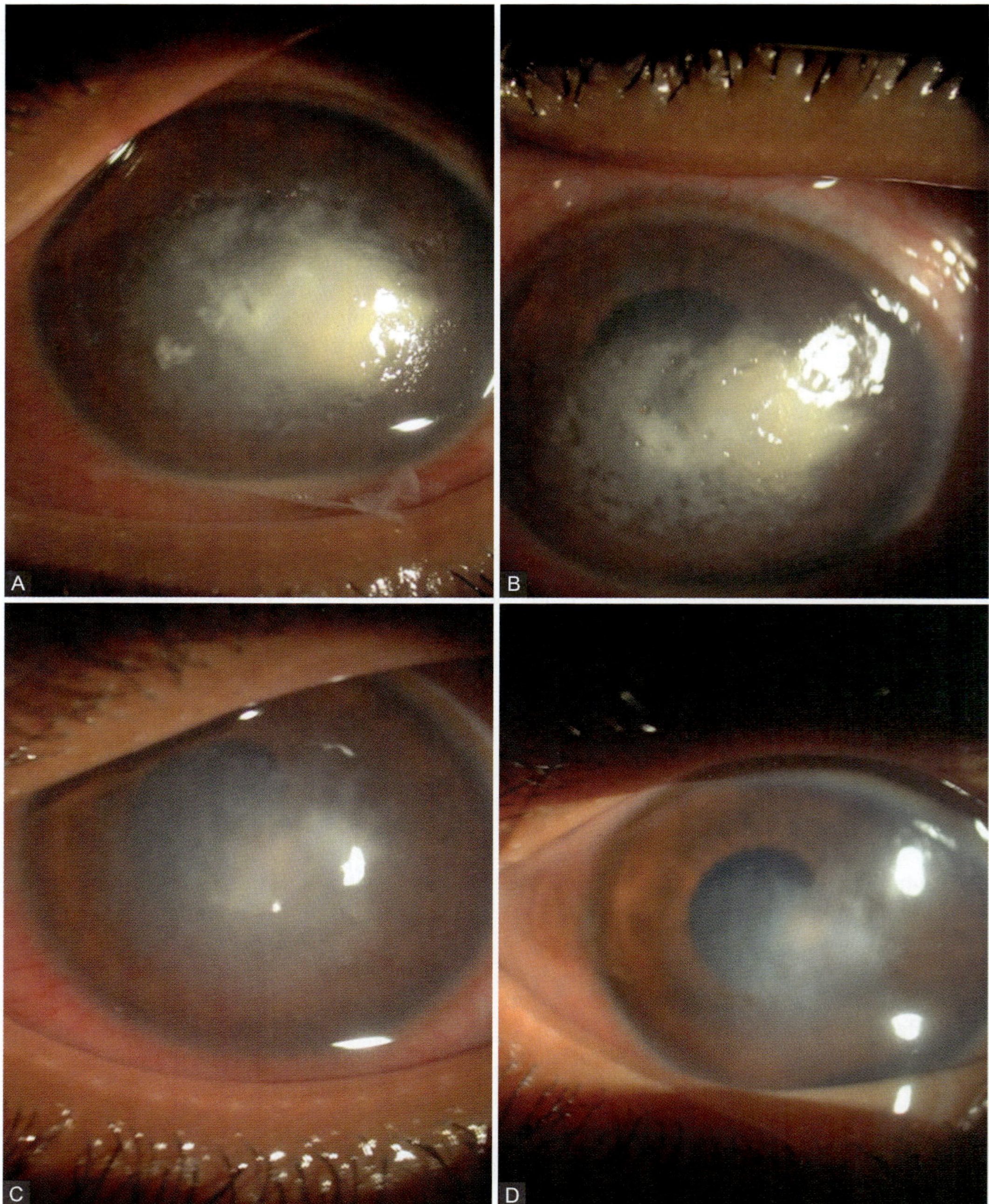

FIGS 5.3.3A to D: Bacterial corneal ulcer photographs. **A.** Stage of progressive infiltration; **B.** Stage of active ulceration; **C.** Stage of regression; **D.** Stage of cicatrization.

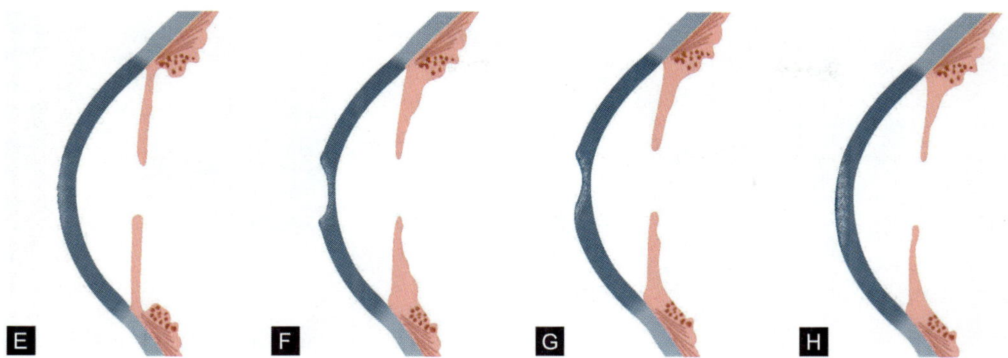

FIGS 5.3.3E to H: Bacterial corneal ulcer diagrammatic representation. **E.** Stage of progressive infiltration; **F.** Stage of active ulceration; **G.** Stage of regression; **H.** Stage of cicatrization.

The uveal tissue, which lies below the cornea or sclera bulges out leading to staphyloma.

5. *Endophthalmitis*: It occurs in case of high virulence of the causative organism because of extension of infection to involve the inner coats and cavities of the eye.
6. *Panophthalmitis*: It also occurs in case of high virulence of the causative organism because of extension of infection to involve all the three coats and cavities of the eye.
7. *Secondary glaucoma*: It is because of inflammatory exudates blocking the trabecular meshwork.
8. *Corneal opacity*: It is the end result of healing of corneal ulcer. The grade of corneal opacity depends on the depth of penetration of the ulcer.

Investigations

1. Corneal scraping for culture and sensitivity is required for definitive diagnosis and treatment according to the sensitivity report. Corneal scraping is done under topical anesthesia using a 26-gauge needle. The material obtained is inoculated on blood agar for bacteria and Sabouraud's agar for fungi. Gram staining and Giemsa's staining are done for bacteria and potassium hydroxide (KOH) mount for fungi.
2. Ocular examination to look for presence of predisposing factors for development of corneal ulcer such as eyelid problems, chronic dacryocystitis, etc.
3. Examination of the corneal ulcer under slit lamp, after staining with fluorescein to study the morphology of corneal ulcer, which may give clues regarding the possible causative agent.

1. Gram-negative bacilli such as *Pseudomonas* are known to produce corneal ulcers with rapid necrosis, presenting as sloughing corneal ulcer. Presence of greenish yellow mucopurulent discharge is typical of pseudomonas infection.
2. Gram-positive cocci such as staphylococci are known to produce localized oval or round grayish white ulcer with distinct margins.
3. Viral corneal ulcers such as herpes simplex viral keratitis cause dendritic ulcer often associated with decreased corneal sensation.
4. Fungal corneal ulcers usually appear dry, grayish white, elevated, feathery margins, sterile immune ring and associated with big hypopyon or endothelial plaque.
5. Acanthamoeba corneal ulcers are usually seen as a complication of contact lens wear present as multiple stromal infiltrates with severe pain because of radial keratoneuritis.

Treatment

Non-specific treatment

Non-specific treatment is done by use of:

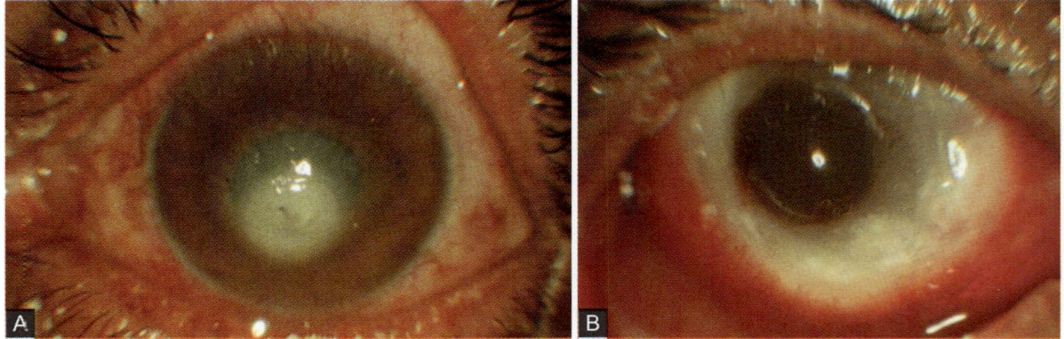

FIGS 5.3.4A and B: Perforated corneal ulcer

1. Cycloplegic agents such as atropine (1%) eye ointment, Homatropine eyedrops or cyclopentolate eyedrops, etc.
2. Oral anti-inflammatory drugs such as diclofenac sodium, ibuprofen, etc. for relief from pain and for treatment of associated inflammatory symptoms.

Role of Atropine in Treatment of General Ulcer*

Atropine decreases pain by relieving ciliary spasm, decreases exudation by reducing hyperemia, prevents formation of synechia because of associated iridocyclitis, increases blood supply to uvea and brings more antibodies to the aqueous humor.

Specific treatment

1. Specific treatment is by use of topical antibiotics in the form of eyedrops and eye ointments. Broad-spectrum antibiotic eyedrops are started initially and later the antibiotic eyedrops are replaced by specific antibiotics according to the culture and sensitivity report. The eyedrops are instilled as frequently as half hourly depending on the severity of the ulcer. Usually, fortified preparations of the eyedrops are preferred over the commercially available preparations. The commonly used fortified preparations are fortified tobramycin (14 mg/mL), fortified cefazolin (75 mg/mL), fortified ceftriaxone (50 mg/mL), etc. as commercially available preparations contain less concentration of the antibiotics compared to fortified preparations.
2. Systemic antibiotics are indicated in patients with total corneal ulcer, marginal corneal ulcer, perforated corneal ulcer, corneal ulcer associated with hypopyon, etc.
3. Corneal ulcers not responding to medical line of management requires evaluation to rule out causes for non-healing corneal ulcer and treatment of causes, if any.
4. Surgical management in the form of therapeutic keratoplasty is indicated for cases not responding to medical line of management.

Non-healing Corneal Ulcer**

Normally, corneal ulcers heal by 2–4 weeks because of formation of granulation tissue; when a corneal ulcer fails to heal within this time, it is referred to as non-healing corneal ulcer.

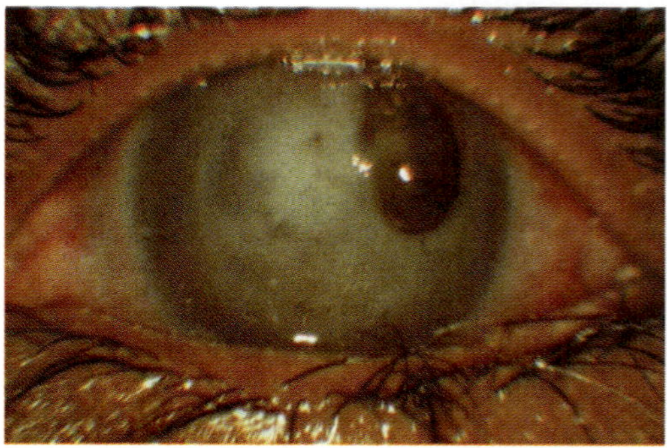

FIG. 5.3.5: Perforated corneal ulcer with iris prolapse

Causes

The causes for non-healing corneal ulcer are:

1. Systemic causes such as uncontrolled diabetes mellitus, treatment with immunosuppressive drugs and steroids, malnutrition, immunosuppressive diseases, etc.
2. Ocular causes such as untreated dacryocystitis, diseases of the cornea, i.e. corneal edema, corneal dystrophies, corneal degenerations, presence of predisposing factors for corneal ulceration such as entropion leading to repeated corneal erosions, ectropion and lagophthalmos leading to exposure keratopathy, etc.
3. Inadequate treatment or wrong treatment.

Treatment

- Evaluation to look for underlying causes for non-healing corneal ulcer and treatment of predisposing causes, if any
- Treatment based on the culture and sensitivity report if not started before
- Mechanical debridement of the ulcer under topical anesthesia
- Cauterization of the ulcer by using thermal cautery or chemical cauterization by using carbolic acid
- Therapeutic keratoplasty in cases not responding to medical line of management.

Perforated Corneal Ulcer**

Extension of corneal ulcer to involve the full thickness of cornea by perforating the Descemet's membrane is called perforated corneal ulcer.

Etiopathogenesis

Bacterial corneal ulcers are the most common corneal ulcers associated with corneal perforation. The other common corneal ulcers associated with corneal perforation are:

- Infective ulcerative keratitis caused by fungi, viruses, etc.
- Ulcerative keratitis-associated systemic collagen vascular diseases
- Post-traumatic corneal ulcers
- Neurotrophic corneal ulcers
- Corneal ulcers associated with keratomalacia, Stevens-Johnson syndrome.

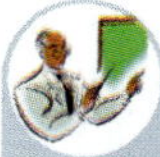

Descemetocele*

The Descemet's membrane offers resistance to the penetration of the necrotic process and it bulges forward as a result of intraocular pressure (IOP). This ectasia of the cornea in which epithelium, Bowman's membrane and stroma are completely destroyed leaving behind Descemet's membrane and endothelium of cornea is called descemetocele.

Descemetocele represents stage of impending perforation and can perforate resulting in perforated corneal ulcer because of strain, IOP or because of extension of the necrotic process.

Treatment of descemetocele is by:

- Asking the patient to avoid straining, sneezing, etc.
- Reducing the IOP by using oral antiglaucoma drugs, i.e. acetazolamide, etc.
- Use of tissue adhesive glues, e.g. cyanoacrylate
- Bandage soft contact lenses
- Therapeutic keratoplasty.

Clinical Features

Symptoms

1. Patient may give history of sudden escape of liquid from the eyes either spontaneously or commonly following straining, violent coughing, rubbing of eyes or squeezing of eyes.
2. Decrease in pain as a result of decrease in IOP and further decrease in visual acuity with perforation.

Signs

Flat anterior chamber, iris prolapse, soft eyeball, etc. are the signs of perforated corneal ulcer.

Sequelae of perforation of corneal ulcer

1. *Iris prolapse*: In case of small perforations, iris can plug the perforated site leading to adherent leukoma after healing of the corneal ulcer. In case of bigger perforations, it can lead to anterior staphyloma.
2. Exudation or anterior dislocation of the lens because of sudden anterior movement of the iris-lens diaphragm.

3. Intraocular extension of infection leading to endophthalmitis or panophthalmitis.

Treatment

Once the corneal ulcer perforates, topical eyedrops should be discontinued and replaced by oral or systemic drugs:

- Small corneal perforation less than 1 mm can be treated by use of tissue adhesive glues such as cyanoacrylate or bandage soft contact lenses
- Bigger corneal perforations more than 5 mm require tectonic keratoplasty.

HYPOPYON CORNEAL ULCER AND CORNEAL ULCER ASSOCIATED WITH HYPOPYON

Corneal Ulcer Associated with Hypopyon

Corneal ulcers caused by virulent microbial organisms or ulcers seen in immunocompromised individuals are usually associated with hypopyon (Fig. 5.3.6).

Hypopyon in corneal ulcers is usually because of associated toxic iritis or because of extension of infection into the anterior chamber. Most of the bacteria cannot penetrate Descemet's membrane; hence, in bacterial corneal ulcers,the hypopyon is usually sterile.

Pneumococcus, Pseudomonas, Staphylococcus, Streptococcus and fungi are the common organisms causing corneal ulcer with hypopyon.

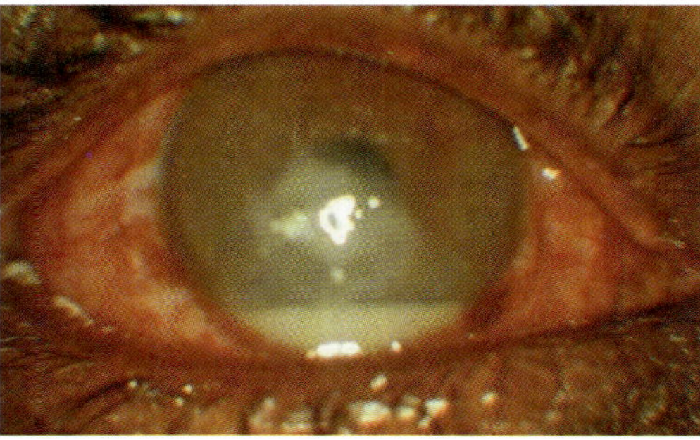

FIG. 5.3.6: Corneal ulcer with hypopyon

Pneumococcus and *Pseudomonas* cause most virulent corneal ulcers with hypopyon resulting in complications more often, hence are considered as most dangerous of all the types of corneal ulcers associated with hypopyon.

The clinical features, investigations and treatment are similar to bacterial corneal ulcer.

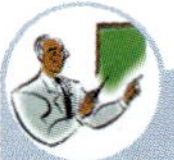

Hypopyon*

Definition

Collection of pus (inflammatory exudates consisting of predominantly leukocytes) in anterior chamber is called hypopyon.

Etiopathogenesis

Hypopyon is seen because of outpouring of polymorphonuclear cells into anterior chamber as a result of severe inflammation or infection. The common causes for hypopyon are:

- Corneal ulcer
- Acute iridocyclitis
- Endophthalmitis
- Panophthalmitis.

Clinical features

Clinical features are seen depending on the cause for hypopyon. Examination shows presence of grayish white pus in the anterior chamber.

Hypopyon remains sterile in acute iridocyclitis and in corneal ulcer in cases where the microbial agent has not penetrated the Descemet's membrane. Since bacteria cannot penetrate Descemet's membrane so hypopyon remains sterile in case of bacterial corneal ulcers, whereas hypopyon shows infective organisms in fungal corneal ulcers, as fungi can penetrate Descemet's membrane.

Differential diagnosis

Hypopyon has to be differentiated from:

1. *Pseudohypopyon*: Collection of malignant cells in intraocular malignant conditions or liquefied cortex in hypermature cataract simulating the appearance of hypopyon.
2. *Inverse hypopyon*: Collection of silicone oil following vitreoretinal surgery done using silicone oil. As silicone oil is lighter than water, it collects in the anterior chamber superiorly; hence, it is called inverse hypopyon.

Treatment

Treatment of hypopyon is done by treating the underlying disease. With the treatment of the underlying disease, hypopyon gets absorbed and disappears.

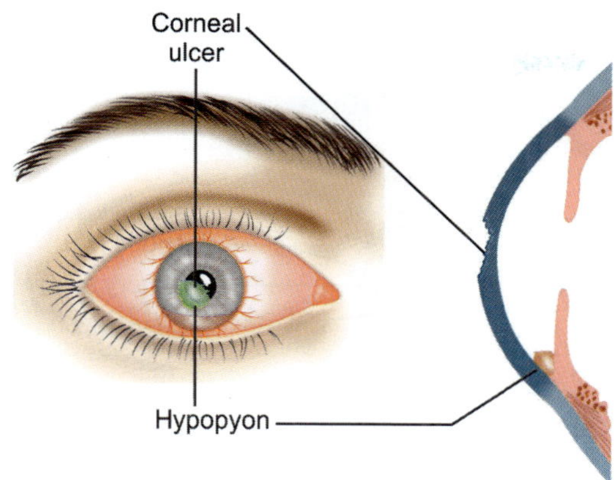

FIG. 5.3.7: Hypopyon corneal ulcer

Hypopyon Corneal Ulcer***

The characteristic corneal ulcer produced by *Pneumococcus* is called hypopyon corneal ulcer (Fig. 5.3.7). It is also called ulcus serpens or serpiginous corneal ulcer.

> The term hypopyon corneal ulcer is reserved for corneal ulcer caused by pneumococci, whereas all others are included in corneal ulcer with hypopyon.

Etiopathogenesis

The corneal ulcer is caused by high-virulent strains in people with decreased immunity, hence more common in immunocompromised patients, elderly debilitated individuals, chronic alcoholics, etc. The development of hypopyon is because of associated toxic iritis leading to exudation and collection of polymorphonuclear cells in anterior chamber.

Clinical Features

Symptoms

Hypopyons are similar to corneal ulcers such as ocular pain, redness, watering, photophobia, diminution of vision, etc.

Signs

The characteristic signs of hypopyon corneal ulcer are:

- Grayish white ulcer with dense infiltration, which spreads over the cornea in a serpiginous fashion with simultaneous presence of healing signs at one end and infiltration at the other end
- Infiltration denser in the deeper layers of cornea, which often leads to posterior corneal abscess or posterior corneal ulcer
- Presence of hypopyon.

Hypopyon corneal ulcer spreads more rapidly and may perforate early as compared to corneal ulcer without hypopyon.

Investigations

The hypopyons are similar to those described under bacterial corneal ulcer.

Treatment

Treatment is similar to that described under bacterial corneal ulcer; however, treatment has to be more aggressive and surgical intervention such as therapeutic keratoplasty should be considered early in cases where ulcer is not responding to medical line of treatment to prevent perforation of corneal ulcer.

Fungal Corneal Ulcer or Mycotic Keratitis***

Pseudomonas Corneal Ulcer

Corneal ulcer caused by *Pseudomonas* is the most dangerous of all the corneal infections. It is a common cause for contact lens-associated bacterial keratitis. It produces rapid necrosis because of production of destructive enzymes such as lipase, protease, etc. resulting in sloughing corneal ulcer. Presence of greenish yellow mucopurulent discharge is typical of pseudomonas infection.

Pseudomonas ulcer progresses rapidly and perforates early; hence aggressive management is needed in pseudomonas corneal ulcer.

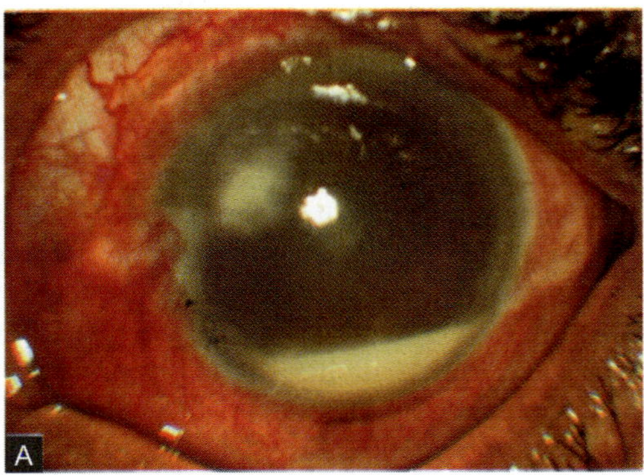

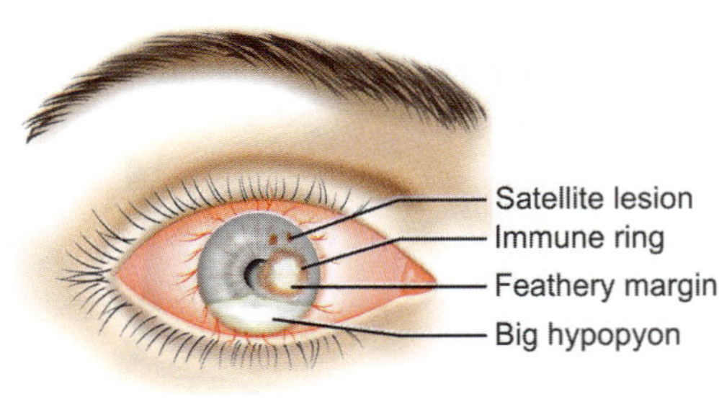

FIGS 5.3.8A and B: Fungal corneal ulcer. **A.** Photograph; **B.** Diagrammatic representation.

Definition

The inflammation of cornea caused by any fungal infection is called mycotic keratitis (Figs 5.3.8A and B).

Etiopathogenesis

Fungal keratitis is less commonly seen in developed countries, but it still continues to be a major type of infective keratitis in developing countries in the tropical region.

In the recent past, there is an increase in the incidence of fungal keratitis because of increase in the incidence of human immunodeficiency virus (HIV) infection, excessive and misappropriate use of antibiotics and steroids, which disturb the symbiosis between bacteria and fungi:

- Filamentous fungi such as *Aspergillus, Fusarium* and yeasts such as *Candida* are the fungi more frequently associated with mycotic keratitis
- Filamentary fungal keratitis is more commonly seen following injury with vegetative matter or injury by animal tail infested by fungi
- Candida keratitis is more commonly seen in people with pre-existing diseases, including ocular surface diseases causing corneal edema, dry eyes and systemic diseases causing immunosuppression.

Unlike bacteria, fungi can invade the Descemet's membrane and reach anterior chamber causing severe infection. Hence, hypopyon in case of mycotic keratitis is not sterile as in bacterial keratitis and contains fungi. Hence, high index of suspicion is necessary to diagnose fungal keratitis and administer appropriate treatment in the initial stages of the disease to prevent devastating complications of mycotic keratitis.

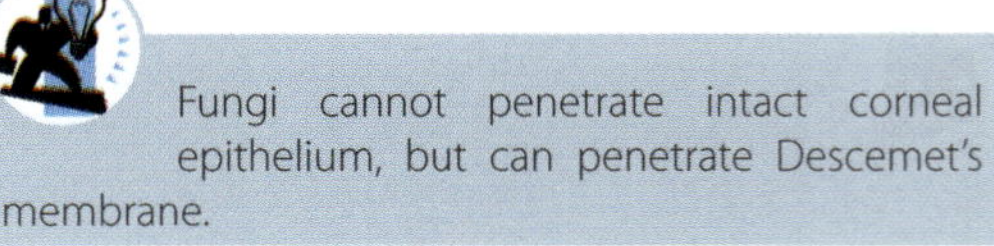
Fungi cannot penetrate intact corneal epithelium, but can penetrate Descemet's membrane.

Clinical Features

Symptoms

The symptoms in case of fungal corneal ulcer are less severe compared to bacterial corneal ulcer and the disease runs a chronic course. The symptoms include ocular pain, redness, watering, photophobia, diminution of vision, etc.

Signs

The signs of typical filamentous fungal corneal ulcer and a typical fungal corneal ulcer caused by *Candida* have been discussed in Table 5.3.5.

Investigations

Fungal corneal ulcer has to be differentiated from other infective keratitis caused by the bacteria, *Acanthamoeba*. History, clinical signs and laboratory investigations such as KOH

TABLE 5.3.5: Signs of typical filamentous fungal corneal ulcer and a typical fungal corneal ulcer caused by *Candida*

A typical filamentous fungal corneal ulcer	*A typical fungal corneal ulcer caused by Candida*
D—**D**ry appearance **E**—**E**levated margins **F**—**F**eathery extensions **G**—**G**rayish white or yellow in color **H**—**B**ig hypopyon or endothelial plaque **I**—**I**mmune ring and independent satellite lesions	Grayish white or grayish yellow oval ulcer with dense infiltration usually affecting a compromised cornea because of pre-existing ocular surface disease

mount (Fig. 5.3.9) and culture on Sabouraud's agar confirm the diagnosis.

Treatment (Table 5.3.6)

- Non-specific treatment is similar to treatment of bacterial corneal ulcer
- Specific treatment is done by using antifungal drugs
- Cases not responding to conventional medical line of management are treated by intracameral amphotericin B (5–10 μg in 0.1 mL)
- Therapeutic keratoplasty is done in refractory cases.

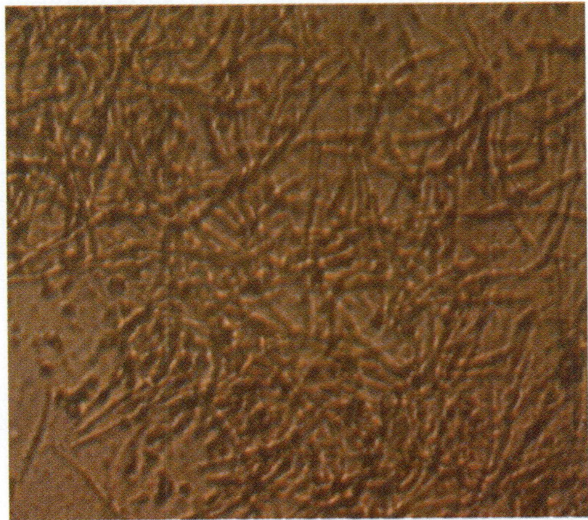

FIG. 5.3.9: Potassium hydroxide (KOH) mount showing fungi

Parasitic or Protozoal Keratitis

Definition

Inflammation of cornea caused by protozoa is called protozoal keratitis. The common protozoa causing keratitis are:
- Acanthamoeba
- Onchocerca
- Microsporidia.

*Acanthamoeba Keratitis***

Etiopathogenesis

Acanthamoeba is a free-living protozoa without human carrier state or insect vector found in soil, air and water. It exists in two forms:
1. Trophozoite.
2. Cystic form.

Trophozoite form is the infective form, which binds to corneal epithelium and penetrates it to enter stroma. In stroma, trophozoite may undergo encystations and exists as cystic form.

Acanthamoeba keratitis (Fig. 5.3.10), though rare, can lead to devastating complications leading to blindness, as it is resistant to treatment.

Acanthamoeba is known to cause amebic encephalitis and disseminated amebic disease in immunocompromised people. It can cause keratitis in immunocompetent people.

TABLE 5.3.6: Treatment for fusarium keratitis and for aspergillus and candida keratitis

Treatment of fusarium keratitis	*Treatment for aspergillus and candida keratitis*
• Natamycin (5%) eyedrops initially hourly and then gradually tapered • Oral fluconazole (100 mg) twice a day in case of deep keratitis • Broad-spectrum topical antibiotic eyedrops to prevent secondary bacterial infection	• Amphotericin B (0.15%) eyedrops • Oral fluconazole (100 mg) twice a day in case of deep keratitis • Broad-spectrum topical antibiotic eyedrops to prevent secondary bacterial infection

Acanthamoeba keratitis is most commonly associated with use of contact lenses in developed countries. In India and other developing countries, the infection occurs more commonly because of exposure to contaminated water combined with ocular trauma. With increase in the use of contact lenses, the incidence of acanthamoeba keratitis following contact lens-associated trauma is increasing in developing countries also.

Clinical features

Patients with acanthamoeba keratitis usually give history of using contact lens with homemade solutions to clean contact lenses or swimming in contaminated water.

Symptoms

- They are similar to bacterial corneal ulcer such as ocular pain, redness, watering, photophobia, diminution of vision, etc.
- Pain is usually out of proportion to the corneal infiltration and it is very severe because of associated infiltration along corneal nerves called keratoneuritis.

Keratoneuritis is a characteristic feature of acanthamoeba keratitis and pseudomonas keratitis.

Signs

- In the initial stages, grayish white infiltration, keratoneuritis, pseudodendritic ulcers are seen
- In later stages, ring abscess, stromal infiltration and eventual corneal melting or opacification are seen.

Laboratory investigations

Acanthamoeba keratitis is often misdiagnosed and it offers as a diagnostic challenge, as it resembles viral keratitis in the initial stages and resembles fungal or bacterial keratitis in later stages, i.e.:

- Staining of the corneal scrapings by calcofluor white, Giemsa, lactophenol cotton blue can show cysts and trophozoites of *Acanthamoeba*
- Potassium hydroxide mount, Gram staining, periodic acid-Schiff can identify acanthamoeba cysts
- Culture on *E. coli* enriched non-nutrient agar yields for the growth of *Acanthamoeba*
- Confocal microscopy is the useful newer diagnostic tool for in vivo diagnosis of *Acanthamoeba*.

Treatment

Treatment is usually required for long duration of 6–12 months, which include:

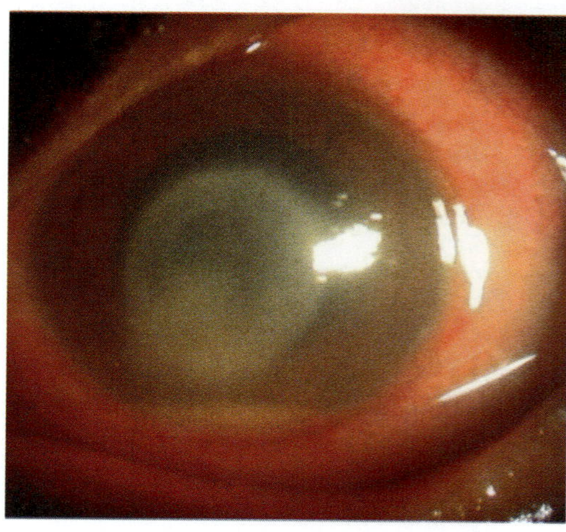

FIG. 5.3.10: Acanthamoeba keratitis

1. Chlorhexidine digluconate and polyhexamethylene biguanide commonly used antiseptic agents are the first-line drugs and they are active against both trophozoite and cysts of *Acanthamoeba*. Propamidine isethionate and neomycin are also effective against *Acanthamoeba*.
2. Azoles such as fluconazole, itraconazole, etc. are used for systemic treatment.
3. Patients not responding to medical line of treatment are treated by surgical treatment in the form of keratoplasty.

Onchocerca Keratitis

Etiopathogenesis

Onchocerca keratitis is caused by protozoal helminth *Onchocerca volvulus*. It is transmitted by bite of black flies belonging to the genus *Simulium,* which are found along fast-flowing rivers, as these flies require well-oxygenated water to mature. Hence, the disease is found along the rivers and it is called river blindness.

> Onchocerca keratitis affects about 18 million people worldwide with more than 90% of them living in Africa. It is the second leading infective cause of blindness next only to trachoma.

Larvae called microfilariae are the infective forms, which enter following the bite from female black flies. The microfilariae migrate through the subcutaneous tissues and mature into adult worms, which become encysted as nodules in the skin. Each adult worm has a life span of about 10 years and during this course, it releases millions of microfilariae, which enter circulation and reach various organs leading to manifestations of the disease.

Clinical features

The ocular manifestations develop later in the disease following skin manifestations. The corneal manifestations are punctate keratitis, sclerosing keratitis, subepithelial opacities and corneal edema. Other ocular manifestations are uveitis, chorioretinitis and optic neuritis.

Investigations

Diagnosis is often difficult and it depends on the isolation of the organism from skin snips. Immunoassay tests are available to identify the *Onchocerca*-specific antigens. Live microfilariae can be seen in the cornea and anterior chamber.

Treatment

Oral ivermectin in a dose of 150 μg/kg is the mainstay of treatment. It is usually given as single dose and it is repeated once in 6 months. The presence of sclerosing keratitis requires treatment by topical steroids. Community mass treatment by ivermectin and vector control is the method employed under Onchocerciasis Control Program.

Microsporidia Keratitis

Microsporidia are one of the commonest parasitic pathogens associated with opportunistic pathogens in HIV infection. Microsporidia keratitis has increased in frequency because of increase in the incidence of HIV infection.

Microsporidia are known to cause stromal keratitis in immunocompetent individuals, and epithelial keratitis is seen in immunocompromised patients. Gram staining, confocal microscopy and electron microscopy are the commonest diagnostic tools employed to identify the organism.

Antifungals such as itraconazole are active against microsporidia. Topical voriconazole, fumagillin and propamidine are also effective against microsporidia.

Viral Keratitis***

Definition

Inflammation of cornea caused by viruses is called viral keratitis. The common viruses causing keratitis are:

- Deoxyribonucleic acid (DNA) viruses such as herpes simplex virus (HSV), varicella-zoster virus, adenovirus, cytomegalovirus, etc.
- Ribonucleic acid (RNA) viruses such as measles virus, mumps virus, arbovirus, etc.

Herpes Simplex Keratitis**

Viral keratitis, specifically herpes simplex viral keratitis is the most common type of infective keratitis in developed countries. Of late, the incidence of herpes simplex keratitis is increasing in developing countries also because of overuse of antibiotics.

Etiopathogenesis

Herpes simplex virus is a DNA virus with humans as the only source of HSV. Herpes simplex virus exists in two forms, i.e. HSV-1 and HSV-2. HSV-1 usually causes infection above the waist and HSV-2 causes infection below the waist. HSV-1 infection is acquired by close contact or by kissing with the infected individual and HSV-2 is transmitted venerally.

Herpes simplex virus infection manifests in two forms:

1. Primary.
2. Recurrent.

Primary infection is acquired early in childhood and the infection remains dormant in ganglionic neurons. The manifestations of primary infection are seen only in 10% of cases and recurrent infection is more common. The recurrent infection is known to occur in conditions associated with decreased systemic immunity, high fever, stress, etc.

Clinical features

Primary ocular herpes

Primary ocular herpes is seen only in 10% of cases and is seen in children between the ages of 6 months and 5 years. Because of protection by the maternal antibodies, the infection is not seen in children below 6 months of age. The ocular manifestations of primary ocular herpes are:

- Vesicular eruptions involving the skin of eyelids
- Acute follicular conjunctivitis
- Corneal lesions such as punctate epithelial keratitis and rarely dendritic keratitis.

Recurrent ocular herpes

Recurrent infection is more common than the primary infection. The ocular manifestations of recurrent ocular herpes are:

- Epithelial keratitis manifesting as punctate epithelial keratitis, dendritic keratitis and geographical keratitis
- Stromal keratitis manifesting as disciform keratitis and necrotizing stromal keratitis
- Endotheliitis manifesting as disciform endotheliitis, diffuse endotheliitis and linear endotheliitis
- Neurotrophic keratopathy.

Epithelial keratitis**

Epithelial keratitis is the inflammation of epithelium of cornea and is infective in nature (Figs 5.3.11A and B, Table 5.3.7).

Dendritic Ulcer*

Typical dendritic ulcer is caused by HSV. It has to be differentiated from pseudodendritic ulcer caused by herpes zoster, drug-induced epithelial toxicity, healing corneal epithelial defect, etc.

TABLE 5.3.7: Manifestations of epithelial keratitis

Punctate epithelial keratitis	*Dendritic keratitis**	*Geographical keratitis*	*Metaherpetic keratitis*
It is the earliest lesion seen involving the epithelium of cornea and it is seen in both primary and recurrent herpes It presents either as fine or diffuse punctate vesicles involving the epithelium of cornea	It is the commonest presentation of herpes simplex virus keratitis and it is seen usually in recurrent herpes, rarely in primary herpes (Fig. 5.3.12) It results because of fusion of vesicles of punctate epithelial keratitis It presents as irregular linear lesion with branches with presence of knobbed ends	It is seen in cases not treated or because of use of topical steroids It is because of enlargement of dendritic ulcer It presents with irregular shape and size, i.e. geographical configuration	It is not an infective disease, but a trophic keratitis caused by decreased corneal sensation, drug toxicity caused by antiviral drugs

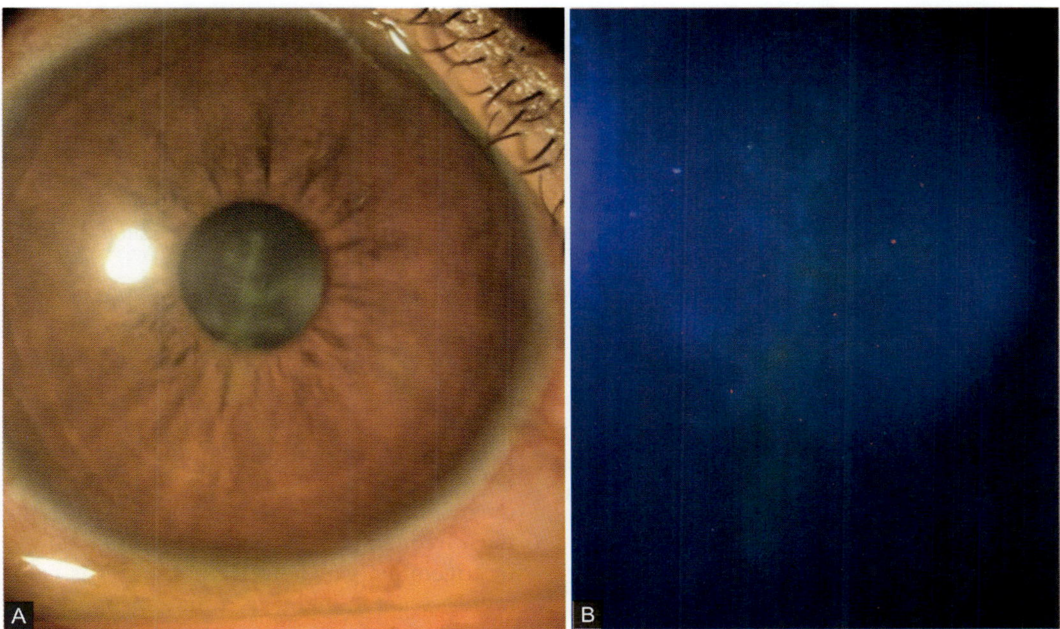

FIGS 5.3.11A and B: Epithelial keratitis

The differences between dendritic ulcer and pseudodendritic ulcer are detailed in Table 5.3.8.

Stromal keratitis

Stromal keratitis is the inflammation of stroma of cornea and it can be immunological or infective in nature.

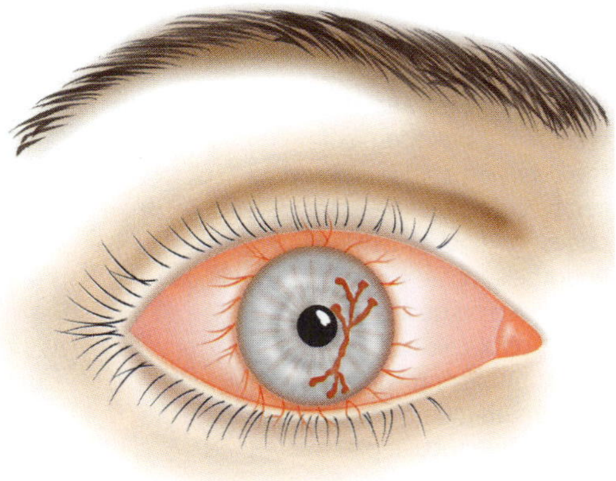

FIG. 5.3.12: Dendritic keratitis

Endotheliitis

Endotheliitis is the inflammation of endothelium of cornea and it is usually immunological in nature (Table 5.3.9).

Investigations

Diagnosis is made by viral culture from the infected specimens, antigen detection by immunofluorescence method or enzyme-linked immunosorbent assay (ELISA), polymerase chain reaction (PCR). However, laboratory investiga-

TABLE 5.3.8: Dendritic ulcer versus pseudodendritic ulcer

Dendritic ulcer	*Pseudodendritic ulcer*
It presents as irregular linear lesion with branches with presence of knobbed ends The ulcer stains prominently with fluorescein and margins stain with rose Bengal	It presents as elevated lesion with absence of knobbed ends It shows little or minimal staining with fluorescein and does not stain with rose Bengal

TABLE 5.3.9: Types of endotheliitis

Disciform endotheliitis	*Diffuse endotheliitis*	*Linear endotheliitis*
It is characterized by presence of keratic precipitates over the endothelium of cornea with disk-shaped stromal edema involving the overlying stroma	It is characterized by presence of keratic precipitates over the endothelium of cornea with diffuse stromal edema involving the overlying stroma	It is characterized by presence of line of keratic precipitates over the endothelium of cornea with edema of the corneal epithelium and stroma involving the overlying stroma

tions are rarely required and typical clinical presentation is sufficient for clinical diagnosis and treatment.

Treatment

Primary herpetic ocular lesions rarely require treatment, as the lesions are self-limiting. Treatment, if required, is done by topical antiviral drugs such as acyclovir applied topically to the lesions.

Recurrent herpetic ocular lesions require treatment invariably and it is done depending on the type of clinical presentation:

1. Infective epithelial keratitis is treated by antiviral drugs. Acyclovir is the commonest drug used for treatment and it is used in the form of 3% eye ointment applied five times per day. The other antiviral drugs used are idoxuridine, vidarabine and trifluridine. Oral acyclovir is indicated in immunocompromised patients and as prophylaxis to prevent recurrences. Oral acyclovir can be used in a dosage of 800 mg up to five times a day.
2. Metaherpetic keratitis is treated by using lubricating artificial tear drops and bandage soft contact lenses.
3. Disciform keratitis is treated by topical steroids under the cover of topical acyclovir eye ointment (Table 5.3.10).
4. Necrotizing stromal keratitis is treated by topical and oral acyclovir (refer Table 5.3.10).
5. Endotheliitis is treated by oral acyclovir and oral steroids.

Herpes Zoster Ophthalmicus**

Herpes zoster is an infection caused by the reactivation of varicella-zoster virus (human herpes virus-3, which causes chicken pox) presenting as painful cutaneous eruptions involving the single or multiple dermatomes. It is also known as shingles.

The lesions are typically unilateral and strictly limited to the dermatome innervated by spinal or cranial sensory ganglion without crossing the midline. Thoracic dermatome (D2–L1) is the most frequently involved dermatome followed by trigeminal ganglion. Herpes zoster is commonly seen in old age, immunosuppressive conditions, poor nutrition, etc.

TABLE 5.3.9: Differences between disciform keratitis and necrotizing keratitis

*Disciform keratitis**	*Necrotizing keratitis*
It is the inflammation of stroma of cornea presenting as a disk-shaped edema (Fig. 5.3.13) It is usually because of delayed hypersensitivity reaction to herpes simplex virus antigen It presents as disk-shaped edema of the corneal stroma with or without edema of the overlying epithelium and keratic precipitates over the corresponding underlying endothelium Decreased corneal sensation, presence of Wesley's autoimmune ring, folds in the Descemet's membrane and elevated intraocular pressure are the associated features often seen in disciform keratitis	It is the inflammation of stroma of the cornea caused by active viral invasion It presents as active corneal ulcer with necrosis of the corneal stroma

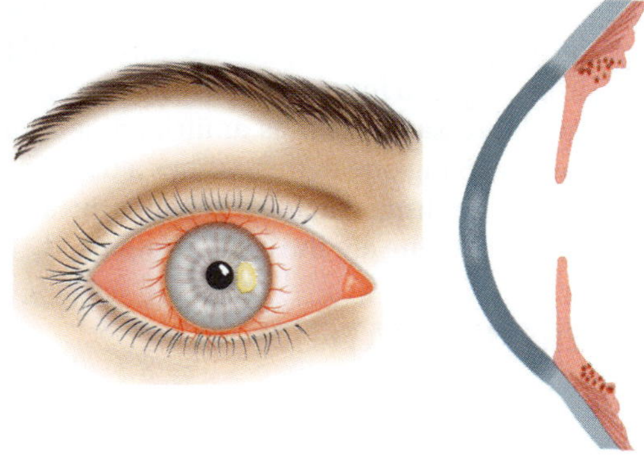

FIG. 5.3.13: Disciform keratitis

The occurrence of herpes zoster in young individuals require evaluation to rule out HIV and other immunosuppressive diseases.

Definition

The reactivation of the varicella-zoster virus in the ophthalmic division of the trigeminal nerve leading to vesicular lesions in the periorbital area is called herpes zoster ophthalmicus (HZO) (Fig. 5.3.14). The HZO can involve one or more branches of the ophthalmic division of the trigeminal nerve, supraorbital, lacrimal and nasociliary branches. It accounts for up to 25% of the cases of herpes zoster.

Etiopathogenesis

Varicella-zoster causes chicken pox in childhood and the same virus remains dormant in the sensory nerve ganglion. The virus gets reactivated and the conditions predisposing to reactivation of the virus are old age, immunosuppressive conditions, poor nutrition, etc.

Clinical features

The clinical features consist of:

1. Systemic features such as fever, malaise, fatigue and mild-to-severe pain along the distribution of the dermatome.
2. Cutaneous features appear within 4–7 days after systemic features and are characterized by appearance of macules along the dermatome, which progress to papules, vesicles and pustules. The cutaneous lesions heal by crusting over 4 weeks. The lesions are typically unilateral and strictly limited to the dermatome innervated by the sensory ganglion without crossing the midline.
3. Ocular involvement is seen in about 30–40% of cases of herpes zoster ophthalmicus. Involvement of the tip of nose by the cutaneous lesions is a useful predictor for ocular involvement and it is called Hutchinson's sign. This is because of nasociliary nerve, which supplies the eye, also innervates the tip of the nose. However, ocular involvement is seen in only 50% of patients with Hutchinson's sign. The ocular features seen are:
   a. Blepharitis.
   b. Conjunctivitis.
   c. Corneal involvement in the form of punctate epithelial keratitis, pseudodendritic ulcer and disciform keratitis.
   d. Episcleritis.
   e. Scleritis.
   f. Uveitis.
   g. Acute retinal necrosis, progressive outer retinal necrosis.
4. Neurological features such as:
   a. Postherpetic neuralgia characterized by pain along the distribution of the affected dermatome seen in about 10% of cases.
   b. Cranial nerve palsies commonly involving the nerves supplying the extraocular muscles and facial nerve.
   c. Optic neuritis.

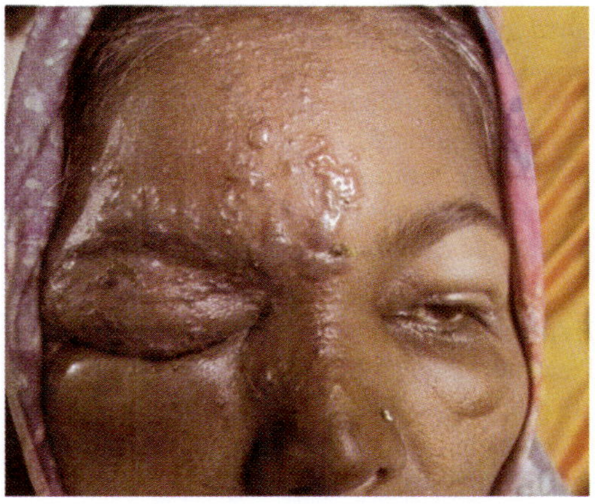

FIG. 5.3.14: Herpes zoster

Investigations

Investigations are not required routinely, as the diagnosis is usually made by typical clinical features. Diagnosis can be confirmed by viral culture, immunofluorescence assay when required.

Treatment

Herpes zoster ophthalmicus is treated by the following methods, as detailed below.

Systemic treatment

1. Antiviral drugs such as oral acyclovir given in a dose of 800 mg for 7–10 days. Acyclovir when started within 72 hours of onset, reduces pain, postherpetic neuralgia and decreases the chances of involvement of cornea. Valacyclovir in a dosage 1,000 mg three times a day or famciclovir 500 mg three times a day for 7 days are the alternative drugs used.
2. Analgesic drugs in the form of non-steroidal anti-inflammatory drugs and opioid drugs are used for pain relief.
3. The use of oral steroids is controversial and when used, they are known to reduce pain and associated inflammation.
4. Intravenous acyclovir is indicated in conditions such as acute retinal necrosis, progressive outer retinal necrosis and optic neuritis.
5. Systemic steroids are indicated in neurological complications such as cranial nerve palsies and optic neuritis.

Local treatment

1. The skin lesions and blepharitis are treated by application of topical antibiotic and steroid ointment.
2. Ocular lesions such as keratitis, scleritis, episcleritis and uveitis are treated by topical steroids and cycloplegic eyedrops under the cover of topical acyclovir eye ointment.

Treatment of postherpetic neuralgia

Treatment is done by:

1. Topical capsaicin application or by application of topical anesthetic agents, i.e. lignocaine.
2. Analgesic drugs in the form of non-steroidal anti-inflammatory drugs and opioid drugs are used for pain relief.
3. Antidepressants such as amitriptyline in a dose of 25 mg one to three times a day. Antiepileptic drugs such as gabapentin and carbamazepine are the other drugs used.

ALLERGIC KERATITIS

Vernal keratitis and phlyctenular keratitis are the common allergic keratitis conditions. They are described under vernal conjunctivitis and phlyctenular conjunctivitis respectively under conjunctiva.

TROPHIC KERATITIS

Definition

Inflammation of cornea secondary to degenerative changes in the corneal epithelium as a result of decreased corneal sensation or drying of cornea leading to altered metabolic activity of the corneal epithelium. Trophic keratitis is of three types (Table 5.3.11):

1. Neurotrophic keratitis.
2. Exposure keratitis.
3. Neuroparalytic keratitis.

Neurotrophic Keratitis**

Definition

Inflammation or ulceration of cornea secondary to degenerative changes in the corneal epithelium as a result of decreased corneal sensation is called neurotrophic keratitis or neurotrophic keratopathy.

Etiopathogenesis

The etiopathogenesis of neurotrophic keratitis is shown in Figure 5.3.15. The causes for decreased corneal sensations are:*

- Familial dysautonomia—also known as Riley-Day syndrome

TABLE 5.3.11: Types of trophic keratitis

Neurotrophic keratitis	*Exposure keratitis*	*Neuroparalytic keratitis*
It is because of decreased corneal sensations	It is because of exposure of cornea leading to drying and desiccation of corneal epithelium	It is because of paralysis of sensory supply of cornea

- Paralysis of trigeminal nerve as a result of surgery, trauma, neoplasms, etc.
- Damage to the sensory nerve endings of cornea as following keratoplasty, refractive corneal surgeries, contact lens wear and herpes simplex keratitis
- Systemic diseases associated with decreased corneal sensation such as diabetes mellitus, leprosy, etc.
- Drug-induced corneal hypoesthesia as seen with long-term use of timolol, betaxolol and ketorolac.

Clinical Features

1. Neutrophic keratitis presents as punctate epithelial erosions in the initial stage, which coalesce together resulting in frank ulcer. If not treated properly, it may result in stromal melting and perforation.

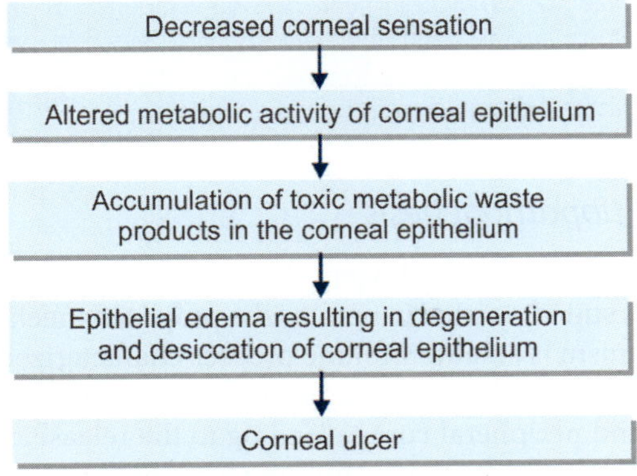

FIG. 5.3.15: Etiopathogenesis of neurotrophic keratitis

2. The characteristic features are absence of pain, lacrimation, decreased corneal sensation and decreased blink rate.

Treatment

- It is done by preservative-free artificial tears in the form of eyedrops or ointments
- Therapeutic soft bandage contact lenses are indicated in non-responsive cases
- Surgical management in the form of amniotic membrane transplantation and keratoplasty are indicated in non-healing corneal ulcers.

Exposure Keratitis**

Definition

Inflammation or ulceration of cornea because of exposure of cornea leading to drying and desiccation of corneal epithelium.

Etiopathogenesis

Exposure keratitis is seen in conditions associated with incomplete closure of the eyelids or infrequent blinking of the eyelids resulting in drying of cornea (Fig. 5.3.16).

The common causes for exposure keratitis are inability to close the eyelids completely as in gross proptosis, severe degree of ectropion, symblepharon, lagophthalmos and comatose state, etc.

Clinical Features

Exposure keratitis presents as punctate epithelial erosions in the initial stage, which coalesce

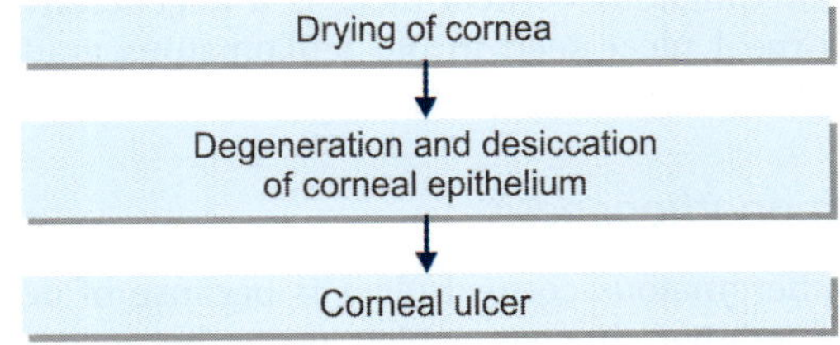

FIG. 5.3.16: Etiopathogenesis of exposure keratitis

together resulting in frank ulcer. The characteristic feature is the presence of lagophthalmos.

Treatment

1. Prophylaxis is by frequent use of artificial tears and taping of the eyelids during sleep to prevent drying of cornea and treatment of the underlying disease responsible for exposure of cornea.
2. Tarsorrhaphy is indicated in patients in whom the underlying cause cannot be treated or the treatment is delayed.

Neuroparalytic Keratitis**

Neurotrophic keratitis and neuroparalytic keratitis are used interchangeably for similar conditions. Neuroparalytic keratitis is similar to neurotrophic keratitis; the only difference being it includes only those causes, which lead to paralysis of the sensory nerve supply of cornea as in paralysis of trigeminal nerve as a result of surgery, trauma, neoplasms, etc.

> Neuroparalytic keratitis can be the first sign of intracranial neoplasms because of paralysis of trigeminal nerve caused by the tumor.

Etiopathogenesis, clinical features and treatment are similar to neurotrophic keratitis; the only difference is that neuroparalytic keratitis tends to be more severe than neurotrophic keratopathy.

Atheromatous Corneal Ulcer

Definition

Atheromatous corneal ulcer is a degenerative corneal ulcer seen in old leukomatous grade corneal opacities.

Etiopathogenesis

Atheromatous corneal ulcer is because of degenerative changes, which occur because of trophic changes in the corneal opacities. It is commonly seen in long-standing eyes with leukomatous grade corneal opacity.

Clinical Features

Atheromatous corneal ulcer are similar to neurotrophic keratitis. Early perforation is seen in untreated cases because of pre-existing corneal scar.

Treatment

The treatment is similar to that of corneal ulcer. Early surgical intervention is indicated in non-responsive cases. In eyes with no visual prognosis, evisceration followed by artificial implant can be done.

IDIOPATHIC KERATITIS

Mooren's Ulcer**

Definition

Mooren's ulcer is a rare type of idiopathic, painful, peripheral, chronic ulcerative keratitis with circumferential and central progression (Figs 5.3.17A and B). It is also known as chronic serpiginous ulcer of the cornea or ulcus rodens.

> Mooren's ulcer was first described by Sir William Bowman, but detailed description was given by Mooren; hence, the name Mooren's ulcer. Bowman was the first to describe Bowman's membrane and to come out with Bowman's probe for probing the lacrimal drainage system.

Etiopathogenesis

The exact etiopathogenesis is not known and it is still idiopathic in nature. The proposed mechanism is an autoimmune process characterized by deposition of immune complexes in limbus and peripheral cornea leading to the release of proteolytic enzymes resulting in ulceration.

The Mooren's ulcer is known to be associated with infections such as helminthiasis,

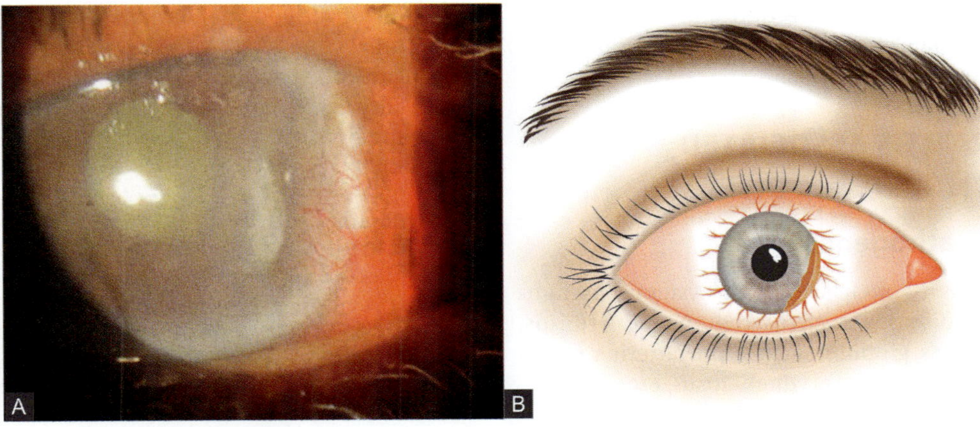

FIGS 5.3.17A and B: Mooren's ulcer. **A.** Photograph; **B.** Diagrammatic representation.

hepatitis C, herpes simplex, herpes zoster, syphilis, tuberculosis, chemical injuries, mechanical injuries, surgeries such as keratoplasty, cataract surgeries, etc.

Clinical Features

1. Mooren's ulcer presents as painful, peripheral corneal ulcer with pain being out of proportion.
2. The ulcer starts as peripheral stromal infiltrates, which coalesce together to form furrow with an epithelial defect.
3. The ulcer spreads circumferentially and centrally with the margins being undermined, hence the name ulcus rodens.
4. One end of the ulcer may show vascularization and healing, while the ulcer spreads by undermining the epithelium at the other end by a characteristic overhanging edge.
5. The ulcer heals by vascularization leaving behind a thin, weak-scarred cornea; the healing process may take 6 months to 1 year. Perforation may be seen rarely usually following minor trauma.

Mooren's ulcer presents in two types as shown in Table 5.3.12.

> Mooren's ulcer is a diagnosis of exclusion and is diagnosed by typical clinical features and absence of secondary systemic diseases that lead to peripheral ulcerative keratitis.

Investigations

Tests are done to rule out systemic diseases such as rheumatoid arthritis, Wegener's granulomatosis, systemic lupus erythematosus and polyarteritis nodosa, etc.

Treatment

1. Topical steroids are mainstay of treatment.
2. Patients not responding to steroids require systemic immunosuppressants in the form of systemic chemotherapy. Cyclophosphamide, methotrexate or azathioprine is the commonly used chemotherapeutic drugs.

TABLE 5.3.12: Types of Mooren's ulcer

Type I Mooren's ulcer	*Type II Mooren's ulcer*
Usually unilateral, seen in elderly individuals, progresses slowly and responds to treatment	Usually bilateral, seen in younger individuals, progresses rapidly and resistant to treatment

3. Conjunctival resection and superficial lamellar keratectomy are carried out in responding patients.

KERATITIS ASSOCIATED WITH SYSTEMIC DISEASES

Etiopathogenesis

Keratitis is often seen with systemic autoimmune diseases such as rheumatoid arthritis, Wegener's granulomatosis, polyarteritis nodosa, systemic lupus erythematosus, etc.

Clinical Features

Keratitis often presents as unilateral or bilateral peripheral corneal ulcer associated with other features such as episcleritis, scleritis, uveitis, etc.

Treatment

Treatment consists of treatment of the underlying systemic disease along with local treatment in the form of topical artificial tears to promote healing, conjunctival resection, etc. Steroids should be better avoided, as they may result in corneal melting.

KERATITIS ASSOCIATED WITH DISEASES OF SKIN

Rosacea Keratitis*

Rosacea is a chronic disease of skin presenting as erythema and pustules affecting the skin of face. It affects the sebaceous glands in the forehead, nose and cheeks.

Corneal involvement is in the form of superficial punctate keratitis and peripheral ulcerative keratitis. Keratitis is seen in about 5% of patients with rosacea. The exact pathogenesis is not known. It is proposed to be because of immunological reaction and associated altered meibomian gland function leading to tear film abnormalities.

Treatment of rosacea keratitis is by topical steroids and by using systemic tetracycline for treatment of altered meibomian gland function. Tetracycline is used for its action of decreasing the bacterial lipase resulting in alteration of fatty acid composition of the secretions of the meibomian gland, thereby increasing the solubility.

Ocular Rosacea

Ocular rosacea is seen in about 40–50% of patients with rosacea. The clinical manifestations of ocular rosacea are:
- Dry eye
- Chronic blepharitis or meibomian gland dysfunction
- Recurrent hordeolum or chalazion
- Chronic conjunctival hyperemia and rarely cicatrizing conjunctivitis
- Rosacea keratitis
- Episcleritis and scleritis.

Treatment is by lid hygiene, systemic tetracycline, topical steroids and artificial tear substitutes.

Peripheral Ulcerative Keratitis

Definition

Inflammation of the periphery of the cornea characterized by stromal infiltration associated with sloughing of corneal epithelium and progressive stromal necrosis (Figs 5.3.18A and B).

Etiopathogenesis

Because of the unique anatomical characteristics such as presence of blood vessels derived from anterior ciliary arteries, the periphery of the cornea is predisposed to develop immunologically mediated diseases. The blood vessels act as a source for collagenolytic and proteolytic enzymes, which are responsible for stromal necrosis.

Underlying systemic diseases, most commonly rheumatoid arthritis, is responsible for peripheral ulcerative keratitis in half of the cases.

The causes for peripheral ulcerative keratitis are:*

- Systemic immunological diseases such as polyarteritis nodosa, rheumatoid arthritis,

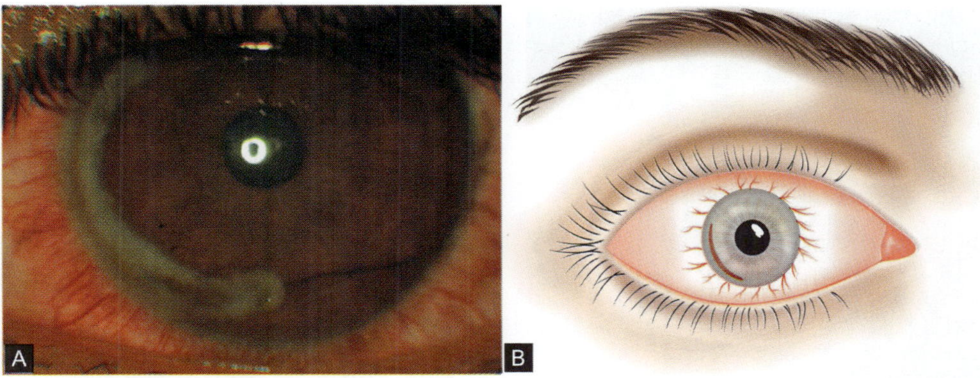

FIGS 5.3.18A and B: Peripheral ulcerative keratitis. **A.** Photograph; **B.** Diagrammatic representation.

systemic lupus erythematosus, Wegener's granulomatosis, etc.

- Ocular immunological diseases such as Mooren's ulcer, rosacea keratitis, marginal keratitis, etc.
- Systemic infectious diseases such as tuberculosis, syphilis, etc.
- Ocular infections caused by bacteria, virus, fungi, etc.

Clinical Features

- Peripheral ulcerative keratitis presents as pain, redness, watering with infiltration in the periphery of the cornea
- Diminution of vision is seen either because of involvement of the central cornea or because of astigmatism induced by thinning of the periphery of the cornea
- The neighboring conjunctiva, episclera and sclera may show signs of inflammation.

Investigations

Investigations are done to rule out underlying systemic immunological and infective diseases and to differentiate ocular infective causes from immunological causes.

Treatment

The main treatment in case of peripheral ulcerative keratitis associated with systemic diseases is by treatment of the underlying disease. The local treatment is by use of artificial tears and topical immunosuppressants, e.g. cyclosporine. Topical steroids are better avoided in cases associated with systemic collagen vascular diseases because of the risk of corneal melting. Systemic tetracycline is used for its collagenase inhibiting action to delay the progression of the disease.

Topical steroids are the mainstay of treatment in cases caused by Mooren's ulcer and rosacea keratitis. The infective causes are treated in similar way as for the infective corneal ulcers.

Marginal Keratitis*

Definition

Marginal keratitis is a type of peripheral ulcerative keratitis associated with chronic staphylococcal blepharitis (Figs 5.3.19A and B).

Etiopathogenesis

Marginal keratitis is a hypersensitive reaction to the exotoxins produced by staphylococci and is characterized by deposition of immune complexes in the peripheral cornea presenting as sterile stromal infiltrates.

Clinical Features

1. Pains, redness, watering with infiltration in the periphery of the cornea are the usually presenting features.

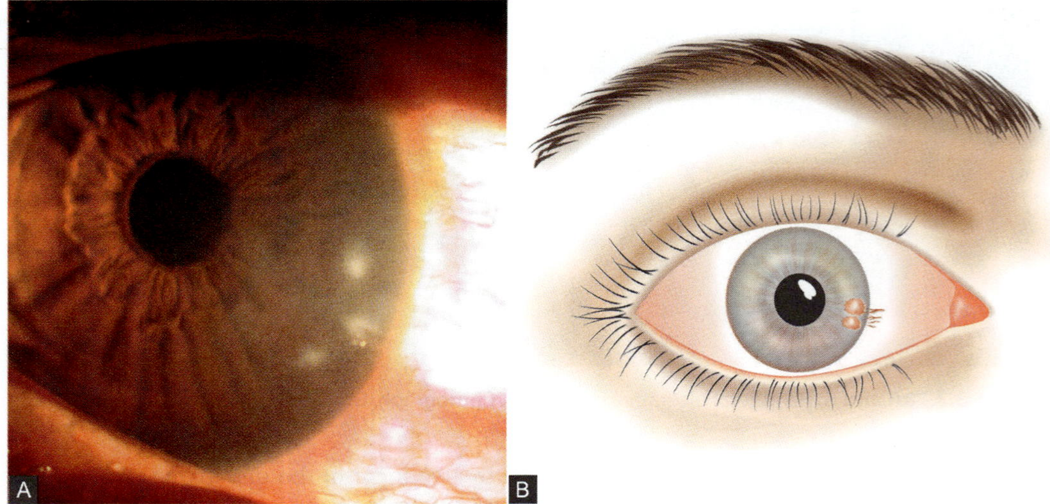

FIGS 5.3.19A and B: Marginal keratitis. **A.** Photograph; **B.** Diagrammatic representation.

2. On examination, grayish white infiltrate is seen in the periphery of the cornea with a clear lucid interval between the infiltrate and the limbus. An associated predisposing condition such as chronic staphylococcal blepharitis is usually seen.

Treatment

- Treatment is by antibiotic steroid eyedrops or eye ointments
- Treatment of the underlying blepharitis is required to prevent recurrences.

RHEUMATOID ARTHRITIS-ASSOCIATED KERATITIS

Rheumatoid arthritis is the most common collagen vascular disease, which affects the cornea. The corneal involvement in rheumatoid arthritis has been discussed in Table 5.3.13.

Other ocular manifestations seen in rheumatoid arthritis are:

- Keratoconjunctivitis sicca
- Scleritis
- Episcleritis
- Uveitis.

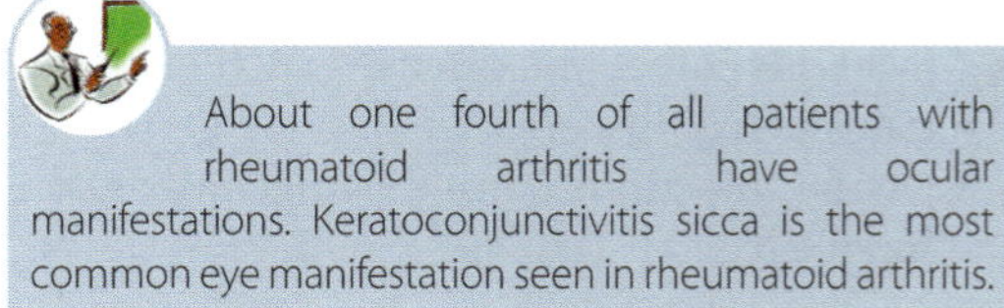

About one fourth of all patients with rheumatoid arthritis have ocular manifestations. Keratoconjunctivitis sicca is the most common eye manifestation seen in rheumatoid arthritis.

NON-ULCERATIVE KERATITIS

Definition

Inflammation of the cornea characterized by stromal infiltration with intact epithelium is called non-ulcerative keratitis. It includes superficial punctate keratitis and interstitial keratitis.

Interstitial Keratitis**

Definition

Interstitial keratitis is the inflammation of corneal stroma without involvement of the epithelium and endothelium. Inflammation is usually nonsuppurative in nature (Figs 5.3.20A and B).

Etiopathogenesis

The inflammation develops because of immune-mediated response to antigens present

TABLE 5.3.13: Corneal involvement in rheumatoid arthritis

Central corneal involvement	*Peripheral corneal involvement*
• Acute stromal keratitis • Sclerosing keratitis	• Peripheral ulcerative keratitis • Peripheral limbal guttering • Keratolysis or corneal melting

in the corneal stroma, most commonly to antigens of the infective microbial agents. The common causes for interstitial keratitis have been discussed in Table 5.3.14.

Clinical Features

Redness, diminution of vision, photophobia and pain are the usual presenting symptoms. On examination, cornea shows stromal infiltration with stromal edema. Vascularization of the stroma is seen in long-standing cases.

Investigations

Investigations are aimed to rule out the underlying diseases as described in Table 5.3.14.

Treatment

Ocular treatment is by topical steroids and cycloplegic agents. Systemic treatment is by treatment of the underlying disease.

Syphilitic Interstitial Keratitis

Definition

Interstitial keratitis caused by immune-mediated reaction to treponemal antigen.

Etiopathogenesis

Syphilis was the commonest cause for interstitial keratitis. With effective treatment of syphilis, the incidence has come down drastically.

Keratitis is more frequently seen in congenital syphilis, which manifests in the age group of

TABLE 5.3.14: Common causes of interstitial keratitis

Causes	*Examples*
Bacterial infections	Syphilis Tuberculosis Leprosy Lyme disease
Viral infections	Herpes simplex virus Herpes zoster
Parasitic infections	Onchocerciasis Leishmaniasis Trypanosomiasis
Systemic diseases	Cogan's syndrome
Collagen vascular diseases	Sarcoidosis Rheumatoid arthritis Wegener's granulomatosis Polyarteritis nodosa
Idiopathic	

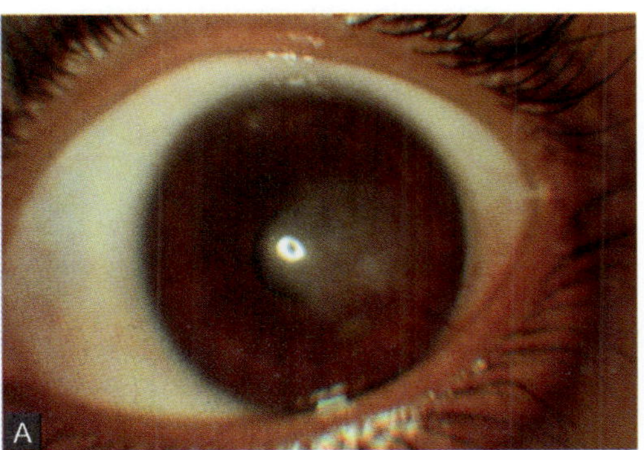

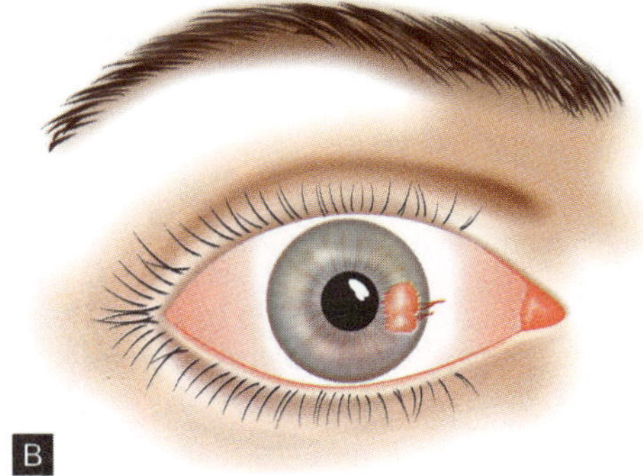

FIGS 5.3.20A and B: Interstitial keratitis. **A.** Photograph; **B.** Diagrammatic representation.

5–15 years. It is because of immune-mediated antigen-antibody reaction directed against the treponemal antigens deposited in the cornea.

Clinical features

Clinical features are same as described under interstitial keratitis. The disease progresses in three stages as follows:

1. The initial stage is characterized by ground-glass appearance of the cornea because of progressive infiltration.
2. The second stage is characterized by deep vascularization with hazy cornea called salmon patch appearance.
3. The late stage is characterized by regression of the inflammation leading to reduction in corneal edema and the blood vessels persist as ghost vessels.

Investigations

Diagnosis is confirmed by serological tests such as fluorescent treponemal antibody absorption test and venereal disease research laboratory test (VDRL).

Treatment

Ocular treatment is by topical steroids and cycloplegic eyedrops. Systemic treatment is by penicillin and oral steroids.

Clinical Manifestations of Congenital Syphilis

Ocular features

Interstitial keratitis, optic atrophy, Argyll Robertson pupil, uveitis, pigmentary retinopathy, etc.

Systemic features

Hutchinson's teeth (small notched and widely spaced teeth), Clutton's joints (symmetrical joint swelling), saddle-shaped nasal deformity (concave nasal bridge), sabre tibia (anterior bowing of the tibia), sensorineural deafness, etc.

Hutchinson's triad

A triad of interstitial keratitis, sensorineural deafness and Hutchinson's teeth.

Cogan's Syndrome

The syndrome is a triad of interstitial keratitis, vestibulocochlear diseases such as vertigo, tinnitus, deafness and autoimmune vasculitis disease such as polyarteritis nodosa, Wegener's granulomatosis, etc.

The syndrome is an autoimmune disease characterized by production of antibodies against the common antigens involving the cornea and the vestibulocochlear apparatus.

Treatment of Cogan's syndrome is by systemic steroids. Interstitial keratitis is treated by topical steroids.

Superficial Non-ulcerative Keratitis

Superficial non-ulcerative keratitis is a group of conditions characterized by non-ulcerative inflammation of the cornea affecting the superficial layers of the cornea including epithelium and anterior parts of the corneal stroma:

- Superficial punctate keratitis
- Superior limbic keratoconjunctivitis
- Thygeson's superficial punctate keratitis
- Filamentary keratitis.

*Superficial Punctate Keratitis***

Definition

Superficial punctate keratitis is defined as inflammation of the superficial layers of cornea involving epithelium and anterior part of the stroma. It presents as multiple, small and discrete lesions (Figs 5.3.21A and B).

Etiopathogenesis

Viral infections are the commonest cause for superficial punctate keratitis. The other causes are dry eye, blepharoconjunctivitis, allergic keratoconjunctivitis, exposure keratitis, contact lenses, drug toxicity, chlamydial infection, etc.

Superior limbic keratoconjunctivitis and Thygeson's superficial punctate keratitis are the idiopathic types of superficial punctate keratitis.

Clinical features

Ocular irritation, photophobia and lacrimation are the presenting symptoms. On examination, punctate epithelial lesions are seen in the epithelium and superficial layers of the stroma. They stain with fluorescein and rose Bengal. The distribution and pattern of punctate lesions depend on the underlying cause:

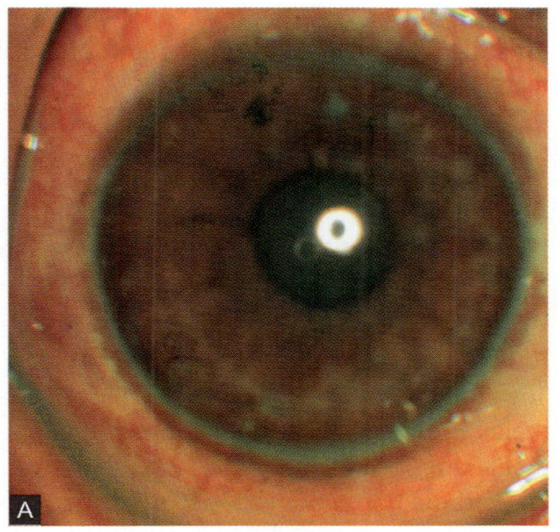

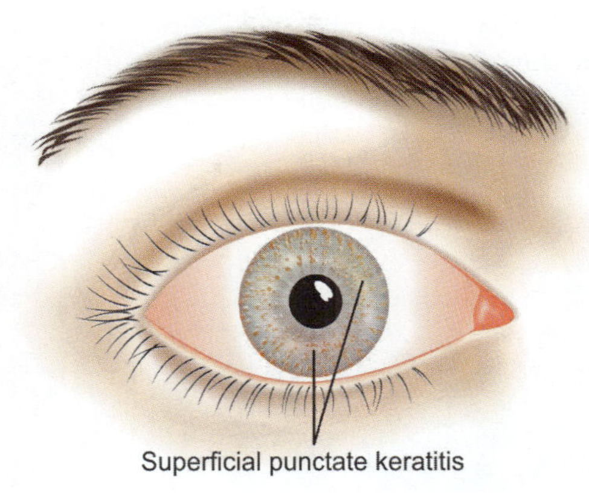

FIGS 5.3.21A and B: Superficial punctate keratitis. **A.** Photograph; **B.** Diagrammatic representation.

- Diffuse pattern is seen in infections and drug toxicity
- Superior distribution is seen in allergic keratoconjunctivitis such as vernal keratoconjunctivitis, chlamydial infection and superior limbic keratoconjunctivitis
- Inferior distribution is seen in exposure keratitis, trichiasis, lagophthalmos
- Central distribution is seen in contact lens wear.

Treatment

Treatment is done by topical steroids and artificial tears, and treatment of the underlying cause. In the infective causes, steroids are used under cover of the appropriate antimicrobial drugs.

Superior Limbic Keratoconjunctivitis

Definition

Superior limbic keratoconjunctivitis is a chronic, recurrent, bilateral inflammation limited to the superior cornea and limbus with papillary hypertrophy of the superior tarsal conjunctiva (Fig. 5.3.22).

Etiopathogenesis

The condition was named by Frederick Theodore, hence called Theodore superior limbic keratoconjunctivitis. It is associated with use of soft contact lenses. Graves' ophthalmopathy and thyroid dysfunction may be seen associated with superior limbic keratoconjunctivitis.

Clinical features

Ocular irritation, photophobia and lacrimation are the presenting symptoms. On examination, it shows hyperemia of the superior bulbar conjunctiva, thickening of the superior limbus and punctate epithelial erosions and filaments involving the superior cornea.

Treatment

The treatment is by artificial tears and topical steroid eyedrops. Non-responding cases may require resection or cauterization of superior bulbar conjunctiva.

Thygeson's Superficial Punctate Keratitis

Definition

The condition is a chronic, recurrent, bilateral, idiopathic superficial punctate keratitis. It is named after Philip Thygeson who first described the condition.

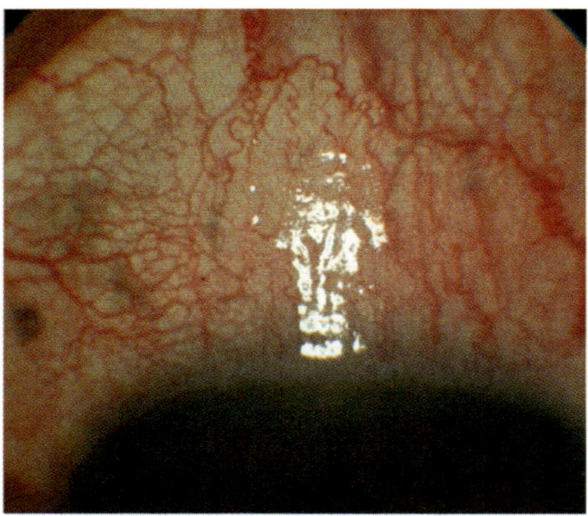

FIG. 5.3.22: Superior limbic keratoconjunctivitis

Clinical features

Ocular irritation, photophobia and watering are the usual presenting symptoms. It presents as multiple, discrete, dot-like intraepithelial superficial corneal opacities with characteristic absence of inflammation of conjunctiva.

Diagnosis

The condition has to be differentiated from other causes of superficial punctate keratitis such as viral conjunctivitis, keratoconjunctivitis sicca, recurrent corneal erosion syndrome, etc. The differentiation is made by typical clinical features and absence of inflammations of the conjunctiva.

Treatment

Treatment is by topical steroids and artificial tears.

*Filamentary Keratitis***

Definition

Filamentary keratitis is a chronic recurrent superficial keratitis characterized by the formation of corneal epithelial filaments.

Etiopathogenesis

The condition occurs because of defective epithelial healing leading to the formation of epithelial threads or filaments.

Keratoconjunctivitis sicca or dry eye is the commonest condition associated with filamentary keratitis. The other conditions associated with filamentary keratitis are use of contact lens, recurrent corneal erosions, surgeries such as keratoplasty and systemic diseases such as diabetes, etc.

Clinical features

Ocular irritation, photophobia and watering are the usual presenting symptoms. On examination, it shows the characteristic presence of filaments on the cornea.

Treatment

Treatment is done by scraping to remove the corneal filaments and use of artificial tear.

Photophthalmia*

Definition

Photophthalmia is a condition characterized by multiple epithelial erosions because of exposure to intense light. It is also called snow blindness or welding keratitis.

Etiopathogenesis

Photophthalmia is seen in conditions involving exposure to ultraviolet rays as in:

- Reflection of light rays from snow surface called snow blindness
- Welding light called welding keratitis
- Short circuit of high-tension electric current.

It is because of desquamation of the epithelial cells of cornea, which usually follows due to the effect of ultraviolet rays.

Contd...

Contd...

Clinical Features

It usually takes 4–6 hours for the onset of the disease following exposure to ultraviolet rays. Patient presents with photophobia, lacrimation, ocular pain and diminution of vision of various degree. On examination, multiple corneal erosions or epithelial defects are seen and they stain with fluorescein.

Treatment

Treatment is by artificial tears and cycloplegic agents. Patching the eyes for 12–24 hours offers symptomatic relief.

Prevention

Prevention is by using protective glasses to prevent exposure to ultraviolet rays.

GIST BOX 5.3

- Inflammatory diseases of cornea are called keratitis.
- Keratitis is classified based on etiology as infective, allergic, traumatic, trophic, idiopathic, etc.; based on morphology as ulcerative and nonulcerative, and based on pathology as suppurative and non-suppurative keratitis.
- Inflammation of cornea caused by infection by microbes is called infective keratitis. It can be caused by bacteria, fungi, viruses, protozoa, spirochetes, chlamydia, etc.
- Bacterial corneal ulcer is the most common type of infective keratitis.
- Corneal ulcer progresses through stage of infiltration, stage of ulceration, stage of regression and stage of cicatrization.
- Normally, corneal ulcers heal by 2–4 weeks because of formation of granulation tissue; when a corneal ulcer fails to heal within this time, it is referred to as non-healing corneal ulcer.
- Extension of corneal ulcer to involve the full thickness of cornea by perforating the Descemet's membrane is called perforated corneal ulcer.
- The characteristic corneal ulcer produced by *Pneumococcus* is called hypopyon corneal ulcer.
- Viral keratitis and specifically herpes simplex viral keratitis are the most common types of infective keratitis in developed countries.
- Vernal keratitis and phlyctenular keratitis are the common allergic keratitis conditions.
- Trophic keratitis is the inflammation of cornea secondary to degenerative changes in the corneal epithelium as a result of decreased corneal sensation or drying of cornea, leading to altered metabolic activity of the corneal epithelium.
- Mooren's ulcer is a rare, idiopathic, painful, peripheral chronic ulcerative keratitis with circumferential and central progression.
- Inflammation of the corneal stroma without involvement of the epithelium and endothelium is called interstitial keratitis.

CHAPTER

5.4

Corneal Dystrophies, Corneal Degenerations and Ectatic Conditions of Cornea

CORNEAL DYSTROPHIES

The word dystrophy is derived from Greek, which means wrong nourishment.

Definition

Corneal dystrophies are a group of non-inflammatory hereditary diseases of cornea presenting bilateral progressive loss of transparency of cornea due to the deposition of abnormal materials within the layers of the cornea.

Classification**

The classification of corneal dystrophies depending on the layer of the cornea affected, is detailed in (Table 5.4.1).

Etiopathogenesis

Corneal dystrophies are because of deposition of abnormal materials in the layers of the cornea. They are usually genetically inherited diseases, most commonly inherited as autosomal inherited diseases.

Autosomal recessively inherited corneal dystrophies are lattice dystrophy type III, congenital hereditary endothelial dystrophy type II, macular dystrophy and gelatinous dystrophy. Sporadic inheritance is seen in Fuchs' endothelial dystrophy.`

TABLE 5.4.1: Classification of corneal dystrophies

Dystrophy types	*Examples*
Epithelial dystrophies	• Epithelial basement membrane dystrophy • Meesmann dystrophy
Bowman's layer dystrophies	• Reis-Buckler dystrophy • Schnyder crystalline dystrophy • Thiel-Behnke dystrophy
Stromal dystrophies	• Lattice dystrophy • Macular dystrophy • Granular dystrophy • Avellino dystrophy • Gelatinous dystrophy
Endothelial dystrophies	• Congenital hereditary endothelial dystrophy • Fuchs' endothelial dystrophy • Posterior polymorphous dystrophy

Epithelial Dystrophies

Epithelial Basement Membrane Dystrophy

Epithelial basement membrane dystrophy is the most common corneal dystrophy. It is characterized by dot-like, fingerprint-like, cyst-like opacities distributed in irregular map-like pattern involving the epithelium of cornea. It is also called map-dot-fingerprint-like dystrophy or Cogan's microcystic dystrophy.

The disease presents in second and third decade with majority of the patients asymptomatic and the disease being diagnosed on casual eye examination. Only 10% of the affected patients present with recurrent corneal erosions. The basic pathology is thickening of the basement membrane of the epithelium.

Management is by treatment of the recurrent corneal erosions by artificial tears and bandage soft contact lenses. Non-responsive cases may require surgical intervention in the form of phototherapeutic keratectomy or anterior stromal puncture.

Meesmann Dystrophy

Meesmann dystrophy is a rare type of corneal dystrophy. It is characterized by clusters of intraepithelial microcysts with onset in 2nd decade. Majority of the patients are asymptomatic. Symptoms, when present, are similar to epithelial basement membrane dystrophy. Treatment is required only in symptomatic cases and it is similar to epithelial basement dystrophy.

Bowman's Layer Dystrophies

Reis-Buckler Dystrophy

Reis-Buckler dystrophy is characterized by polygonal opacities involving the Bowman's membrane of the cornea. It presents with symptoms of recurrent corneal erosions. Treatment is by phototherapeutic keratectomy or by anterior lamellar keratoplasty.

Schnyder Crystalline Dystrophy

Schnyder crystalline dystrophy is characterized by deposition of cholesterol resulting in characteristic crystalline opacities involving the Bowman's membrane of the cornea. Treatment is by phototherapeutic keratectomy.

Thiel-Behnke Dystrophy

Thiel-Behnke dystrophy is characterized by polygonal opacities arranged in honeycomb pattern; hence, it is also called honeycomb dystrophy. Clinical presentation and treatment are similar to Reis-Buckler dystrophy.

Stromal Dystrophies

Lattice Dystrophy

Lattice dystrophy is characterized by opacities in the form of branching lines involving the stroma of the cornea because of deposition of amyloid. It is of three subtypes:

1. *Lattice type I*: It is characterized by deposition of lattice lines in the center of the cornea sparing the periphery. It is called Biber–Haab–Dimmer syndrome or dystrophy.
2. *Lattice type II*: It is characterized by deposition of lattice lines in the cornea associated with progressive facial palsy and it is called Meretoja syndrome.
3. *Lattice type III*: It is characterized by deposition of lattice lines extending from limbus to limbus.

Treatment is by lamellar keratoplasty or penetrating keratoplasty.

Macular Dystrophy

Macular dystrophy is characterized by deposition of glycosaminoglycans in corneal stroma presenting as white, poorly demarcated dense spots. Treatment is by lamellar keratoplasty or penetrating keratoplasty (PK).

Granular Dystrophy

Granular dystrophy is characterized by deposition of hyaline in corneal stroma presenting as white, sharply delineated spots resembling snowflakes. Treatment is by lamellar keratoplasty or PK. It is also called Groenouw type I dystrophy.

Avellino Dystrophy

Avellino dystrophy is characterized by features of both macular dystrophy and granular dystrophy with deposition of both hyaline and glycosaminoglycans. Treatment is by lamellar keratoplasty or PK. It is also called Groenouw type II dystrophy.

Gelatinous Dystrophy

Gelatinous dystrophy is characterized by deposition of amyloid presenting as mulberry-like appearance resembling gelatinous drop-like appearance. Treatment is by superficial keratectomy as lamellar keratoplasty or PK results in repeated recurrences.

Endothelial Dystrophies

Congenital Hereditary Endothelial Dystrophy

Congenital hereditary endothelial dystrophy is characterized by dystrophic presence of corneal endothelium or absence of corneal endothelium presenting as bilateral corneal edema. The disease usually presents in first decade.

The dystrophy is of two types, type I is autosomal dominant and type II is autosomal recessive. Type II variety is more severe with onset at birth. The dystrophy has to be differentiated from congenital glaucoma, which presents with corneal edema associated with raised intraocular pressure (IOP) and other causes of congenital corneal opacity. Treatment is by penetrating keratoplasty.

Posterior Polymorphous Dystrophy

Posterior polymorphous dystrophy is a rare type of endothelial dystrophy characterized by dysplastic corneal endothelium, which leads to transformation of corneal endothelial cells into keratinized cells resembling epithelial cells. It presents as multiple vesicular lesions in the posterior part of the corneal stroma.

Treatment is required in cases presenting with significant corneal opacity and it is done by keratoplasty.

Fuchs' Endothelial Dystrophy

Fuchs' endothelial dystrophy is one of the common type corneal endothelial dystrophy. It is characterized by late onset usually presenting in fifth to seventh decade with progressive and often asymmetrical corneal edema.

Fuchs' dystrophy occurs due to the production of abnormally thickened Descemet's membrane as a result of defective endothelial cells. Fuchs' endothelial dystrophy presents in four stages:

1. Stage I is asymptomatic stage and is usually detected by slit-lamp examination with findings of presence of corneal guttata in the central cornea and sometimes showing beaten metal appearance
2. Stage II presents with early morning blurring of vision due to edema of the corneal epithelium because of decreased tear evaporation during nighttime as a result of closed eyelids.
3. Stage III presents with moderate-to-severe diminution of vision because of total corneal edema and epithelial bullae.
4. Stage IV presents with severe diminution of vision with scarring of cornea.

Fuchs' endothelial dystrophy has to be differentiated from other endothelial dystrophies, bullous keratopathy, etc.

Treatment is by medical management in the form of topical hypertonic saline in earlier stages. Advanced disease is managed by endothelial keratoplasty or PK.

Corneal Guttata

Corneal guttata are the earliest lesions seen in Fuchs' endothelial dystrophy. Irregular thickening or excrescences of the Descemet's membrane are called corneal guttata.

They are seen in other conditions as in old age following uveitis. The presence of corneal guttata indicates poor endothelial function and is a risk factor for development of corneal edema following intraocular surgeries as in cataract surgery.

Contd...

Contd...

Presence of corneal guttata in the periphery is normal age-related change and they are called Hassall-Henle bodies.

ECTATIC CONDITIONS OF CORNEA

The ectatic conditions of cornea are a group of diseases characterized by progressive thinning of cornea. The ectatic conditions are:

- Keratoconus
- Iatrogenic keratectasia
- Keratoglobus
- Pellucid marginal degeneration.

Keratoconus***

Definition

Keratoconus is defined as bilateral, but often asymmetrical, non-inflammatory progressive thinning and conical protrusion of cornea.

The condition is called keratoconus because of conical protrusion of the thinned cornea. The word keratoconus is derived from Greek, meaning kerato—cornea and conus—cone.

Etiopathogenesis

The incidence of keratoconus is about 1 in 2,000 people and 10% of them have family history. It is more commonly seen in females and the onset is in the first to second decade and the disease progresses till third to fourth decade. It is associated with various systemic and ocular diseases; the most common conditions being vernal catarrh and other atopic diseases, which are associated with repeated eye rubbing. The exact etiology is not known, the various proposed mechanisms are:

- Genetic abnormalities because of association with trisomy 21 and Turner's syndrome
- Collagen abnormalities because of association with Marfan's syndrome
- Metabolic abnormalities because of the association with increased level of lysosomal enzymes and decreased levels of inhibitors of proteolytic enzymes.

Keratoconus is known to be associated with systemic and ocular diseases as discussed in Table 5.4.2.

The basic pathological features seen in keratoconus are increased activity of proteases leading to increased breakdown of the collagen cross-linking leading to progressive thinning of cornea.

Clinical Features

Symptoms

- Diminution of vision gradually progressive and painless in nature because of progressive myopic astigmatism is the most common symptom, monocular diplopia or polyopia is seen rarely
- Pain, redness, photophobia and watering are seen in acute hydrops, a complication of keratoconus.

Signs

- Munson's sign—protrusion of the lower lid margin when the patient looks down is called Munson's sign and it is seen in advanced stage of keratoconus (Figs 5.4.1A to C).
- Examination of cornea shows:
  - Steepening of cornea, most commonly inferior steepening with conical protrusion of the thinned cornea
  - Fleischer's ring—a ring formed because of deposition of iron in the epithelium at the base of the cone

TABLE 5.4.2: Diseases associated with keratoconus

Systemic diseases	*Ocular diseases*
• Marfan's syndrome • Down syndrome • Ehlers-Danlos syndrome • Osteogenesis imperfecta • Asthma • Atopic dermatitis	• Vernal conjunctivitis • Floppy eyelid syndrome • Leber's congenital amaurosis • Retinitis pigmentosa • Retinopathy of prematurity • Congenital cataract • Aniridia

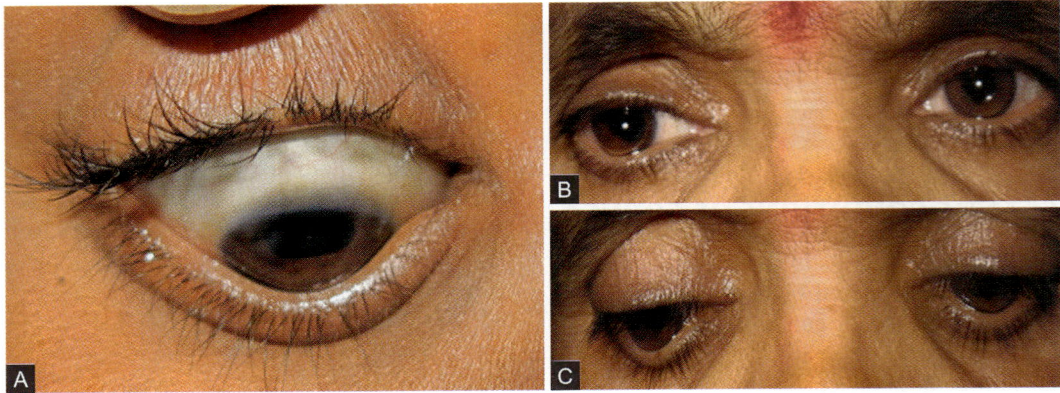

FIGS 5.4.1A to C: Keratoconus and Munson's sign

- Vogt's striae—vertical lines at the level of Descemet's membrane and deeper stroma because of stretching of cornea, which disappears with external pressure on the globe
- Corneal scarring usually at the level of Descemet's membrane is seen following healing of ruptured Descemet's membrane as in acute hydrops
- Rizzuti's sign—illumination of cornea from temporal side leads to illumination of nasal sclera.

- *Retinoscopy*: It shows scissoring of the retinoscopic reflex
- *Placido disk test*: It shows distortion of the mires of the placido's disk.
- *Keratometry*: It shows irregular astigmatism
- *Distant direct ophthalmoscopy*: It shows oil droplet reflex and it is called Charleaux's sign (Fig. 5.4.2).

As the keratoconus progresses, the thickness of cornea decreases and it may lead to acute hydrops and healing by scar formation or corneal perforation.

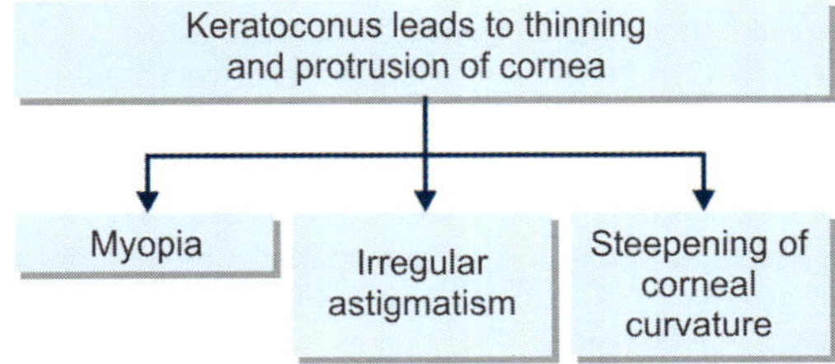

FIG. 5.4.2: Clinical features of keratoconus

Based on the pathological changes in cornea because of keratoconus, it is classified into four stages as detailed below.

Classification of Keratoconus

Modified Krumeich classification is used to classify keratoconus (Table 5.4.3).

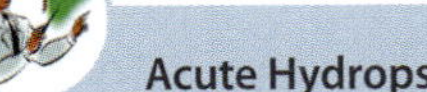

Acute Hydrops

Acute hydrops is a rare complication of keratoconus characterized by corneal edema as a result of spontaneous breaks in the Descemet's membrane and thus allowing the aqueous humor to enter the stroma of cornea.

Acute hydrops is also seen in other ectatic conditions of cornea such as keratoglobus and pellucid marginal degeneration. It is seen in about 5% of cases of keratoconus. Acute hydrops presents with sudden onset of pain, photophobia, watering and gross diminution of vision. On examination, corneal edema is seen with pre-existing keratoconus.

Treatment is by topical hyperosmotic agents to reduce corneal edema, aqueous suppressants such as acetazolamide to decrease secretion of aqueous, cycloplegics such as homatropine for pain relief and steroids for decreasing inflammation.

Acute hydrops usually leads to corneal opacity involving the full thickness of cornea; hence, it requires full thickness keratoplasty for treatment of the residual corneal opacity.

TABLE 5.4.3: Modified Krumeich classification of keratoconus

Clinical features	*Stage I*	*Stage II*	*Stage III*	*Stage IV*
Myopia/Astigmatism	< 5 D	5–8 D	8–10 D	Not measurable
Radius of curvature of cornea	< 48 D	48–53 D	53–55 D	> 55 D
Thickness of cornea	Normal	> 400 µm	200–400 µm	< 200 µm
Corneal scar	Absent	Absent	Absent	Present

Complications

- Progressive myopia
- Irregular astigmatism
- Acute hydrops
- Corneal perforation
- Corneal scar.

Investigations

Corneal topography is the investigation of choice in patients with suspected keratoconus. It shows characteristic inferior steepening of cornea.

Differential Diagnosis

Keratoconus has to be differentiated from keratoglobus and pellucid marginal degeneration.

*Treatment***

The management of keratoconus has undergone rapid advancement with newer diagnostic and therapeutic methods. However, the older and conventional methods are still practiced. The treatment options available are:

1. *Spectacles*: They are indicated in early or mild cases of keratoconus, which have got minimal astigmatism.
2. *Contact lenses*: They are indicated in moderate degree of keratoconus where the spectacle correction is unsatisfactory. Usually, spectacles fail to correct astigmatism of more than 4 D. Rigid gas permeable lenses are the contact lens of type preferred in keratoconus. Piggyback contact lenses consisting of wearing rigid lenses over soft lenses may be required in few patients.
3. *Corneal ring segments* (*INTACS—intracorneal ring segments*): It consists of insertion of polymethyl methacrylate arcs into the corneal stroma through incisions made on the steeper corneal axis. The corneal ring segments act by arc shortening, thereby flattening the central cornea. The flattening effect is proportional to the thickness and diameter of the ring segment.
4. *Corneal collagen cross-linking with riboflavin (C3R)*: It is indicated in cases of keratoconus with progression. It is done by topical application of riboflavin and its activation by exposure to ultraviolet A light. The activation of riboflavin results in increased cross-linking of collagen, which increases the strength of cornea that helps to decrease the progression of keratoconus.
5. *Phakic intraocular lens*: It is indicated to correct high myopia. It is done by insertion of intraocular lens over and above the natural lens.
6. *Lamellar keratoplasty*: It is indicated in cases with scars involving the anterior stroma with intact endothelium and Descemet's membrane.
7. *Optical full thickness keratoplasty*: It is indicated in cases with scars involving the whole thickness of cornea and in cases where all other methods fail to give satisfactory vision.

Iatrogenic Keratectasia

Iatrogenic keratectasia is defined as corneal ectasia as a complication of incisional refractive or excimer laser ablation refractive corneal surgery.

Laser-assisted in situ keratomileusis (LASIK) and other refractive surgeries are contraindicated in cases with decreased corneal thickness and in keratoconus. With the increase in incidence of refractive surgeries, the incidence of iatrogenic keratectasia or LASIK-induced keratectasia has increased in incidence. The treatment of iatrogenic keratectasia is similar to keratoconus.

Pellucid Marginal Degeneration

Pellucid marginal degeneration is a rare ectatic condition of cornea characterized by thinning of the peripheral inferior cornea with protrusion of cornea superior to the area of thinning. In keratoconus, the thinned cornea protrudes and it is usually inferocentral in location. It is commonly seen in males and in third to fourth decade, whereas keratoconus is commonly seen in females with onset in first to second decade.

The clinical features are similar to keratoconus, except for the fact that in pellucid marginal degeneration, the cornea tends to be clear and it causes diminution of vision in advanced stages. Treatment is similar to keratoconus.

Keratoglobus

Keratoglobus is a rare ectatic condition of cornea characterized by generalized thinning and protrusion of whole of the cornea. It exists in two forms, congenital and acquired. The congenital type is associated with Ehlers-Danlos syndrome. The clinical features and treatment are similar to keratoconus.

CORNEAL DEGENERATIONS

Definition

Corneal degenerations are defined as age-related degenerative conditions involving the cornea occurring as a result of age-related changes or because of pathological conditions such as inflammation, trauma and chronic exposure to ultraviolet rays.

The differences between corneal dystrophies and corneal degenerations have been mentioned in Table 5.4.4.*

Classification

Corneal degenerations are classified based on the location and underlying cause as detailed below:

1. Central corneal degenerations.
2. Peripheral corneal degenerations.

Central Corneal Degenerations (Table 5.4.5)

Crocodile Shagreen

Crocodile shagreen is age-related change affecting the stroma of cornea and presents as polygonal opacities in the center of the cornea with each opacity being separated by clear spaces. It is called crocodile shagreen, as the appearance resembles to crocodile skin. It rarely interferes with vision; hence, treatment is usually not required.

Cornea farinata

Cornea farinata is also age-related change affecting the posterior part of the stroma and presents as fine dust- or flour-like opacities involving the posterior part of the stroma. It is called farinata because of its resemblance to wheat flour. It rarely interferes with vision; hence, treatment is usually not required.

Amyloid degeneration of cornea

Amyloid degeneration is a rare type of corneal degeneration characterized by deposition of amyloid secondary to injury or inflammation of cornea. Primary amyloid deposition in cornea is seen in lattice and gelatinous corneal dystrophies and they are associated with familial amyloidosis.

Hyaline degeneration of cornea

Hyaline degeneration is a type of corneal degeneration characterized by the deposition of hyaline in cornea. The deposition is seen usually secondary to injury or inflammation. Primary hyaline deposition in cornea is seen in granular and Avellino dystrophies.

Salzmann's nodular degeneration of cornea

Salzmann's nodular degeneration is a corneal degeneration characterized by deposition of

TABLE 5.4.4: The differences between corneal dystrophies and corneal degenerations

Corneal dystrophies	*Corneal degenerations*
Hereditary with genetic inheritance	Nonhereditary
Bilateral	Unilateral or bilateral
Noninflammatory	They follow pathological conditions, i.e. following inflammation, trauma, chronic exposure to ultraviolet (UV) rays
Age or presentation is in younger age and middle age	Elderly age group

TABLE 5.4.5: Central corneal degenerations

Central age-related corneal degenerations	*Central pathological degenerations*
Crocodile shagreen Cornea farinata	Amyloid degeneration Hyaline degeneration Salzmann's nodular degeneration Spheroidal degeneration Band-shaped keratopathy Lipid keratopathy

elevated grayish nodules in the anterior part of the cornea. It is because of hyalinization of the anterior part of the cornea. It is seen in cornea with chronic inflammation such as trachoma and vernal keratitis. Treatment of the condition is by lamellar keratoplasty.

Spheroidal degeneration of cornea*

Spheroidal degeneration is a common corneal degeneration characterized by deposition of amber colored or brownish yellow granules in the anterior part of the cornea (Fig. 5.4.3).

The degeneration is commonly seen in people with chronic exposure to UV rays. It is also called climatic droplet keratopathy/Bietti's nodular corneal degeneration/Labrador keratopathy/Fisherman's keratopathy. The degeneration begins in the periphery involving the 3 O'clock and 9 O'clock positions and gradually encroaches to involve the central part of the cornea.

Treatment is required in cases with visual impairment and it is done by superficial keratectomy or by anterior lamellar keratoplasty.

Band-shaped keratopathy of cornea*

Band-shaped keratopathy is a common degenerative condition of cornea characterized by formation of a band on the cornea due to deposition of calcium (Fig. 5.4.4). It occurs in ocular conditions such as chronic uveitis, chronic keratitis, phthisis bulbi, etc. It can occur in systemic conditions associated with elevated serum calcium such as hyperparathyroidism, excessive intake of vitamin D, renal failure, sarcoidosis, etc.

Degeneration begins in the periphery involving the 3 O'clock and 9 O'clock positions and gradually encroaches to involve the central part of the cornea, similar to spheroidal degeneration.

Treatment is required in cases with visual impairment and it is done by chelation using ethylene diamine tetra-acetic acid (EDTA) or by superficial keratectomy or by anterior lamellar keratoplasty.

Lipid keratopathy of cornea

Lipid keratopathy is a type of corneal degeneration characterized by deposition of cholesterol and lipids presenting as deposition of yellowish opacities with feathery margins in corneal stroma. It occurs in ocular conditions such as chronic inflammation of cornea because of vascularization and in systemic conditions associated with altered lipid metabolism.

Treatment is by argon laser photocoagulation of the vessels of cornea to prevent deposition of lipids. The established cases are treated by keratoplasty.

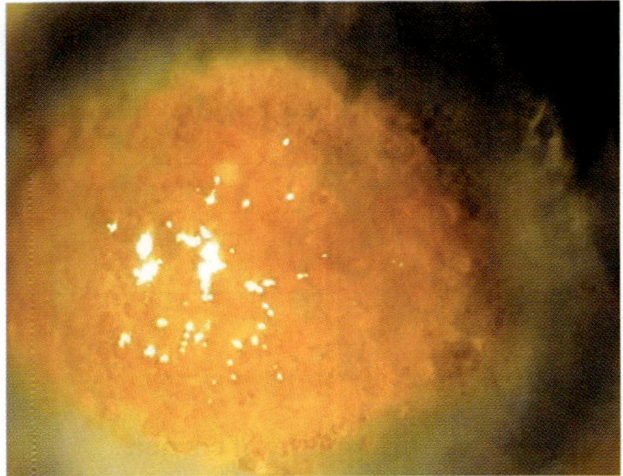

FIG. 5.4.3: Spheroidal degeneration

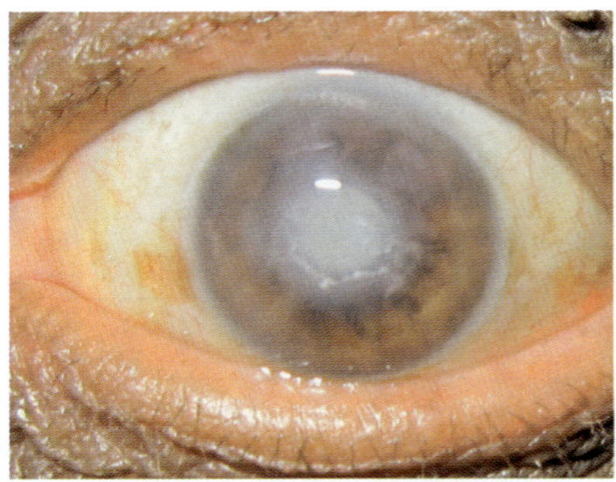

FIG. 5.4.4: Band-shaped keratopathy

Peripheral Corneal Degenerations (Table 5.4.6)

Arcus Senilis*

Arcus senilis is the most common type of corneal degeneration. It is characterized by deposition of grayish white ring-like opacity in the periphery of the cornea. It is because of deposition of lipids in the corneal stroma (Fig. 5.4.5).

Arcus senilis begins in the superior and inferior portions of the peripheral cornea and then progresses gradually to form a band of 0.5–1 mm, separated by the limbus by a clear area called lucid interval of Vogt. Treatment is not required, as the condition does not cause any symptoms.

Arcus senilis is usually a bilateral condition and presence of unilateral arcus senilis should arouse suspicion of vascular obstruction such as carotid stenosis on the contralateral side.

Presence of arcus in younger patients with age lesser than 50 years is called arcus juvenilis and it requires evaluation to rule out hyperlipoproteinemia and carotid artery disease.

Vogt limbal girdle

Vogt limbal girdle is an age-related peripheral corneal degeneration characterized by grayish white arc-shaped crescentic opacity along the limbus usually along the horizontal meridian.

TABLE 5.4.6: Peripheral corneal degenerations

Peripheral age-related corneal degenerations	*Peripheral pathological degenerations*
Arcus senilis Vogt's limbal girdle Furrow degeneration Hassall-Henle bodies	Terrien's marginal degeneration Mooren's ulcer

Furrow degeneration

Furrow degeneration is an age-related peripheral corneal degeneration usually affecting corneas with arcus senilis, characterized by thinning of the clear cornea between the limbus and the arcus.

Evaluation should be made to rule out systemic diseases such as rheumatoid arthritis

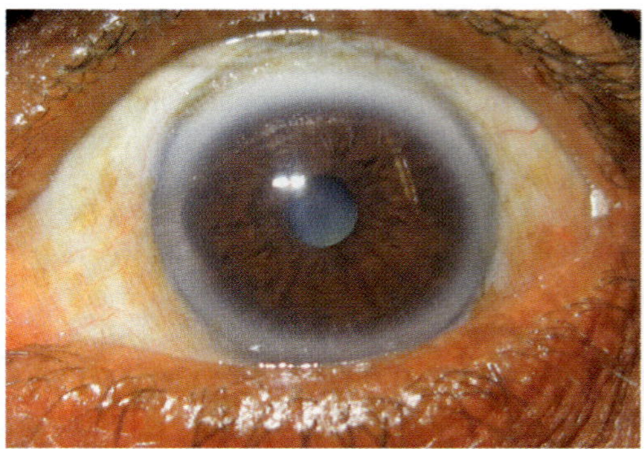

FIG. 5.4.5: Arcus senilis

and other collagen vascular diseases, which show peripheral corneal thinning.

Hassall-Henle bodies

The presence of corneal guttata in the periphery because of age-related changes is called Hassall-Henle bodies. Corneal guttata is described under Fuchs' endothelial dystrophy.

Terrien's marginal degeneration

- It is peripheral corneal degeneration characterized by peripheral corneal thinning, lipid deposition with vascularization and corneal opacification
- It usually affects middle-aged people with males being affected more than females
- It leads to astigmatism because of corneal thinning
- It usually begins in the upper part of cornea, may progress circumferentially leading to corneal perforation
- Treatment is by correction of astigmatism in early stages and advanced stage of disease may require keratoplasty.

Mooren's ulcer

Mooren's ulcer is described under idiopathic keratitis.

GIST BOX 5.4

- Corneal dystrophies are a group of non-inflammatory hereditary diseases of cornea presenting with bilateral progressive loss of transparency of cornea due to the deposition of abnormal materials within the layers of the cornea.
- Depending on the layer of the cornea affected, corneal dystrophies are classified as epithelial dystrophies, Bowman's layer dystrophies, stromal dystrophies and endothelial dystrophies.
- The ectatic conditions of cornea are a group of diseases characterized by progressive thinning of cornea. The ectatic conditions are keratoconus, iatrogenic keratectasia, keratoglobus and pellucid marginal degeneration.
- Keratoconus is defined as bilateral, but often asymmetrical, non-inflammatory progressive thinning and conical protrusion of cornea.
- Corneal degenerations are defined as age-related degenerative conditions involving the cornea occurring as a result of age-related changes or because of pathological conditions such as inflammation, trauma, chronic exposure to UV rays, etc.
- Corneal degenerations are classified into central and peripheral corneal degenerations. Spheroidal degeneration, band-shaped keratopathy and lipid keratopathy are the common central corneal degenerations and arcus senilis and Vogt's limbal girdle are common peripheral corneal degenerations.

CHAPTER

5.5 Diseases Affecting Corneal Transparency

Normal cornea is a transparent structure, the diseases of cornea result in loss of corneal transparency. The diseases affecting corneal transparency are:

- *Congenital causes* are described under congenital anomalies of cornea
- *Inflammatory causes* include both infective and non-infective keratitis
- Dystrophies and degenerations of cornea.

The common pathogenic pathways involved in loss of corneal transparency are:

- Corneal edema
- Corneal vascularization
- Corneal opacity.

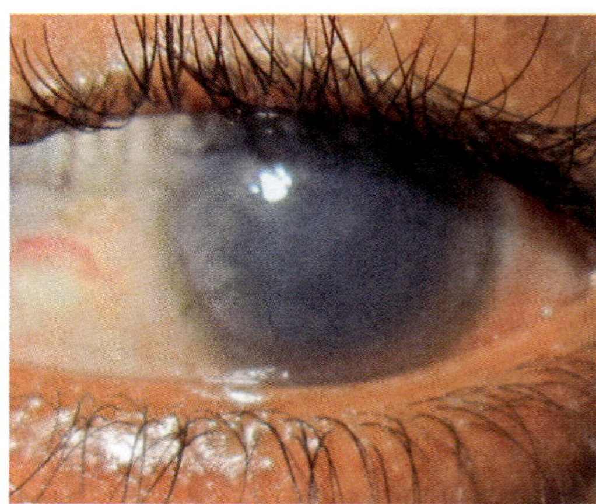

FIG. 5.5.1: Corneal edema

CORNEAL EDEMA**

Definition

Corneal edema is a condition characterized by increased hydration of cornea as a result of disturbances in the normal physiological mechanisms, which keep cornea in a state of relative dehydration (Fig. 5.5.1).

Etiopathogenesis

Normally, cornea is maintained in a state of relative dehydration by a balance between the factors, which lead to hydration of cornea such as stromal swelling pressure and intraocular pressure (IOP) and the factors, which prevent hydration of cornea such as epithelium, which acts by barrier action and endothelium, which acts by metabolic pump mechanism. The causes for corneal edema are:

- Acute raise of IOP as in acute angle closure glaucoma lens-induced glaucoma, etc.
- Damage to corneal epithelium secondary to injuries, inflammations, contact lens-induced trauma, dystrophies and degenerations of cornea, etc.
- Damage to corneal endothelium secondary to inflammations, intraocular surgeries, endothelial dystrophies, etc.

Clinical Features

- Diminution of vision, colored halos, watering, photophobia, ocular pain, etc. are the usual presenting symptoms.
- Examination of cornea shows hazy cornea with signs of the primary disease leading to corneal edema.

Treatment

Hypertonic agents such as 5% sodium chloride eyedrops or eye ointments are used for dehydrating the cornea.

Treatment of the underlying causes such as control of raised IOP and control of inflammation by appropriate drugs. Chronic longstanding corneal edema can lead to bullous keratopathy (Fig. 5.5.2).

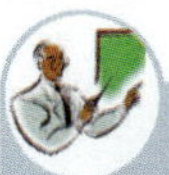

Bullous Keratopathy

Bullous keratopathy is a condition seen as a complication of untreated corneal edema characterized by the irreversible corneal edema with epithelial bullae.

The commonest cause for bullous keratopathy was a complication of cataract surgery. Aphakic bullous keratopathy was more common than pseudophakic bullous keratopathy. With the recent advances in techniques of cataract surgery, the incidence of postoperative bullous keratopathy following cataract surgery has come down drastically.

Presently, glaucoma surgeries and endothelial corneal dystrophies are the common causes for bullous keratopathy. It is a painful condition and presents with sever ocular pain, watering, photophobia and gross diminution of vision. Treatment is by keratoplasty.

CORNEAL VASCULARIZATION OR NEOVASCULARIZATION**

Definition

Corneal vascularization is defined as a condition characterized by presence of blood vessels in the cornea (Figs 5.5.3A to D).

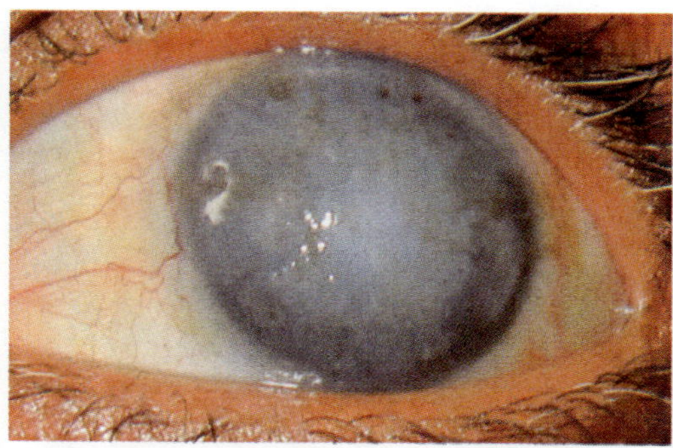

FIG. 5.5.2: Bullous keratopathy

Etiopathogenesis

Normally, cornea is an avascular structure and avascularization plays an important role in maintenance of corneal transparency. This avascularization is because of presence of vasoinhibitory substances in cornea and because of compact arrangement of corneal lamellae, thus preventing the invasion of blood vessels from the surrounding vascular limbus.

Vascularization of cornea is seen in inflammatory conditions, probably because of release of vasostimulatory factors or in conditions associated with chronic long-standing corneal edema because of loosening of the compactness of the cornea.

Clinical Features

Corneal vascularization can be asymptomatic and it may lead to visual symptoms when it involves the central part of the cornea. The symptoms of underlying cause may be seen.

Corneal vascularization is of two types:

1. Superficial vascularization.
2. Deep vascularization.

Superficial Vascularization

Superficial vascularization is seen in conditions causing keratoconjunctivitis such as trachoma, phlyctenular keratoconjunctivitis and in contact lens wearers. It is usually subepithelial in

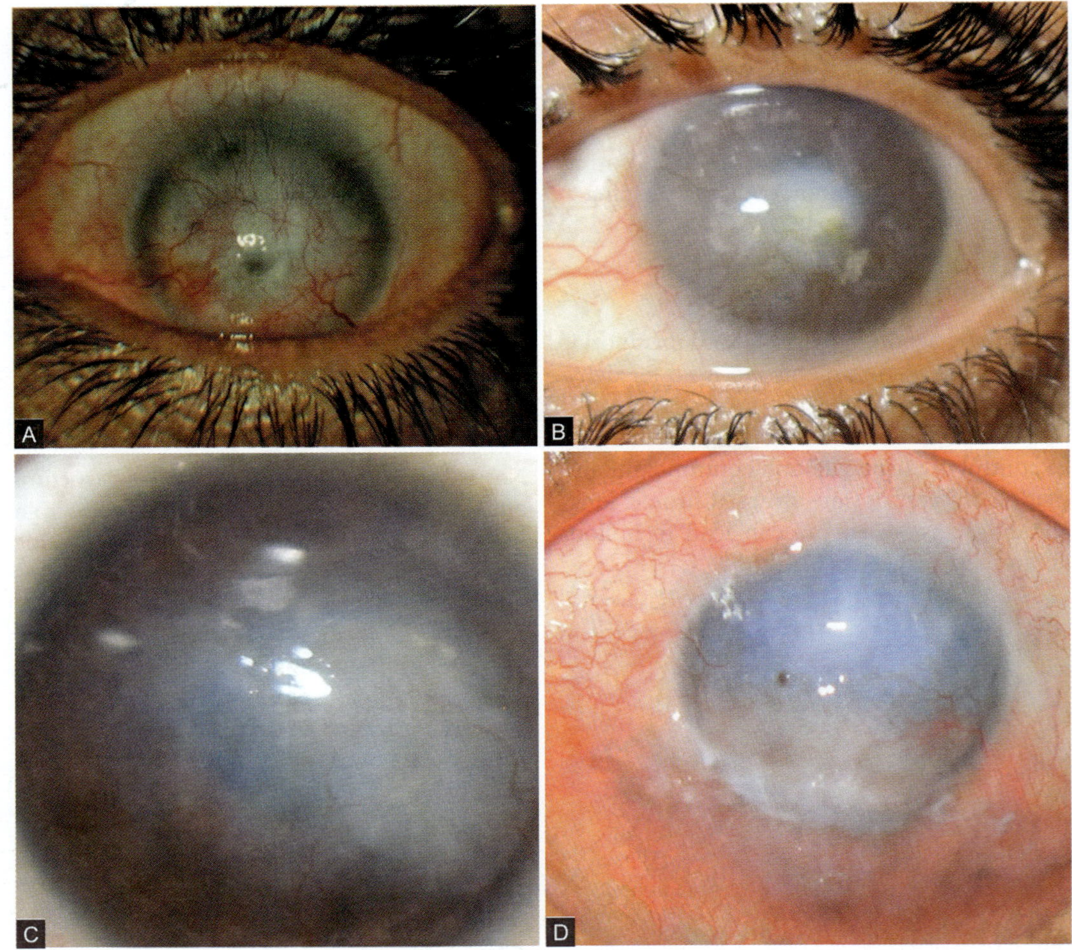

FIGS 5.5.3A to D: Vascularization of cornea

location and the vessels can be traced onto the conjunctival vessels. The vessels in superficial vascularization show multiple branching and arborizing patterns, with source being conjunctival vessel.

> **Pannus**
>
> Infiltration by inflammatory cells associated with superficial vascularization is called pannus.

Deep Vascularization

Deep vascularization is seen in diseases of corneal stroma such as interstitial keratitis, disciform keratitis, sclerosing keratitis. It is usually located in the stroma and the vessels are derived from anterior ciliary vessels, hence they are not continuous with conjunctival vessels. The vessels in deep vascularization are straighter with minimal branching.

> Deep vascularization associated with hazy cornea seen in syphilitic interstitial keratitis is called salmon patch.

Corneal vascularization can be helpful by the fact that the vessels carry antibodies and antibiotics to the site and help in healing of corneal ulcer.

Complications

Corneal vascularization can lead to lipid keratopathy and other secondary corneal degenerations, corneal opacity and intrastromal bleeding.

Treatment

- Medical treatment is by use of topical steroids and treatment of the underlying disease
- Argon laser photocoagulation of vessels is a recent mode of treatment to photocoagulate the vessels
- Cases associated with corneal opacity are treated by keratoplasty.

Presence of vascularization is a risk factor for graft rejection.

CORNEAL OPACITY**

Definition

Corneal opacity is a condition characterized by opaque cornea replacing the transparent cornea as a result of loss of transparency of cornea.

Etiopathogenesis

Corneal opacity is caused by a variety of conditions including congenital and acquired causes:

- The congenital causes are described under congenital anomalies of cornea
- The acquired causes are healing of inflammations of cornea and ocular trauma involving cornea.

The corneal opacity is because of disturbance in the regular lattice arrangement of the corneal lamellae caused by inflammations or injuries of cornea.

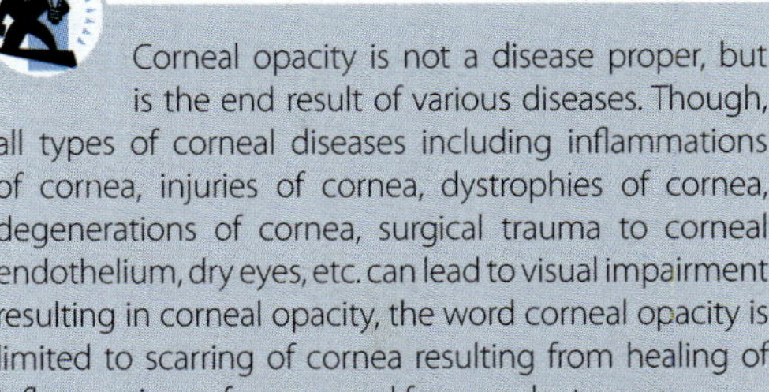

Corneal opacity is not a disease proper, but is the end result of various diseases. Though, all types of corneal diseases including inflammations of cornea, injuries of cornea, dystrophies of cornea, degenerations of cornea, surgical trauma to corneal endothelium, dry eyes, etc. can lead to visual impairment resulting in corneal opacity, the word corneal opacity is limited to scarring of cornea resulting from healing of inflammations of cornea and from ocular trauma.

Corneal opacity is one of the leading causes of blindness globally and it accounts for about 4% of all cases of blindness.

Clinical Features

Clinical features depend on the site and size of the corneal opacity. The corneal opacities in the central optical area of cornea lead to visual impairment, whereas opacities in the periphery only cause cosmetic disfigurement.

Classification of Corneal Opacity*

Corneal opacity will not have inflammatory symptoms such as pain, redness, watering, photophobia, etc. as corneal opacity is a non-inflammatory condition and in fact is the result of healing of corneal inflammation. Visual symptoms in corneal opacity are because of astigmatism or because of obstruction to the path of light when it is present in the visual axis. Classification of corneal opacity has been discussed in Table 5.5.1.

A small nebular grade of corneal opacity in the visual axis will lead to more visual impairment because of diffraction of light resulting in glare.

Treatment*

Treatment depends on the site of corneal opacity and its effect on the vision. Localized corneal

TABLE 5.5.1: Classification of corneal opacity

Types	*Features*
Nebular grade	Corneal opacity involving less than one third of corneal thickness involving the epithelium and Bowman's membrane (Fig. 5.5.4)
Macular grade	Corneal opacity involving one third to half of corneal thickness
Leukomatous grade	Corneal opacity involving more than half of corneal thickness (Fig. 5.5.5)
Adherent leukoma	Leukomatous corneal opacity with incarceration of iris into the opacity (Fig. 5.5.6)

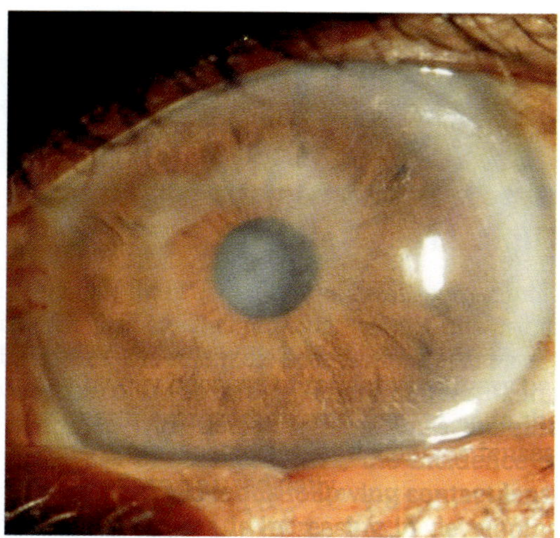

FIG. 5.5.4: Central nebular grade corneal opacity

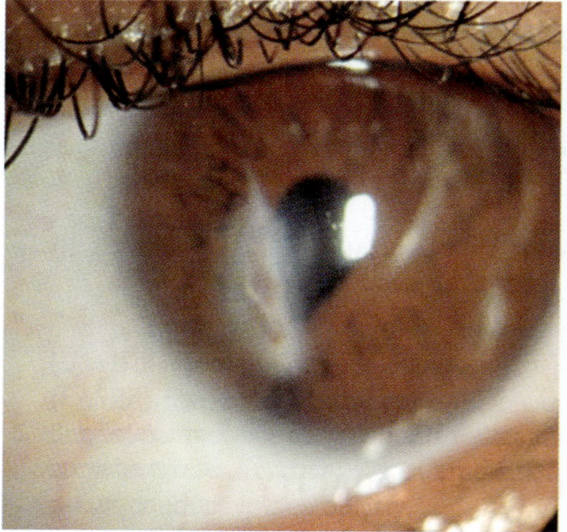

FIG. 5.5.6: Adherent leukoma

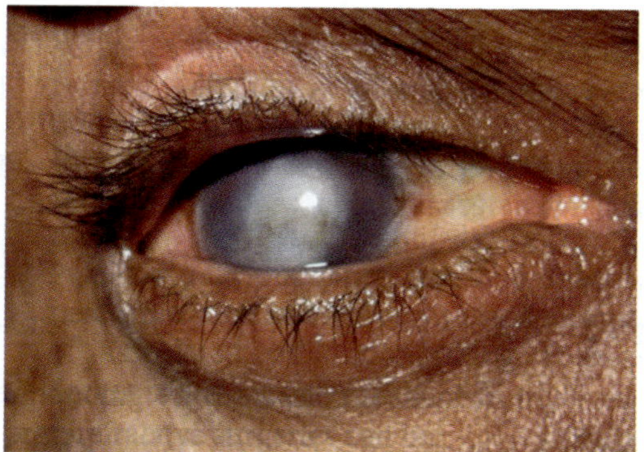

FIG. 5.5.5: Leukomatous grade corneal opacity

opacity in the periphery will not cause any visual impairment as they are away from the visual axis and hence treatment may not be necessary. However, treatment can be done for cosmetic purposes by corneal tattooing or by cosmetic contact lenses.

Localized corneal opacity in the visual axis: Treatment as follows:

1. *Optical iridectomy:* This is done in the iris below the clear cornea to improve the vision by allowing the light rays to pass through clear cornea.
2. *Rotational autograft:* It consists of trephining the scarred cornea and suturing it back

by rotating it so that opaque cornea directs away from the visual axis.

Diffuse corneal opacities: Treatment as follows:

1. Nebular grade corneal opacity is treated by phototherapeutic keratectomy (PTK).
2. Macular grade corneal opacity is treated by lamellar keratoplasty.
3. Leukomatous grade corneal opacity is treated by deep anterior lamellar keratoplasty (DALK) or penetrating keratoplasty.
4. Adherent leukoma is treated by penetrating keratoplasty.

Corneal opacity with no visual prognosis: Treatment as follows:

1. Tattooing of corneal opacity using gold chloride and platinum chloride.
2. Cosmetic contact lenses.
3. Cosmetic keratoplasty.

GIST BOX 5.5

- Normal cornea is a transparent structure; the diseases of cornea result in loss of corneal transparency. Congenital diseases, inflammations, dystrophies and degenerations are the common causes for loss of corneal transparency.
- Corneal edema, corneal vascularization and corneal opacity are the common pathogenic pathways involved in the loss of corneal transparency.
- Corneal edema is a condition characterized by increased hydration of cornea as a result of disturbances in the normal physiological mechanisms, which keep cornea in a state of relative dehydration.
- Corneal vascularization is defined as a condition characterized by presence of blood vessels in the cornea.
- Corneal opacity is a condition characterized by opaque cornea replacing the transparent cornea as a result of loss of transparency of cornea.

CHAPTER

5.6 Eye Banking and Keratoplasty

EYE BANKING

Definition

Eye banking is the process of creating awareness of eye donation, procurement, processing, preserving and distribution of donor's eyes or corneas for therapeutic use or research and training of personnel (Fig. 5.6.1).

Eye bank training centers are established for a population of 50 lakhs and cater to the needs of about 4–8 eye banks. They are involved in training of the personnel and research activities.

Eye banks are established for a population of 10–15 lakhs and cater to the needs of 4–8 eye donation centers. They procure process, preserve and distribute the donor eyes for therapeutic use.

Eye donation centers are established for a population of 2–4 lakhs. They are meant for collection of the eyes. The eyes collected in eye donation centers are transferred to eye banks for processing, preserving and distribution for use.

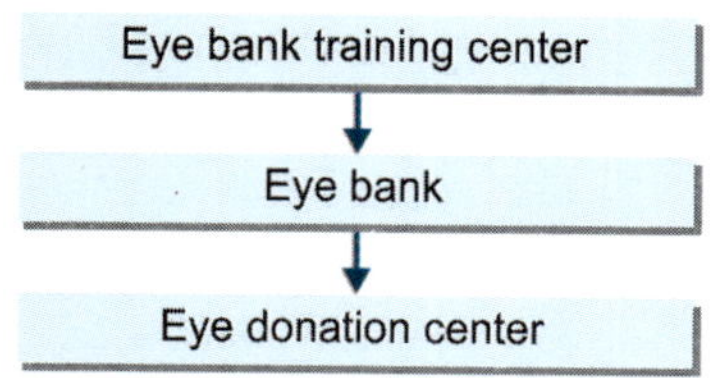

FIG. 5.6.1: Organization chart of eye banking

Corneal blindness is one of the leading causes of preventable blindness globally and in India. The only way of curing corneal blindness is by corneal transplantation and the only source of cornea being the cornea harvested from eye donors. There are about 1.1 million corneal blind people in India with about 30,000 new cases of corneal blindness being added to the list every year. Every year, only about 30,000–40,000 eyes are collected by eye donation as against a requirement of 1 lakh corneas to cure corneal blindness.

Hence, there is a need to create awareness for eye donation. To create awareness, September 8 of every year is celebrated as National Eye Donation Day and National Eye Donation Fortnight is celebrated between August 25 and September 8.

EYE BANK*

Definition

Eye bank is defined as a non-profitable voluntary organization, which procures, processes, preserves and distributes the donor's eyes for therapeutic use.

Composition

1. Each eye bank should have a:
   - Medical Director
   - Eye bank technician trained in collecting, processing and preserving donor eyes

- Grief counselor
- Vehicle with driver and a dedicated telephone line.

2. Eye bank should have equipments such as:
   - Enucleation set necessary for collecting the eyes by enucleation
   - Storage media for preserving the collected corneas
   - Operation theater for excising the corneal button
   - Refrigerator with uninterrupted power supply for storing the corneas
   - Microbiology facilities for carrying out serological blood tests
   - Slit lamp and preferably specular microscope for evaluation of the corneas.

EYE DONORS

There is no contraindication for eye donation; however, there are certain conditions where the donor tissue cannot be used for corneal grafting and they are mentioned below. There is no upper age limit for eye donation, all individuals with clear cornea can donate eye. The lower limit for eye donation is not clearly defined; however, corneas from children less than 1 year are not used because of delicate nature and thin corneas.

Conditions for Use of Donor Tissue in Eye Donation

1. *Ocular*: Intrinsic eye diseases such as intraocular tumors, intraocular inflammations, corneal degenerations, corneal dystrophies, corneal opacity, etc.
2. *Systemic*:
   a. Acquired immunodeficiency syndrome (AIDS) or human immunodeficiency virus (HIV) seropositivity, rabies, Creutzfeldt-Jakob disease, viral hepatitis.
   b. Death from unknown cause.
   c. Septicemia.
   d. Malignancies such as leukemia and lymphoma.

Eye Donation

1. Pledging is done when a person is alive and eye donation is done only after death, and it requires the consent of the family members of the deceased person irrespective of the fact whether the deceased person has done pledging for eye donation or not.
2. On death of a person, the family members should call the nearest eye bank and the eye bank team will reach the spot and collects eyes at free of cost.
3. On arrival, the eye bank team looks for the contraindications for eye donation, takes a valid written consent from the family members and collects medical records if any, notes cause of death, time of death and collect 2 mL of blood for serological testing to rule out HIV and hepatitis B surface antigen (HBsAg).
4. The eye collection should be done within 6 hours of death; a further delay may lead to suboptimal quality cornea because of drying. In the meantime, before the eyes are collected, precaution should be taken to prevent drying of the cornea by closing the eyelids and placing cotton dipped in water over the closed eyelids.
5. Usually, whole eyeball is collected from the donor and the eyeball is placed in the container and transported to the eye bank.
6. The eyeball is examined and graded in the eye bank by slit-lamp examination and preferably by the specular microscopic examination.
7. Only cornea and rim of sclera are used for transplantation and rest of the eye is used for research purposes. Corneas, which are not found to be fit for transplantation are used for research purposes.
8. Corneas found suitable for human use are preserved for use in corneal transplantation.

Eye banks and corneal transplantation in India are governed by Human Organ Transplantation Act, 1994.

Methods of Corneal Preservation*

- *Short-term storage* (up to 48 hour):
  - Moist chamber method
  - McCarey-Kaufman medium.
- *Intermediate-term storage* (up to 2 week):
  - K-Sol medium
  - Dexol medium
  - Optisol medium
  - Corneal storage medium.
- *Long-term storage*:
  - Organ culture method (up to 35 day)
  - Cryopreservation for indefinite period of time.

EYE BANK ASSOCIATION OF INDIA

The Eye Bank Association of India was established in the year 1989 to act as a resource center for the eye banks. The aims and objectives of the association are to create awareness about eye donation and to implement uniform medical standards for corneal transplantation.

Hospital Cornea Retrieval Program

Hospital cornea retrieval program (HCRP) was initiated under Eye Bank Association of India to increase the collection of eyes in the year 1991. It targets at the collection of corneas in deaths occurring in hospitals. It is done by grief counselors, who approach the relatives of the deceased person and motivate them for eye donation.

KERATOPLASTY**

Definition

Keratoplasty is also known as corneal transplantation. It is a surgical procedure in which the diseased host or patient's cornea is replaced by healthy donor cornea by excising the diseased cornea and suturing the healthy donor cornea. Keratoplasty is the most commonly performed organ transplantation (Fig. 5.6.2).

Classification

1. Based on indications, keratoplasty is classified as detailed below:*
   a. Optical keratoplasty: This is done for improvement of vision as for corneal opacity, corneal dystrophies and corneal degenerations.
   b. Therapeutic keratoplasty: This is done as a part of treatment as in treatment of non-healing corneal ulcer, which may ultimately end in perforation.
   c. Tectonic keratoplasty: This is done to restore integrity of eyeball and to provide structural support as in perforated corneal ulcer.
   d. Cosmetic keratoplasty: This is done only for cosmetic purpose without any visual prognosis as in anterior staphyloma or corneal opacity without any chance of visual impairment.
2. Based on the morphology, keratoplasty is classified as shown in Table 5.6.1.

Procedure

1. Keratoplasty is performed under local anesthesia; general anesthesia is indicated in pediatric cases and in uncooperative adults.
2. The donor corneal button is trephined and kept ready before starting the surgery on the patient. Usually, the size of donor cornea is taken 0.5 mm more than the recipient's cornea.

TABLE 5.6.1: Classification of keratoplasty on the basis of morphology

Types	*Features*
Penetrating keratoplasty	Full thickness of cornea is transplanted
Lamellar keratoplasty	Partial thickness of cornea is transplanted
Keratoepithelioplasty	Transplantation of only epithelium is done

3. The recipient's cornea is trephined and it is replaced by donor cornea. It is sutured by intermittent or continuous sutures.
4. Postoperatively, antibiotic eyedrops are used till the epithelium defect heals; steroid eyedrops are used hourly in the initial period after keratoplasty and they are tapered over 3–6 months.

The postoperative complications of keratoplasty are detailed in Table 5.6.2.

Lamellar Keratoplasty

Lamellar keratoplasty is further classified as:

1. *Anterior lamellar keratoplasty:* Only anterior portion of cornea excluding Descemet's membrane and endothelium is transplanted. It is indicated in diseases involving only anterior part of the cornea such as stromal dystrophies of cornea, keratoconus, etc. It is of two types:
   a. *Anterior lamellar keratoplasty (ALK):* Here, epithelium, Bowman's membrane and anterior part of the stroma are transplanted.
   b. *Deep anterior lamellar keratoplasty (DALK):* Here, except endothelium and Descemet's membrane, rest of the cornea is transplanted.

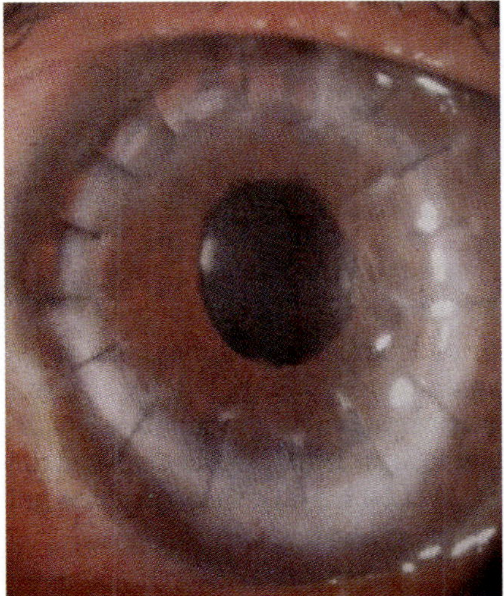

FIG. 5.6.2: Appearance of cornea after keratoplasty

2. *Posterior lamellar keratoplasty:* Only posterior portion of cornea involving endothelium and Descemet's membrane is transplanted. It is indicated in diseases involving only the endothelium such as endothelial dystrophies of cornea. It is also called endothelial keratoplasty or Descemet's stripping endothelial keratoplasty (DSEK) or deep lamellar endothelial keratoplasty (DLEK).

Keratoepithelioplasty

Keratoepithelioplasty is a surgical procedure for treatment of persistent epithelial defect by using donor corneal epithelium. It is indicated in patients with recurrent or persistent epithelial defects as in chemical injuries.

Keratoprosthesis

Keratoprosthesis is a surgical procedure in which the diseased patient's cornea is replaced by artificial cornea. It is indicated in cases of corneal blindness in which the corneal grafting is failed or associated with high risk of corneal graft failure as in corneal opacity associated with severe dry eye, which is seen in conditions such as Stevens-Johnson syndrome, chemical burns, etc. The commonly

TABLE 5.6.2: Postoperative complications of keratoplasty

Early postoperative complications	*Late postoperative complications*
Shallow anterior chamber	Graft rejection
Wound leak	Epithelial downgrowth
Wound dehiscence	Fibrous ingrowth
Iris prolapse	Astigmatism
Epithelial defects	Glaucoma
Hyphema	Recurrence of the disease
Graft edema	
Primary graft failure	
Acute elevated intraocular pressure	
Graft infection	
Endophthalmitis	

used keratoprosthesis are osteo-odonto-keratoprosthesis and Boston keratoprosthesis.

Because of the high risk of infections and other complications following keratoprosthesis, the use of keratoprosthesis is limited to end stage corneal blindness, which cannot be treated by keratoplasty. Following keratoprosthesis, patient requires lifelong follow-up at frequent intervals and patient is advised with antibiotic eyedrops daily to prevent infections.

GIST BOX 5.6

- Eye banking is the process of creating awareness of eye donation, procurement, processing, preserving and distribution of donor eyes/corneas for therapeutic use/research and training of personnel.
- Eye bank is defined as a non-profitable voluntary organization, which procures, processes, preserves and distributes the donor eyes for therapeutic use.
- Keratoplasty is also known as corneal transplantation. It is a surgical procedure in which the diseased host or patient's cornea is replaced by healthy donor cornea by excising the diseased cornea and suturing the healthy donor cornea.
- Keratoplasty is the most commonly performed organ transplantation.

FREQUENTLY ASKED QUESTIONS (FAQs)

*Short Answers

1. Histology of cornea.
2. Nerve supply of cornea.
3. Metabolism of cornea.
4. Mention the factors responsible for transparency of cornea.
5. Microcornea.
6. Megalocornea.
7. Differential diagnosis of megalocornea.
8. Role of atropine in the treatment of corneal ulcer.
9. Descemetocele.
10. Hypopyon.
11. Dendritic keratitis or dendritic ulcer.
12. Disciform keratitis.
13. Mention the causes for decreased corneal sensation.
14. Rosacea keratitis.
15. Marginal keratitis.
16. Mention the causes for peripheral ulcerative keratitis.
17. Photophthalmia.
18. Mention the differences between corneal dystrophies and corneal degenerations.
19. Spheroidal degeneration of cornea.
20. Band-shaped keratopathy of cornea.
21. Arcus senilis.
22. Define and classify corneal opacity.
23. Treatment of corneal opacity.
24. Mention the indications for keratoplasty.
25. Eye bank.
26. Mention the methods of preservation of cornea in eye bank.

**Short Essays

1. Mention the causes for congenital corneal opacity.
2. Describe the complications of corneal ulcer.
3. Non-healing corneal ulcer.
4. Perforated corneal ulcer.
5. Acanthamoeba keratitis.
6. Herpes simplex keratitis.
7. Epithelial keratitis.
8. Herpes zoster ophthalmicus.
9. Neurotrophic keratitis.
10. Exposure keratitis.
11. Neuroparalytic keratitis.
12. Mooren's ulcer.
13. Interstitial keratitis.
14. Superficial punctate keratitis.
15. Filamentary keratitis.
16. Treatment of keratoconus.
17. Define and classify corneal dystrophies.
18. Corneal edema.
19. Corneal vascularization.
20. Corneal opacity.
21. Keratoplasty.

***Long Essays

1. Define corneal ulcer or ulcerative keratitis. Describe the etiology, pathogenesis, clinical features and management of bacterial corneal ulcer.
2. Define and classify keratitis. Describe etiology, clinical features and management of hypopyon corneal ulcer.
3. Describe etiology, clinical features and management of mycotic keratitis or fungal corneal ulcer.
4. Mention the causes for viral keratitis. Describe the clinical features and treatment of herpes simplex keratitis.
5. Mention the ectatic conditions of cornea. Describe the clinical features, differential diagnosis and treatment of keratoconus.

BIBLIOGRAPHY

1. Agrawal PK. The pathology of cornea (a histopathological study). Indian J Ophthalmol. 1983;31(5):662-5.
2. Akpek KE. A case of peripheral ulcerative keratitis associated with ocular rosacea. [online]. Available from www.uveitis.org/docs/dm/rosacea_and_puk.pdf
3. Al-Aqaba MA, Fares U, Suleman H, et al. Architecture and distribution of human corneal nerves. Br J Ophthalmol. 2010;94(6):784-9.
4. Dubey AK, Jaisankar TJ, Thappa DM. Clinical and morphological characteristics of herpes zoster in south India. Indian J Dermatol. 2005; 50:203-7.
5. Dutta LC. Modern Ophthalmology, 3rd edition. New Delhi: Jaypee Brothers Medical Publishers (P) Ltd; 2005.
6. Elliott JH, Feman SS, O'Day DM, et al. Hereditary sclerocornea. Arch Ophthalmol. 1985;103(5):676-9.
7. Etya'ale D. Vision 2020: Update on onchocerciasis. Community Eye Health. 2001; 14(38):19-21.
8. Garg P, Rao GN. Corneal ulcer: diagnosis and management. Community Eye Health. 1999; 12(30):21-3.
9. Goldman JN, Benedek GB. The relationship between morphology and transparency in the nonswelling corneal stroma of the shark. Invest. Ophthalmol. 1967;6(6):574-600.
10. Gore DM, Shortt AJ, Allan BD. New clinical pathways for keratoconus. Eye (Lond). 2013; 27(3):329-39.
11. Judge J, Waring GO, Blocker RJ. Congenital and neonatal corneal abnormalities. Corneal Disorders Clinical Diagnosis and Management, 2nd edition. Philadelphia: WB Saunders; 1998.
12. Liu C, Paul B, Tandon R, et al. The osteo-odonto-keratoprosthesis (OOKP). Semin Ophthalmol. 2005;20(2):113-28.
13. Perez MK, Hannush SB, Waring GO. Congenital and neonatal corneal abnormalities. Duane's Foundations of Clinical Ophthalmology.
14. Preez V. Interstitial keratitis. [online]. Available from www.uveitis.org/docs/dm/interstial_keratitis.pdf
15. Ranjakumar. Parasitic keratitis. Kerala Journal of Ophthalmology. 2008;XX(4).
16. Rautaraya B, Sharma S, Kar S, et al. Diagnosis and treatment outcome of mycotic keratitis at a tertiary eye care center in eastern India. BMC Ophthalmol. 2011;11:39.
17. Sangwan VS, Zafirakis P, Foster CS. Mooren's ulcer: current concepts in management. Indian J Ophthalmol. 1997;45(1):7-17.
18. Shaikh S, Ta CN. Evaluation and management of herpes zoster ophthalmicus. Am Fam Physician. 2002;66(9):1723-30.
19. Tsai CK, Lai IC, Kuo HK, et al. Anterior megalophthalmos. Chang Gung Med J. 2005;28(3):191-5.
20. Vajpyee RB. Corneal transplantation, 2nd edition. New Delhi: Jaypee Brothers Medical Publishers (P) Ltd; 2010.
21. Vantieghem G, Maudgal PC. Neuroparalytic keratopathy as the first sign of a cerebral meningioma. Bull Soc Belge Ophtalmol. 2007;303:81-6.

SECTION 6

Sclera

CHAPTER

6.1 Anatomy of Sclera

Sclera is the outermost layer of the eyeball. It accounts for posterior five sixths of the outer fibrous coat, remaining one sixth being constituted by cornea.

GROSS ANATOMY

Sclera covers the posterior five sixths of the eyeball. Sclera encloses whole of the eyeball with two openings, anteriorly for cornea and posteriorly for optic nerve.

The outer surface of sclera is covered by Tenon's capsule and bulbar conjunctiva. Sub-Tenon's space lies between Tenon's capsule and outer surface of sclera, which is the site for giving sub-Tenon's injection. The inner surface of sclera is separated from choroid by suprachoroidal space. Accumulation of fluid in suprachoroidal space can lead to choroidal detachment.

The thickness of sclera varies from 1 to 0.3 mm. Sclera is thickest posteriorly, surrounding the entry of optic nerve and is thinnest at the insertion of the recti muscles.

Apertures in Sclera

The sclera is pierced by three sets of apertures, which are as follows:

1. Anterior apertures situated near the limbus for the entry of anterior ciliary vessels and nerves.
2. Middle apertures situated 4 mm behind the equator for the entry of vortex veins.
3. Posterior apertures near the optic nerve for the entry of long and short posterior ciliary nerves and vessels.

Histology

Sclera shows three layers from outside inwards, which are as follows:

1. Episclera: It is a vascularized connective tissue, which covers the sclera.
2. Sclera proper: It consists of irregularly arranged collagen fibers and it is avascular.
3. Lamina fusca: It is the innermost layer of the sclera, which becomes continuous with suprachoroidal lamina.

FUNCTIONS

- Sclera being the tough fibrous layer, maintains the structural integrity and shape of the eyeball
- It provides site for insertion of extraocular muscles.

EMBRYOLOGY

Sclera develops from mesenchyme, which is derived from neural crest.

Why Sclera is Involved in Collagen Vascular Diseases and Arthritis?

Sclera is a connective tissue and it develops from same embryological layer as connective tissue elsewhere in the body, cartilage, tendons and ligaments. Hence one of the most common etiological basis for scleritis are collagen vascular diseases and arthritic diseases.

Lamina Cribrosa

Lamina cribrosa is a mesh-like structure present behind the optic disk in the sclera. It allows the fibers of the optic nerve to pass through it and it acts as a pressure barrier between the intraocular space and the retrobulbar space. The pores in the lamina cribrosa are visible as lamellar dot sign in advanced glaucomatous atrophy.

Scleral Spur

Scleral spur is a circular ridge of sclera present on the inner side of corneoscleral junction. It is visible on gonioscopy above the ciliary body band as a white line.

GIST BOX 6.1

- Sclera is the outermost layer of the eyeball. It accounts for posterior five sixths of the outer fibrous coat.
- Sclera being the tough fibrous layer, maintains the structural integrity and shape of the eyeball.
- The thickness of sclera varies from 1 to 0.3 mm. Sclera is thickest posteriorly, surrounding the entry of optic nerve and is thinnest at the insertion of the recti muscles.

CHAPTER

6.2 Inflammatory Diseases of Episclera and Sclera

EPISCLERITIS**

Definition

Inflammation of episclera is called episcleritis (Figs 6.2.1A and B). The inflammation is benign, recurrent and self-limiting in nature.

Etiopathogenesis

1. Episcleritis is seen more commonly in females. It is seen in younger and middle age group.
2. Episcleritis is idiopathic in nature. It may be found in association with underlying systemic disorders, e.g. gout, rheumatoid arthritis, Wegener's granulomatosis, polyarteritis nodosa and rosacea. Episcleritis may be a manifestation of systemic infective diseases, e.g. tuberculosis, syphilis.
3. The inflammatory response is limited to episcleral tissue and the inflammatory response may be diffused, called simple episcleritis or localized, called nodular episcleritis.

Clinical Features

1. Redness of the eye, mild-to-moderate pain and watering are the presenting symptoms.
2. On examination, one of the following clinical types may be seen:
   a. Simple episcleritis: It is characterized by diffuse involvement of the episclera involving more than one quadrant of the eye. The inflammation is deeper and lies

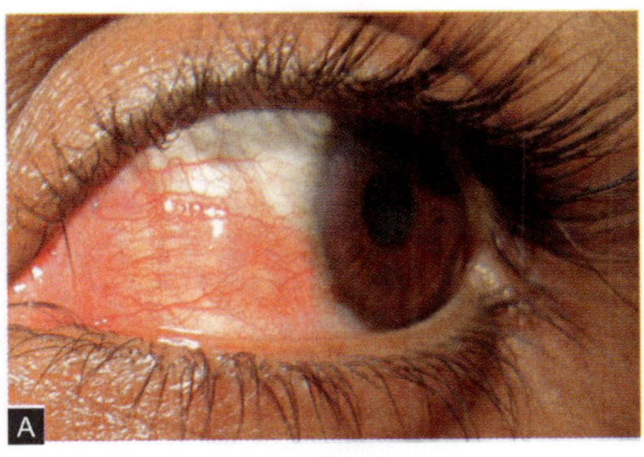

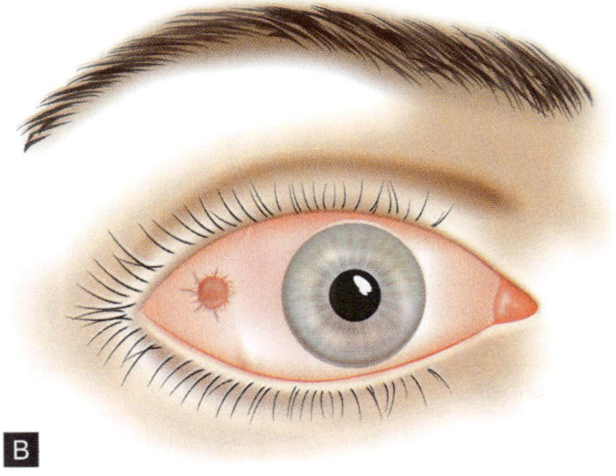

FIGS 6.2.1A and B: Episcleritis. **A**. Photograph; **B**. Diagrammatic representation.

below the conjunctiva, thus differentiating from conjunctival congestion.

b. Nodular episcleritis: It is characterized by nodular inflammation of the episclera.

Simple episcleritis usually resolves spontaneously over a period of 1–3 weeks. Nodular episcleritis is usually more symptomatic than simple episcleritis and takes longer time to resolve.

Differential Diagnosis

Episcleritis has to be differentiated from:

1. Conjunctivitis: It is characterized by discharge, which is absent in episcleritis and in conjunctivitis, congestion is superficial, and shows features of conjunctival congestion.
2. Scleritis (Table 6.2.1).

Investigations

Laboratory investigations are not required in all the patients. They are indicated in a small group of patients who show recurrent episcleritis or have a history of underlying autoimmune or collagen vascular or metabolic diseases as described in etiology. Investigations are similar to those described under scleritis.

Treatment

- Treatment is by topical steroids, i.e. eyedrops such as prednisolone or dexamethasone or fluorometholone
- Oral non-steroidal anti-inflammatory drugs such as indomethacin 75 mg or diclofenac 50 mg are prescribed for pain relief and control of inflammation
- Oral steroids are indicated in non-responsive cases.

Episcleritis Periodica Fugax*

- It is a type of episcleritis characterized by recurrence at regular intervals
- It is diffuse episcleritis with clinical features and treatment similar to simple episcleritis.

SCLERITIS*

Definition

Inflammation of sclera is called scleritis. The disease runs a chronic course and causes significant visual impairment.

TABLE 6.2.1: Differences between episcleritis and scleritis*

Features	*Episcleritis*	*Scleritis*
Definition	Benign recurrent inflammation of episclera	Chronic inflammation of sclera
Etiology	Seen in younger or middle age group and more common in females	Seen in elderly age group and more common in females
Association with underlying systemic diseases	Uncommon	Common with 50% of patients showing underlying systemic disease
Clinical features	Mild pain and sectoral congestion	Severe pain and scleral congestion
Visual prognosis	Good	Poor in necrotizing scleritis and posterior scleritis
Complications	Rare	Commonly seen in necrotizing scleritis
Treatment	Topical steroids, oral anti-inflammatory drugs	Topical steroids, oral anti-inflammatory drugs, oral steroids and immunosuppressive drugs

Etiopathogenesis

- It is more common in middle-aged and elderly patients; usually more in females than males
- Exact etiology is not known
- It is more commonly seen in association with underlying systemic diseases, such as:
  - Collagen vascular diseases, e.g. systemic lupus erythematosus, polyarteritis nodosa, Wegener's granulomatosis, rheumatoid arthritis, giant cell arteritis, etc.
  - Chronic granulomatous bacterial infective diseases, e.g. syphilis, tuberculosis, etc.
  - Metabolic diseases, e.g. gout, etc.
  - Surgery-induced scleritis following ocular surgeries, e.g. cataract surgery, trabeculectomy, pterygium surgery, squint surgery, etc.
  - Infectious scleritis caused by pyogenic bacteria such as *Staphylococcus aureus* or viruses such as varicella zoster virus because of contiguous spread of infection from surrounding structures such as infective keratitis.

Pathology

Pathology of scleritis is characterized by granulomatous inflammation with fibrinoid necrosis with infiltration by epithelioid cells along with polymorphonuclear cells, lymphocytes and plasma cells.

Classification of Scleritis**

Based on the anatomical site of inflammation and associated pathological features, scleritis is classified into:

- Anterior scleritis (Figs 6.2.2A and B):
  - Necrotizing:
    - Necrotizing scleritis with inflammation
    - Necrotizing scleritis without inflammation (scleromalacia perforans).
  - Non-necrotizing:
    - Diffuse non-necrotizing scleritis
    - Nodular non-necrotizing scleritis.
- Posterior scleritis.

Anterior Necrotizing Scleritis with Inflammation

The condition is the most severe form of scleritis.

Etiology

The condition is usually associated with underlying systemic vascular disorders.

Clinical features

- Redness of the eye, severe pain and watering are the presenting symptoms

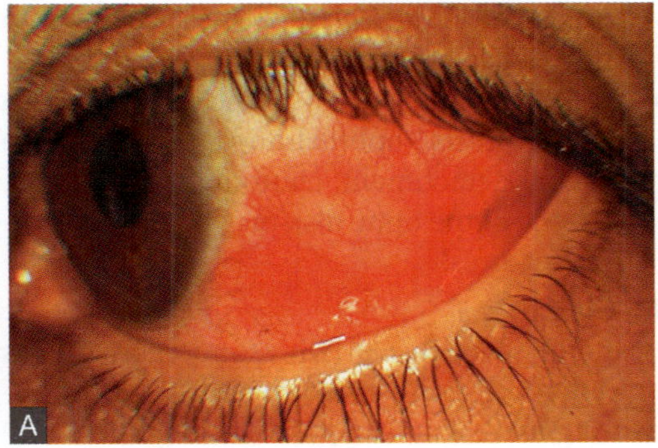

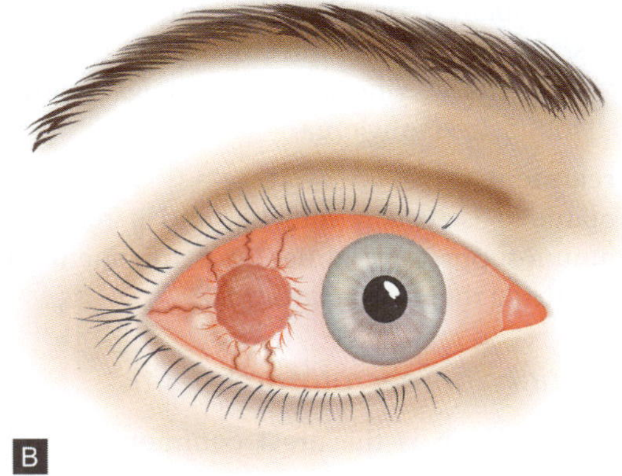

FIGS 6.2.2A and B: Anterior scleritis. **A**. Photograph; **B**. Diagrammatic representation.

- On examination, severe inflammation of the sclera associated with scleral necrosis is seen
- Sclera thins out ultimately resulting in staphyloma and loss of vision.

Treatment
- Treatment is by oral steroids, 1–2 mg/kg body weight
- Immunosuppressive drugs such as cyclophosphamide or cyclosporine are indicated in cases not responding to steroids
- Topical steroids are subconjunctival steroid injections, which should be preferably avoided, as they may lead to scleral thinning and scleral perforation.

*Anterior Necrotizing Scleritis Without Inflammation/ Scleromalacia Perforans**

The condition is also known as scleromalacia perforans.

Etiology
The condition is seen in elderly females with rheumatoid arthritis. It is usually bilateral.

Clinical features
- Patient usually presents with minimal symptoms and pain is usually absent
- On examination, it presents with appearance of yellow anterior scleral nodules, which gradually develop a necrotic slough eventually separating from the underlying sclera, leaving behind thin sclera through which underlying uveal tissue bulges out resulting in staphyloma.

Treatment
Treatment is usually difficult, and it requires immunosuppressive drugs and treatment of underlying rheumatoid arthritis.

Anterior Non-necrotizing Scleritis

The condition is the most common type of scleritis.

Clinical features
- It presents with redness, moderate-to-severe pain and watering similar to episcleritis, but the degree of pain is more severe compared to episcleritis
- On examination, one of the following clinical types may be seen:
  - Diffuse scleritis: It is characterized by diffuse involvement of the sclera involving more than one quadrant of the eye
  - Nodular scleritis: It is characterized by nodular inflammation of the sclera.

Treatment
- Treatment is by topical steroids such as prednisolone eyedrops or dexamethasone eyedrops or fluorometholone eyedrops
- Oral non-steroidal inflammatory drugs such as indomethacin 75 mg or diclofenac 50 mg are prescribed for pain relief and control of inflammation
- Oral steroids are indicated in non-responsive cases.

Posterior Scleritis

Inflammation of sclera behind the equator of the globe is called posterior scleritis. Because of varied clinical presentations, it is one of the most commonly misdiagnosed diseases in ophthalmology.

Clinical features
- Posterior scleritis alone presents with pain and diminution of vision; redness is absent unless posterior scleritis is associated with anterior scleritis
- Complications of posterior scleritis such as proptosis, ophthalmoplegia, exudative retinal detachment, choroidal detachment, edema of the optic disk may be the presenting features.

Investigations
Bi-modal scan (B-scan) ultrasonography shows fluid in the Tenon's space characteristically appearing as T-sign. Computed tomography (CT)

scan is also useful as it shows thickening of the posterior sclera.

Differential diagnosis

Posterior scleritis should be differentiated from choroidal tumor, exudative retinal detachment, pseudotumor of the orbit, central serous chorioretinopathy, Vogt-Koyanagi-Harada syndrome and posterior uveitis.

Treatment

- Posterior scleritis is treated by oral non-steroidal anti-inflammatory drugs, oral steroids and periocular steroid injections
- Immunosuppressive drugs are indicated in non-responsive cases.

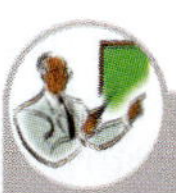

Investigations Required for Evaluation of Scleritis

- Complete blood count (CBC).
- Erythrocyte sedimentation rate (ESR).
- C-reactive protein (CRP).
- Rheumatoid factor to rule out rheumatoid arthritis.
- Serum uric acid to rule out gout.
- Venereal disease research laboratory (VDRL), fluorescent treponemal antibody absorption (FTA-ABS) to rule out syphilis.
- Antinuclear antibody (ANA) to rule out systemic lupus erythematosus.
- Antineutrophil cytoplasmic antibody (ANCA) to rule out Wegener's granulomatosis.
- Chest X-ray and Mantoux test to rule out tuberculosis.
- B-scan, CT scan and fundus fluorescein angiography in posterior scleritis.

Complications of Scleritis*

Complications are most commonly seen in anterior necrotizing scleritis and posterior scleritis.

- Anterior necrotizing scleritis is associated with complications such as:
  - Corneal involvement in the form of peripheral corneal thinning, corneal ulceration, sclerokeratitis
  - Uveal involvement, i.e. uveitis of the type anterior/posterior or panuveitis
  - Staphyloma formation with loss of vision is the end result of scleritis.
- Posterior scleritis can cause complications such as:
  - Macular edema
  - Exudative retinal detachment
  - Choroidal detachment.

Treatment of Scleritis*

- Scleritis is treated mainly by medical line of management such as:
  - Topical steroids, e.g. prednisolone or dexamethasone or fluorometholone and oral non-steroidal anti-inflammatory drugs such as indomethacin or flurbiprofen are indicated in anterior non-necrotizing scleritis
  - Oral steroids and immunosuppressive drugs are indicated in anterior necrotizing scleritis and posterior scleritis
  - Topical steroids should be used with precaution in necrotizing scleritis and periocular injections of steroids are contraindicated in necrotizing scleritis because of risk of sclera thinning and sclera perforation.
- Surgical management of scleritis:
  - Surgical management in the form of sclera grafting is indicated in cases of extensive scleral thinning or scleral perforation. Donor sclera or autologous periosteum can be used as grafts.

GIST BOX 6.2

- Inflammation of episclera is called episcleritis. The inflammation is benign, recurrent and self-limiting in nature.
- Episcleritis is seen more commonly in females. It is seen in younger and middle age group.
- Inflammation of sclera is called scleritis. The disease runs a chronic course and causes significant visual impairment. It is more common in middle-aged and elderly patients; usually more in females than males.

CHAPTER

6.3 Staphyloma

STAPHYLOMA*

Definition

Abnormal protrusion of uveal tissue through weak outer coat of the eyeball.

Etiopathogenesis

Staphyloma is secondary to localized or diffuse thinning of the outer coat of eyeball, cornea or sclera. The uveal tissue, which lies below the cornea or sclera, bulges out leading to staphyloma.

Clinical Features

Clinical features depend on the subtype of staphyloma. Depending on the anatomical site of involvement, staphyloma is divided into:

1. Anterior staphyloma: It is the abnormal protrusion of iris through weak and thinned out cornea. It usually follows perforated corneal ulcer or perforating corneal injury.
2. Intercalary staphyloma: It is the abnormal protrusion of root of the iris through weak and thinned out limbus. It usually follows perforated peripheral corneal ulcer or perforating injury involving limbus.
3. Ciliary staphyloma: It is the abnormal protrusion of ciliary body through weak and thinned out sclera in the ciliary zone, which lies 3 mm away from limbus. It usually follows scleritis or perforating injury involving the ciliary zone.
4. Equatorial staphyloma: It is the abnormal protrusion of choroid through weak and thinned outer sclera in the equatorial region. It usually follows scleritis.
5. Posterior staphyloma**: It is the abnormal protrusion of choroid through weak and thinned out sclera behind the equator. It usually follows pathological myopia and posterior scleritis.
6. Different types of staphyloma are shown in Figures 6.3.1A to H.

Staphyloma presents with diminution of vision and cosmetic disfigurement (excluding posterior staphyloma). Staphyloma usually follows primary causative disease or event, e.g. perforated corneal ulcer, penetrating injury or may be associated with conditions such as pathological myopia.

Treatment

Anterior staphyloma and intercalary staphyloma with visual prognosis are treated by staphylectomy and keratoplasty. Staphyloma with no visual prognosis are treated by evisceration or enucleation of the eye followed by artificial prosthetic eye for cosmetic indication.

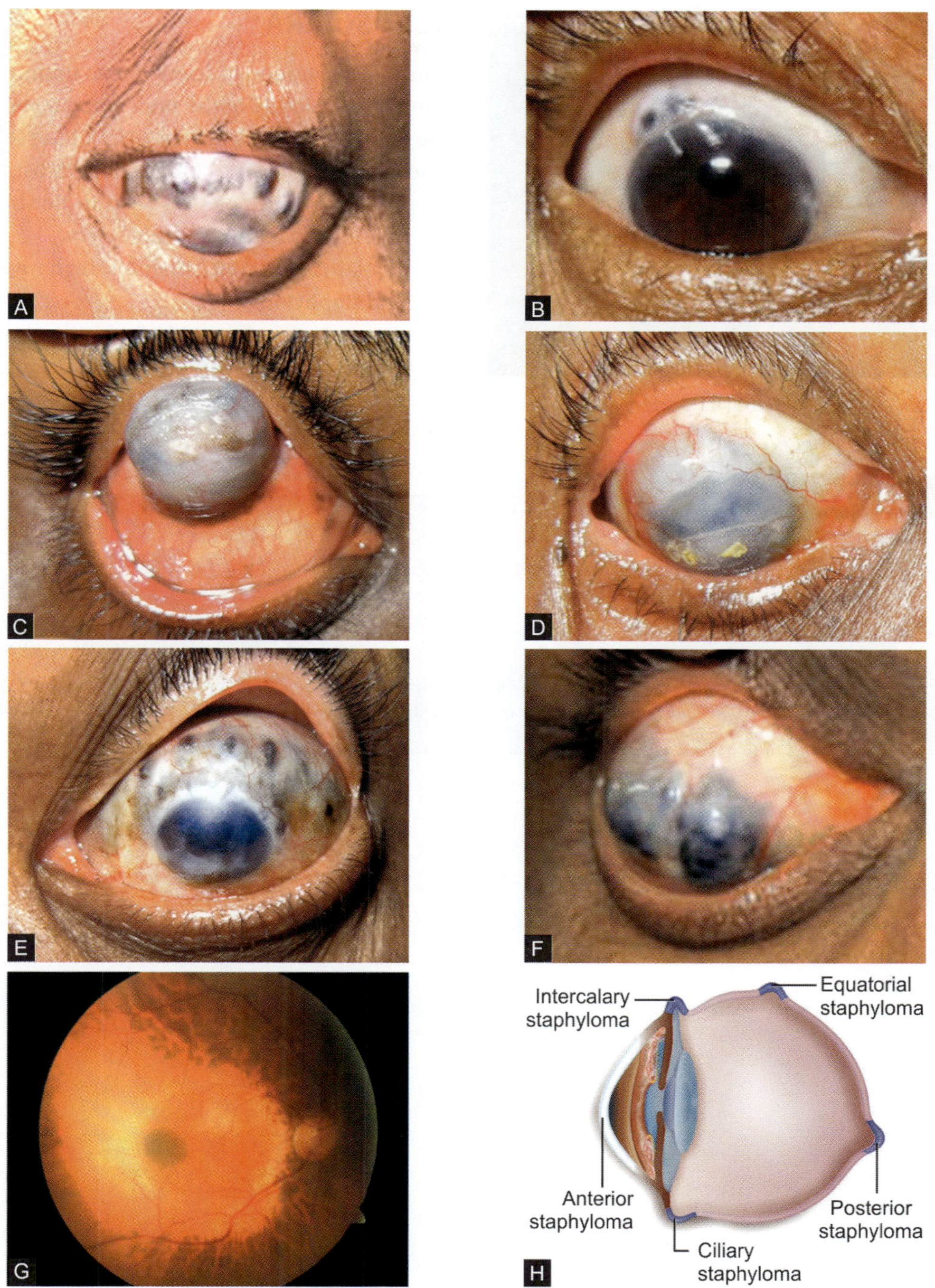

FIGS 6.3.1A to H: Staphyloma. **A.** Diffuse staphyloma; **B.** Localized staphyloma; **C.** Anterior staphyloma; **D.** Intercalary staphyloma; **E** and **F.** Ciliary staphyloma; **G.** Posterior staphyloma; **H.** Diagrammatic representation.

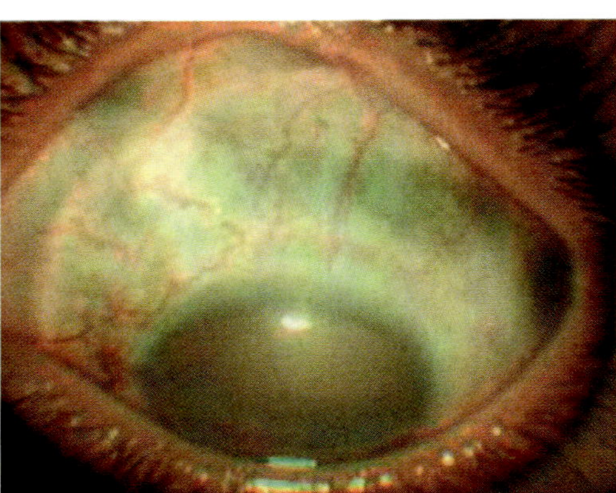

FIG. 6.3.2: Blue sclera

BLUE SCLERA*

Bluish discoloration of sclera due to thinning of sclera and visibility of the underlying uveal tissue is called blue sclera (Fig. 6.3.2). Blue sclera is seen in the following conditions such as:

1. Normally blue sclera is seen in newborns and infants because of thin sclera.
2. Ocular causes: Buphthalmos, high myopia and staphyloma.
3. Systemic causes: Marfan's syndrome, Ehlers-Danlos syndrome, pseudoxanthoma elasticum and osteogenesis imperfect.

GIST BOX 6.3

- Abnormal protrusion of uveal tissue through weak outer coat of the eyeball.
- Staphyloma occurs secondary to localized or diffuse thinning of the outer coat of the eyeball, cornea or sclera. The uveal tissue, which lies below the cornea or sclera, bulges out leading to staphyloma.
- Depending on the anatomical site, staphyloma is classified into anterior, intercalary, ciliary, equatorial and posterior staphyloma.
- Anterior staphyloma and intercalary staphyloma with visual prognosis are treated by staphylectomy and keratoplasty. Staphyloma with no visual prognosis is treated by evisceration or enucleation of the eye followed by artificial prosthetic eye for cosmetic indication.

FREQUENTLY ASKED QUESTIONS (FAQs)

*Short Essays

1. Episcleritis.
2. Scleritis.
3. Staphyloma.

**Short Answers

1. Episcleritis periodica fugax.
2. Classification of scleritis.
3. Mention the systemic diseases associated with scleritis.
4. Mention the complications of scleritis.
5. Treatment of scleritis.
6. Mention the differences between scleritis and episcleritis.
7. Scleromalacia perforans.
8. Posterior staphyloma.
9. Blue sclera.

BIBLIOGRAPHY

1. Akpek EK. Necrotizing scleritis: diagnosis and therapy. [online]. Available from www.uveitis.org/docs/dm/necrotizing_scleritis_diagnosis_therapy.pdf
2. Biswas J, Mittal S, Ganesh SK, et al. Posterior scleritis: clinical profile and imaging characteristics. Indian J Ophthalmol. 1998;46(4):195-202.
3. Goldstein DA, Tessler HH. Section 5: Scleral and episcleral diseases. In: Yanoff M, Duker JS (Eds). Ophthalmology, 3rd edition. Mosby.
4. Kanski JJ. Episclera and sclera. Clinical Ophthalmology, 5th edition. Butterworth Heinemann; 2003.

SECTION 7

Uvea

CHAPTER

7.1 Anatomy of Uvea

- The word 'uvea' is derived from a Latin word 'uva' meaning grape. It is called so because uveal tissue appears black in color resembling a grape on dissection of the eye.
- Uvea is the middle vascular coat of the eye. It is divided into three parts—iris, ciliary body and choroid from anterior to posterior.

PARTS OF UVEA

Iris

The anterior portion of the uvea is called iris. Iris is a pigmented layer of the eye with variable degrees of pigmentation due to melanin. Because of its pigmentation, iris gives color to the eye varying from dark brown to blue. Iris resembles a circular disk situated in between corneal endothelium and lens separating the anterior chamber from the posterior chamber of the eye. Pupil is an aperture in the center of iris, which is called gateway to the brain and it regulates the amount of light reaching retina by constriction and dilatation.

Gross Anatomy

Anterior surface of the iris is divided into two zones, pupillary zone and ciliary zone. Pupillary zone is located in the center surrounding the pupil and ciliary zone is located in the periphery. Pupillary zone is smooth in appearance whereas ciliary zone shows ridges and crypts because of underlying radial blood vessels. The junction between the two zones is called collarette.

Histology

Iris has got five layers from anterior to posterior.

1. Anterior limiting layer: It is the condensed part of the iris stroma and it continues as corneal endothelium.
2. Iris stroma: It is composed of melanocytes, collagen and nerves.
3. Smooth muscles: Sphincter pupillae situated in the pupillary zone, responsible for constriction of pupil and it is supplied by parasympathetic supply via oculomotor nerve. Dilator pupillae situated in the ciliary zone, responsible for dilation of the pupil and it is supplied by sympathetic supply.
4. Anterior pigment epithelium.
5. Posterior pigment epithelium.

Ciliary Body

The middle portion of the uvea is called ciliary body. Ciliary body consists of two parts, pars plicata and pars plana.

Gross Anatomy

Pars plicata

Pars plicata is the anterior one-third portion of the ciliary body. It consists of ciliary processes and ciliary muscle. Ciliary processes are projections on the pars plicata about 70 in number and are the sites of aqueous production.

Ciliary muscle: It is a smooth muscle consisting of longitudinal, circular and radial fibers. Circular fibers are responsible for accommodation. Longitudinal and radial fibers are inserted into trabecular meshwork and contraction of these fibers leads to increase in aqueous outflow. Nerve supply of ciliary muscles is by parasympathetic fibers via short ciliary nerves.

Pars plana

Pars plana is the posterior two-third portion of the ciliary body.

> *Pars plana:* It is 5 mm wide temporally and 3 mm wide nasally. It is relatively avascular and is the safe route for posterior segment surgeries.

Histology

The histology of ciliary body shows five layers from inside to outwards:

1. Internal limiting membrane.
2. Non-pigmented epithelium.
3. Pigmented epithelium.
4. Stroma consisting of collagen and ciliary muscle.
5. Supraciliary lamina.

Choroid

The posterior portion of uvea is called choroid.

Gross Anatomy

Gross Anatomy is the vascular layer of the eyeball extending from optic disk to ora serrata. It lies between sclera and retina with inner surface in contact with retinal pigment epithelium and outer surface in contact with sclera.

Histology

From outside to inwards choroid shows:

1. Suprachoroid lamina lying outside towards sclera separated by a potential space called suprachoroidal space.
2. Stroma of the choroid: Stroma is formed by three layers of vessels. The outer vessel layer consisting of larger vessels is called Haller's layer. The middle layer consists of medium vessels is called Sattler's layer. The inner most choriocapillaris form the innermost layer.
3. Bruch's membrane: It is the innermost layer separating the choriocapillaris from retinal pigment epithelium.

BLOOD SUPPLY OF UVEA

Arterial blood supply of uvea comes from three sets of arteries:

1. Short posterior ciliary arteries.
2. Two long posterior ciliary arteries.
3. Anterior ciliary arteries.

Venous drainage is by four vortex veins, which drain into superior and inferior ophthalmic veins, which eventually drain into cavernous sinus.

FUNCTIONS OF UVEA

Iris

1. Iris gives color to the eye.
2. Sphincter pupillae and dilator pupillae control the size of pupil thereby controlling the amount of light entering the eye.

Ciliary Body

1. Secretion of aqueous humor by ciliary processes of pars plicata of ciliary body.
2. Ciliary muscle of ciliary body takes part in accommodation.

Choroid

Blood supply to outer four layers of retina.

GIST BOX 7.1

- Uvea is the middle vascular coat of the eye. It is divided into three parts, i.e. iris, ciliary body and choroid from anterior to posterior.
- The anterior portion of the uvea is called iris. Iris is pigmented layer of the eye with variable degrees of pigmentation due to melanin. It resembles a circular disk situated in between corneal endothelium and lens separating the anterior chamber from the posterior chamber of the eye. Pupil is an aperture in the center of the iris, which is called gateway to the brain and it regulates the amount of light reaching the retina by constriction and dilatation.
- The middle portion of the uvea is called ciliary body. Ciliary body consists of two parts, pars plicata and pars plana. Pars plicata is the anterior one-third portion of the ciliary body. Pars plicata consists of ciliary processes and ciliary muscle. Pars plana is the posterior two-third portion of the ciliary body.
- The posterior portion of the uvea is called choroid. It is the vascular layer of the eyeball extending from optic disk to ora serrata.

CHAPTER

7.2 Congenital Anomalies of Uvea

EMBRYOLOGY OF UVEA

1. Uvea consisting of iris, ciliary body and choroid develops from mesoderm and neuroectoderm.
2. Epithelium of iris, epithelium of ciliary body and muscles of iris (sphincter pupillae and dilator pupillae) are developed from neuroectoderm.
3. Stroma of iris, stroma of ciliary body, ciliary muscle and choroid are developed from mesoderm.

CONGENITAL ANOMALIES OF UVEA

Aniridia

1. Aniridia is a rare hereditary disorder characterized by hypoplasia of iris. The term aniridia is a misnomer because at least a rudimentary iris is always present.
2. It is due to developmental arrest of neuroectoderm and associated mesoderm. Hence in aniridia development of all other structures of the eye, which develop from neuroectoderm and associated mesoderm is arrested, thus making it a pan ocular disorder.
3. Associated ocular anomalies involve macular hypoplasia, optic nerve hypoplasia, cataract, corneal changes such as corneal opacification because of limbal stem cell deficiency and glaucoma because of anomalies of the angle of anterior chamber.
4. Characteristic clinical features of aniridia include a child presenting with poor vision and nystagmus caused by one or more of the above said anomalies, with examination of the anterior chamber showing complete absence of iris or presence of rudimentary iris, which is visible only by gonioscopy.

The WAGR syndrome is a rare genetic syndrome caused by mutation of chromosome 11. It is characterized by:

- **W**ilms' tumor of kidneys
- **A**niridia
- **G**enitourinary anomalies
- Mental **R**etardation.

Coloboma of Uveal Tract*

Definition

Localized absence of uveal tract as a result of incomplete closure of choroidal fissure is called coloboma of uveal tract.

Pathogenesis

1. Normally choroidal fissure also known as fetal fissure fuses by 7th week of intrauterine life, failure of which results in persistence of the cleft resulting in coloboma.

2. A coloboma can involve only iris or it may extend to involve ciliary body or choroid or both.

Types of Coloboma

Typical coloboma

Coloboma of iris occurring in the inferonasal quadrant of iris is called typical coloboma and it is due to persistence of choroidal fissure (Figs 7.2.1A and B). Typical coloboma can be complete or incomplete:

1. Complete coloboma extends from iris to optic nerve involving ciliary body, choroid and optic disk. Complete coloboma is usually bilateral and it is often seen in association with microphthalmos (Figs 7.2.2A and B).
2. Incomplete coloboma will not extend upto optic disk and may fall short.

Atypical coloboma

Occurrence in any other site of iris is called atypical coloboma. The cause for atypical coloboma is not related to closure of choroidal fissure. Persistence of fibrovascular sheath of lens is indicated as probable cause for atypical coloboma.

Ocular and systemic associations of coloboma:

1. Ocular associations of coloboma involve microcornea and microphthalmos.
2. Systemic associations of coloboma involve skeletal anomalies, e.g. thumb hypoplasia and genitourinary anomalies like horseshoe kidney; craniofacial anomalies such as cleft lip may be associated with coloboma.

Clinical Features and Treatment

1. Isolated iris colobomas present as photophobia, which can be treated by cosmetic contact lenses. Surgical iridoplasty may be done as an alternative option.
2. Colobomas involving optic nerve and macula present with low vision and nystagmus, treatment of which is usually unsatisfactory.

Albinism

Definition

Albinism is a group of hereditary diseases caused by decreased levels or complete absence of melanin resulting in hypopigmentation of skin, hair and eyes. It can be oculocutaneous albinism, involving skin and eyes or ocular albinism involving only eyes.

Oculocutaneous albinism shows autosomal recessive inheritance, whereas ocular albinism shows sex-linked or autosomal recessive inheritance.

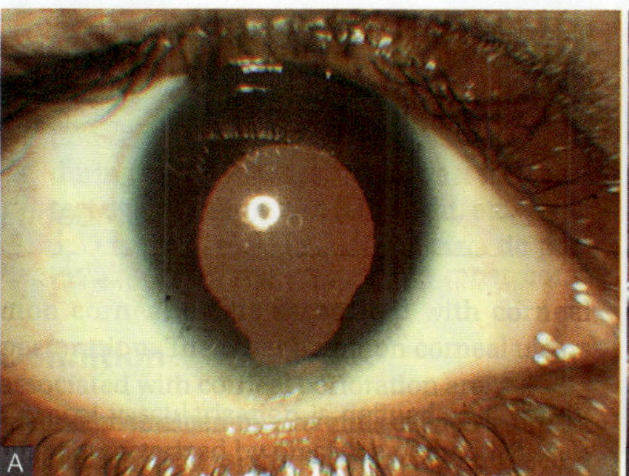

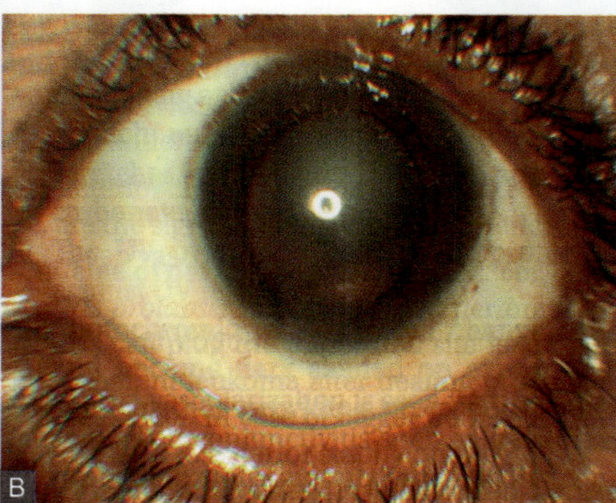

FIGS 7.2.1A and B: Coloboma of iris

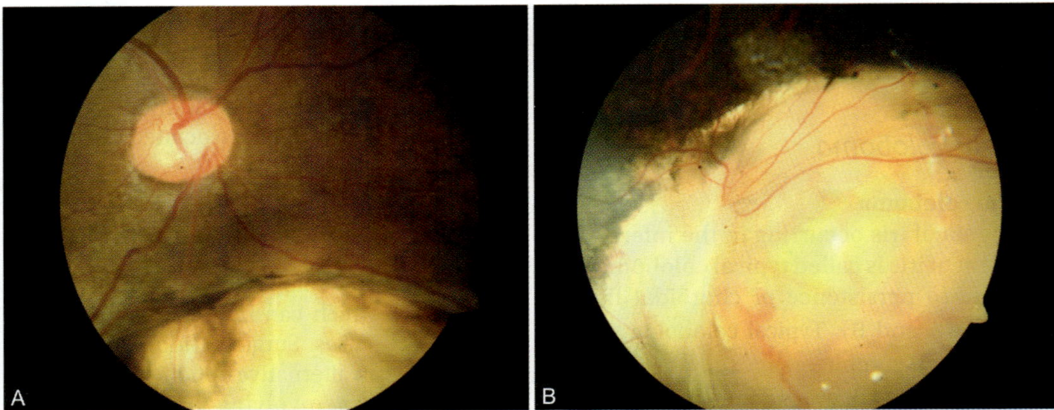

FIGS 7.2.2A and B: Coloboma involving retina and choroid

Pathogenesis

Pathogenesis is due to defective synthesis of melanin, which is synthesized from amino acid tyrosine in melanosomes by the enzyme tyrosinase. Based on the activity of this enzyme, albinism can be:

- Type 1 tyrosinase negative
- Type 2 tyrosinase positive.

Clinical Features

Both oculocutaneous albinism and ocular albinism show similar ocular features such as:

- Hypopigmentation of iris
- Translucency of iris
- Decreased pigmentation of retinal pigment epithelium (Figs 7.2.3A and B)
- Hypoplasia of fovea
- Congenital nystagmus.

Patient usually presents with white-colored eyelashes and eyebrows (Fig. 7.2.4), light-colored iris, decreased visual acuity and moderate to severe photophobia and varying degrees of skin and hair hypopigmentation depending on the subtype.

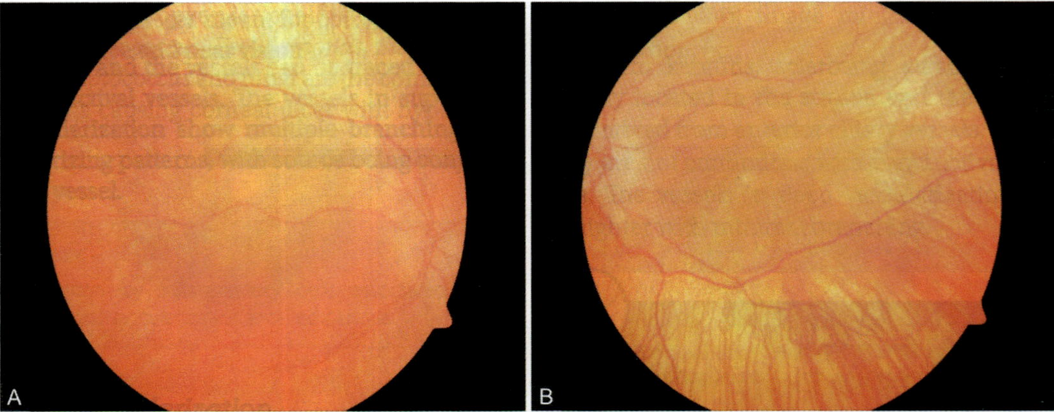

FIGS 7.2.3A and B: Fundus picture in albinism

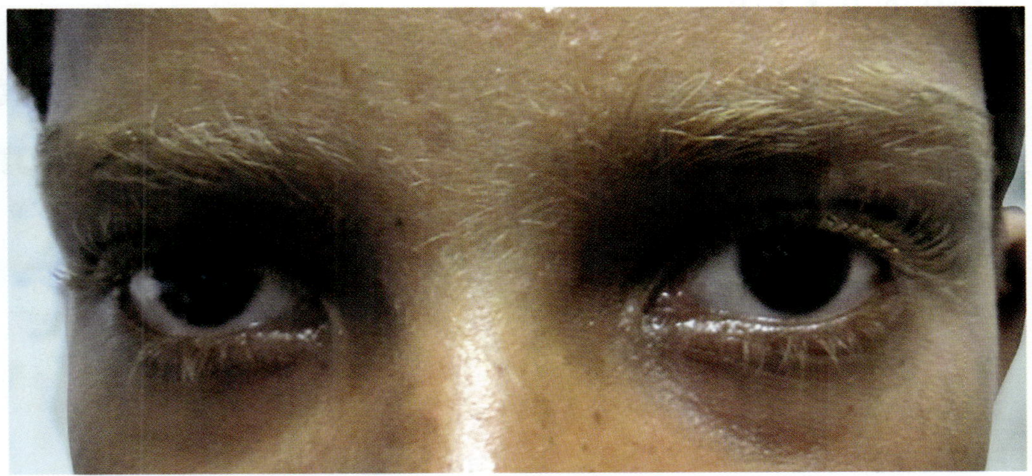

FIG. 7.2.4: A patient with albinism

Treatment

Treatment of the ocular features is mainly aimed at reducing photophobia by using iris color contact lenses or photochromic glasses. Low visual aids are advised for decreased visual acuity.

Associated Systemic Syndromes for Albinism

- Hermansky-Pudlak syndrome characterized by albinism, bleeding disorder, lung fibrosis and colitis.
- Chédiak-Higashi syndrome characterized by albinism, increased susceptibility to bacterial infections and prolonged bleeding time.
- Waardenburg syndrome characterized by albinism and deafness.

GIST BOX 7.2

- Aniridia is a rare hereditary disorder characterized by hypoplasia of iris. It is due to developmental arrest of neuroectoderm and associated mesoderm. Hence, in aniridia development of all other structures of the eye, which develop from neuroectoderm and associated mesoderm is arrested, thus making it a panocular disorder. Associated ocular anomalies involve macular hypoplasia, optic nerve hypoplasia, cataract, corneal changes such as corneal opacification because of limbal stem cell deficiency, glaucoma because of anomalies of the angle of the anterior chamber, etc.
- Coloboma of iris is localized absence of uveal tract as a result of incomplete closure of choroidal fissure. Normally, choroidal fissure also known as fetal fissure fuses by 7th week of intrauterine life, failure of which results in persistence of the cleft resulting in coloboma. A coloboma can involve only iris or they may extend to involve ciliary body or choroid or both.

CHAPTER

7.3

Uveitis: Definition and Classification

DEFINITION

Inflammation of a part or whole of the uveal tract is called uveitis.

CLASSIFICATION**

Anatomical Classification (Table 7.3.1)

TABLE 7.3.1: Anatomical classification of uveitis

Types	*Features*
Anterior uveitis	Inflammation of iris (iritis) and anterior part of ciliary body, i.e. pars plicata (anterior cyclitis); usually iris and pars plicata of ciliary body are involved together resulting in iridocyclitis
Intermediate uveitis	Inflammation of posterior part of ciliary body, i.e. pars plana and the surrounding peripheral retina and choroid
Posterior uveitis	Inflammation of the choroid Usually the surrounding retina is invariably involved resulting in chorioretinitis
Panuveitis	Inflammation involving whole of the uvea, i.e. iris, ciliary body and choroid

Pathological Classification (Table 7.3.2)

TABLE 7.3.2: Pathological classification of uveitis

Types	*Features*
Granulomatous uveitis	Chronic uveitis seen in chronic inflammations usually caused by tuberculosis, leprosy and sarcoidosis
Non-granulomatous uveitis	Acute uveitis seen in infective pyogenic microbial causes, allergic and idiopathic causes

Etiological Classification (Table 7.3.3)

TABLE 7.3.3: Etiological classification of uveitis

Types	*Features*
Microbial/ Infective	• Bacteria: Pyogenic bacteria such as streptococci, staphylococci, pneumococci: – Bacteria causing granulomatous inflammation such as *Mycobacterium tuberculosis (M. tuberculosis), M. leprae* and *Treponema pallidum* • Viruses such as herpes simplex, herpes zoster, cytomegalovirus • Fungi such as *Candida, Histoplasma*

Contd...

Contd...

Types	*Features*
	• Parasites such as *Toxoplasma, Toxocara* • *Rickettsia*
Immunological	• Associated with allergic reactions, microbial allergy, atopic allergy, autoimmune diseases
Traumatic	• May follow mechanical trauma or surgical trauma
Toxic	• Endocular toxins as seen in intraocular tumors • Exogenous toxins, e.g. drug-induced uveitis caused by drugs • Topically used drugs, e.g. metipranolol, miotic agents • Systemically used drugs, e.g. sulfonamides, rifabutin
Idiopathic	• About one third to half of all the cases belong to this category in which definitive etiological evidence cannot be determined
Lens-induced uveitis	• Phacotoxic uveitis, phacoanaphylactic endophthalmitis
Uveitis associated with systemic diseases	• Respiratory diseases, e.g. sarcoidosis, tuberculosis • Diseases of skin, e.g. psoriasis • Metabolic diseases, e.g. diabetes, gout • Gastrointestinal diseases, e.g. ulcerative colitis • Systemic septic conditions, e.g. meningitis, pneumonia, cholecystitis

Clinical Classification (Table 7.3.4)

TABLE 7.3.4: Clinical classification of uveitis

Types	*Features*
Acute uveitis	Uveitis with sudden onset, lasting for 6 week or less
Chronic uveitis	Uveitis with insidious onset, extending for more than 3 month
Recurrent uveitis	Recurrent episodes of uveitis with periods of inactivity in between, lasting for 3 month or more

ETIOPATHOGENESIS

Etiology is described above in etiological classification. The etiology of uveitis is very extensive; almost any infective organism, any systemic disease, any type of allergy can cause uveitis. This also includes 30% of the cases, which are labeled as idiopathic in which a cause cannot be identified.

Inflammation of the uveal tissue is characterized by the basic mechanisms seen elsewhere in the body such as vascular dilation, increased vascular permeability resulting in the outpouring of exudates and migration of inflammatory cells.

PATHOLOGY OF UVEITIS

Pathology of uveitis is classified into suppurative inflammation and non-suppurative inflammation. Non-suppurative inflammation is further classified into granulomatous and nongranulomatous (Table 7.3.5).

TABLE 7.3.5: Differences between granulomatous and non-granulomatous uveitis

*Granulomatous uveitis***	*Non-granulomatous uveitis*
Chronic uveitis seen in chronic inflammations usually caused by tuberculosis, leprosy, viruses, fungi and parasites	Acute uveitis seen in infective pyogenic microbial causes, allergic and idiopathic causes
Chronic mild-grade inflammation	Moderate to severe inflammation and presents as acute red eye
Inflammatory cells include large mononuclear cells, which aggregate to become nodules on the iris and mutton-fat keratic precipitates over endothelium of cornea	Inflammatory cells include lymphocytes and plasma cells resulting in aqueous flare, cells in anterior chamber, hypopyon and fine keratic precipitates over the endothelium of cornea

Suppurative inflammation is seen in endophthalmitis and panophthalmitis caused by pyogenic bacteria. It is characterized by infiltration by neutrophils and other polymorphonuclear cells resulting in necrosis of the ocular tissue and accumulation of pus in the cavities of the eyeball.

GIST BOX 7.3

- Inflammation of the part or whole of the uveal tract is called uveitis.
- Uveitis is classified anatomically as anterior uveitis, intermediate uveitis, posterior uveitis and panuveitis.
- Uveitis is classified pathologically as granulomatous and non-granulomatous uveitis.
- Uveitis is classified clinically as acute uveitis, chronic uveitis and recurrent uveitis.

CHAPTER

7.4 Anterior Uveitis

DEFINITION***

Anterior uveitis involves inflammation of iris alone (iritis) or inflammation of anterior part of ciliary body alone (cyclitis) or inflammation of both (iridocyclitis). It is the most common type of uveitis.

SYMPTOMS

Patient with acute anterior iridocyclitis presents with:

1. Pain: It is usually due to ciliary muscle spasm or secondary rise of intraocular pressure (IOP) because of inflammatory glaucoma.
2. Redness: It is due to circumcorneal congestion, which is because of hyperemia of ciliary vessels.
3. Blurring of vision: It is caused by turbidity of aqueous and induced myopia caused by ciliary muscle spasm.
4. Diminution of vision: It is caused in the acute stages because of corneal edema and fibrinous exudates in the anterior chamber. In later stages complicated cataract, secondary glaucoma and cystoid macular edema are responsible for diminution of vision.
5. Photophobia: It is caused by corneal edema and ciliary muscle spasm.
6. Blepharospasm: It is due to reflex between the trigeminal nerve, sensory for eye and facial nerve, motor for blinking.
7. Watering: It is due to reflex between the trigeminal nerve, sensory for eye and facial nerve, secretomotor for lacrimation.

SIGNS

1. *Lid edema*: Depending on the severity of inflammation varying degrees of lid edema is present.
2. *Conjunctiva*: It shows circumcorneal ciliary congestion.
3. *Cornea*: It shows varying degrees of corneal edema and keratic precipitates: Corneal edema is because of toxic endotheliitis or because of secondary rise of IOP.

Keratic Precipitates

Keratic precipitates (KPs) are cellular deposits over the corneal endothelium (Fig. 7.4.1).

Types of KPs

Mutton-fat KPs: They are composed of lymphoplasmacytic inflammatory cells with epithelioid cells.
Small- and medium-sized KPs: They are composed of lymphoplasmacytic inflammatory cells.
Old KPs: They are seen in old healed iridocyclitis.
Red KPs: They are seen in hemorrhagic uveitis, where red blood cells are also part of cellular deposits.
Fresh KPs: They are round, white, fluffy and have hydrated appearance. Old KPs are shrunken, faded, pigmented and have crenated edges.

Distribution of KPs

Normally KPs are seen in the inferior part of the cornea in a base down triangular fashion called Arlt's triangle. Aqueous currents in the anterior chamber are responsible for distribution of KPs in triangular fashion. Diffuse distribution of KPs all over the cornea is seen in Fuchs heterochromic iridocyclitis and herpetic uveitis.

ANTERIOR CHAMBER

1. Aqueous cells and/or aqueous flare are seen in the anterior chamber.
2. Hypopyon, collection of pus in anterior chamber is seen in infectious causes, endophthalmitis and in Behçet's disease.
3. Hyphema, collection of blood in anterior chamber is seen in hemorrhagic uveitis caused by gonococci.
4. Depth of anterior chamber is shallow in cases of formation of anterior synechiae and deep, and irregular in cases of posterior synechiae formation.

Aqueous Cells and Aqueous Flare (Fig. 7.4.2)*

1. Aqueous cells are due to cellular infiltration of the anterior chamber. Aqueous flare is due to protein exudation into anterior chamber.
2. Aqueous cells and aqueous flare are visible due to Tyndall effect (scattering of light suspended in clear liquid medium).
3. Aqueous cells and flare are seen by directing the slit lamp obliquely to the plane of the iris with intensity and magnification of the slit lamp set at maximum, and width and length of slit set at 1 mm.
4. Aqueous cells are the earliest sign of iridocyclitis. Aqueous flare is more marked in non-granulomatous uveitis and is minimal in granulomatous uveitis.

Grading of aqueous cells and flare

Grade	*Cells/Field*	*Flare*
-	0	No flare
1+	1–10	Faint or just detectable
2+	11–20	Moderate with clear details of iris and lens visible
3+	21–50	Marked with hazyview of iris and lens
4+	> 50	Fixed and aplastic aqueous with no view of iris and lens

Iris

1. Normal color of the iris is changed and it usually becomes muddy in active phase-and may show hypopigmented atrophic patches in healed phase of the disease.
2. Normal pattern of iris is affected because of edema in the active phase and may show atrophic patches in healed phase of the disease.

Iris nodules are accumulation of leukocytes on the anterior iris. Koeppe's nodules

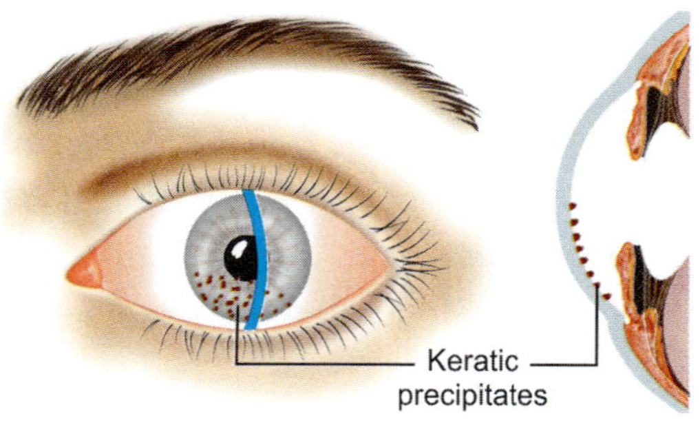

FIG. 7.4.1: Keratic precipitates

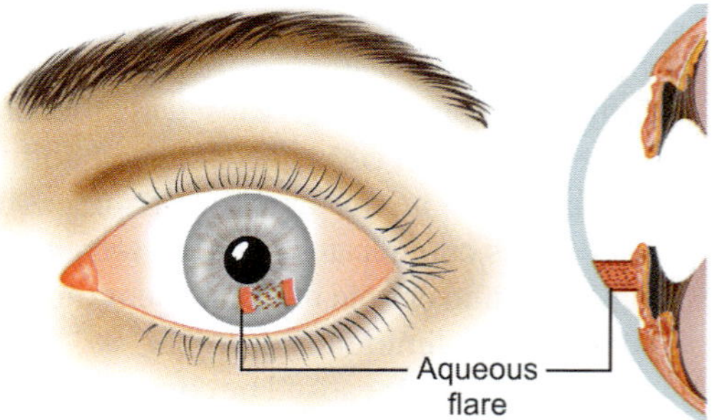

FIG. 7.4.2: Aqueous flare

are seen at the pupillary border and Busacca's nodules are seen away from the iris stroma. Iris nodules are usually seen in granulomatous iridocyclitis (Fig. 7.4.3).*

3. Presence of synechiae.
4. Neovascularization or rubeosis iridis seen in chronic iridocyclitis and in Fuchs heterochromic iridocyclitis.

Synechiae (Figs 7.4.4 to 7.4.6A to C)*

1. Synechiae are adhesions of iris to other intraocular structures.
2. Anterior synechiae refers to adhesion of iris to structures in front of it, e.g. corneal endothelium.
3. Peripheral anterior synechiae refers to adhesion of iris root to trabecular meshwork. It is made out by gonioscopy and it can result in synechial angle closure.
4. Posterior synechiae refers to adhesion of iris to structures behind the iris, e.g. lens.
5. Posterior synechiae can be segmental, annular or total:
   a. Segmental posterior synechiae is adhesion of iris to lens at some segments.
   b. Annular posterior synechiae is adhesion of entire pupillary margin to anterior capsule of lens, thus preventing the circulation of aqueous humor from posterior chamber to anterior chamber resulting in seclusio pupillae.

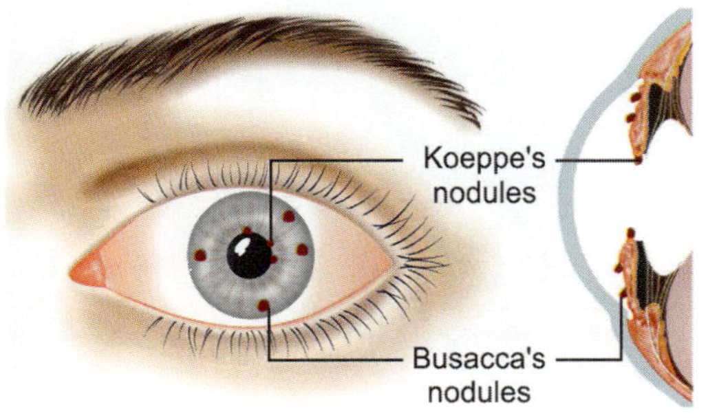

FIG. 7.4.3: Iris nodules

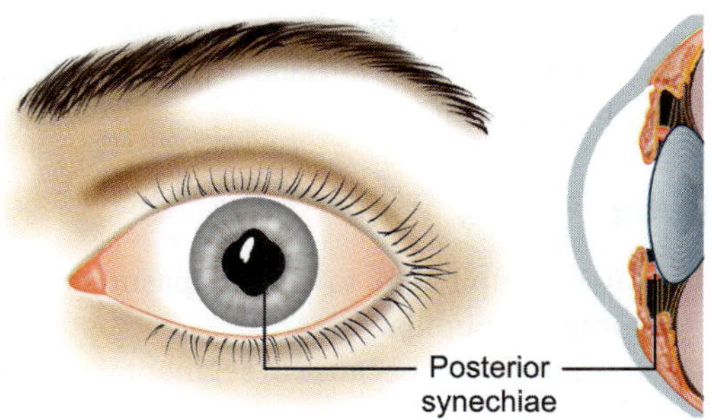

FIG. 7.4.4: Posterior synechiae

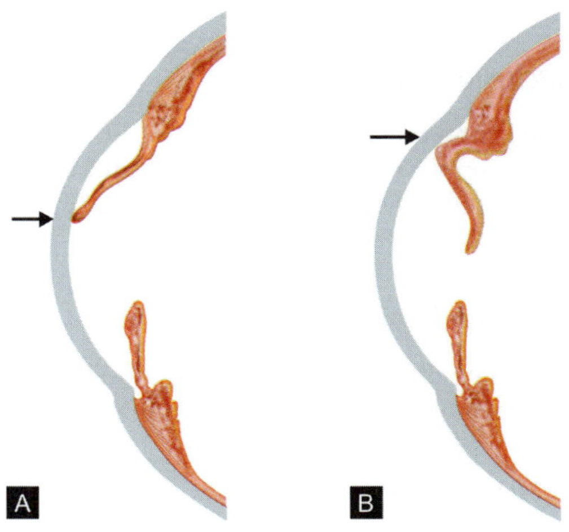

FIGS 7.4.5A and B: Anterior synechiae. **A.** Central anterior synechiae; **B.** Peripheral anterior synechiae.

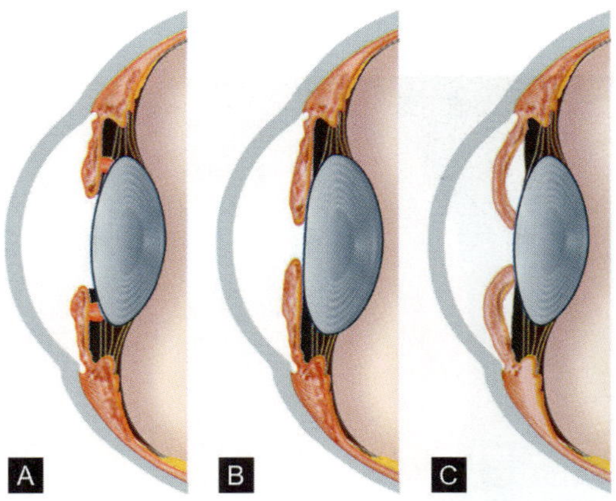

FIGS 7.4.6A to C: Posterior synechiae. **A.** Segmental posterior synechiae; **B.** Total posterior synechiae; **C.** Annular posterior synechiae.

c. Total posterior synechiae is adhesion of total posterior surface of iris to anterior capsule of lens.

Pupil

1. Miotic pupil due to reflex spasm of the sphincter pupillae.
2. Irregular pupil because of segmental posterior synechiae.
3. Sluggish or absent pupillary reaction due to edema of the iris.

*Seclusio Pupillae**

Fixed, non-reactive pupil because of annular posterior synechiae as a result of adhesion of entire pupillary margin to the anterior capsule of lens.

*Occlusio Pupillae**

Occlusion of the pupil (Fig. 7.4.7) by inflammatory membrane completely covering the pupil.

Festooned Pupil

Irregular-shaped pupil seen after dilatation of pupil with mydriatic drugs in a patient with segmental posterior synechiae.

Ectropion Uveae

Eversion of the pupillary border of the iris due to shrinkage or contraction of the fibrovascular membrane on the anterior surface of iris.

Lens

1. Pigments on the anterior capsule of lens.
2. Complicated cataract.

Anterior Vitreous

Anterior vitreous shows vitreous haze and vitreous cells (Figs 7.4.8 to 7.4.10).

COMPLICATIONS OF ANTERIOR IRIDOCYCLITIS (Figs 7.4.11 to 7.4.14A and B)**

Complicated Cataract

Cataract formation occurs as a sequence of inflammatory process and it is more common in chronic or long-standing uveitis.

Secondary Glaucoma

Secondary glaucoma is a common complication of anterior iridocyclitis and it is caused by two mechanisms:

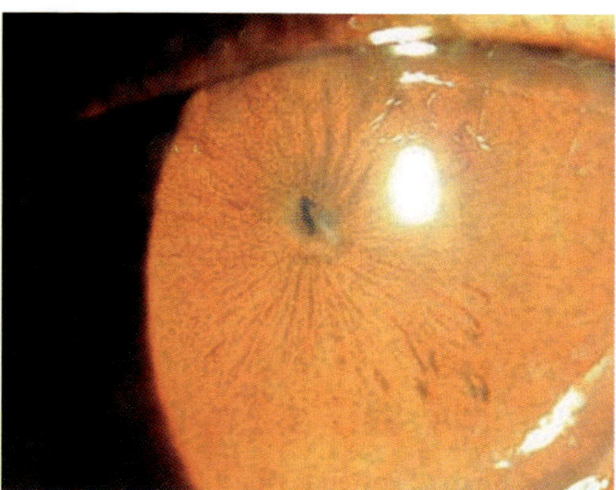

FIG. 7.4.7: Occlusive pupillae (*Note:* Occlusion of pupil completely due to exudates)

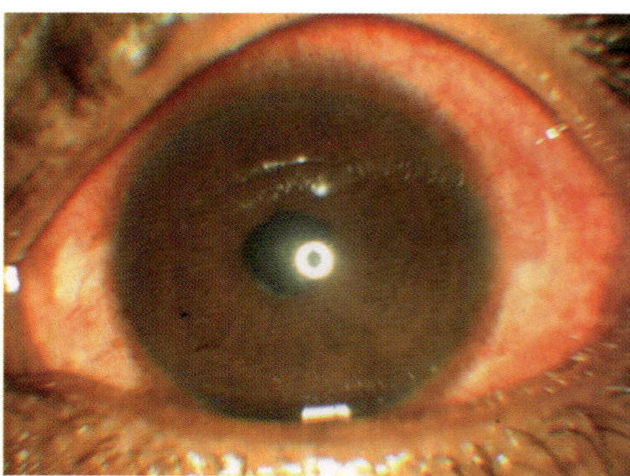

FIG. 7.4.8: Acute iridocyclitis

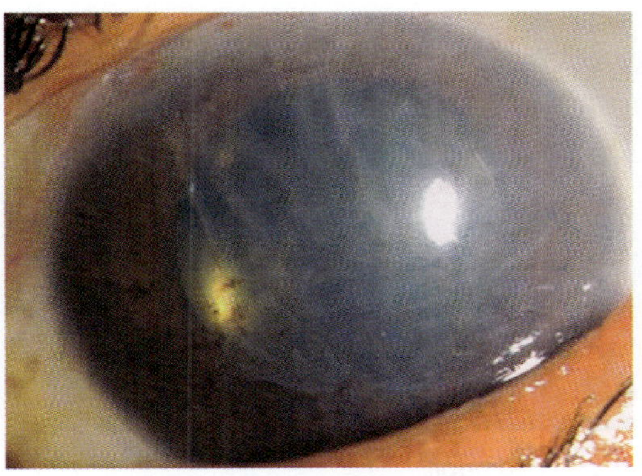

FIG. 7.4.9: Keratic precipitates

1. Clogging of the trabecular meshwork by inflammatory cells as seen in active iridocyclitis (open-angle glaucoma).
2. Synechial closure of the angle of the anterior chamber, secondary to formation of peripheral anterior synechiae, which usually follows iris bombe and seclusio pupillae (angle-closure glaucoma). It is usually seen in the late phase of iridocyclitis or in chronic cases.

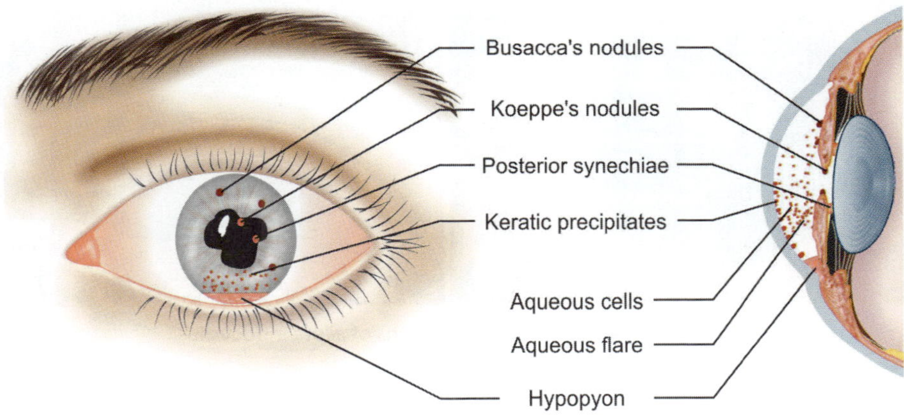

FIG. 7.4.10: Signs of acute iridocyclitis

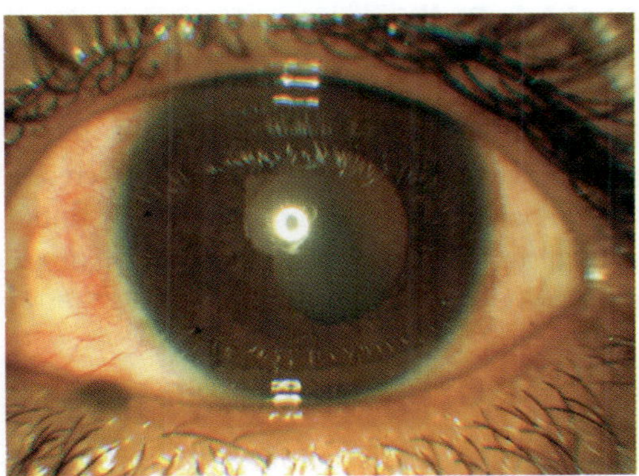

FIG. 7.4.11: Chronic iridocyclitis

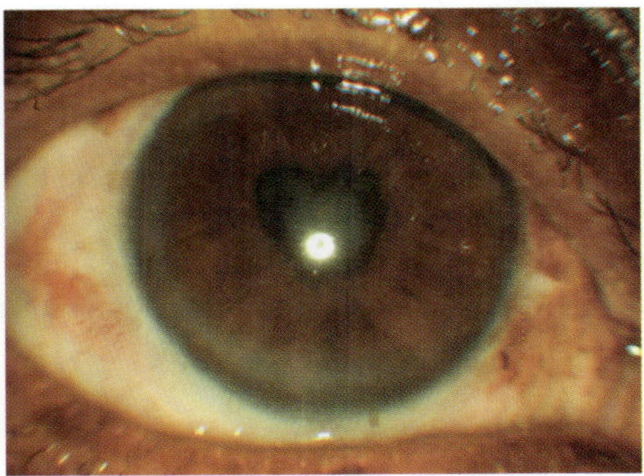

FIG. 7.4.12: Posterior synechiae

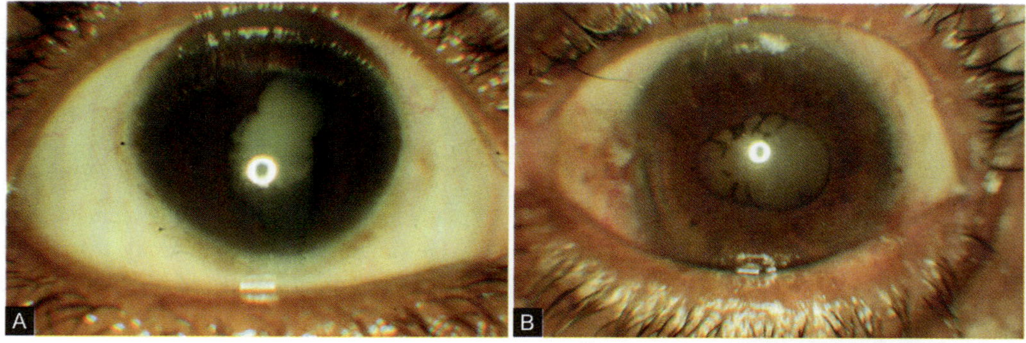

FIGS 7.4.13A and B: Festooned pupil

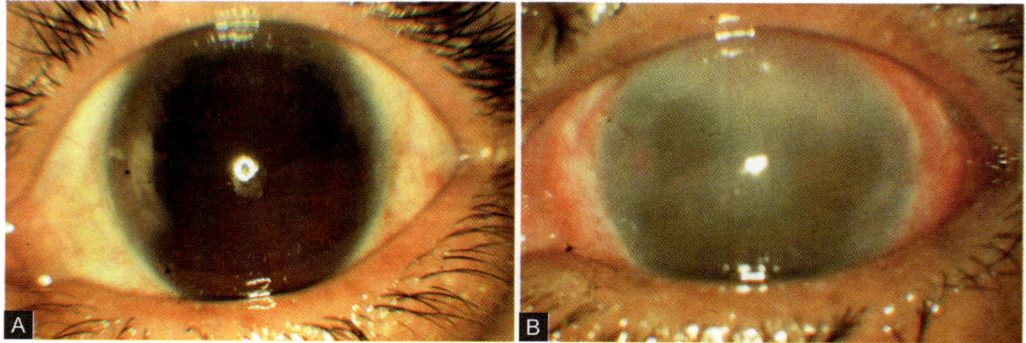

FIGS 7.4.14A and B: Complications of acute iridocyclitis

Band-shaped Keratopathy

Band-shaped keratopathy is characterized by the formation of a band across the central part of cornea due to deposition of calcium salts in Bowman's layer of cornea.

Posterior Segment Complications

Long-standing anterior uveitis may result in posterior segment complications such as cystoid macular edema, choroiditis, retinitis, retinal detachment, disk edema and vascular sheathing.

Cyclitic Membrane

Cyclitic membrane is due to fibrosis of exudates over ciliary body seen in chronic iridocyclitis. Cyclitic membrane may cause detachment of the ciliary body resulting in hypotony because of decreased aqueous production and decreased IOP.

Phthisis Bulbi

Phthisis bulbi is the end result of prolonged hypotony seen in chronic uveitis. As ciliary body is detached and aqueous production is decreased the eyeball becomes soft, shrunken and undergoes disorganization resulting in formation of phthisis bulbi.

DIFFERENTIAL DIAGNOSIS

Acute iridocyclitis should be differentiated from other causes of **acute red eye***** (Table 7.4.1), acute conjunctivitis and acute congestive glaucoma.

Investigations*

Approach to a Patient with Uveitis

Since causes for uveitis are very exhaustive before ordering the investigations, following approach is followed. Systemic approach to a patient with uveitis includes:

- Detailed history with uveitis questionnaire.
- Ocular examination.
- Physical examination.
- Tailored laboratory investigations.

Routine Screening Tests

- Complete blood count (total count) and differential count (DC)—will show inflammatory response
- Erythrocyte sedimentation rate (ESR) and CRP (C-reactive protein)
- Chest radiograph to rule out tuberculosis
- Mantoux test
- Serological tests to rule human immunodeficiency virus (HIV) and syphilis
- Urine examination.

Specific test tailored according to the history and physical examination:

- Tests to rule out autoimmune diseases—antinuclear antibody (ANA), rheumatoid factor (RF)
- Radiological examination of spine, sacroiliac joints (to rule out ankylosing spondylitis), computed tomography (CT) scan of chest (to rule out sarcoidosis)
- Human leukocyte antigen (HLA)
- Serological tests for toxoplasmosis.

TABLE 7.4.1: Differential diagnosis of acute red eye

Features	*Acute iridocyclitis*	*Acute conjunctivitis*	*Acute congestive glaucoma*
Symptoms			
• Onset	Insidious in onset	Sudden in onset	Sudden in onset
• Diminution of vision	Present	Vision is not affected	Marked impairment of vision
• Pain	Moderate to severe	Mild or nil	Severe
• Redness	Circumcorneal congestion	Conjunctival congestion	Circumcorneal congestion
• Discharge	Absent	Mucoid, mucopurulent or purulent	Absent
• Watering	Present	Present	Present
Signs			
• Congestion	Deep ciliary congestion	Superficial conjunctival	Deep ciliary congestion
• Cornea	Clear or may show keratic precipitates (KPs)	Usually clear	Shows corneal edema
• Anterior chamber	Shows aqueous cells, flare, hypopyon, depth may be normal or deep or irregular	Normal	Shallow
• Iris	Muddy	Normal	Edematous
• Pupil	Small, irregular and sluggishly reactive	Normal	Mild dilated oval and non-reactive
• Intraocular pressure	Increased or decreased or normal	Normal	Markedly raised
Treatment	Steroids and cycloplegics	Antimicrobial drugs	Antiglaucoma drugs

TREATMENT*

The main goals of treatment are elimination of inflammation, pain relief, prevention of complications and restoration of vision.

Non-specific Treatment

Non-specific treatment is by corticosteroids for elimination of inflammation and cycloplegics for pain relief.

Corticosteroids

1. Corticosteroids are the drug of choice in iridocyclitis. They act by decreasing the inflammatory response by inhibiting the cyclooxygenase pathway. Topical steroids are the most common form of treatment. Commonly used topical steroids are prednisolone acetate 1% and dexamethasone 0.1% eyedrops. They are usually started as frequently as one drop hourly initially and tapered slowly depending on the severity of inflammation.
2. Periocular injections/subconjunctival injections are required in severe disease.
3. Systemic steroids are indicated in non-responsive cases, bilateral iridocyclitis and in posterior uveitis.
4. Posterior sub-Tenon's injection of long-acting steroids such as triamcinolone acetate is usually indicated in intermediate and posterior uveitis.

Non-steroidal Anti-inflammatory Drugs

Non-steroidal anti-inflammatory drugs (NSAIDs) such as flurbiprofen, ketorolac and diclofenac are used in cases of contraindications of steroids or in cases of complications of steroids.

Immunosuppressive Drugs

Cyclosporine and methotrexate are used in steroid-resistant cases or as steroid-sparing drugs where steroids are required for a long time. Immunosuppressive drugs are required in severe types of anterior uveitis in which it is associated with Behçet's disease, autoimmune diseases.

*Cycloplegic Drugs**

Cycloplegic drugs act in uveitis by:
- Relief from pain by immobilizing iris
- Prevent the formation of synechiae
- Stabilize the blood aqueous barrier thereby preventing protein leakage and reduce exudation.

Commonly used cycloplegic drugs are atropine eye ointment 1%, Homide eyedrops and cyclopentolate eyedrops.

Specific Treatment

Specific treatment is done in cases where the underlying cause for uveitis is found out such as treatment of tuberculosis, toxoplasmosis, etc.

Treatment of Complications

Complicated Cataract

Complicated cataract is treated by cataract extraction and intraocular lens (IOL) implantation after the inflammation is controlled. Cataract surgery is performed once the eye is free from inflammation for at least a period of 3 months. Systemic steroids are started 3 days prior to surgery and continued for 6 weeks following surgery.

Secondary Glaucoma

Secondary glaucoma is treated by control of inflammation by using steroids and reduction of IOP by antiglaucoma drugs. Non-responsive cases and chronic cases with synechial angle closure usually require surgical management, trabeculectomy.

Cystoid Macular Edema

Cystoid macular edema is the most common posterior segment complication. It is managed by topical NSAIDs, systemic steroids. Non-responsive cases may require posterior sub-Tenon's injection and intravitreal steroids.

Band Keratopathy

Band keratopathy is treated by control of inflammation, superficial debridement and chelation of the band keratopathy.

Phthisis Bulbi

Phthisis bulbi is treated by enucleation or evisceration and implantation of artificial eye. Indications for removal of the phthisical eye are painful blind eye and cosmetic disfigurement.

SPECIFIC CLINICAL TYPES OF ANTERIOR UVEITIS

Idiopathic Specific Anterior Uveitis Syndromes

*Fuchs Heterochromic Iridocyclitis**

Definition: Anterior uveitis is idiopathic, unilateral, non-granulomatous anterior iridocyclitis occurring in young and middle-aged adults characterized by heterochromia of iris.

Etiopathogenesis: Idiopathic in nature, probably immunologically mediated occlusion of the iris vessels because of abnormal hyalinization resulting in ischemia, iris stromal atrophy and hypochromia of iris of the affected eye leading to heterochromia of the iris.

Clinical features: As follows:

1. Heterochromia of iris with affected eye being lighter color because of iris atrophy.
2. Fine non-pigmented keratic precipitates with diffuse distribution all over the endothelium of cornea.
3. Iris and angle of the anterior chamber usually show new vessels.
4. Diminution of vision is usually because of cataract and glaucoma.
5. Posterior synechiae formation is not seen.

Treatment: Fuchs heterochromic iridocyclitis is treated by corticosteroids. Cycloplegics are not required because of absence of posterior synechiae.

*Posner-Schlossman Syndrome (Glaucomatocyclitic Crisis)**

Definition: Posner-Schlossman syndrome is idiopathic, unilateral, non-granulomatous anterior iridocyclitis occurring in middle-aged adults characterized by recurrent episodes of markedly elevated IOP. It is also called glaucomatocyclitic crisis.

Etiopathogenesis: Recurrent mild inflammation of the anterior segment results in obstruction of the aqueous outflow in the trabecular meshwork resulting in episodes of elevated IOP.

Clinical features: As detailed below:

1. Usually unilateral affecting the middle-aged adults.
2. Ocular discomfort, colored halos and diminution of vision are presenting complaints.
3. Mild corneal edema with the fine keratic precipitates.
4. Posterior synechiae is absent.
5. Markedly raised intraocular pressure in the range of 40–60 mm Hg.
6. On examination, eye is quiet, anterior chamber is normal to deep, angle of anterior chamber is open with normal visual fields and normal optic disk, thus differentiating it from angle closure and open-angle glaucoma.

Treatment: It is by corticosteroids and antiglaucoma drugs to lower raised IOP.

Human Leukocyte Antigen (HLA-B27) Iridocyclitis

1. Human leukocyte antigen-B27 iridocyclitis is acute, but recurrent non-granulomatous iridocyclitis seen in relation with HLA-B27. It usually affects young males.
2. More than 50% of the patients with HLA-B27 positivity have seronegative spondyloarthropathies and enteroarthropathies such as:
   a. Ankylosing spondylitis: It is a chronic inflammatory condition characterized by articular inflammation involving the sacroiliac joints and axial skeleton.

b. Reiter's syndrome: It is characterized by triad of arthritis, urethritis and conjunctivitis.
c. Psoriatic arthritis: It is characterized by psoriatic skin changes and arthritis involving mainly small joints of hands and feet.
d. Inflammatory bowel diseases: It is a chronic immunologically mediated disorder of the intestinal tract characterized by recurrent abdominal pain and diarrhea.

3. Young patients presenting with recurrent acute non-granulomatous anterior uveitis with history of the above told spondyloarthropathies or enteroarthropathies such as history of back pain, pain of small joints in hands and feet, dysuria and gastrointestinal (GI) symptoms should be investigated for the presence of HLA-B27.
4. Treatment is done by corticosteroids and cycloplegics, and appropriate evaluation, and treatment of the specific underlying disease.

Anterior Uveitis Associated with Juvenile Rheumatoid Arthritis

1. Juvenile rheumatoid arthritis is defined as chronic, seronegative, and peripheral arthritis occurring in children below 16 years.
2. It is the most common arthritic disorder seen in children and it is the most common systemic disease associated with anterior uveitis in this age group.
3. Uveitis is most commonly seen in pauciarticular type of juvenile rheumatoid arthritis.
4. Anterior uveitis is bilateral non-granulomatous and recurrent in nature.
5. Majority of the patients are asymptomatic and present with white and quiet eye with uveitis detected only on slit-lamp examination.
6. Band keratopathy is the most common complication seen in association with uveitis with juvenile rheumatoid arthritis.

Traumatic Iridocyclitis

1. Traumatic iridocyclitis is commonly seen following blunt injury because of disruption of blood aqueous barrier.
2. It presents with non-granulomatous iridocyclitis.
3. It is usually self-limiting condition and treated by cycloplegic drugs to relieve ciliary spasm.

Lens-induced Iridocyclitis

Lens-induced iridocyclitis is of two types:

1. Phacogenic uveitis: It is the mild non-granulomatous inflammation induced by lens protein.
2. Phacoanaphylactic uveitis: It is a granulomatous inflammation induced by the lens antigen, when lens antigen is liberated into anterior chamber following disruption of lens capsule.

Treatment is by cycloplegics and corticosteroids followed by extraction of lens.

Postoperative Uveitis

1. Postoperative uveitis is the uveitis seen following surgery of the eye.
2. It is because of breakdown of blood aqueous barrier following intraocular surgery.
3. It may be seen because of anaphylactic reaction to lens antigen following cataract surgery.

Herpetic Iridocyclitis

1. Herpetic iridocyclitis is a granulomatous iridocyclitis seen secondary to herpes simplex or herpes zoster infection of the eye.
2. The diagnosis is usually made by clinical examination. Corneal disciform keratitis may be seen in association with uveitis in case of herpes simplex infection.

Masquerade Syndromes

- Masquerade syndrome consist of a group of diseases, which clinically resemble anterior iridocyclitis, but have an underlying primary cause, neoplastic or nonneoplastic.

Causes

1. Malignant diseases such as retinoblastoma, uveal melanoma, leukemia, metastatic carcinoma of the eye, etc.
2. Non-neoplastic conditions such as retinal detachment, juvenile xanthogranuloma and pigment dispersion syndrome.

GIST BOX 7.4

- Anterior uveitis involves inflammation of iris alone (iritis) or inflammation of anterior part of ciliary body alone (cyclitis) or inflammation of both (iridocyclitis). It is the commonest type of uveitis.
- Patient with acute anterior iridocyclitis presents with pain, redness, blurring of vision, diminution of vision, photophobia, blepharospasm, watering, etc.
- The signs of acute anterior uveitis are lid edema, circumcorneal congestion, corneal edema, keratic precipitates, aqueous cells and flare, hyphema, hypopyon, synechiae, etc.
- The complications of anterior uveitis are complicated cataract, secondary glaucoma, band-shaped keratopathy, cyclitic membrane, cystoid macular edema, phthisis bulbi, etc.
- Acute iridocyclitis should be differentiated from other causes of acute red eye, acute conjunctivitis and acute congestive glaucoma.
- Non-specific treatment is by corticosteroids for elimination of inflammation and cycloplegics for pain relief.
- Specific treatment is done in cases where the underlying cause for uveitis is found out such as treatment of tuberculosis, toxoplasmosis, etc.
- Fuchs heterochromic iridocyclitis is an idiopathic unilateral non-granulomatous anterior iridocyclitis occurring in young and middle-aged adults characterized by heterochromia of iris.
- Posner-Schlossman syndrome is an idiopathic unilateral non-granulomatous anterior iridocyclitis occurring in middle-aged adults characterized by recurrent episodes of markedly elevated intraocular pressure. It is also called glaucomatocyclitic crisis.

CHAPTER

7.5 Intermediate Uveitis and Posterior Uveitis

INTERMEDIATE UVEITIS**

Definition

Inflammation of pars plana of ciliary body and the surrounding peripheral retina, choroid and anterior vitreous is called intermediate uveitis. It is also called pars planitis/cyclochorioretinitis/basal uveoretinitis/chronic cyclitis.

Epidemiology

Epidemiology accounts for 10–18% of all types of uveitis. It is usually seen in middle-aged adults in second to fourth decade.

Etiology

Majority of the causes are idiopathic; in few cases the underlying cause may be:
- Sarcoidosis
- Multiple sclerosis
- Lyme disease.

Clinical Features

Symptoms

1. Symptoms are usually minimal. Pain and redness of the eye is not seen in majority of cases.
2. Floaters are the presenting complaint of the disease.
3. Blurring of vision and mild photophobia are occasionally seen.
4. Diminution of vision is seen in case of complications such as complicated cataract and cystoid macular edema.

Signs

1. Examination of the pars plana by indirect ophthalmoscopy and sclera depression shows accumulation of inflammatory aggregates in the pars plana called vitreous snow banks, the characteristic feature of pars planitis.
2. Retinal changes such as periphlebitis of the peripheral retinal veins, neovascularization and retinal detachment are seen less often.

Complications

- Complicated cataract
- Secondary glaucoma
- Cystoid macular edema
- Retinal vasculitis
- Retinal detachment
- Vitreous hemorrhage.

Treatment

Treatment is done in a stepwise approach as described below:

1. *Step I*: Posterior sub-Tenon's injection of long-acting steroids, e.g. triamcinolone acetate. Generally injections are repeated once in 4 weeks and intermediate uveitis requires three to four injections.
2. *Step II*: If the disease is not responding to local steroids, oral steroids are indicated.
3. *Step III*: Immunosuppressive treatment by using drugs such as azathioprine, cyclosporine, etc.
4. *Step IV*: Cryotherapy to destroy the vascular component of the peripheral retinitis, to eliminate the inflammatory mediators.
5. *Step V*: Cases not responsive to all above methods are treated by vitrectomy.

POSTERIOR UVEITIS**

Definition

Posterior uveitis is defined as inflammation of the choroid alone or choroid and the surrounding retina. It is also called choroiditis or chorioretinitis.

Etiology

1. Infectious causes such as toxoplasmosis, toxocariasis, cysticercosis, onchocerciasis, tuberculosis, syphilis, cytomegalovirus (CMV) infection, human immunodeficiency virus (HIV)-related eye diseases, etc.
2. Non-infectious causes such as sarcoidosis, acute posterior multifocal placoid pigment epitheliopathy (APMPPE), birdshot choroidopathy and punctate inner choroidopathy.

Clinical Features

Symptoms

1. Inflammatory symptoms such as pain and redness are absent.
2. Floaters are more often seen in the peripheral lesions involving periphery of retina similar to pars planitis.
3. Diminution of vision is seen in the central lesions involving macula.

Signs

1. Anterior segment examination is normal.
2. Examination of posterior segment shows:
   a. Vitreous opacities, which may be fine or coarse or snowball opacities.
   b. Choroiditis, focal or multifocal, characterized by pale white or yellow patch with well-demarcated margins.
   c. Retinitis, focal or multifocal, characterized by patches of white cloudy areas with indistinct margins (Figs 7.5.1A and B).

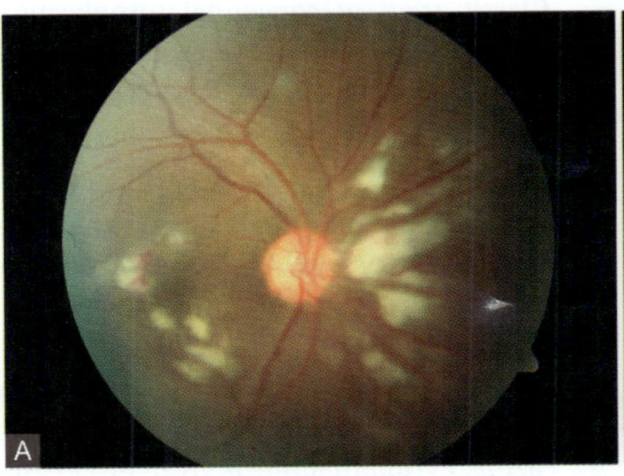

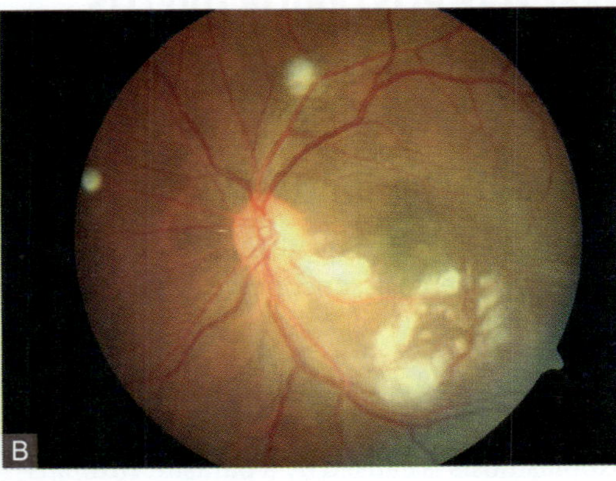

FIGS 7.5.1A and B: Multifocal chorioretinitis

Complications

- Cystoid macular edema
- Periphlebitis
- Vitreous hemorrhage
- Exudative retinal detachment
- Neuroretinitis or optic neuritis.

Investigations

Fundus fluorescein angiography, ultrasonography, optical coherence tomography and tailored laboratory investigations depending on the etiology suspected are required for confirmation of diagnosis and to find out the etiological agent in case of infectious etiology.

Treatment

1. Non-infective posterior uveitis is treated by local and systemic steroids along with immunosuppressive drugs in non-responsive cases.
2. Infective conditions are treated initially with the specific anti-infective agents followed by steroids. Steroids are started after 3 days of initiating the specific anti-infective treatment.

SPECIFIC CLINICAL TYPES OF POSTERIOR UVEITIS

INFECTIVE POSTERIOR UVEITIS

Infective causes include parasitic causes, viral causes, bacterial causes and fungal causes.

Parasitic Posterior Uveitis

Parasitic causes include toxoplasmosis, toxocariasis, cysticercosis, onchocerciasis, etc.

Toxoplasmosis

Etiology

Toxoplasmosis is caused by a parasite *Toxoplasma gondii*, which has worldwide distribution. Approximately one third of the world population is exposed to infection by this parasite.

Pathogenesis

Definite hosts are cats; human beings and all warm-blooded animals are intermediate hosts. Toxoplasma exists in three forms, oocyst is found in definitive hosts, cats and it is shed in feces of cats. Tachyzoite and bradyzoite are seen in intermediate hosts.

Human beings acquire infection by ingesting bradyzoite (tissue cysts) by eating raw or undercooked flesh from other intermediate hosts or by ingesting oocyst from the environment. Congenital infection occurs because of transplacental transmission of infection, when mother is infected during gestation.

Ocular toxoplasmosis

Ocular toxoplasmosis is seen only in congenital infection. Ocular toxoplasmosis is because of congenital infection or because of reactivation of old healed congenital infection.

Clinical features

Ocular toxoplasmosis presents as:

- Focal retinitis adjacent to an old pigmented atrophic retinal scar (Figs 7.5.2A and B)
- Severe vitritis giving the appearance of headlight in the fog appearance on fundoscopy (Figs 7.5.3 and 7.5.4)
- Papillitis
- Retinal vasculitis.

Classic triad of congenital toxoplasmosis consists of hydrocephalus, intracerebral calcification and chorioretinitis.

Peripheral chorioretinal scar of toxoplasmosis

Investigations

Toxoplasmosis is diagnosed by enzyme-linked immunosorbent assay (ELISA), indirect fluorescent antibody test and hemagglutination tests.

Treatment

1. Treatment is done by antitoxoplasma drugs such as pyrimethamine and sulfadiazine. Pyrimethamine is given in a loading dose of 75 mg followed by maintenance

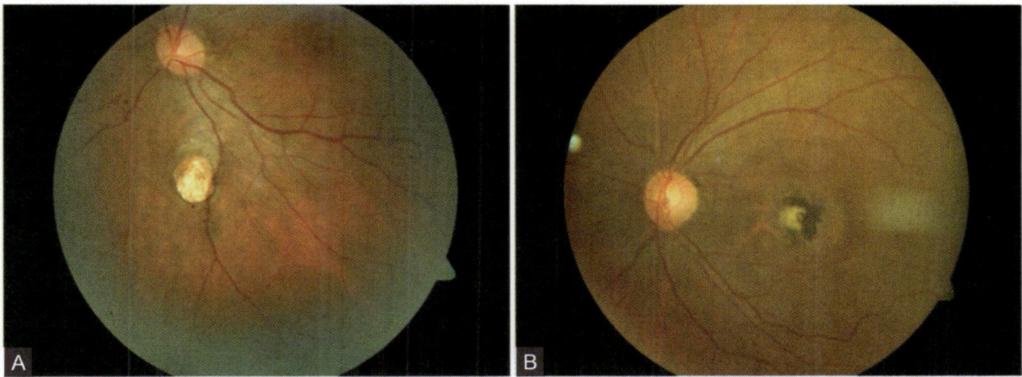

FIGS 7.5.2A and B: Peripheral and macular toxoplasmic chorioretinal scar

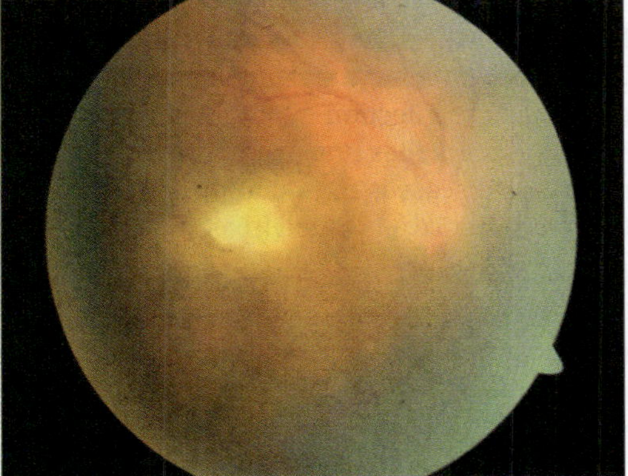

FIG. 7.5.3: Headlight in the fog appearance

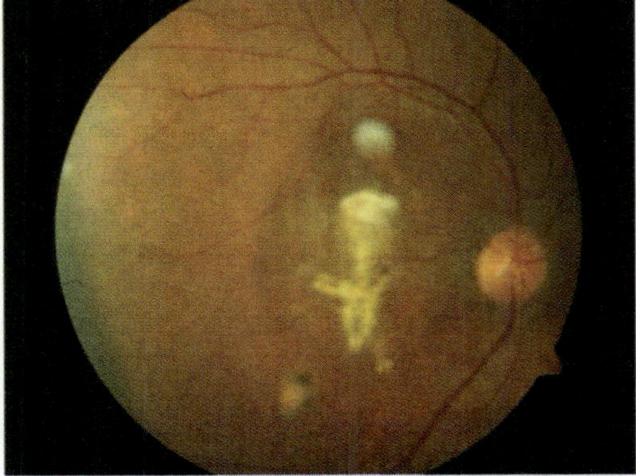

FIG. 7.5.4: Toxoplasma retinitis

dose of 25 mg daily for 4 weeks. Sulfadiazine is given in a loading dose of 2 g followed by maintenance dose of 1 g daily for 4 weeks.

2. Clindamycin 300 mg four times a day for 3 weeks, cotrimoxazole twice daily for 4 weeks is the other effective antitoxoplasma drug.
3. Systemic steroids are indicated in vision-threatening conditions such as involvement of optic nerve and macula in immunocompetent patients.

Toxocariasis

Etiology

Toxocariasis is caused by roundworm [*Toxocara canis* (*T. canis)* (dog roundworm) or *Toxocara cati* (*T. cati*) (cat roundworm)].

Pathogenesis

The *T. canis* completes its lifecycle only in dogs and *T. cati* only in cats. Human beings acquire infection by ingestion of eggs found in soil.

Clinical features

Ocular toxocariasis presents as:

1. Granuloma either in periphery of retina or in posterior pole of retina. Granuloma is formed after the larva of *Toxocara* gets lodged in choroid and becomes encysted. Tractional retinal detachment may be seen in later stages of the disease because of traction of the granuloma on the retina (Figs 7.5.5A and B).
2. Chronic endophthalmitis.
3. Usually presents in children < 10 years and is one of the differential diagnoses for

leukocoria. Other common causes of leukocoria such as retinoblastoma, retinopathy of prematurity should be ruled out.

Investigations

Toxocariasis is diagnosed by ELISA, by identifying the antibodies against the organism.

Treatment

1. Medical treatment is by anthelmintic drugs such as thiabendazole or diethylcarbamazine. Steroids are used to reduce the secondary inflammatory response.
2. Surgical treatment in the form of pars plana vitrectomy is indicated for granuloma with retinal traction or for tractional retinal detachment.

Cysticercosis

Etiology

Cysticercosis is caused by larval form of pork tapeworm, *Taenia solium* (*T. solium*).

Pathogenesis

The adult worms of *T. solium* lives in the intestine and usually will not cause any symptoms. The larval stage, cysticercus cellulosae develops following ingestion of eggs of *T. solium* along with vegetables or following consumption of inadequately cooked pork containing cysticercus cellulosae.

Clinical features

Ocular cysticercosis presents as translucent white cyst with a dense spot corresponding to the scolex of the cysticercus cellulosae. Ocular cysticercosis usually involves vitreous cavity or subretinal space.

Treatment

Treatment is by surgical excision of the cyst.

Onchocerciasis

Etiology

Onchocerciasis is caused by filariae, *Onchocerca volvulus (O.* Volvulus).

Pathogenesis

Humans are the definitive hosts. Black flies of the genus *Simulium* are the intermediate hosts. Humans acquire infection by bite of the black flies. Since the black flies breed along the fast-flowing rivers, the disease is most commonly seen along the rivers; hence it is called 'river blindness'.

Clinical features

Ocular lesions seen in onchocerciasis are:

- Chorioretinitis
- Sclerosing keratitis
- Anterior iridocyclitis.

Treatment

Diethylcarbamazine is used for treatment of microfilariae. Suramin and ivermectin are the other drugs used.

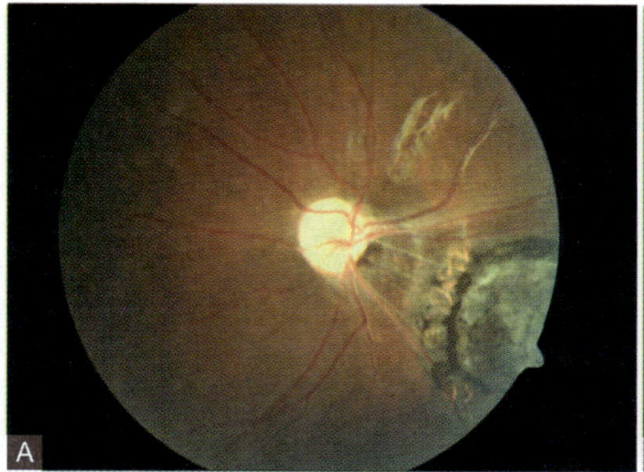

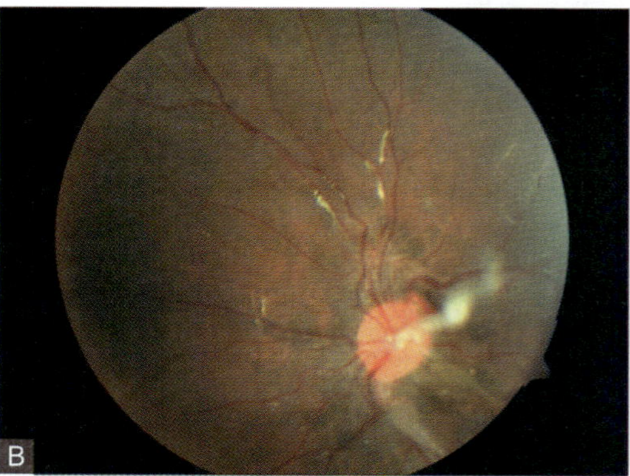

FIGS 7.5.5A and B: Toxocara granuloma

Viral Posterior Uveitis

Viral causes include CMV retinitis, acute retinal necrosis, progressive outer retinal necrosis.

Cytomegalovirus Retinitis (Figs 7.5.6A to D)

Etiology

Cytomegalovirus retinitis is caused by CMV, a member of the herpes virus family.

Pathogenesis

The primary infection in immunocompetent hosts is usually asymptomatic and the virus remains in a latent stage. The virus becomes reactivated in immunocompromised hosts.

Clinical features

Cytomegalovirus retinitis is seen in patients with CD4 count less than 50 cells/mm. It is acquired immunodeficiency syndrome (AIDS) defining disease and it is the most common ocular opportunistic infection seen in AIDS.

Cytomegalovirus retinitis presents as:

1. Fulminating necrotizing retinitis presenting as yellow-white areas of retinal necrosis with hemorrhages. It is called 'pizza pie' appearance or 'cottage cheese with ketchup' appearance.
2. Indolent granular retinitis characterized by granular appearance of retinal necrosis with no or few hemorrhages.
3. Perivascular retinitis called 'frosted branch angiitis' because of its resemblance to frosted branches of a tree.

Treatment

Treatment is done by anti-CMV drugs such as ganciclovir, valganciclovir, foscarnet and cidofovir.

Acute Retinal Necrosis (Fig. 7.5.7)

Etiology

Acute retinal necrosis is caused by herpes zoster virus, herpes simplex type 1 and type 2 virus, and CMV.

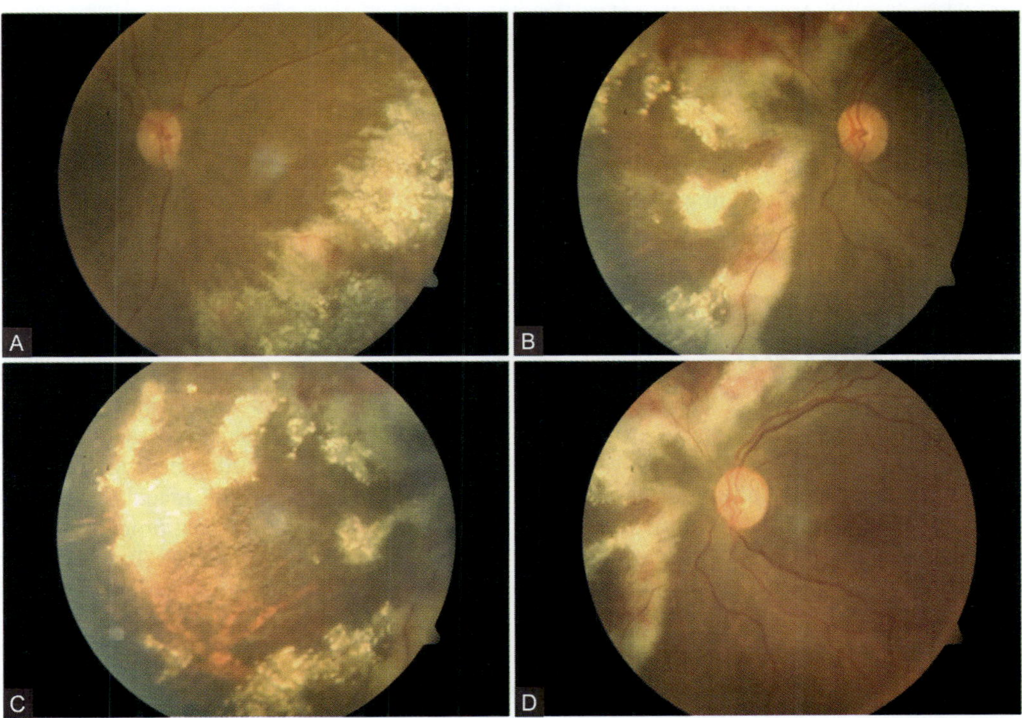

FIGS 7.5.6A to D: Cytomegalovirus retinitis

Clinical Features

Acute retinal necrosis is seen in both immunocompromised and immunocompetent patients. It presents with severe vitritis and yellowish white retinal necrotic lesions.

Treatment

Treatment is done using antiviral drugs acyclovir.

Progressive Outer Retinal Necrosis

Etiology

Progressive outer retinal necrosis is caused by varicella zoster virus.

Clinical features

Progressive outer retinal necrosis is seen in immunocompromised patients. It is characterized by yellowish white retinal necrotic lesions.

Treatment

Treatment is done by antiviral drugs such as acyclovir and ganciclovir.

Bacterial Posterior Uveitis

Bacterial causes include syphilis, tuberculosis, etc.

Fungal Posterior Uveitis

Endogenous endophthalmitis caused by candidiasis. Candidia is the most common fungi causing fungal posterior uveitis. Fungal endophthalmitis is described under endophthalmitis.

NON-INFECTIVE POSTERIOR UVEITIS (Table 7.5.1)

Multiple Evanescent White Dot Syndrome

Multiple evanescent white dot syndrome (MEWDS) is idiopathic self-limiting inflammatory disease usually affecting females more than males and is characterized by small, deep, discrete white lesions involving the posterior pole.

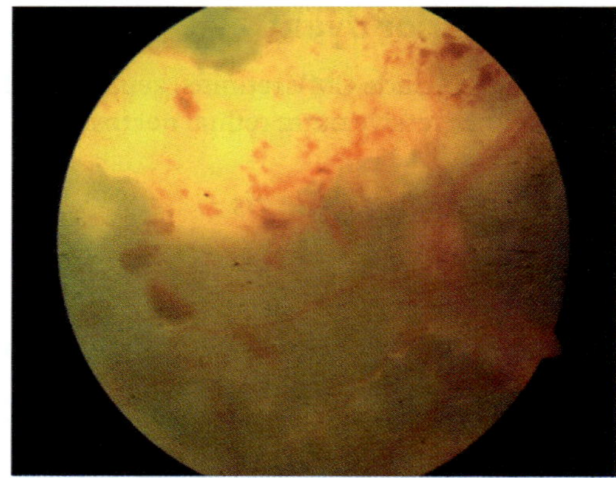

FIG. 7.5.7: Acute retinal necrosis

Acute Posterior Multifocal Placoid Pigment Epitheliopathy

Acute posterior multifocal placoid pigment epitheliopathy is idiopathic, bilateral, self-limiting inflammatory disease characterized by presence of multiple yellowish white plaques such as lesions involving the posterior pole.

Acute Retinal Pigment Epithelitis

Acute retinal pigment epithelitis is idiopathic, inflammatory, self-limiting condition. It is characterized by gray spots at the level of retinal pigment epithelium (RPE). No treatment is required as it is self-limiting condition.

Serpiginous Choroiditis

Serpiginous choroiditis is idiopathic bilateral progressive disease characterized by presence of yellow white subretinal infiltrates with fuzzy appearance and hazy borders. Since the lesions spread in a snake-like manner starting near the optic disk and extending towards the macula, it is called 'serpiginous choroiditis.' Visual prognosis is poor because of involvement of fovea. Treatment is by systemic steroids and immunosuppressive drugs such as azathioprine and cyclosporine.

TABLE 7.5.1: Non-infectious posterior uveitis

Disease	*Etiology*	*Unilateral/Bilateral*	*Visual prognosis*	*Treatment*
Multiple evanescent white dot syndrome (MEWDS)	Young women in 3rd–4th decade	Unilateral	Good	Not required
Acute posterior multifocal placoid pigment epitheliopathy (APMPPE)	3rd–4th decade	Bilateral	Good	Not required
Acute retinal pigment epitheliitis	3rd–4th decade	Unilateral or bilateral	Good	Not required
Serpiginous choroiditis	4th–6th decade	Bilateral	Poor	Systemic steroids, azathioprine and cyclosporine
Birdshot retinochoroidopathy	HLA* A29	Bilateral	Poor	Systemic steroids and cyclosporine
Punctate inner choroidopathy	Young myopic females	Bilateral	Poor	Systemic steroids

*HLA, human leukocyte antigen

Birdshot Retinochoroidopathy

Birdshot retinochoroidopathy is bilateral chronic inflammatory disease characterized by discrete poorly defined cream-colored spots at the level of choroid. Visual prognosis is poor because of involvement of fovea. Treatment is by systemic steroids and immunosuppressive drugs, e.g. cyclosporine.

Punctate Inner Choroidopathy

Punctate inner choroidopathy is idiopathic, bilateral inflammatory disease typically affecting myopics. It is characterized by presence of multiple yellow indistinct lesions involving the posterior pole. Visual prognosis is poor in patients with foveal involvement. Treatment is by systemic steroids.

GIST BOX 7.5

- Intermediate uveitis is the inflammation of pars plana of ciliary body and the surrounding peripheral retina, choroid and anterior vitreous. Majority of the causes are idiopathic; in few cases, the underlying cause may be sarcoidosis, multiple sclerosis, Lyme disease, etc. Symptoms are usually minimal. Pain and redness of the eye is not seen in majority of cases. Floaters are the presenting complaint of the disease. Examination of the pars plana by indirect ophthalmoscopy and sclera depression shows accumulation of inflammatory aggregates in the pars plana is called vitreous snow banks, the characteristic feature of pars planitis.
- Posterior uveitis is defined as inflammation of the choroid alone or choroid and the surrounding retina. It is also called choroiditis or chorioretinitis. Infectious causes are toxoplasmosis, toxocariasis, cysticercosis, onchocerciasis, tuberculosis, syphilis, cytomegalovirus, HIV-related eye diseases, etc. Non-infectious causes are sarcoidosis, acute posterior multifocal placoid pigment epitheliopathy, birdshot choroidopathy, punctate inner choroidopathy, etc.

CHAPTER

7.6 Panuveitis

DEFINITION

Panuveitis is defined as inflammation involving whole of the uvea, i.e. iris, ciliary body and choroid.

Etiology*

The common causes of panuveitis are:
- Tuberculosis.
- Sarcoidosis.
- Vogt-Koyanagi-Harada (VKH) syndrome.
- Sympathetic ophthalmitis.
- Behçet's disease.
- Syphilis.

CLINICAL FEATURES

Panuveitis shows all the symptoms and signs of anterior and posterior uveitis together:
1. Anterior segment shows signs of anterior uveitis such as aqueous cells and flare, keratic precipitates, etc.
2. Posterior segment shows signs of posterior uveitis such as vitreous cells, choroiditis, retinitis, etc.

INVESTIGATIONS

All the laboratory tests as described for both anterior uveitis and posterior uveitis are required based on the history and examination findings.

TREATMENT

Non-specific treatment is by:
1. Corticosteroids administered through topical, local and systemic route.
2. Cycloplegic drugs to relieve ciliary muscle spasm and to prevent synechiae formation.
3. Immunosuppressive drugs in cases, which are nonresponsive to steroids or in cases where steroids are contraindicated.

Specific treatment depends on the cause.

SPECIFIC TYPES OF PANUVEITIS

Tuberculosis

Tuberculosis is caused by *Mycobacterium tuberculosis* (*M. tuberculosis*). It is one of the most common infective diseases worldwide particularly in developing and underdeveloped countries. In the recent years it has re-emerged as a serious public health problem because of increase in the incidence of acquired immune deficiency syndrome (AIDS).

Ocular tuberculosis: It is most often results from hematogenous spread. Primary ocular infection is very rare. The ocular manifestations are:
- Granulomatous iridocyclitis
- Choroiditis
- Choroidal granuloma
- Retinal periphlebitis
- Phlyctenular keratoconjunctivitis
- Scleritis.

Sarcoidosis

Definition

Sarcoidosis is a granulomatous inflammatory disorder involving multiple organs, with lungs being involved predominantly. Skin, lymph nodes, eyes, salivary glands, liver, spleen, musculoskeletal system and central nervous system are the other predominantly involved organs.

Etiopathogenesis

Sarcoidosis shows impaired cell-mediated and humoral immunity leading to impaired response to antigens. Impaired cellular immune response to antigens leads to development of granulomas in the target organs.

Histologically sarcoidosis is characterized by the presence of non-caseating granulomas. The granulomas persisting for a longer time result in fibrosis and scarring in the involved tissues. The exact etiology of sarcoidosis is unknown, an immunological basis for the disease has been proposed.

Clinical Features

Sarcoidosis usually affects young and middle-aged adults. Lungs are affected in more than 90% of patients and presents with respiratory system complaints. Bilateral hilar lymphadenopathy is the earliest sign of involvement with progression of the disease causing parenchymal involvement of the lungs and late stage of the disease characterized by pulmonary fibrosis:

1. Ocular involvement:
   a. Ocular involvement is seen in 25–60% of patients with sarcoidosis.
   b. Uveitis is the most common ocular manifestation. Sarcoidosis can cause anterior uveitis, posterior uveitis or panuveitis:
      - Anterior uveitis is usually chronic granulomatous type classically presenting with iris nodules and mutton-fat keratic precipitates, whereas young patients may present with acute granulomatous uveitis
      - Posterior uveitis characteristically showing:
        - Vitreous involvement in the form of snowball opacities
        - Vascular involvement in the form of peripheral retinal periphlebitis with candle wax drippings along the retinal veins
        - Choroidal granulomas
        - Optic disk involvement in the form of optic neuropathy, granuloma involving the optic disk and neovascularization of the optic disk.

Investigations

1. Chest X-ray and thoracic computed tomography (CT) scan will show enlarged hilar lymph nodes.
2. Serum angiotensin-converting enzyme (ACE) is usually elevated in patients with active disease.
3. Kveim skin test is positive.
4. Biopsy of the suspicious lesions showing non-caseating granulomas.

Treatment

Treatment is done by topical and periocular steroids in cases of anterior iridocyclitis. Systemic steroids and immunosuppressive drugs, e.g. cyclosporine, are indicated in posterior uveitis.

Sympathetic Ophthalmitis**

Definition

Sympathetic ophthalmitis is defined as bilateral granulomatous panuveitis, which occurs following penetrating ocular injury or surgery with incarceration of uveal tissue in the wound.

The injured eye is called exciting eye and the eye, which develops inflammation is called sympathizing eye.

Pathogenesis

Sympathetic ophthalmitis is usually seen after few days or weeks following penetrating injury or surgery with the peak incidence after 4 weeks. Trauma leads to drainage of antigen from the eye via lymphatics leading to development of delayed hypersensitivity resulting in granulomatous inflammation of the uveal tract. The antigen responsible is presumed to be retinal S antigen.

Pathology

Histopathology of sympathetic ophthalmitis is characterized by granulomatous inflammation with infiltration of lymphocytes, plasma cells, epithelioid cells and giant cells. The characteristic lesions are Dalen-Fuchs nodules composed of aggregation of epithelioid cells, lymphocytes and histiocytes in the choroid.

Clinical Features

Inflammation in the sympathizing eye following inflammatory symptoms in the exciting eye:

1. Exciting eye: It shows features of chronic persistent panuveitis.
2. Sympathizing eye: As follows:
    a. In the early stages minimal pain, photophobia and diminution of vision for near because of weakening of accommodation are the earliest symptoms.
    b. Ciliary congestion and aqueous flare are the earliest signs. In later stages, it progresses to granulomatous iridocyclitis with mutton-fat keratic precipitates.
    c. Posterior segment shows multiple yellow lesions in the posterior pole because of choroidal thickening. Other posterior segment findings are vitritis, retinal vasculitis and papillitis.

Treatment

Sympathetic ophthalmitis can be prevented by:

1. Meticulous repair of the injured eye or the surgical wound to prevent incarceration of uveal tissue in the wound.
2. Early enucleation of the badly injured eye with no visual prognosis.

Sympathetic ophthalmitis is treated by corticosteroids and immunosuppressive drugs.

Vogt-Koyanagi-Harada Syndrome**

Definition

Vogt-Koyanagi-Harada (VKH) syndrome is an autoimmune disease characterized by bilateral panuveitis with exudative retinal detachment and frequently associated with neurological, auditory and dermatological manifestations.

The syndrome consists of two distinct entities:

1. *Vogt-Koyanagi syndrome*: It is bilateral chronic anterior uveitis associated with dermatological and auditory manifestations.
2. *Harada syndrome*: It is bilateral posterior uveitis with exudative retinal detachment associated with neurological manifestations.

Vogt-Koyanagi-Harada syndrome is named after ophthalmologists Alfred Vogt, Yoshizo Koyanagi and Einosuke Harada, who described the clinical disorder independently. Since both these syndromes overlap in many features they are described together as VKH syndrome.

Etiopathogenesis

Females are more affected compared to males. It is more common in darkly pigmented races such as Asians, native Americans, etc. It is more common in Japanese among Asians. It is said to be because of cell-mediated immunity against melanocytes of uveal tissue, meninges and cutaneous tissues.

Clinical Features

1. *Neurological features:* Neck stiffness because of meningeal irritation, headache and cranial nerve palsies.
2. *Dermatological features:* Vitiligo and poliosis.
3. *Auditory features:* Vertigo and tinnitus.
4. *Ocular features:* They are described in four stages:

a. *Prodromal stage:* This stage is characterized by orbital pain and extraocular features such as headache, stiff neck, tinnitus and vertigo and it lasts for few days to weeks.
b. *Uveitis stage:* It presents as bilateral posterior uveitis or granulomatous panuveitis.
c. *Convalescent stage:* It is characterized by depigmentation of the skin and choroidal tissue. Choroid shows areas of chorioretinal atrophy leading to the typical appearance of orange-red color called sunset-glow appearance. Dermatological changes include poliosis of eyelashes, eyebrows, vitiligo.
d. *Recurrent stage:* It is characterized by recurrent anterior or posterior uveitis.

Treatment

Treatment is done by systemic steroids and patients who are unresponsive to steroids may require immunosuppressive drugs such as cyclosporine, azathioprine or cyclophosphamide.

Behçet's Disease

Definition

Behçet's disease is a multisystemic inflammatory disorder characterized by the triad of oral ulcers, genital ulcers and ocular lesions. It is named after Hulusi Behçet, a dermatologist who first described the disease.

Etiopathogenesis

Behçet's disease is more common in young males. It is associated with human leukocyte antigen (HLA) B5 and HLA-B51. It is most commonly seen in Japanese and in people from Middle East. The exact pathogenesis is not known. It is because of abnormal autoimmune response leading to obliterative vasculitis.

Clinical Features

1. *Ocular features:*
   a. Anterior segment features such as hypopyon anterior iridocyclitis.
   b. Posterior segment involvement in the form of retinal vasculitis, vitritis, optic neuropathy.
   c. Other ocular manifestations are episcleritis, conjunctivitis and keratitis.
2. *Systemic features:*
   a. Oral ulcers.
   b. Skin involvement in the form of erythema nodosum, acneiform lesions, etc.
   c. Genital ulcers.
   d. Other features such as arthritis, intestinal ulcers, epididymitis.

Treatment

Treatment is done by topical and systemic steroids. Cytotoxic drugs (e.g. chlorambucil) may be used in unresponsive cases or as steroid-sparing drugs.

Syphilis

Definition

Syphilis is an infectious disease caused by *Treponema pallidum.*

Etiopathogenesis

The incidence of syphilis, which was decreased after the availability of penicillin has increased again because of high-risk sexual activity and human immunodeficiency virus (HIV) infection. It is transmitted through sexual contact and transplacentally from infected mother to newborn during pregnancy.

Clinical Features

Syphilis is called great masquerader or great imitator as it can mimic number of other diseases because of its varied presentations.

Syphilis presents in four stages:

1. Primary syphilis is characterized by chancre at the site of contact.
2. Secondary syphilis is characterized by skin rashes, and involvement of lymph nodes and mucous membranes.
3. Latent syphilis is the stage without any symptoms.
4. Tertiary syphilis is characterized by gumma involving skin or bones, neurological lesions such as tabes dorsalis, Argyll Robertson pupil and cardiovascular lesions, e.g. aortitis.

Ocular Manifestations

Ocular manifestations are most commonly seen in secondary and tertiary stages of the disease.

Anterior segment: As follows:

- Anterior granulomatous iridocyclitis
- Episcleritis, scleritis
- Keratitis.

Posterior segment: As follows:

- Posterior uveitis
- Chorioretinitis
- Neuroretinitis (Fig. 7.6.1)
- Argyll Robertson pupil
- Pseudoretinitis pigmentosa.

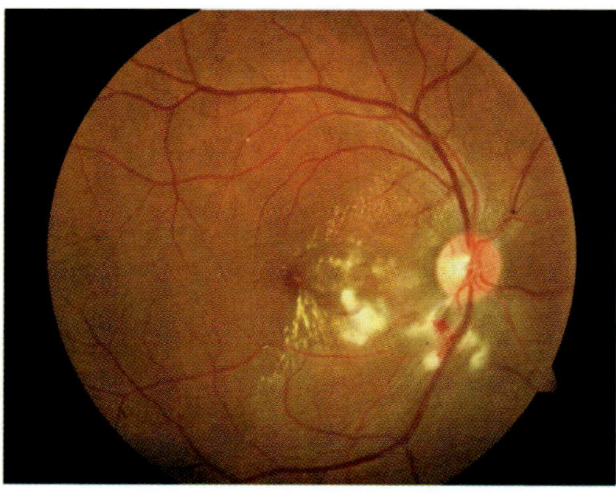

FIG. 7.6.1: Syphilitic neuroretinitis

Investigations

Commonly done serological tests are Venereal Disease Research Laboratory (VDRL) test, fluorescent treponemal antibody absorption (FTA-ABS).

Treatment

1. Intramuscular procaine penicillin 2.4 million units and oral probenecid 2 g for 15 days.
2. Patients who are allergic to penicillin are treated by erythromycin 500 mg four times a day for 1 month.

GIST BOX 7.6

- Panuveitis is defined as inflammation involving whole of the uvea, i.e. iris, ciliary body and choroid. The common causes of panuveitis are tuberculosis, sarcoidosis, Vogt-Koyanagi-Harada syndrome, sympathetic ophthalmitis, Behçet's disease, syphilis, etc.
- Sympathetic ophthalmitis is defined as bilateral granulomatous panuveitis, which occurs following penetrating ocular injury or surgery with incarceration of uveal tissue in the wound.
- Vogt-Koyanagi-Harada syndrome is an autoimmune disease characterized by bilateral panuveitis with exudative retinal detachment and frequently associated with neurological, auditory and dermatological manifestations.
- Behçet's disease is a multisystemic inflammatory disorder characterized by the triad of oral ulcers, genital ulcers and ocular lesions.

CHAPTER

7.7 Endophthalmitis and Panophthalmitis

ENDOPHTHALMITIS***

Definition

Endophthalmitis is defined as severe inflammation of inner coats (uvea and retina) and the intraocular cavities (anterior chamber and vitreous chamber).

Etiology

The endophthalmitis may be infective or non-infective:

1. Infective endophthalmitis is due to entry of infective microbial organism into the eye from exogenous route (following trauma or surgery) or endogenous route (hematogenous spread from distant site). Bacteria and fungi are the etiological agents in majority of cases. Parasites and viruses are less common causes.
2. Non-infective or sterile causes include phacoanaphylactic endophthalmitis, toxic inflammation to agents used for sterilization of intraocular lens (IOL) and inflammation following necrosis of intraocular tumors.

Clinical Features

Symptoms

Symptoms depend on the type of endophthalmitis; common symptoms include:

- Usually unilateral condition
- Pain, redness and diminution of vision
- Acute and sudden onset in acute postoperative endophthalmitis, chronic and insidious onset in chronic endophthalmitis.

Signs

- Lid edema
- Circumcorneal congestion
- Gross diminution of vision
- Keratic precipitates
- Anterior chamber aqueous cells and flare, hypopyon
- Vitreous exudates
- Yellowish white reflex in the pupillary area because of vitreous exudates
- Initially raised intraocular pressure (IOP) because of inflammatory glaucoma, later decreased IOP because of ciliary shutdown
- Phthisis bulbi with complete loss of vision is the end result.

Investigations

Microbiological diagnosis is done from microscopy and culture of the samples from aqueous tap from anterior chamber or vitreous tap from vitreous chamber.

Clinical Types (Table 7.7.1)

TABLE 7.7.1: Clinical types of endophthalmitis

Type	*Clinical features*	*Common causative organisms*
Postoperative endophthalmitis		
• Acute postoperative endophthalmitis (Fig. 7.7.1)	Infection within 6 week of surgery	*Staphylococcus aureus (S. aureus)* *Streptococcus* species
• Chronic endophthalmitis	Infection > 6 week of surgery	*Propionibacterium acnes, Staphylococcus epidermidis, Corynebacterium* species, fungi, etc.
• Bleb-associated endophthalmitis	Infection following filtering surgery	*S. aureus, Streptococcus* species, *Haemophilus*
Traumatic endophthalmitis	Infection following open-globe injury or following retained intraocular foreign body	*Streptococcus* species, *Bacillus* species
Endogenous endophthalmitis	Infection secondary to systemic infection	*Candida* species, *Escherichia coli*

Differential Features (Table 7.7.2)

TABLE 7.7.2: Differences between endophthalmitis and panophthalmitis

Features	*Endophthalmitis*	*Panophthalmitis*
Definition	Severe purulent inflammation involving inner coats and cavities of eyeball	Severe purulent inflammation involving all the three coats and cavities of eyeball
Vision	Depends on the severity of inflammation rarely perception of light (PL) negative	Complete loss of vision PL negative
Cornea	Transparent with keratic precipitates	Hazy and necrotic cornea
Anterior chamber	Shows aqueous cells, flare and hypopyon	Filled with pus
Examination of eye	Yellowish white pupillary reflex, vitreous exudates	Cornea is hazy and entire eye is filled with pus
Extraocular movements	Full	Limited
Treatment	Medical line of management with intravitreal injections and vitrectomy	Medical line of management is rarely successful
	Enucleation is indicated for non-responsive cases	Evisceration is required in most of the cases and enucleation is contraindicated because of risk of spread of infection to intracranial cavity along the cut ends of the optic nerve

Treatment

Antibiotics

Antibiotics are the mainstay of treatment of endophthalmitis. Antibiotics are administered through topical route, systemic route and intravitreal route:

1. *Topical antibiotics*: Fortified tobramycin (14 mg/mL) and fortified Cefazolin (50 mg/mL) eyedrops are used.

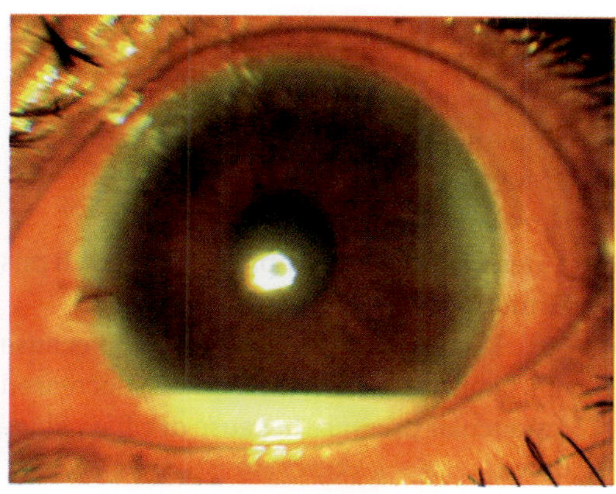

FIG. 7.7.1: Acute endophthalmitis

2. *Systemic antibiotics*: Drugs, which cross blood retinal barrier such as ciprofloxacin (500–750 mg 12th hourly), Cefazolin and ceftazidime (2 g intravenously 8th hourly) are the preferred antibiotics.
3. *Intravitreal antibiotics*: Usually ceftazidime (2.25 mg/0.1 mL) for gram-negative organisms and vancomycin (1 mg/0.1 mL) for gram-positive organisms are preferred for intravitreal injection.

Corticosteroids

1. Corticosteroids are indicated to decrease the inflammation. Corticosteroids are administered by topical route (prednisolone acetate eyedrops 1%), oral route (prednisolone 1 mg/kg), intravitreal route (dexamethasone 400 μg).
2. Corticosteroids are contraindicated in fungal endophthalmitis.
3. Topical steroids are started from the time of diagnosis and oral steroids are started under cover of antibiotics, a day after intravitreal antibiotics.

Antifungals

- Antifungals are indicated in fungal endophthalmitis
- *Topical antifungals:* Natamycin eyedrops
- *Oral antifungals:* Ketoconazole or fluconazole for 4-6 weeks
- *Intravitreal antifungals:* Amphotericin B (5 μg).

Cycloplegics

Atropine 1% eye ointment is given for relief of pain.

Vitrectomy

Vitrectomy is indicated in:

- No improvement clinically after 48 hours of conservative management
- Advanced stage on initial presentation with complete absence of red reflex and presenting visual acuity of less than hand movements
- Endophthalmitis associated with retained intraocular foreign body
- Chronic endophthalmitis
- Fungal endophthalmitis.

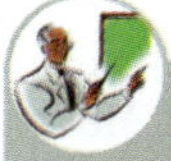

Recommendations of Endophthalmitis Vitrectomy Study

- Conservative management with antibiotics in patients with initial presentation of visual acuity of better than hand movements.
- Surgical management in the form of vitrectomy in patients with initial presentation of visual acuity of less than hand movements.

PANOPHTHALMITIS (Fig. 7.7.2)**

Definition

Panophthalmitis is defined as severe inflammation of all the three coats of the eye (cornea and sclera, uvea, retina) and the intraocular cavities (anterior chamber and vitreous chamber).

Etiopathogenesis

Panophthalmitis usually follows penetrating intraocular injuries or postoperative infections.

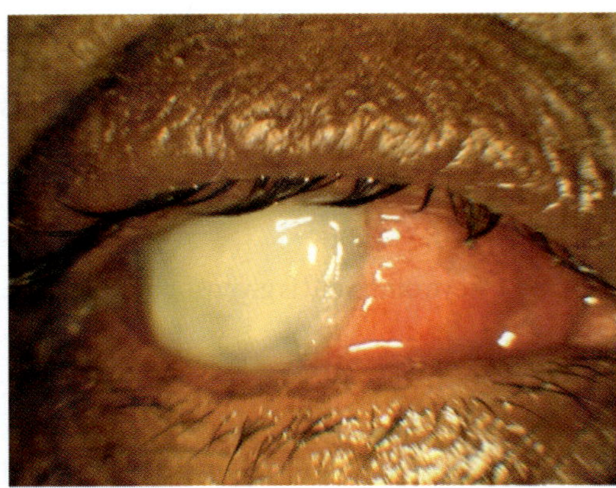

FIG. 7.7.2: Panophthalmitis

Staphylococcus, Streptococcus, Pseudomonas, E. coli are the common causative agents. Panophthalmitis is characterized by marked suppurative inflammation with necrosis affecting all the layers of the eyeball.

Clinical Features

Symptoms

- Constitutional symptoms such as fever, headache, etc.
- Severe ocular pain, redness, complete loss of vision, etc.

Signs

- Lid edema
- Circumcorneal congestion and chemosis
- Loss of vision
- Hazy and necrotic cornea
- Anterior chamber completely filled with pus
- Limited extraocular movements
- Initially raised intraocular pressure because of inflammatory glaucoma, later decreased intraocular pressure because of ciliary shutdown
- Phthisis bulbi with complete loss of vision is the end result.

Complications

Uncontrolled panophthalmitis may spread to surrounding structures resulting in orbital cellulitis, cavernous sinus thrombosis, meningitis, etc.

Treatment

Medical line of treatment is usually not successful; evisceration of eye is required in most of the cases (refer Table 7.7.2).

GIST BOX 7.7

- Endophthalmitis is defined as severe inflammation of inner coats (uvea and retina) and the intraocular cavities (anterior chamber and vitreous chamber).
- Panophthalmitis is defined as severe inflammation of all the three coats of the eye (cornea and sclera, uvea, retina) and the intraocular cavities (anterior chamber and vitreous chamber).

CHAPTER

7.8

Dystrophies and Degenerations of Uveal Tract

IRIDOCORNEAL ENDOTHELIAL SYNDROME*

Definition

Iridocorneal endothelial syndrome (ICE) includes a group of diseases characterized by abnormalities of corneal endothelium and iris.

It includes three conditions:

1. **I**ris nevus syndrome.
2. **C**handler's syndrome.
3. **E**ssential iris atrophy (Fig. 7.8.1).

Etiopathogenesis

Iridocorneal endothelial syndrome is usually a unilateral condition seen typically in middle-aged women.

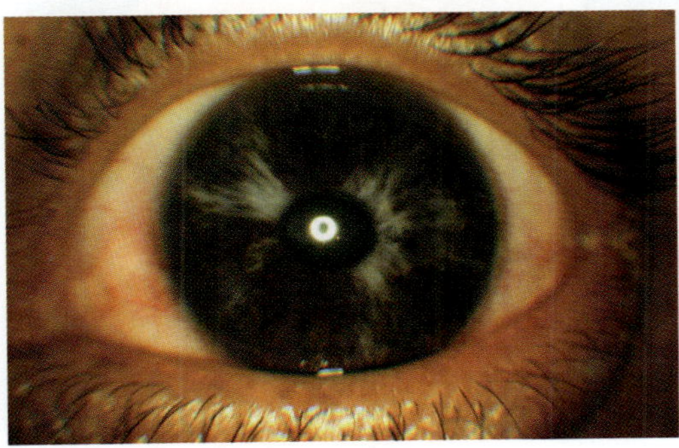

FIG. 7.8.1: Essential iris atrophy

It is because of abnormal corneal endothelial layer, which proliferates involving the angle of the anterior chamber and iris.

The underlying cause for the disease is not known. It is suspected to be a viral infection caused by herpes simplex viral infection.

Clinical Features

Iridocorneal endothelial syndrome depends on one of the three components with considerable overlap of the features:

1. *Iris nevus syndrome*: It is characterized by diffuse nevus of iris or pigmented iris nodules. It is also called Cogan-Reese syndrome.
2. *Chandler's syndrome*: It is characterized by corneal edema because of endothelial abnormalities.
3. *Essential iris atrophy*: It is characterized by iris atrophy, displacement of pupil and iris hole formation.

About 50% of patients may develop glaucoma because of formation of peripheral anterior synechiae resulting in synechial closure of the angle of anterior chamber.

Treatment

Treatment is required in patients developing glaucoma. Surgical management of glaucoma in the form of trabeculectomy or artificial drainage devices is required as usually medical management of glaucoma is ineffective.

GYRATE ATROPHY (Figs 7.8.2A and B)

Definition

Gyrate atrophy is an autosomal recessive condition due to the deficiency of the enzyme, ornithine aminotransferase.

Ornithine aminotransferase is required for conversion of ornithine to proline. Deficiency of this enzyme results in hyperornithinemia.

Clinical Features

1. The disease usually presents in the second decade.
2. It is characterized by progressive chorioretinal atrophy appearing as scalloped areas starting from periphery of retina presenting as progressive loss of peripheral vision and night vision.
3. Fovea is involved later in the disease hence patient will have good central vision until late stage.

Treatment

Oral supplementation of vitamin B_6 may help by decreasing hyperornithinemia.

Arginine-restricted diet to decrease the level of ornithine (arginine is precursor of ornithine) by avoiding arginine-rich foods such as sea foods, nuts, yolk of the eggs and whole wheat.

Visual prognosis is poor with most of the patients reaching legal blindness by sixth decade.

CHOROIDEREMIA (Fig. 7.8.3)

Definition

Choroideremia is an X-linked recessive disease affecting only males with females as carriers, characterized by choroidal atrophy.

Etiopathogenesis

Choroideremia is caused by mutation in the choroideremia gene on the X chromosome leading to absence of Rab escort protein 1, which is essential for intracellular vesicular transport.

Clinical Features

1. It is seen in males in first decade presenting with progressive loss of night vision.
2. It presents with areas of chorioretinal atrophy starting in the equatorial region of the retina and progressing toward macula with involvement of macula later.

ANGIOID STREAKS (Fig. 7.8.4)*

Definition

Angioid streaks is a crack-like dehiscence in the Bruch's membrane of the choroid.

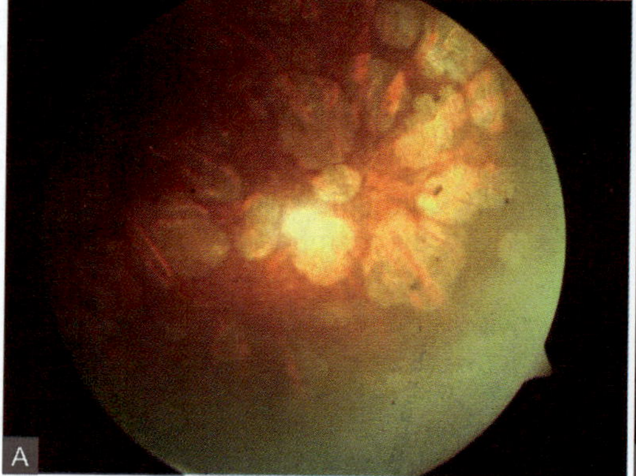

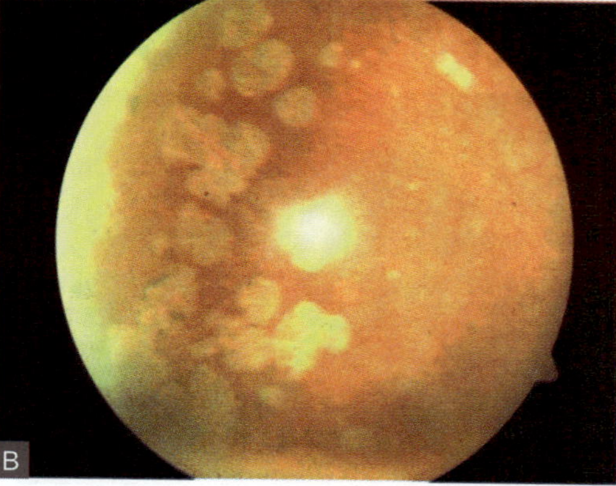

FIGS 7.8.2A and B: Gyrate atrophy

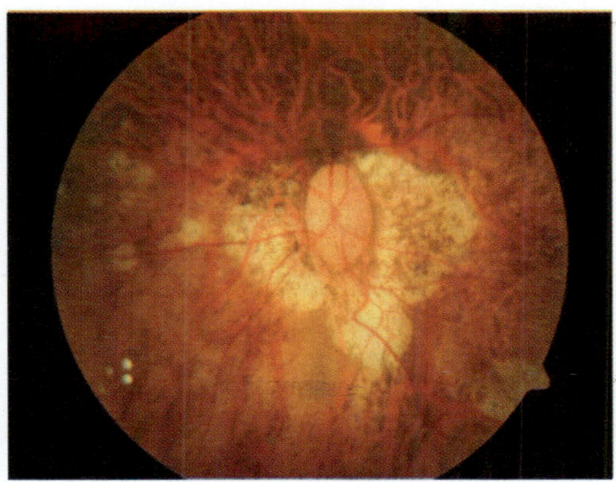

FIG. 7.8.3: Choroideremia

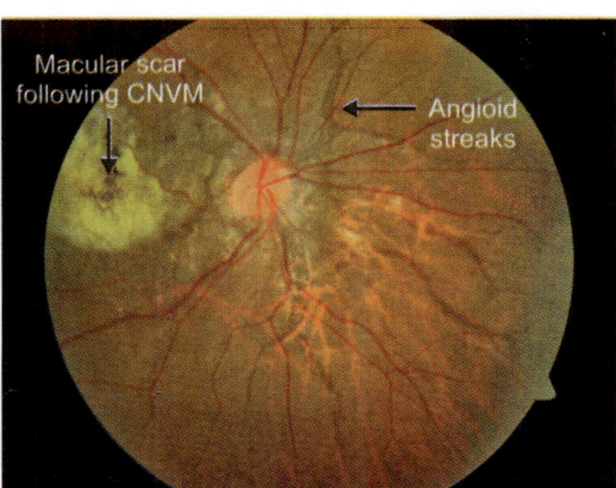

FIG. 7.8.4: Angioid streaks (CNVM, choroidal neovascularization membrane)

Etiopathogenesis

Angioid streaks are because of degeneration of Bruch's membrane, and deposition of calcium and iron. Angioid streaks are called so because of resemblance to blood vessels.

Angioid streaks are found in association with systemic diseases such as pseudoxanthoma elasticum, Paget's disease, Ehlers-Danlos syndrome and sickle cell disease.

Clinical Features

Angioid streaks present as lines reddish brown in color with irregular serrated edges, radiating outwards from the peripapillary area giving the appearance of orange skin (Peau d'orange).

Visual impairment is seen because of involvement of macula by choroidal neovascularization membrane (CNVM) leading to macular scar.

Treatment

Treatment is not required in asymptomatic cases. Treatment is required in cases of choroidal neovascularization. Treatment options are laser photocoagulation, photodynamic therapy and intravitreal injections of antivascular endothelial factors (e.g. ranibizumab).

GIST BOX 7.8

- Iridocorneal endothelial syndrome (ICE syndrome) includes a group of diseases characterized by abnormalities of corneal endothelium and iris. It includes three conditions, iris nevus syndrome, Chandler's syndrome and essential iris atrophy.
- Gyrate atrophy is an autosomal recessive condition due to the deficiency of the enzyme ornithine aminotransferase.
- Choroideremia is an X-linked recessive disease affecting only males, with females as carriers, characterized by choroidal atrophy.
- Angioid streaks are crack-like dehiscence in the Bruch's membrane of the choroid because of degeneration of Bruch's membrane and deposition of calcium and iron.

FREQUENTLY ASKED QUESTIONS (FAQs)

*Short Answers

1. Coloboma of uveal tract.
2. Keratic precipitates.
3. Aqueous cells and aqueous flare.
4. Synechiae.
5. Seclusio pupillae.
6. Occlusio pupillae.
7. Iris nodules.
8. Mention the treatment of acute iridocyclitis.
9. Mention the treatment and investigations for acute red eye.
10. Mention the role of atropine in the treatment of cycloplegic drugs.
11. Fuchs heterochromic iridocyclitis.
12. Posner-Schlossman syndrome.
13. Mention the causes for panuveitis.
14. Iridocorneal endothelial syndromes.
15. Angioid streaks.

**Short Essays

1. Classify uveitis.
2. Granulomatous uveitis.
3. Mention the complications of acute iridocyclitis.
4. Pars planitis.
5. Posterior uveitis.
6. Sympathetic ophthalmitis.
7. Panophthalmitis.
8. Vogt-Koyanagi-Harada syndrome.

***Long Essays

1. Discuss the differential diagnosis of acute red eye. Describe the etiology, clinical features and management of acute iridocyclitis.
2. Describe the etiology, clinical features and management of granulomatous iridocyclitis.
3. Describe the etiology, clinical features and management of endophthalmitis.

BIBLIOGRAPHY

1. Agrawal RV, Murthy S, Sangwan V, et al. Current approach in diagnosis and management of anterior uveitis. Indian J Ophthalmol. 2010;58(1):11-9.
2. Babu BM, Rathinam SR. Intermediate uveitis. Indian J Ophthalmol. 2010;58(1):21-7.
3. Bansal R, Gupta V, Gupta A. Current approach in the diagnosis and management of panuveitis. Indian J Ophthalmol. 2010;58(1):45-54.
4. Dutta LC. Modern Ophthalmology, Vol. 3, 3rd edition. New Delhi: Jaypee Brothers Medical Publishers; 2005.
5. Gregory-Evans CY, Williams MJ, Halford S, et al. Ocular coloboma: a reassessment in the age of molecular neuroscience. J Med Genet. 2004;41(12):881-91.
6. Grønskov K, Ek J, Brondum-Nielsen K. Oculocutaneous albinism. Orphanet J Rare Dis. 2007;2:43.
7. Kanski JK. Clinical Ophthalmology, 5th edition. Philadelphia: Butterworth-Heinemann; 2003.
8. Mosuro A, Baiyeroju A. A report of a case of bilateral iris coloboma in a 9 year old boy. The Internet Journal of Ophthalmology and Visual Science. 2009;7(1).
9. Rohatgi J, Singal A. Ocular manifestations of Behcet's disease in Indian patients. Indian J Ophthalmol. 2003;51(4):309-13.
10. Rothova A. Ocular involvement in sarcoidosis. Br J Ophthalmol. 2000;84(1):110-6.
11. Sudharshan S, Ganesh SK, Biswas J. Current approach in the diagnosis and management of posterior uveitis. Indian J Ophthalmol. 2010;58(1):29-43.

SECTION 8

Lens

8.1 Anatomy and Physiology of Lens
8.2 Congenital Anomalies of Lens
8.3 Cataract
8.4 Cataract Surgeries
8.5 Lens-induced Glaucoma
8.6 Ectopia Lentis

CHAPTER

8.1 Anatomy and Physiology of Lens

ANATOMY OF LENS

Lens is a transparent refractive element of the eye accounting for one third of refractive power of the eye.

Gross Anatomy

Lens is a biconvex crystalline structure situated in the anterior segment of the eye between iris and vitreous body in a fossa called patellar fossa.

Dimensions of Lens (Table 8.1.1)

TABLE 8.1.1: Dimensions of lens

Radius of curvature: • Anterior surface • Posterior surface	 10 mm 6 mm
Equatorial diameter	10 mm
Refractive index	1.39
Refractive power	16 diopter (D)

Histology of Lens (Fig. 8.1.1)*

Histologically, lens consists of lens capsule, lens epithelium and lens substance.

Lens Capsule

Lens capsule is a thick elastic basement membrane, which surrounds the lens completely. The thickness of capsule varies according to the region of the lens and it is thickest anteriorly and posteriorly in the pre-equator region (approximately measures about 21 μm and 23 μm respectively), followed by at the equator measuring about 17 μm and followed by anterior pole measuring about 14 μm. It is thinnest at the posterior pole where it measures about 4 μm.

Lens Epithelium

Only anterior lens epithelium is present and the corresponding posterior lens epithelium is absent as the posterior epithelium cells elongate to form the lens fibers in the embryonic nucleus. Anterior lens epithelium consists of a single layer of cuboidal cells, which lies beneath the anterior capsule. The anterior epithelial cells do not divide. The epithelial cells change to columnar cell subtype in the pre-equatorial and equatorial region, which actively divide throughout life to form new lens fibers.

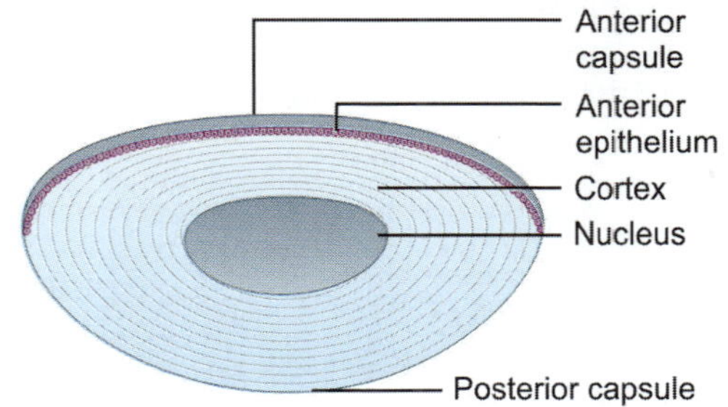

FIG. 8.1.1: Histology of human lens

Lens Substance

Lens substance consists of the lens fibers. The lens fibers are produced from the posterior lens epithelium during embryonic life and in adults they are produced from equatorial lens epithelium. The lens fibers are arranged in nucleus and cortex. The nucleus is in the central part of the lens and it consists of various zones depending on the time of formation of the lens fibers (Table 8.1.2). The cortex is the peripheral part of the lens consisting of the recently formed lens fibers. The infantile and adult nucleus, which lies outside the hard embryonic and fetal nucleus is called epinucleus.

Ciliary zonules also called zonules of Zinn are the suspensory ligaments, which suspend the lens and keep it in its position. They arise from ciliary body and extend to the lens equator in continuous circumferential fashion. These ciliary zonules are responsible for accommodation by the action of ciliary muscle. Lens does not have blood supply or nerve supply.

TABLE 8.1.2: Formation of lens fibers in nucleus

Embryonic nucleus	Lens fibers formed in the first 3 month of gestation
Fetal nucleus	Lens fibers formed from 3 month of gestation to birth
Infantile nucleus	Lens fibers formed from birth to puberty
Adult nucleus	Lens fibers formed after puberty

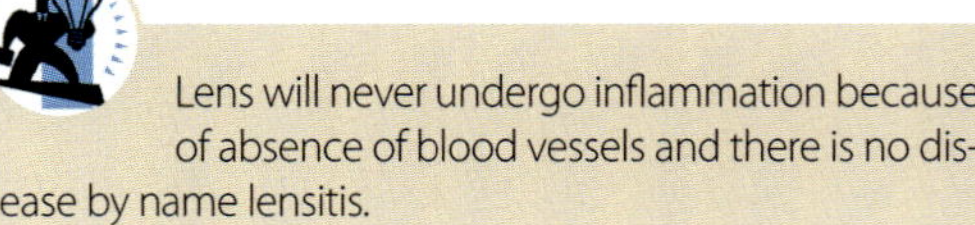

Lens will never undergo inflammation because of absence of blood vessels and there is no disease by name lensitis.

Metabolism of Lens*

Since the lens is an avascular structure, it is dependent on the aqueous humor for its metabolic requirements. Glucose is the main source of energy and it enters into the lens from aqueous humor by simple diffusion.

The important metabolic pathways of glucose in lens are:

- Anaerobic glycolysis, accounting for 80%
- Hexose monophosphate shunt accounting for 10–15%
- Sorbitol pathway accounting for less than 5%
- Krebs cycle accounting for less than 1%.

GIST BOX 8.1

- Lens is a transparent refractive element of the eye accounting for one third of refractive power of the eye. It is a biconvex crystalline structure situated in the anterior segment of the eye between iris and vitreous in a fossa called patellar fossa.
- Histologically, lens consists of lens capsule, lens epithelium and lens substance.
- Ciliary zonules also called zonules of Zinn are the suspensory ligaments, which suspend the lens and keep it in its position.
- The important metabolic pathways of glucose in lens are anaerobic glycolysis, hexose monophosphate shunt, sorbitol pathway and Krebs cycle.

CHAPTER

8.2

Congenital Anomalies of Lens

EMBRYOLOGY*

Lens develops from surface ectoderm:

- It starts as thickening of the surface ectoderm overlying the optic vesicle to form lens placode
- The lens placode sinks into the optic cup and forms lens vesicle
- The cells lining the posterior wall of the lens vesicle elongate and form the primary lens fibers
- The cells lining the anterior wall of the lens will continue as anterior lens epithelium. Since, cells lining the posterior wall are utilized in the development of primary lens fibers, posterior epithelium is absent.

The equatorial cells of the anterior epithelium form the secondary lens fibers. These cells remain active throughout the life and are named depending on the period of development (Fig. 8.2.1):

- Embryonic nucleus refers to secondary lens fibers formed during first 3 months of life
- Fetal nucleus refers to secondary lens fibers formed between 3 months and birth
- Infantile nucleus refers to secondary lens fibers formed between birth to puberty
- Adult nucleus refers to secondary lens fibers formed after puberty.

Hence, in congenital and developmental cataract only the particular lens fibers, which are being formed are affected.

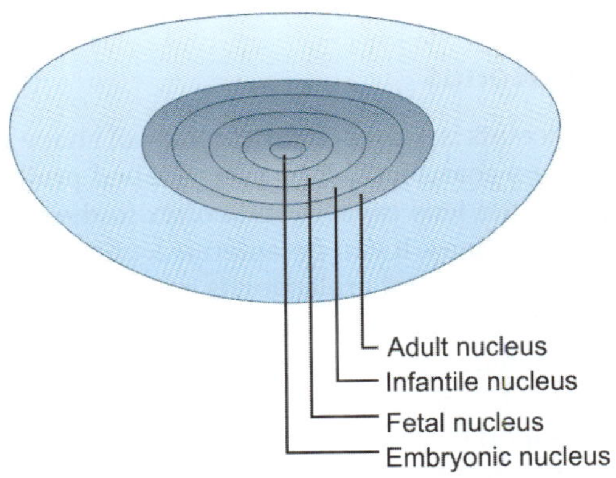

FIG. 8.2.1: Different nuclear zones of lens

CONGENITAL ANOMALIES OF LENS

Microspherophakia*

Microspherophakia is a rare congenital anomaly of the lens in which lens is small in size (micro) and spherical in shape (spherical shape is due to increase in anteroposterior diameter and decrease in equatorial diameter):

1. It may occur as an isolated anomaly or it may be associated with systemic diseases such as Marfan's syndrome, Weill-Marchesani syndrome, hyperlysinemia and congenital rubella.
2. It causes index lenticular myopia because of increase in anteroposterior diameter of

the lens. Hence, child will have decreased distant vision due to myopia. On examination with dilated pupil, zonules will be visible all around and subluxation of the lens is common due to weak zonules.

3. Microspherophakia causes glaucoma because of the pupillary block caused by small spherical lens. This is called inverse glaucoma as it is aggravated by miotic agents and relieved by mydriatic drugs.
4. Management of this condition is by the treatment of index myopia by refraction and correction. Inverse glaucoma can be prevented by prophylactic iridectomy and avoiding the use of mydriatic drugs.

Lenticonus

Lenticonus is a congenital anomaly of shape of the lens characterized by cone-shaped projection of the lens capsule and cortex in the center of the lens. It can be anterior lenticonus in which the conical projection is anterior or posterior lenticonus in which the conical projection is posterior:

1. Lenticonus anterior is usually a part of Alport's syndrome (characterized by progressive renal failure due to nephritis, sensorineural deafness and ocular manifestations). Lenticonus posterior is usually an isolated anomaly of the eye.
2. Lenticonus gives the appearance of oil droplet reflux on retinoscopy due to high index myopia in the center part of the lens.
3. Treatment of this condition is by refraction and correction of the index myopia.

Coloboma of Lens*

Coloboma of lens is a rare autosomal dominant inherited condition. In coloboma of lens there is no defect in the lens as in coloboma of uveal tissue or retina (Figs 8.2.2A and B):

1. Lens shows characteristic notch-shaped defect usually in the inferior position. This notch-shaped appearance is because of flattening of the lens surface due to maldevelopment of the zonules of the lens. The lens, which is deprived of its normal pull in the defective region becomes thicker and spherical, appearing as if there is loss of lens substance.
2. Coloboma of the lens is usually found in association with Marfan's syndrome and other connective tissue disorders.

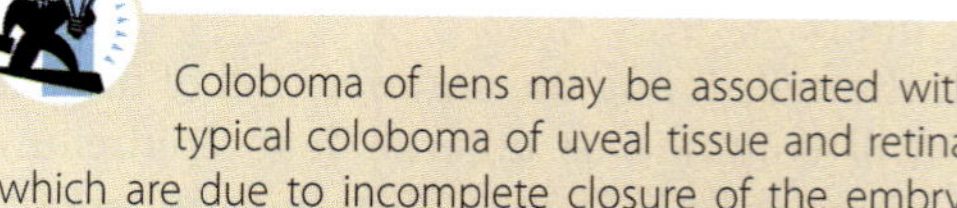

Coloboma of lens may be associated with typical coloboma of uveal tissue and retina, which are due to incomplete closure of the embryonic fissure of the optic vesicle. Since lens vesicle closes

Contd...

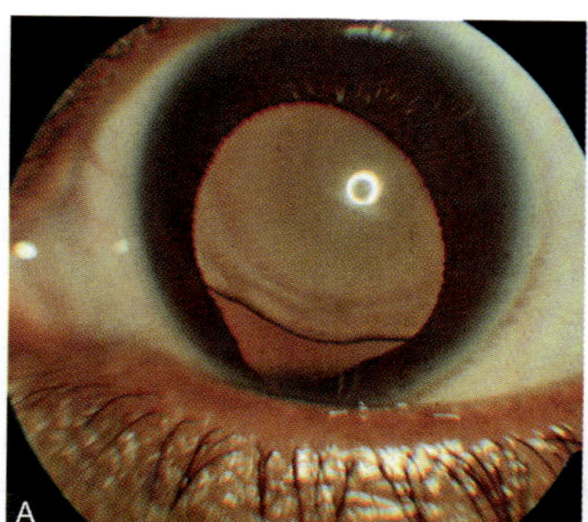

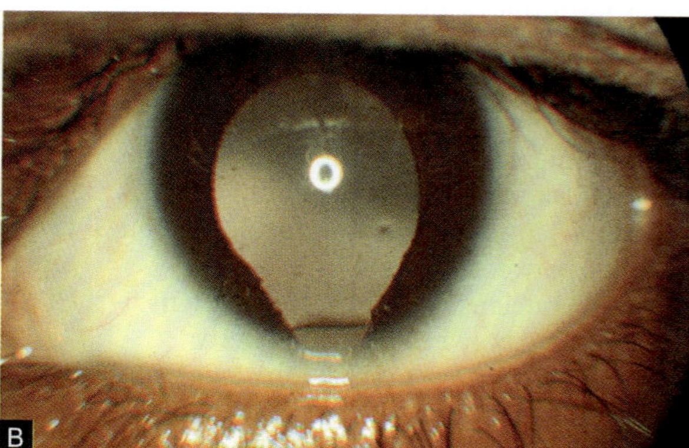

FIGS 8.2.2A and B: Coloboma of lens

Contd...

independent of the closure of the embryonic fissure, coloboma of the lens is not because of defective closure of the embryonic fissure.

Congenital cataract and congenital ectopia lentis are the most common congenital anomalies of lens. They are described in detail in Chapters 8.3 and 8.6 'Cataract' and 'Ectopia Lentis'.

GIST BOX 8.2

- Microspherophakia is a rare congenital anomaly of the lens in which lens is small in size (micro) and spherical in shape (spherical shape is due to increase in anteroposterior diameter and decrease in equatorial diameter).
- Lenticonus is a congenital anomaly of shape of the lens characterized by cone-shaped projection of the lens capsule and cortex in the center of the lens.
- Coloboma of lens is a rare autosomal dominant inherited condition. In coloboma of lens, there is no defect in the lens as in coloboma of uveal tissue or retina. Lens shows characteristic notch-shaped defect usually in the inferior position. This notch-shaped appearance is because of flattening of the lens surface due to maldevelopment of the zonules of the lens.

CHAPTER

8.3 Cataract

DEFINITION***

Cataract is defined as opacification of lens and/or its capsule congenital or acquired, progressive or stationary, partial or complete, with or without visual impairment.

The word 'cataract' is derived from a Latin word 'cataracta' meaning waterfalls. The word cataract is used to indicate the white appearance of mature cataract similar to waterfall. It also implies that vision of a patient with cataract is foggy as if he/she seeing through a glass covered with water droplets in early stages of cataract.

Cataract is the most common cause for avoidable blindness worldwide and in India. In India, it accounts for about 62% of the blindness.

CLASSIFICATION OF CATARACT**

Etiological Classification

Based on the etiology, cataract is classified into:

- Congenital and developmental cataract
- Acquired cataract, which is further classified into:
  - Senile cataract
  - Presenile cataract
  - Complicated cataract
  - Metabolic cataract
  - Traumatic cataract
  - Toxic cataract
  - Electric cataract
  - Radiation cataract
  - Cataract associated with any systemic syndromes
  - Dermatogenic cataract
  - Cataract associated with osseous diseases.

Morphological Classification

- Capsular cataract: Anterior capsular and posterior capsular cataract
- Subcapsular cataract: Anterior subcapsular and posterior subcapsular cataract
- Cortical cataract
- Supranuclear cataract
- Nuclear cataract
- Polar cataract: Anterior polar and posterior polar cataract.

Classification with Respect to Maturity

- Incipient cataract
- Immature cataract
- Mature cataract
- Hypermature cataract.

Classification with Respect to Age of Onset

- Congenital cataract
- Infantile cataract
- Juvenile cataract
- Presenile cataract
- Senile cataract.

CONGENITAL AND DEVELOPMENTAL CATARACT***

Congenital and developmental cataracts account for majority of pediatric or childhood cataracts. Pediatric cataracts include cataracts from birth to adolescence.

Cataracts in this age group along with reducing vision also interfere with the normal visual development. Hence, its management requires treatment for cataract and management of amblyopia.

Congenital cataract is cataract with onset at birth. In true congenital cataract the lens opacity is present in the embryonic or fetal nucleus.

Developmental cataract is cataract with onset after birth till puberty. The opacity is present in the infantile nucleus.

Etiology

1. Idiopathic: Most of the unilateral cataracts are of unknown etiology. Bilateral cataracts are more likely to be associated with underlying ocular or systemic cause.
2. Heredity: Chromosomal abnormalities in the form of genetic mutations are the common cause for hereditary cataracts. Autosomal inheritance is the most common type of inheritance.
3. Intrauterine infections: Toxoplasmosis, other (syphilis, varicella-zoster, parvovirus B19), rubella, cytomegalovirus and herpes infections (TORCH):
   a. Intrauterine exposure to drugs such as steroids, thalidomide, etc.
   b. Intrauterine exposure to radiation, e.g. X-rays.
   c. Maternal malnutrition and deficiency of vital nutrients such as vitamin D deficiency, hypocalcemia, etc.
   d. Fetal hypoxia, birth trauma, malnutrition, etc.
   e. Congenital diseases such as galactosemia, Lowe's syndrome, Alport's syndrome, Norrie's disease, myotonic dystrophy, Stickler's syndrome, congenital ichthyosis, incontinentia pigmenti, etc.
   f. Chromosomal syndromes such as Down syndrome, Turner's syndrome, etc.

Clinical Features

- Congenital and developmental cataracts present as leukocoria or white pupillary reflex as noticed by the parents
- Long-standing cataracts show associated features such as poor vision, amblyopia, squint, nystagmus, etc.

Investigations**

The laboratory investigations should be carried out in all cases of congenital and developmental cataract. All cases should be evaluated by complete history to find out the associated underlying cause. The laboratory investigations include:
- Vertically transmitted infection—TORCH screening
- Urine assay for reducing substances (to rule out galactosemia), amino acids (to rule out Lowe's syndrome)
- Plasma calcium and phosphorus
- Blood sugar.

Ocular examination is performed to rule out associated ocular anomalies. The ocular examination includes visual acuity assessment and fundus examination. Visual acuity in neonates and infants is assessed by fixation reflex, optokinetic nystagmus test and visual evoked potential.

Systemic examination is done by a pediatrician to rule out systemic syndromes.

Clinical Types of Congenital Cataract (Figs 8.3.1 to 8.3.5)**

Punctate cataract or blue dot cataract or cataracta punctata cerulea
It is characterized by the presence of bluish opaque dots scattered in the peripheral cortex of the lens. It is one of the most common types of congenital cataract. It usually does not affect vision and hence treatment is not required.
Cataracta centralis pulverulenta
It is characterized by the presence of powdery opacities in the embryonic nucleus. It usually does not affect vision and hence treatment is not required.
Coronary cataract
It is characterized by the presence of club-shaped opacities in the peripheral cortex. It usually does not affect vision and hence treatment is not required.
Coralliform cataract
It is characterized by the presence of fusiform-shaped opacities in the peripheral cortex. It usually does not affect vision and hence treatment is not required.
Sutural cataract
It is characterized by the presence of opacities situated around the sutural lines of the lens. It usually does not affect vision and hence treatment is not required.
*Lamellar cataract or zonular cataract***
It is characterized by the presence of a disk-shaped opacity involving the fetal nucleus surrounded by a clear cortex. The presence of small radial opacities resembling spokes of a wheel called riders, is the characteristic feature of lamellar cataract. It is the most common type of congenital cataract. The genetic form is inherited as autosomal dominant trait. Intrauterine rubella infection and intrauterine metabolic disturbances affecting the calcium metabolism as seen in deficiency of vitamin D are the other causes for lamellar cataract. It causes moderate to severe visual impairment and requires surgery.
Anterior polar cataract
It is characterized by the presence of small opacity involving the anterior pole. The opacity involves anterior capsule and the superficial cortex. The congenital anterior polar cataract is seen in anterior chamber cleavage syndrome. The acquired form is seen following perforation of corneal ulcer. It rarely affects vision.
Posterior polar cataract
It is characterized by the presence of small opacity involving the posterior pole with the opacity involving posterior capsule and the underlying cortex. It is because of persistence of remnants of posterior hyaloid artery called Mittendorf dot. A true posterior pole cataract is associated with high incidence of posterior capsular tear during surgery. Hydrodissection should be avoided in posterior polar cataract surgery as this may lead to posterior capsular rent as the opacity involves the posterior capsule.

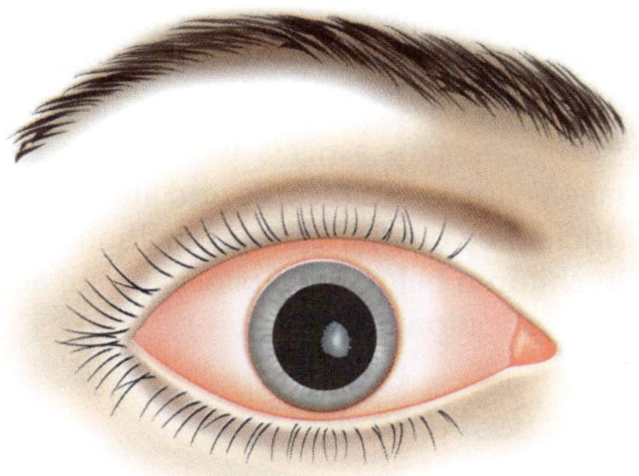

FIG. 8.3.1: Cataracta centralis pulverulenta

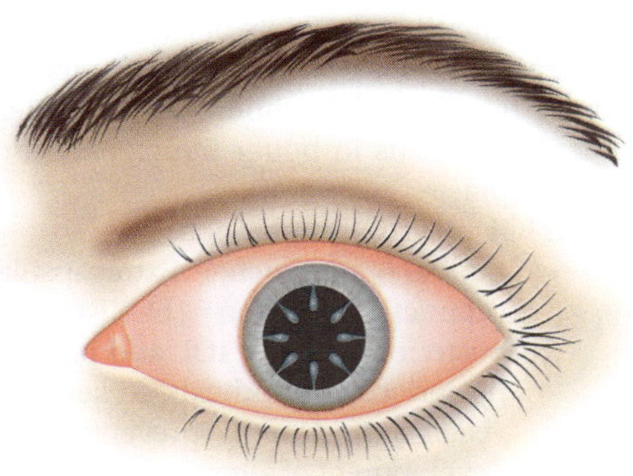

FIG. 8.3.2: Coronary cataract

Treatment/Management**

The indications for cataract surgery are:

- Visually significant cataracts
- Cataracts associated with squint and the nystagmus.

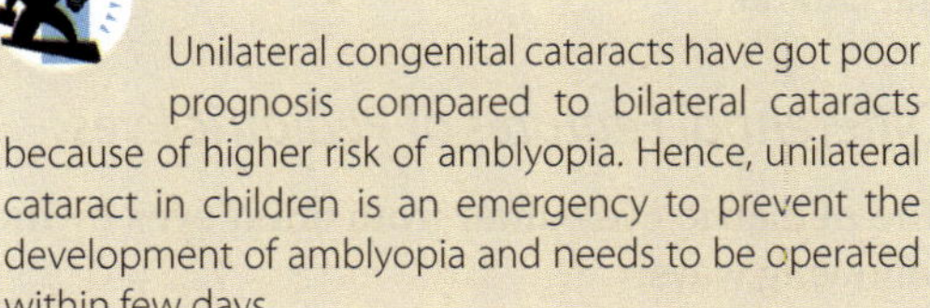

Unilateral congenital cataracts have got poor prognosis compared to bilateral cataracts because of higher risk of amblyopia. Hence, unilateral cataract in children is an emergency to prevent the development of amblyopia and needs to be operated within few days.

Poor Prognostic Factors

The poor prognostic factors associated with pediatric cataracts are given below:

- Late presentation or late treatment.
- Unilateral dense cataract.
- Cataract associated with ocular and systemic type of anomalies.

Timing of Surgery in Congenital Cataract

Congenital cataract, unilateral or bilateral, should be operated as early as possible within few days to weeks of birth.

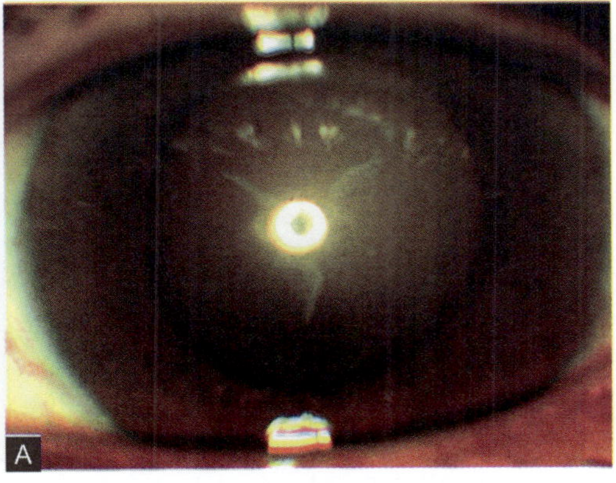

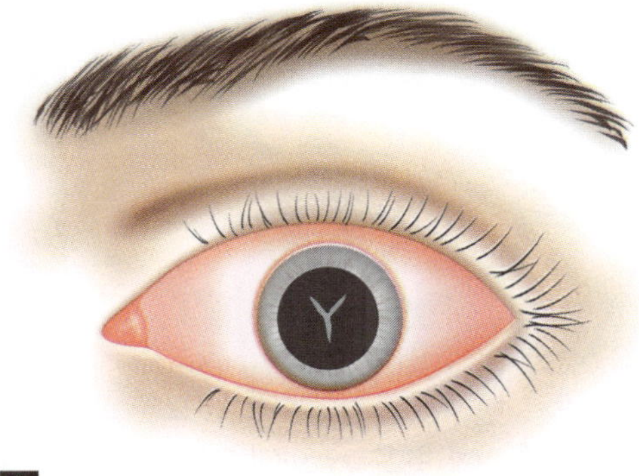

FIGS 8.3.3A and B: Congenital cataract subtype—sutural cataract. **A.** Photograph; **B.** Diagrammatic representation.

Unilateral cataract should be operated within few days of birth as early as possible, till the time of surgery on the cataractous eye; the normal eye has to be occluded to prevent amblyopia in the cataractous eye. Unilateral congenital cataract is associated with more incidence of amblyopia when compared to bilateral congenital cataract.

Differential Features of Pediatric Eyes

The pediatric eyes differ from adult eyes by the following ways:

1. The eyes are smaller and softer than adult eyes and they are more prone for postoperative inflammation.

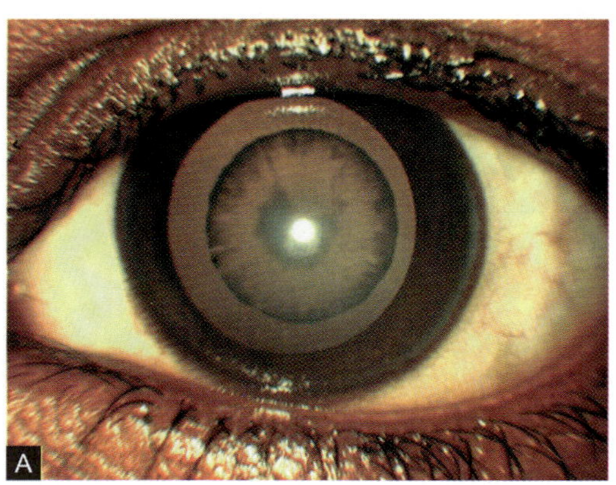

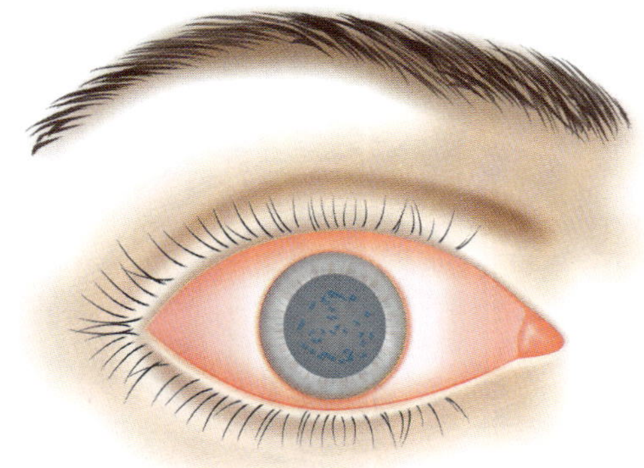

FIGS 8.3.4A and B: Congenital cataract subtypes. **A.** Photograph of lamellar cataract; **B.** Diagrammatic representation of blue dot cataract.

2. The scleral rigidity is lower and vitreous pressure is higher thus making the surgery difficult.
3. Two important aspects which have to be taken care are amblyopia and after cataract (incidence of after cataract is almost 100% in children below 2 years because of active multiplication of lens fibers).

Surgery: Based on Age

The surgery based on age is a type of surgery which depends on the age of the patient and it is described as follows.

Below 2 years of age

1. Intraocular lens (IOL) insertion below 2 years of age is still controversial as it is more difficult technically because of small structures of the eye. Hence not practiced by all, but if possible should be most ideal because it helps in better management of amblyopia:
   a. If IOL insertion is planned:
      - Limbal approach: Extracapsular cataract extraction (ECCE) with posterior chamber IOL and primary posterior capsulorhexis, to keep the visual axis clear by preventing the development of after cataract.
   b. If IOL insertion is not planned:
      - Limbal approach: ECCE without IOL implantation

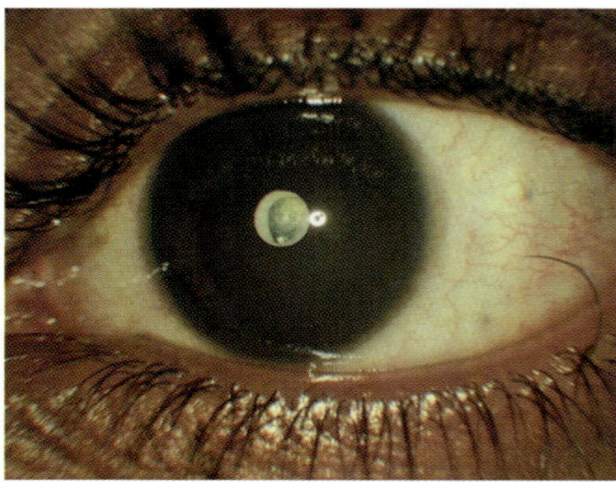

FIG. 8.3.5: Developmental cataract

- Pars plana approach: It is done through pars plana, 3.5 mm behind the limbus.

2. Through pars plana, lensectomy and vitrectomy is done and later once the age of the patient crosses 2 years, IOL is inserted through limbal approach.

Above 2 years of age

1. In children above 2 years of age, the eye would have reached nearly adult size hence the surgery of choice is through limbal approach.
2. Extracapsular cataract extraction with posterior chamber IOL implantation.
3. Primary posterior capsulorhexis is not compulsory as the incidence of after cataract decreases after 2 years and if at all it develops it can be treated by yttrium-aluminum-garnet (YAG) capsulotomy as the child will be cooperative to sit at the slit lamp by this age.

Guidelines for Choosing Intraocular Lens (IOL) Power in Pediatric Cataract

Below 2 year old	*2–8 year old*	*Above 8 year old*
Biometry is done and it is under corrected by 20%, i.e. only 80% of the power required is implanted	Biometry is done and it is under corrected by 10%, i.e. only 90% of the power required is implanted	Same as adults

Treatment to Prevent Amblyopia

1. If IOL is implanted spectacles for astigmatism induced by surgery as calculated by refraction are given by 4 months onward.
2. Bifocals with near addition for reading are given by 3 years onward.
3. Cases of bilateral pseudophakia are followed closely to detect and treat amblyopia.
4. Cases of unilateral pseudophakia are given occlusion therapy starting from 4 months to 4 years and then gradually reduced till the age of the child is 12 years.
5. If IOL is not implanted aphakic correction has to be given immediately from next day of surgery and rest is same as in the case of IOL implantation.

SENILE CATARACT***

Senile cataract is the most common type of cataract and it accounts for 90% of cataracts seen in clinical practice.

Definition

Senile cataract is defined as opacification of lens and/or its capsule because of age-related changes with characteristic absence of secondary and other specific causes of cataract.

Etiology

The proposed etiological factors for senile cataract are as follows.

Hereditary factors: The hereditary factors play an important role in the age of onset of senile cataract. Presence of family history of cataract increases the chances of cataract formation at an earlier age compared to those with negative family history.

Dietary factors: Deficiency of proteins and amino acids, essential elements—copper, zinc, calcium and vitamins—vitamin C and vitamin E, are associated with senile cataract.

Dehydration crisis: This crisis because of diarrhea, heat stroke, etc. are known to be associated with onset and maturation of cataract.

Ultraviolet radiation: Exposure to this radiation from exposure to sunlight is one of the commonly implicated factors for senile cataract.

Pathogenesis

The pathogenesis of senile cataract depends on the type of cataract. Senile cataract is broadly classified into:

1. Cortical cataract: Affecting the cortex of the lens predominantly.

2. Nuclear cataract: Affecting the nucleus of the lens predominantly.

Mechanism of formation of cortical cataract: Cortical cataract is formed due to decreased levels of proteins and amino acids with increasing age that leads to increased permeability of lens capsule resulting in increased levels of sodium causing increased hydration. Increased hydration of the lens leads to opacification of lens fibers. The cortical cataract is because of overhydration and is called soft cataract.

Mechanism of formation of nuclear cataract: Nuclear cataract is because of dehydration and it is called hard cataract. The mechanism of formation of nuclear cataract is from dehydration leading to increase in water insoluble proteins and compaction of nucleus.

Nuclear cataract may be associated with deposition of urochrome or melanin derived from amino acids.

Cortical Cataract

Cortical cataract is the most common type of senile cataract and it accounts for up to 80% of senile cataract. It is of two types.

Types

Cuneiform cortical cataract

Cuneiform cortical cataract begins at the periphery and gradually progresses toward the center (Figs 8.3.6A to C).

Cupuliform cataract

Cupuliform cataract begins at the center in the posterior cortex; hence it is also called posterior subcapsular cataract (Figs 8.3.7A to C).

Clinical Features

Symptoms

- Gradually progressive painless diminution of vision
- Colored halos
- Glare
- Uniocular polyopia in incipient stage.

Signs

The signs depend on the stage of cataract. The stages of cataract formation are:

1. *Stage of lamellar separation:* It is characterized by demarcation of the cortical lens fibers by hydration.
2. *Stage of incipient cataract:* It is characterized by the formation of lens opacities. The lens opacities appear in the peripheral cortex in cuneiform cataract and they appear in the center in the cupuliform cataract.
3. *Immature cataract:* It is characterized by progression of the lens opacities, but few transparent lens fibers are left behind. The signs of cataract depend on the stage of cataract:
   - *Visual acuity:* 6/6 to counting fingers close to face
   - *Color of the lens:* Grayish white
   - *Iris shadow:* Present
   - *Purkinje's images:* All four are present.
4. *Mature cataract:* It is characterized by opacification of all the lens fibers (Figs 8.3.8A and B). The signs of cataract depend on the stage of cataract:
   - *Visual acuity:* Hand movements
   - *Color of the lens:* Pearly white
   - *Iris shadow:* Absent
   - *Purkinje's images:* Fourth Purkinje's image absent.
5. *Hypermature cataract:* It is the result of hypermaturity of cataract. The signs of cataract depend on the stage of cataract:*
   - *Visual acuity:* Perception of light
   - *Color of the lens:* Milky white
   - *Iris shadow:* Absent
   - *Purkinje's images:* Fourth Purkinje's image absent.

   It is of two types:

a. *Morgagnian cataract:* It is a type of hypermature cataract characterized by liquefaction of the cortex and the brownish nucleus sinks to the bottom of the capsular bag (Fig. 8.3.9).

b. *Hypermature sclerotic cataract:* It is a type of hypermature cataract characterized by loss of fluid resulting in shrunken and wrinkled appearance (Fig. 8.3.10).

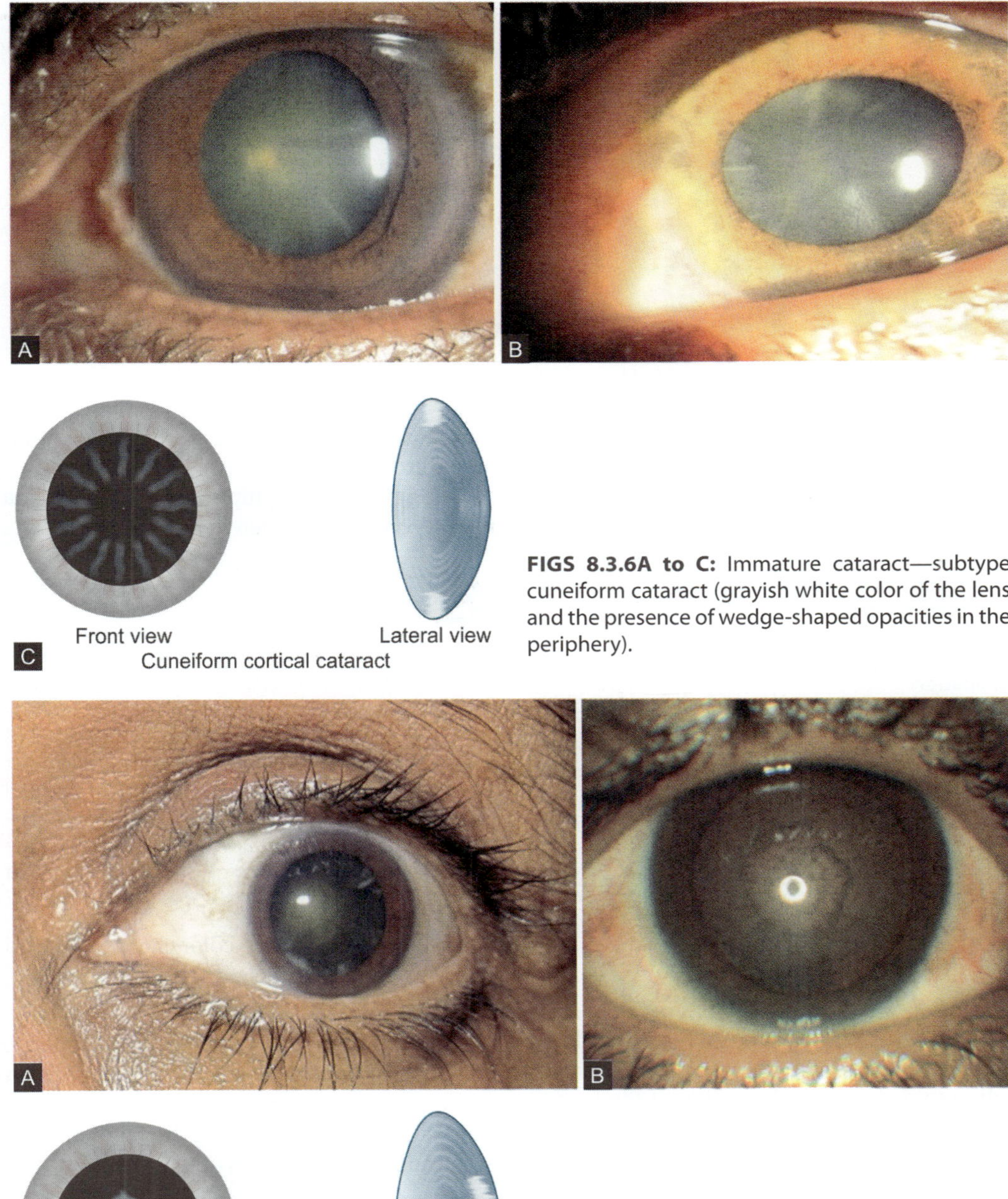

FIGS 8.3.6A to C: Immature cataract—subtype cuneiform cataract (grayish white color of the lens and the presence of wedge-shaped opacities in the periphery).

Front view
Lateral view
C
Cupuliform cortical cataract

FIGS 8.3.7A to C: Immature cataract—subtype posterior subcapsular cataract or cupuliform cataract (grayish white color of the lens and the presence of opacity in the center of the posterior cortex).

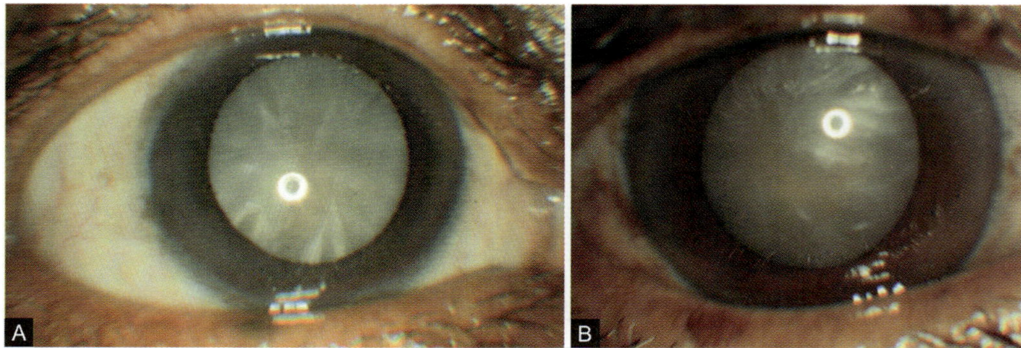

FIGS 8.3.8A and B: Mature cataract (pearly-white color of the lens)

Intumescent Cataract*

It is characterized by progressive hydration of lens leading to swelling of the lens. It can occur in immature or in mature cataract stage. It may lead to secondary angle closure in individuals with shallow angle.

Iris Shadow

Crescentic shadow of pupillary margin of iris formed on the grayish opacity of the lens when an oblique beam of light is thrown on the pupil is called iris shadow. Iris shadow is seen when lens is partly transparent and partly opaque, hence it is seen in immature cataract. When lens is completely transparent or opaque no iris shadow is formed (Figs 8.3.11A and B).

Nuclear Cataract**

Nuclear cataract accounts for 20% of senile cataract. Nuclear cataract is because of age-related sclerosis thus making the lens inelastic and hard leading to decrease in the ability of the lens to accommodate and to transmit rays. Nuclear cataract can be:

- Cataracta brunescens: Brown cataract (Fig. 8.3.12)
- Cataracta rubra: Red cataract
- Cataracta nigra: Black cataract (Fig. 8.3.13).

Clinical Features

Symptoms: The symptoms are similar to cortical cataract, i.e. gradually progressive painless diminution of vision, colored halos, glare, etc.

Along with the symptoms of cortical cataract, second sight is seen in nuclear cataract.

Second Sight

Improvement of near vision in patients with nuclear sclerosis due to progressive index myopia is called second sight. This is because of neutralization of the plus power of presbyopia by the minus power of myopia, which is because of index myopia as a result of increase in the refractive index of the lens caused by nuclear sclerosis. Hence, a person who was wearing reading glasses for near vision will be able to see near things without reading glasses with the onset of nuclear sclerosis.

Signs: The nucleus shows color changes depending on the grade of nuclear sclerosis.

Nuclear sclerosis

It is the hardness of the nucleus. It is found in both cortical and nuclear cataracts, and in immature or mature cataract. Nuclear sclerosis can be graded by examining the color and size of the lens after dilatation of the pupil.

Grading of nuclear sclerosis

- Grade I: Yellow (Fig. 8.3.14)
- Grade II: Orange (Fig. 8.3.15)
- Grade III: Brown (Fig. 8.3.16)
- Grade IV: Black.

Nuclear sclerosis has to be differentiated from nuclear cataract. The differences are described below in differential diagnosis.

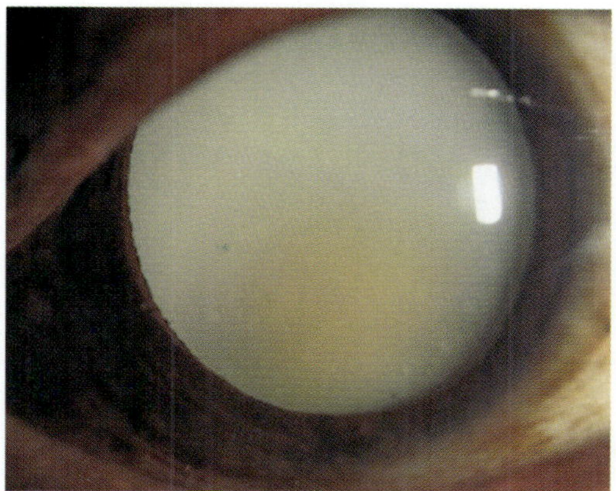

FIG. 8.3.9: Hypermature cataract—subtype morgagnian cataract (the presence of milky-white color of the lens with nucleus sinking at the bottom of lens capsule as indicated by brown tinge inferiorly).

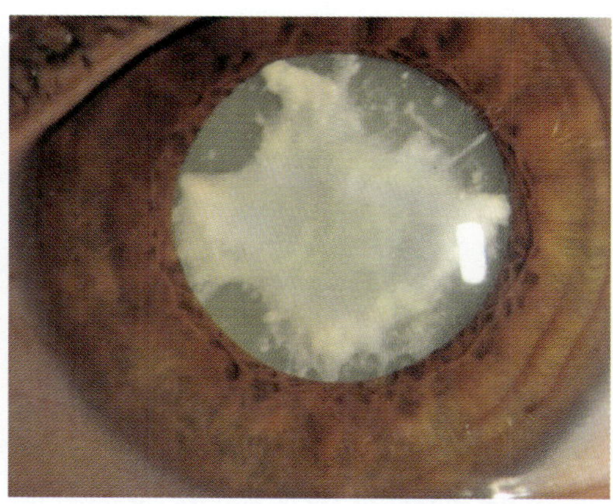

FIG. 8.3.10: Hypermature cataract with calcification of anterior capsule—subtype sclerotic hypermature cataract (milky-white color of the lens with calcification of anterior capsule).

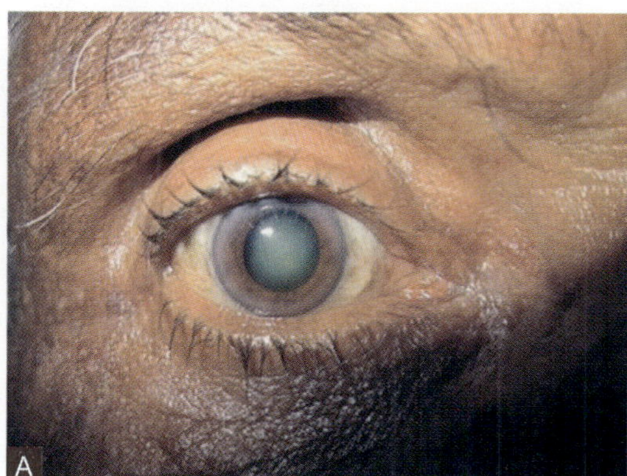

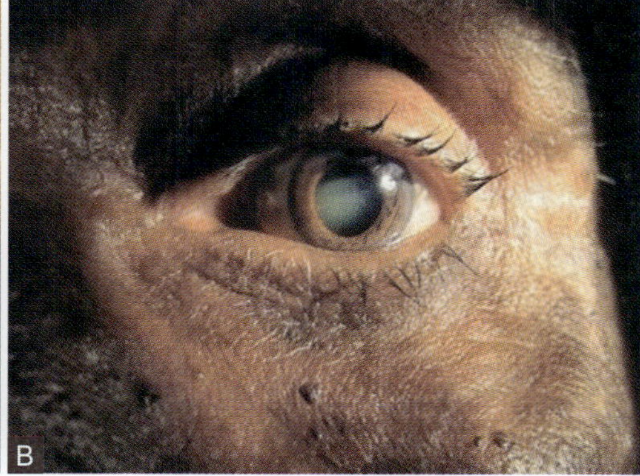

FIGS 8.3.11A and B: Demonstration of iris shadow (the presence of crescentic shadow of the iris in second photograph on the temporal side when light is shown on the eye from temporal side).

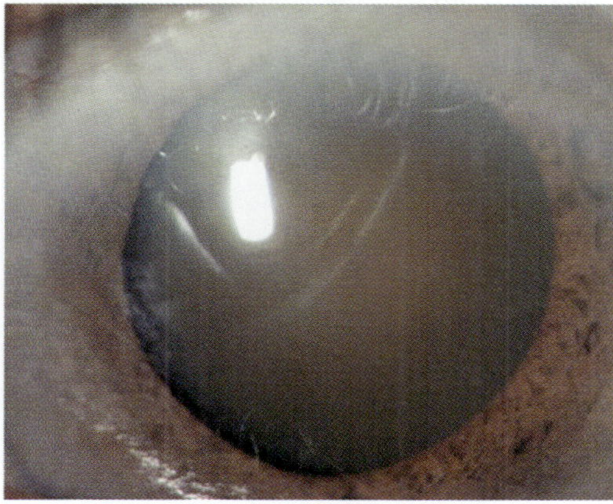

FIG. 8.3.12: Cataracta brunescens

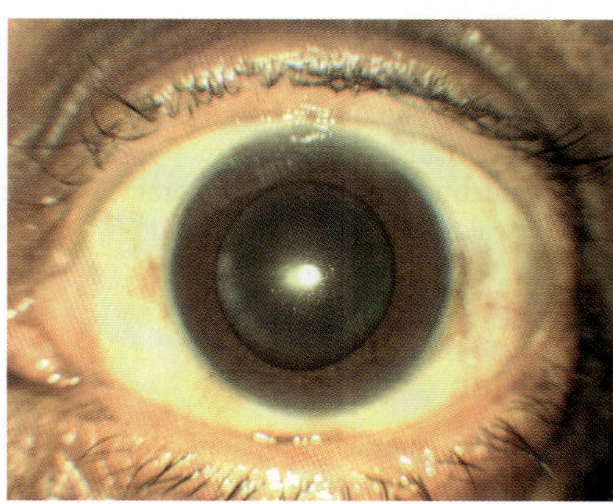

FIG. 8.3.13: Cataracta nigra

> The importance of increase in grade of nuclear sclerosis indicates increase in hardness of the lens. Thus, a grade IV or cataracta nigra indicates that the lens is very hard and this requires more phaco energy during phacoemulsification. During manual small incision cataract surgery, cataracta nigra requires a larger incision to deliver the nucleus without causing damage to the corneal endothelium.

Differential Diagnosis

Differential diagnosis for immature cataract: Immature cataract has to be differentiated from nuclear sclerosis (Table 8.3.1).

Differential diagnosis of mature and hypermature cataract: Mature and hypermature cataract has to be differentiated by pseudoglioma (Table 8.3.2).

Differential diagnosis for nuclear cataract: Nuclear cataract has to be differentiated from nuclear sclerosis (Table 8.3.3).

The investigations and treatment of senile cataract are described under cataract surgeries in the Chapter 8.4 'Cataract Surgeries'.

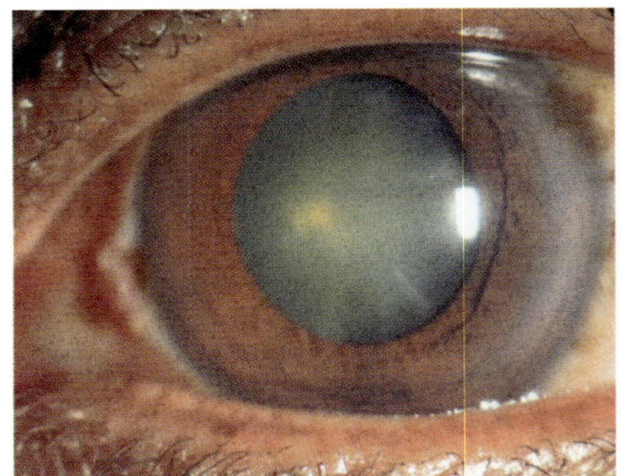

FIG. 8.3.14: Grade I nuclear sclerosis with immature cataract

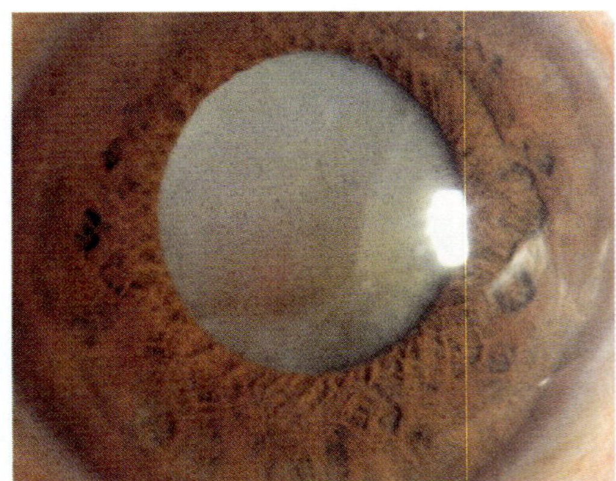

FIG. 8.3.15: Grade II nuclear sclerosis with mature cataract

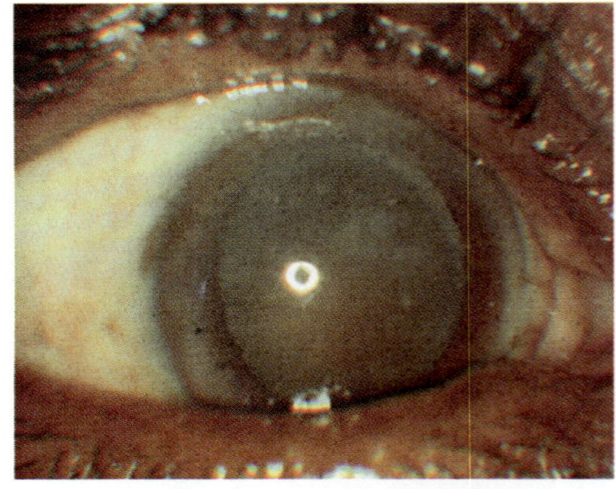

FIG. 8.3.16: Grade III nuclear sclerosis with mature cataract

PRESENILE CATARACT**

Cataract formation because of age-related changes in people aged less than 50 years is called presenile cataract.

In all cases of presenile cataract other causes for cataract have to be ruled out, i.e. trauma, metabolic diseases (diabetes), intraocular diseases causing complicated cataract, drug intake such as corticosteroids and other drugs causing cataract, skin diseases causing cataract, etc.

The treatment of presenile cataract is similar to senile cataract.

COMPLICATED CATARACT**

Definition

Complicated cataract is opacification of lens secondary to a primary ocular disease.

TABLE 8.3.1: Differential diagnosis for immature cataract

Clinical features	*Immature cataract*	*Nuclear sclerosis*
Vision	Diminution of vision, painless and progressive in nature No improvement with pinhole	Diminution of vision, painless and progressive in nature Improvement with pinhole
Anterior segment examination	Grayish white color of the lens Iris shadow present	Color varies according to the grade of nuclear sclerosis; the color of the lens can be gray to amber or brown Iris shadow absent
Distant direct ophthalmoscopy	Black spots against red background	Red glow

TABLE 8.3.2: Differential diagnosis for mature and hypermature cataract

Clinical features	*Mature and hypermature cataract*	*Pseudoglioma*
Vision	Decreased, painless and progressive in nature	Decreased, nature of diminution of vision depends on the cause
Pupil	White color	White color and pupil is usually semidilated
Anterior segment examination	Cataractous lens Fourth Purkinje's image absent	Clear lens Opacity behind the lens Fourth Purkinje's image present
B-scan	Normal	Vitreous/Retinal pathology seen

TABLE 8.3.3: Differential diagnosis for nuclear cataract

Clinical features	*Nuclear cataract*	*Nuclear sclerosis*
Vision	Diminution of vision, painless and progressive in nature No improvement with pinhole	Diminution of vision, painless and progressive in nature Improvement with pinhole
Anterior segment examination	Color of the lens depends on the grade of nuclear sclerosis and it will be grayish yellow or grayish orange or brown or black Iris shadow present	Color varies according to the grade of nuclear sclerosis Iris shadow absent
Distant direct ophthalmoscopy	Black spots against red background	Red glow

Complicated cataract is also called secondary cataract (Figs 8.3.17A and B).

Etiopathogenesis

The cause for cataract is because of disturbances in the nutrition of the lens as a result of primary ocular disease.

The common primary ocular diseases causing complicated cataract are:

1. Inflammatory conditions of the eye such as uveitis including iridocyclitis, intermediate uveitis, choroiditis and endophthalmitis, keratitis.
2. Diseases of the retina such as long-standing retinal detachment, retinitis pigmentosa, gyrate atrophy, Leber's congenital amaurosis.

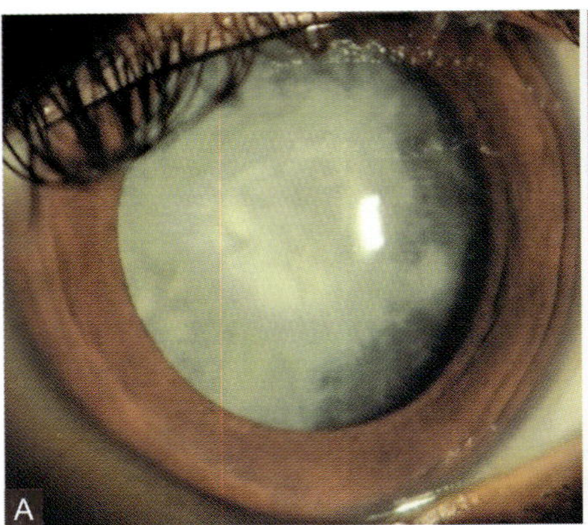

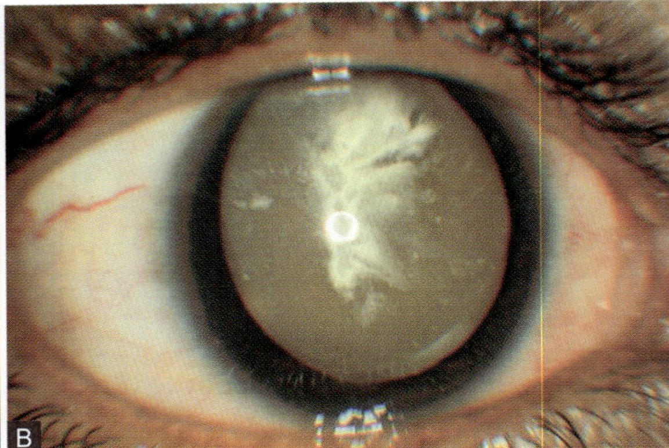

FIGS 8.3.17A and B: Complicated cataract

3. Glaucoma including primary and secondary glaucoma.
4. Pathological myopia.
5. Intraocular tumors including primary tumors such as retinoblastoma, melanoma and metastatic tumors.

Clinical Features

1. Complicated cataract presents with symptoms of cataract, e.g. diminution of vision along with the symptoms of the primary ocular disease.
2. Complicated cataract usually begins in the posterior cortex as posterior subcapsular opacity.
3. Bread crumb appearance and polychromatic luster are the characteristic features of complicated cataract.

Treatment

Treatment is similar to senile cataract, but the surgery has to be performed after the treatment for the primary ocular disease wherever possible. Before surgery inflammation and intraocular pressure has to be controlled and brought under control.

The surgical steps are difficult when compared to senile cataract because of pre-existing ocular diseases and sequelae like synechiae, decompensation of corneal endothelium, etc.

The visual prognosis is usually poor, because of pre-existing conditions caused by primary ocular diseases.

DIABETIC CATARACT**

Definition

Cataract seen as a result of metabolic changes associated with diabetes is called diabetic cataract.

Etiopathogenesis

Diabetes is usually associated with about three to five times increase in the prevalence of cataracts. Diabetic cataract can be associated with:

- True diabetic cataract
- Early onset of senile cataract.

True Diabetic Cataract

True diabetic cataract is usually seen in type I diabetes with poor glycemic control. The mechanisms involved in the formation of true diabetic cataract are:

- Aldose reductase and sorbitol pathway and non-enzymatic glycosylation of the lens proteins

- The excess glucose in the lens is converted into sorbitol by the aldose reductase. The resultant sorbitol increases the osmolarity of the lens resulting in overhydration and cataract formation.

Clinical features: True diabetic cataract resembles snowflake in the form of multiple white dot-like opacities in the cortex of the lens. Hence, a true diabetic cataract is called snowflake cataract.

Management of diabetes with cataract is discussed in detail in Author's textbook '*Clinical Methods in Ophthalmology*'.

DRUG-INDUCED CATARACT*

Definition

Cataract seen as a result of toxic effects of the drugs used either topically or systemically is called drug-induced cataract. Drug-induced cataracts are also called toxic cataract.

Etiopathogenesis

1. Posterior subcapsular cataracts are associated with prolonged use of steroids.
2. Anterior subcapsular cataracts are associated with long-term use of miotics such as pilocarpine, echothiophate and demecarium chloride.
3. Amiodarone, thioridazine, phenothiazine, chlorpromazine, busulfan are some other drugs associated with the development of cataract.

The mechanism of steroid-induced cataract is related to activation of glucocorticoid receptors in the lens and aberrant migration of lens epithelial cells.

Clinical Features

Posterior subcapsular opacities are typically found in steroid-induced cataract and anterior subcapsular opacities are found with long-term use of miotics.

Treatment

Treatment is by stopping the offending drug in the initial stages and by surgery similar to senile cataract in advanced cases.

Prophylaxis is by judicious use of drugs with frequent examination to look for the adverse effects.

METABOLIC CATARACT**

Definition

Cataract seen as a result of metabolic changes is called metabolic cataract. It is seen in metabolic diseases such as diabetes, galactosemia, Wilson's disease, Lowe's syndrome, etc. Metabolic cataract can be seen in all the age groups.

Etiology

In neonates: The common causes for metabolic cataracts are:

- Lowe's syndrome
- Zellweger syndrome
- Galactosemia
- Hypocalcemia.

In adults: The common causes for metabolic cataracts are:

- Diabetes mellitus
- Hypoparathyroidism
- Wilson's disease
- Gyrate atrophy.

Galactosemia

It is an inborn error of galactose metabolism due to deficiency of the enzyme galactose-1-phosphate uridyl transferase called classic galactosemia or because of deficiency of galactokinase leading to mild variety of the disease.

Due to the deficiency of the above mentioned enzymes the lens metabolism is affected leading to the production of dulcitol, similar to sorbitol seen in diabetic cataract. The increased osmotic pressure leads to overhydration and lens opacity.

The treatment of the condition is by avoiding consumption of foods containing galactose such as milk and milk products.

Lowe's Syndrome

It is an X-linked recessive syndrome, which affects the metabolism of the amino acids. It is characterized by congenital cataract, mental retardation, renal tubular acidosis and aminoaciduria, hence called oculocerebral renal syndrome.

Zellweger Syndrome

It is a peroxisome biogenesis disorder characterized by cerebral, hepatic, renal abnormalities along with eye abnormalities as in cataract.

Wilson's Disease

It is an autosomal recessive disease, which affects the metabolism of copper characterized by hepatolenticular degeneration.

Kayser-Fleischer ring (K-F ring) is the most characteristic sign seen and it is because of deposition of copper in the Descemet's membrane. The cataract seen in Wilson's disease is called sunflower cataract because of its appearance.

Clinical Features

Metabolic cataracts differ from congenital and senile cataracts by the fact that they show rapid progression and they show specific features depending on the underlying metabolic disease (Table 8.3.4).

HEAT CATARACT*

Definition

A cataract seen as a result of chronic exposure to increased temperature and infrared rays is called heat cataract.

Etiopathogenesis

Heat cataract is seen in industrial workers who are exposed to high temperature, e.g. furnace workers, etc.

Since it was first described in glassblowers it is called glassblower's cataract.

TABLE 8.3.4: Some specific types of cataracts and their causes

Type	*Cause*
Oil-droplet cataract	Galactosemic cataract
Snowflake cataract	Diabetic cataract
Sunflower cataract	Inborn errors of copper metabolism as in Wilson's disease

Heat cataract is because of the effect of infrared rays, which are absorbed by pigments of the iris, which affect the lens fibers resulting in opacification.

Clinical Features

The cataract begins as a honeycomb-shaped opacity in the posterior cortex and appears as posterior subcapsular opacity. True exfoliation of the lens capsule may be seen as an associated feature.

Treatment

Treatment is similar to senile cataract.

OTHER COMMON TYPES OF CATARACTS

Syndermatotic Cataract

Syndermatotic cataract is associated with skin diseases such as atopic dermatitis, psoriasis, etc. and it is also called dermatogenic cataract.

Electric Cataract

Electric cataract is cataract seen because of electric shock. The mechanism involved is coagulation of lens proteins caused by electric shock.

Traumatic Cataract

Traumatic cataract is described in detail under ocular trauma.

GIST BOX 8.3

- Cataract is defined as opacification of lens and/or its capsule congenital or acquired, progressive or stationary partial or complete, with or without visual impairment.
- Cataract is the commonest cause for avoidable blindness worldwide and in India.
- Based on the etiology, cataract is classified into congenital/developmental cataract and acquired cataract.
- Senile cataract is the most common type of cataract and it accounts for 90% of cataracts seen in clinical practice.
- Cortical cataract is the most common type of senile cataract and it accounts for up to 80% of senile cataract.
- Cataract formation because of age-related changes in people aged less than 50 years is called presenile cataract.
- Complicated cataract is opacification of lens secondary to a primary ocular disease.

CHAPTER

8.4 Cataract Surgeries

Cataract surgery is the most commonly performed eye surgery and it is one of the most commonly performed surgeries worldwide.

INDICATIONS FOR CATARACT SURGERY

Optical

The most common indication in clinical practice is to improve vision when cataract is causing visual impairment.

Therapeutic

When lens itself is acting as source of disease as in lens-induced glaucoma or in phacoanaphylactic uveitis or lens is causing difficulties in the treatment of posterior segment problems such as diabetic retinopathy, retinal detachment is used.

INVESTIGATIONS BEFORE CATARACT SURGERY***

Investigations are required for:

- Confirmation of diagnosis
- To rule out coexisting ocular diseases
- To tell about the visual prognosis following surgery
- To prevent those blinding postoperative complications
- To confirm fitness of the patient for surgery
- Investigations are must more so because of the involvement of the medicolegal aspects if any untoward complications occur.

The routinely carried out investigations at our hospital and most other hospitals are given below.

Systemic Investigations to Confirm Fitness for the Surgery

1. Urine sugar/random blood sugar to rule out diabetes mellitus. If the patient is known diabetic, fasting and postprandial blood sugar has to be done.
2. Blood pressure measurement to rule out hypertension.
3. Electrocardiogram (ECG) to know the cardiac status.
4. If the patient is known to have chronic disorders such as chronic obstructive pulmonary disease (COPD), ischemic heart disease (IHD), etc. they have to be controlled before posting the patient for surgery.
5. Human immunodeficiency virus (HIV) and surface antigen of the hepatitis B virus (HBsAg) to take safety precautions if the patient is seropositive.
6. Rule out any potential source of infection, such as infected abscess, open infected wound, which may act as a foci for development of endophthalmitis.

7. Xylocaine test dose to rule out hypersensitivity to Xylocaine.

Ocular Investigations

- Rule out any ocular infections such as conjunctivitis, stye, chronic dacryocystitis, etc. and inflammatory diseases in case of active uveitis, etc.
- Lacrimal syringing to rule out chronic dacryocystitis
- Intraocular pressure (IOP) measurement by tonometry
- Retinal and macular function tests to know visual prognosis
- Biometry for calculation of intraocular lens (IOL) power, which includes keratometry and A-scan.

Along with the above mentioned investigations, following should be done in examination:

- Slit-lamp examination/Anterior segment examination to rule out corneal disorders such as dystrophies, degenerations, etc. pterygium encroaching the pupillary area
- Retinoscopy to rule out refractive error
- Ophthalmoscopic examination of retina (fundoscopy), to look for retinal pathologies such as age-related macular degeneration, chorioretinal degeneration, optic atrophy, etc.
- Intraocular pressure measurement to rule out ocular hypertension and glaucoma.

Retinal and Macular Function Tests**

Retinal Function Tests

1. *Projection of rays*: The patient is asked to identify the direction of light by which light is coming by projecting light from various directions. Each eye is tested separately with the other eye being closed. If the patient can identify the direction from which light is coming, it indicates good retinal function. Usually projection of rays is tested in the four quadrants to check for the retinal function in the four quadrants of retina.
2. *Entoptic visualization*: It is done by placing a point source of light against the closed eyelids and asking the patient if he/she can perceive the retinal vascular pattern. The presence of entoptic visualization indicates good retinal function.
3. *Test for Marcus-Gunn pupil:* Presence of Marcus-Gunn pupil indicates afferent pathway defect.
4. *B-scan*: To detect anatomical state of retina and vitreous.
5. Electroretinogram.
6. Electro-oculogram.
7. Visual evoked potential.

Macular Function Tests

1. *Cardboard test/Two-point discrimination test:* Patient is asked to see through a cardboard with two holes close to each other with light behind the holes if two lights are appreciated, it indicates good macular function.
2. *Maddox rod test:* Patient is asked to look through a Maddox rod at a bright light, if the patient sees continuous unbroken and undistorted red line it indicates that the macula is normal and if the line is broken it indicates diseases of macula.
3. *Amsler grid test:* It can be used in eyes with better vision. Patient is asked to close one eye and to see at Amsler chart with the other eye holding at normal reading distance. Patient is asked to look for any distortion in the grid, while looking at the central fixing dot when present distortion indicates macular pathology. The test is repeated in the other eye.
4. *Laser interferometry*: It is done by laser interferometer, an instrument used to detect visual acuity in the presence of opaque media.
5. *Potential acuity meter*: It is done by projecting a slit-lamp miniature Snellen's chart into the eye and the macular function can be judged by lines read.

CALCULATION OF INTRAOCULAR LENS POWER***

Calculation of IOL power is the most important step before cataract surgery. Implantation of IOL of correct power leads to good vision. This has undergone rapid progress from the days of using standard lens power to the days of biometry.

Without Biometry

Without biometry calculation of IOL power was practiced in the past, but currently not done because of inaccurate measurements:

- Using standard power +19 D
- Based on basic refraction.

Basic refraction is the refractive error present before formation of cataract. The power of the IOL is calculated by the formula:

P = +19 D + (1.25 R)

where,

P is implant power;

R is basic refractive error.

With Biometry

Using regression formula:

- Sanders-Retzlaff-Kraff (SRK)-I
- SRK-II
- SRK/T
- Modified SRK-II
- Holladay.

SRK formulae are most commonly used:

P = A – 2.5 L – 0.9 K

where,

P is implant power; A is constant; L is axial length; K is corneal power in diopter; A is constant, for posterior chamber (PC) -IOL 118.2 and for anterior chamber (AC) -IOL it is 114 (the value of constant varies with the type of lens).

ANESTHESIA FOR CATARACT SURGERY

General Anesthesia

General anesthesia is indicated in children and mentally-retarded patients.

Local Anesthesia

Local anesthesia is the preferred mode of anesthesia for cataract surgery.

Retrobulbar anesthesia, peribulbar anesthesia, sub-Tenon's anesthesia, topical anesthesia are the most commonly used methods of anesthesia.

Because of increased incidence of complications retrobulbar anesthesia has become less popular and it almost replaced by peribulbar anesthesia.

Different techniques of anesthesia are described in Author's textbook *Clinical Methods in Ophthalmology* in the chapter 'Common Ophthalmic Surgeries'.

DIFFERENT TECHNIQUES OF CATARACT SURGERY***

The techniques for cataract surgery have undergone evolution starting from couching, which was practiced in the ancient times to the modern cataract surgery by phacoemulsification.

Couching**

1. Couching was the ancient technique of cataract surgery.
2. It was practiced from 5th century BC till 19th century.
3. Sushruta, Father of Indian surgery was one among the first to practice couching. It was described in the book '*Sushruta Samhita*'. A curved needle was used to apply pressure on the lens and push the lens into the back portion of the eye.
4. Couching was followed in Egypt, Greek, Rome, Arab, Europe, etc.
5. Couching was described in 'Code of Hammurabi', Hammurabi was a ruler from Babylonian dynasty from Mesopotamia.
6. Because of poor vision and high risk of complications couching is no longer followed. But it is still followed in poor African countries and it is practiced by traditional healers.

Principle

The principle of couching is applying pressure on the eyeball to dislocate the intact lens into vitreous chamber, so that patient becomes aphakic and will have aphakic vision, which is better than vision with mature and hypermature cataracts.

Technique

The technique consists of two methods.

Sharp method: This method uses sharp objects to perforate the cornea, enter the anterior chamber and lens is pushed backwards into the vitreous chamber.

Blunt method: This method includes applying pressure on the eye by blunt method without causing perforation of cornea to dislocate the intact lens into vitreous chamber.

Complications

Endophthalmitis, phacogenic uveitis, phacoanaphylactic uveitis, lens-induced glaucoma, poor vision, etc.

Intracapsular Cataract Extraction**

Intracapsular cataract extraction (ICCE) was first performed by Smith in 1880. It was practiced till 1980, now it is not performed. It is not performed because of increased rate of complications and availability of better surgical techniques.

Definition

Intracapsular cataract extraction is a surgical procedure for cataract where entire cataractous lens is removed along with intact capsule.

Indications

The only indication for ICCE now is dislocated lens into anterior chamber.

Procedure (Steps of Intracapsular Cataract Extraction)

1. Local anesthesia peribulbar block is the preferred one.
2. Preparation of the eyeball by painting the eye with povidone-iodine draping the eye with eye towel.
3. Insertion of the wire speculum to keep the eyelids apart (Fig. 8.4.1A).
4. Superior rectus stitch or bridle suture for fixation of the globe (Fig. 8.4.1B).
5. Conjunctival peritomy and cauterization of the bleeding vessels (Fig. 8.4.1C).
6. Partial thickness limbal groove 10–12 mm.
7. Corneoscleral section and entry into anterior chamber (Fig. 8.4.1D).
8. Injection of viscoelastic into the anterior chamber.
9. Lens delivery by cryoextraction or tumbling. In cryoextraction the lens is removed by applying cryoprobe onto the surface of lens (Fig. 8.4.1E). In tumbling lens is removed by applying pressure and counter pressure at 6 O'clock and 12 O'clock position respectively.
10. Peripheral iridectomy (Fig. 8.4.1F).
11. The anterior chamber IOL insertion (refer Fig. 8.4.1F).
12. Formation of anterior chamber by balanced salt solution.
13. Closure of the corneoscleral incision by 9-0 or 10-0 nylon suture (refer Fig. 8.4.1F).
14. Closure of conjunctiva.
15. Subconjunctival injection of antibiotic with steroid.
16. Pad and bandage.

Advantages

Intracapsular cataract extraction was done in the past and it was very popular particularly for mass eye camps as it does not require microscope, can be under naked eye thus making it a

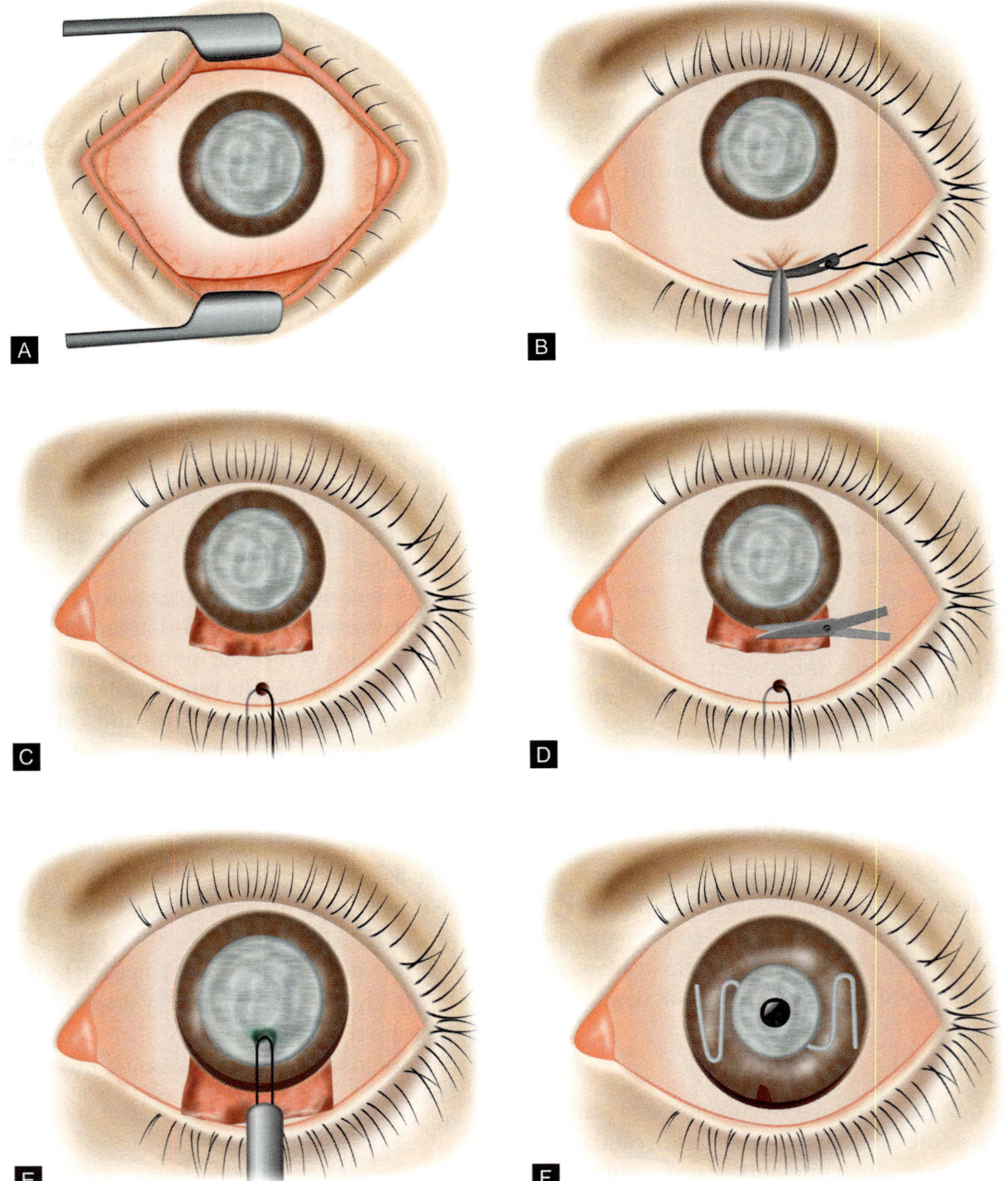

FIGS 8.4.1A to F: Steps of cataract surgery. **A.** Insertion of wire speculum; **B.** Bridle suture; **C.** Conjunctival peritomy; **D.** Corneoscleral section; **E.** Lens delivery by cryoextraction; **F.** Peripheral iridectomy, anterior chamber intraocular lens insertion and closure of the corneoscleral incision.

cheaper and quick surgical procedure suitable for mass camps.

Intracapsular cataract extraction is not done nowadays and it has become obsolete because of increased incidence of postoperative complications such as:

- Vitreous-related complications, e.g. vitreous touch syndrome, etc.
- Inability to insert posterior chamber IOL after ICCE.
- High-postoperative astigmatism because of large incision.

Extracapsular Cataract Extraction***

Jacques Daviel was the first one to perform extracapsular cataract extraction (ECCE). He performed the surgery through inferior incision in the year 1747 von Graefe was the first to perform the surgery through superior incision.

Intraocular lenses were first used by Sir Harold Ridley in the year 1949. They were posterior chamber IOLs and were called Ridley's IOLs.

Definition

Extracapsular cataract extraction is a surgical procedure for cataract where cataractous lens is removed leaving behind intact posterior capsule.

Types

- Conventional ECCE
- Small incision cataract surgery (SICS)
- Phacoemulsification.

Procedure (Steps of Conventional Extracapsular Cataract Extraction)

1. Anesthesia: Local anesthesia in the form of peribulbar anesthesia.
2. Preparation of the eyeball by painting the eye with povidone-iodine and draping the eye with eye towel.
3. Insertion of the wire speculum.
4. Superior rectus stitch or bridle suture for fixation of the globe.
5. Conjunctival peritomy and cauterization of the bleeding vessels.
6. Partial thickness limbal groove 8–10 mm.
7. Corneoscleral section.
8. Injection of viscoelastic into the anterior chamber.
9. Capsulotomy or capsulorhexis: It is the most important step in ECCE, which differentiates it from ICCE. This step removes the anterior capsule and leaves behind the posterior capsule:
    a. Capsulotomy: It is done by using a bent 26-gauge needle called cystitome. Multiple radial punctures are made in the anterior capsule in a circular fashion of approximately 6–7 mm in diameter. Capsulotomy is completed by joining these cuts and removing the part of anterior capsule. This is also called can-opener capsulotomy or multipuncture capsulotomy (Figs 8.4.2A and B).
    b. Capsulorhexis: It is done either by a cystitome or a capsulorhexis forceps. This is done by tearing the capsule in a circular fashion of 6–7 mm diameter. Capsulorhexis is better than capsulotomy and preferred as this can be stretched for in the bag IOL insertion.
10. Enlarging the corneoscleral section.
11. Hydrodissection: This is done by injecting the fluid under the anterior capsule to separate the cortex and nucleus from capsule.
12. Removal of nucleus by pressure and counter pressure method or by using vectis (Fig. 8.4.2C).
13. Removal of cortical matter by irrigation and aspiration (Fig. 8.4.2D).
14. Insertion of the posterior chamber IOL (Fig. 8.4.2E).
15. Formation of anterior chamber by balanced salt solution.
16. Closure of the corneoscleral incision.
17. Closure of conjunctiva.
18. Subconjunctival injection of antibiotic with steroid.
19. Pad and bandage.

Advantages and Disadvantages of Conventional Extracapsular Cataract Extraction

The advantages and disadvantages of conventional ECCE are given in Table 8.4.1.

Due to increased postoperative astigmatism and time required for healing of the bigger incision, thus delaying visual rehabilitation conventional ECCE is replaced by SICS and phacoemulsification.

TABLE 8.4.1: Advantages and disadvantages of conventional ECCE*

Advantages	*Disadvantages*
• Implantation of posterior chamber IOL† can be done • Fewer incidences of vitreous-related complications	• Requires microscope and other micro instruments, hence expensive compared to older ICCE‡ • The incision requires suturing, hence increased postoperative astigmatism compared to other recent techniques

*ECCE, extracapsular cataract extraction; †IOL, intraocular lens; ‡ICCE, intracapsular cataract extraction.

Small Incision Cataract Surgery***

Small incision cataract surgery is one of the popular techniques of cataract surgery and widely practiced all over the world.

Principle of Small Incision Cataract Surgery

The principle of SICS is construction of a self-sealing sclerocorneal tunnel. This was first described by Richard Kartz.

The size of the incision is 5.5–6.5 mm. The incision differs from the ECCE conventional by the fact that here a self-sealing sclerocorneal tunnel is created. This is a two-step incision with external scleral wound and the internal corneal wound connected by a tunnel, thus making it self-sealing thus avoiding the need of suturing the wound, thus reducing the astigmatism. The second principle of SICS is reduction in the size of the nucleus by separating the inner harder nucleus from epinucleus by hydrodelineation. Hydrodelineation is separation of outer soft epinucleus from inner hard nucleus by injecting fluid into the cortical layer of the lens. This step enables to remove the nucleus through a smaller incision.

Procedure (Steps of Small Incision Cataract Surgery)

1. Anesthesia: Local anesthesia in the form of peribulbar block or sub-Tenon's anesthesia. Peribulbar block is the preferred one.
2. Preparation of the eyeball by painting the eye with povidone-iodine and draping the eye with eye towel.
3. Insertion of the wire speculum.
4. Superior rectus stitch or bridle suture for fixation of the globe.
5. Conjunctival peritomy and cauterization of the bleeding vessels.
6. Scleral groove and sclerocorneal tunnel construction using crescent blade (Figs 8.4.3A and B).
7. Paracentesis or side port entry into anterior chamber: It is made by using a paracentesis needle and it is self-sealing as the dimension is less than 1 mm. This is made at 90° to the main incision. The main purpose of side port incision is to remove the subincisional cortical matter. This can also be used to do capsulotomy/capsulorhexis, injection of viscoelastic, etc. because of easy maneuverability (Fig. 8.4.3C).
8. Injection of viscoelastic into anterior chamber.

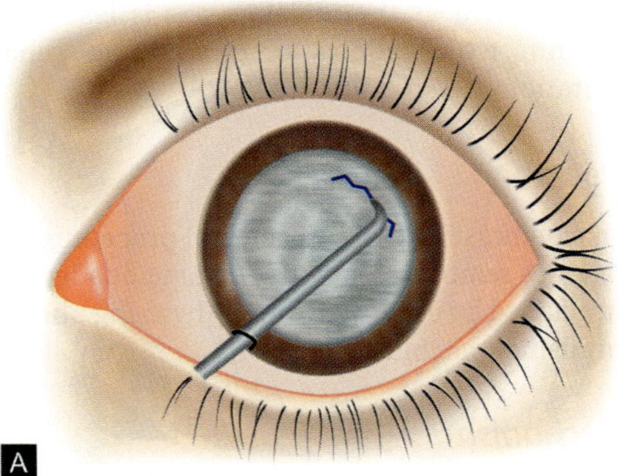

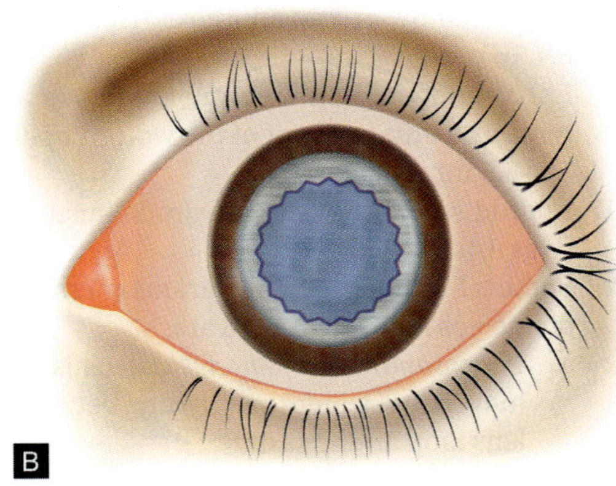

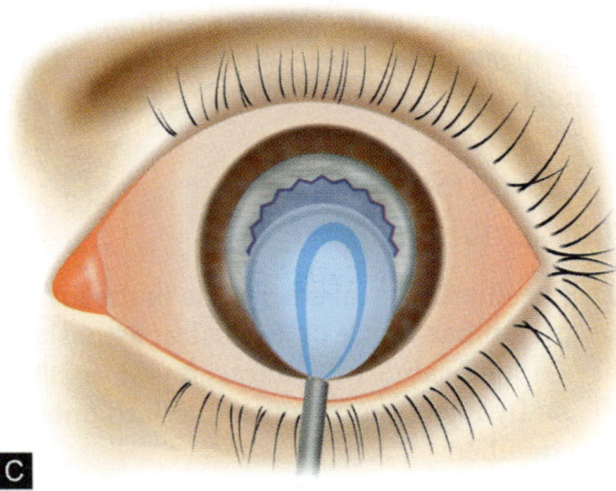

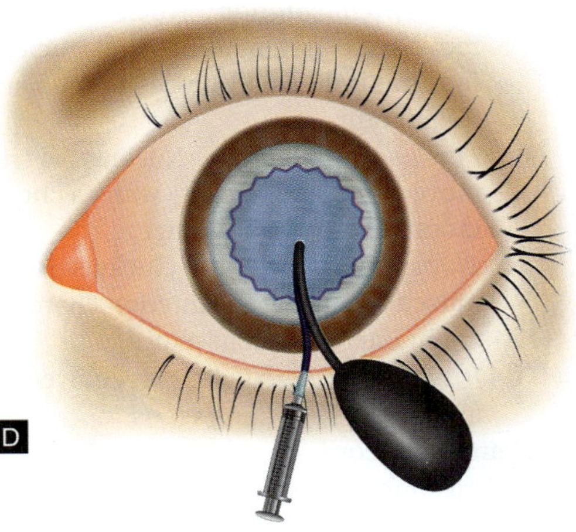

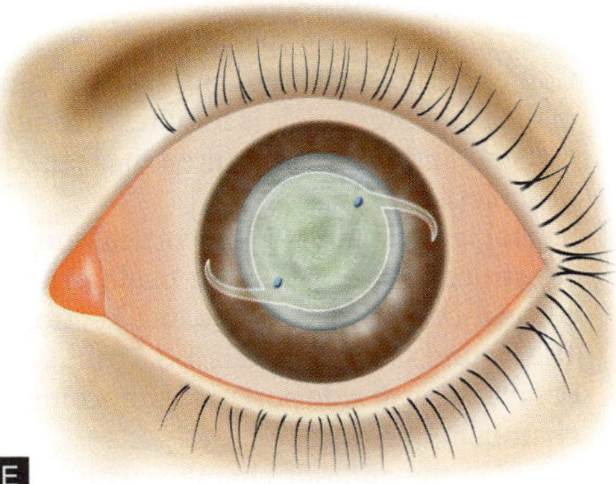

FIGS 8.4.2A to E: Steps of conventional extracapsular cataract extraction. **A.** Initiation of capsulotomy; **B.** Capsulotomy completed; **C.** Removal of nucleus; **D.** Removal of cortical matter by irrigation and aspiration; **E.** Posterior chamber insertion with closure of corneoscleral incision.

9. Capsulotomy or capsulorhexis (refer Fig. 8.4.3C).
10. Entry into anterior chamber with keratome and enlargement of the wound up to 5.5–6.5 mm (Fig. 8.4.3D).
11. Hydrodissection and hydrodelineation (Figs 8.4.3E and F).
12. Removal of nucleus: The various methods of nucleus removal in SICS are:*
    a. *Phacosandwich method:* Nucleus is removed by squeezing tightly between lens loop and spatula.
    b. *Phacofracture:* Nucleus is removed by cutting it into two or more pieces.
    c. *Phacofragmentation:* Nucleus is removed by fragmenting the nucleus into multiple small pieces by nucleus fragmentor.
    d. *Fish-hook technique:* Nucleus is removed by hooking it with a hook mounted on a 1 mL syringe.
    e. *Blumenthal technique:* Nucleus is removed by using an anterior chamber maintainer and a lens glide.
    f. *Irrigating vectis:* Nucleus is removed by inserting an irrigating vectis.
13. Removal of cortical matter and epinucleus by irrigation and aspiration.
14. Posterior chamber IOL insertion.
15. Formation of anterior chamber and closure of conjunctiva.
16. Subconjunctival injection of antibiotic with steroid.
17. Pad and bandage.

Advantages and Disadvantages

The advantages and disadvantages of SICS is given in Table 8.4.2.

Phacoemulsification***

Phacoemulsification is the most popular surgery and is considered as the gold standard surgical procedure for cataract (Figs 8.4.4A and B). It was first introduced by Charles D Kelman in 1967. It is the most preferred mode of treatment as the incision size is less than 3.5 mm, which allows for quick visual rehabilitation. It uses foldable IOL.

Definition

Phacoemulsification is a surgical procedure for cataract removal where the cataractous lens is emulsified by ultrasonic energy by using phacoemulsifier machine.

Mechanism

Phaco handpiece consists of piezoelectric crystals, which convert electrical energy into mechanical vibration. The phaco needle vibrates at about 40,000 times per second, thus emulsifying the nucleus.

Procedure (Steps of Phacoemulsification)

1. Anesthesia: Local anesthesia in the form of peribulbar block or topical anesthesia by 4% lignocaine with intracameral anesthesia by injection of lignocaine into anterior chamber.
2. Preparation of the eyeball by painting the eye with povidone-iodine and draping the eye with eye towel.
3. Insertion of the wire speculum.
4. Conjunctival peritomy and cauterization of the bleeding vessels is required in limbal incision and it is not required in clear corneal incision.
5. Scleral groove and sclerocorneal tunnel construction using crescent blade or clear corneal incision is made using keratome. The wound size required is 3–3.5 mm.
6. Paracentesis or side port entry into anterior chamber.
7. Forming the anterior chamber with viscoelastic.
8. Capsulorhexis: It is compulsory as phacoemulsification requires a stable capsular bag.
9. Hydrodissection and hydrodelineation.
10. Emulsification of nucleus: The various methods of emulsification of nucleus are:

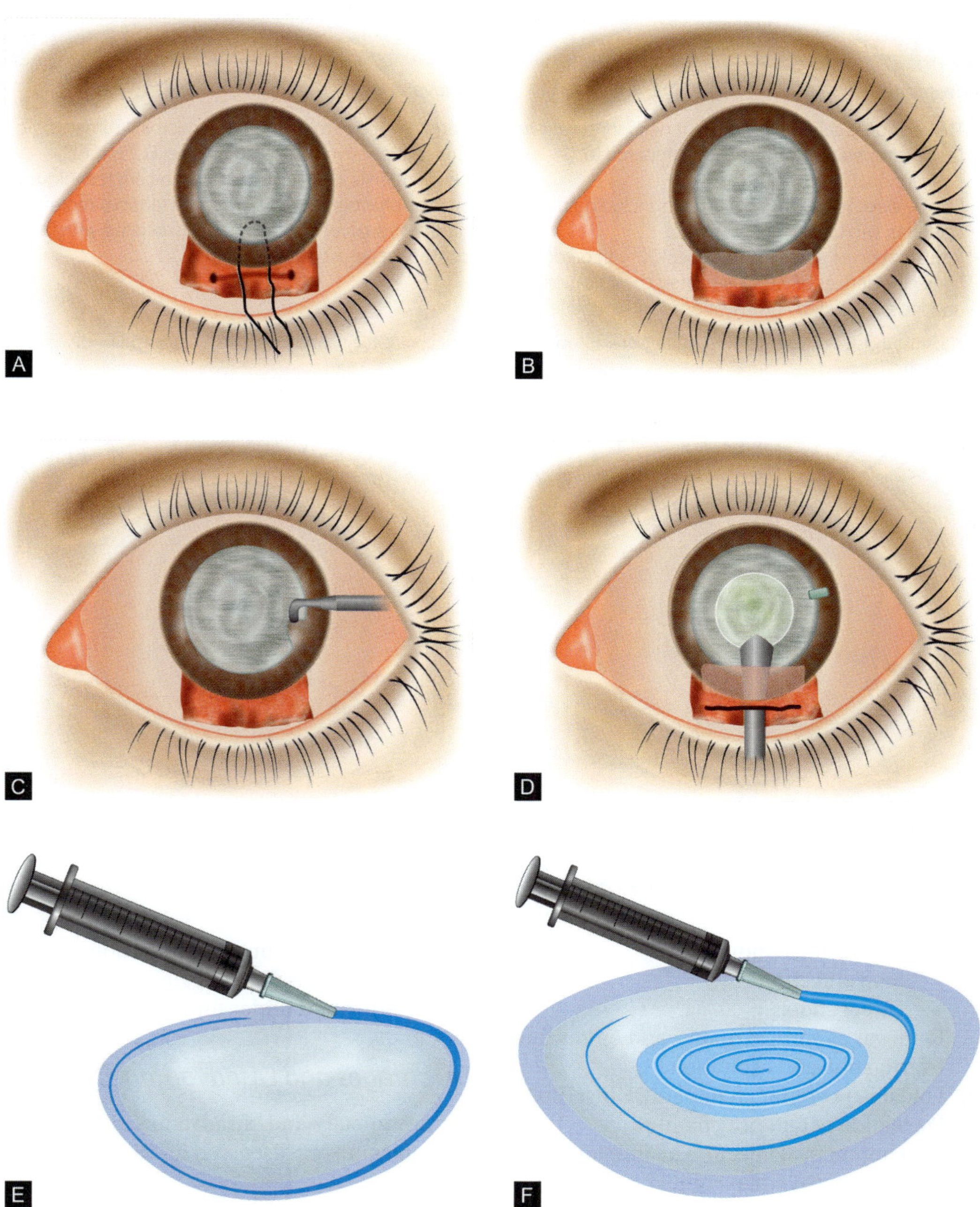

FIGS 8.4.3A to F: Steps of small incision cataract surgery. **A.** Scleral incision; **B.** Sclerocorneal tunnel construction; **C.** Side port incision and capsulorhexis; **D.** Entry into anterior chamber with keratome; **E.** Hydrodissection; **F.** Hydrodelineation.

TABLE 8.4.2: Advantages and disadvantages of SICS*

Advantages	*Disadvantages*
• The incision is self-sealing without need for suturing • Less postoperative astigmatism compared to conventional ECCE† • Can be done in all types of cataracts including nuclear cataracts, subluxated cataracts, etc. • Implantation of posterior chamber IOL‡ can be done • Fewer incidences of vitreous-related complications and incision-related complications, e.g. wound leak	• Requires microscope and other microinstruments, hence expensive compared to older ECCE, ICCE§ • The incision is bigger compared to recent techniques such as phacoemulsification hence requires more time for visual rehabilitation and associated with more postoperative astigmatism

*SICS, small incision cataract surgery; †ECCE, extracapsular cataract extraction; ‡IOL, intraocular lens; §ICCE, intracapsular cararact extraction.

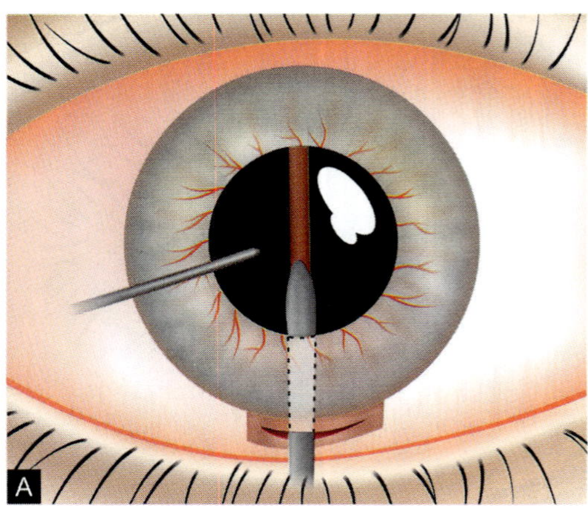

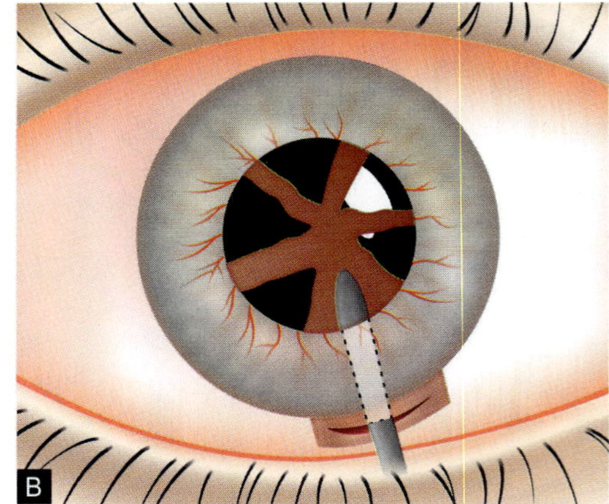

FIGS 8.4.4A and B: Phacoemulsification of nucleus

- Divide and conquer
- Stop and chop
- Direct chop.

11. Removal of cortical matter and epinucleus by irrigation and aspiration.
12. Foldable posterior chamber IOL insertion.
13. Formation of anterior chamber.
14. Subconjunctival injection of antibiotic with steroid is given when surgery is performed under local anesthesia, antibiotic steroid eyedrops is applied topically when surgery is performed under topical anesthesia.
15. Pad and bandage is done when surgery is performed under local anesthesia and patient walks out of operation theater with postoperative goggles when surgery is performed under topical anesthesia.

*Advantages and Disadvantages**

The advantages and disadvantages of phacoemulsification are discussed in Table 8.4.3.

Comparison between various techniques of cataract surgery is described in the chapter 'Common Ophthalmic Surgeries' in Author's textbook *Clinical Methods of Ophthalmology.*

RECENT ADVANCES IN CATARACT SURGERY**

The cataract surgery has undergone rapid advancement from the last century, from couching to intracapsular surgery, from intracapsular to extracapsular surgery. The extracapsular surgery, which started with conventional type requiring sutures advanced into sutureless surgeries in the phacoemulsification and small incision cataract surgery.

In the present century cataract surgery has undergone further advancement in the form of microincisional cataract surgery (MICS).

Microincisional Cataract Surgery

Microincisional cataract surgery includes cataract surgery performed through an incision less than 2.2 mm in size:

- Coaxial MICS
- Bimanual MICS.

Coaxial MICS is performed through incision of 2.2 mm in size. It uses a phaco tip of lesser dimension compared to the conventional phacoemulsification phaco tips, which measure about 3–3.5 mm.

Bimanual MICS is also called phakonit and it uses two incisions of about 1 mm in size. A sleeveless phaco tip without infusion sleeve is used through one incision and infusion sleeve is used separately through another incision.

Phakonit

Phakoemulsification with **n**eedle opening via small **i**ncision with sleeveless ultrasound **t**ip. The size of the incision is 0.9 mm.

Microphakonit

Microphakonit is performed through an incision of 0.7 mm. It is also called ultrasmall incision cataract surgery.

Laser-assisted Cataract Surgery

Laser-assisted cataract surgery uses femtosecond laser along with phacoemulsification. Femtosecond laser is used to perform capsulorhexis, lens fragmentation and corneal incision. The later steps of emulsifying the nucleus and insertion of IOL are similar to phacoemulsification.

POSTOPERATIVE MANAGEMENT AFTER CATARACT SURGERY**

1. Postoperatively dressing is removed after 6 hours of surgery.
2. Antibiotic-steroid eyedrops, such as ofloxacin-prednisolone acetate, gatifloxacin-prednisolone acetate, etc. are prescribed for 6 weeks in tapering dosage:
    - Six times per day in 1st week
    - Five times per day in 2nd week

TABLE 8.4.3: Advantages and disadvantages of phacoemulsification

Advantages	*Disadvantages*
• Can be done under topical anesthesia; thus, avoiding the need for injections for anesthetic injections • The incision size is small without the need for sutures and associated with quick visual rehabilitation • Implantation of foldable posterior chamber IOL* can be done • Surgery can be done through clear corneal incision; thus, avoiding conjunctival incision • Fewer postoperative complications	• Costlier compared to other methods as it requires the use of phacoemulsifier, foldable IOLs • Surgeon requires training for mastering the technique as this includes use of phacoemulsifier machine • Difficult to do in hard nuclear cataracts, subluxated cataracts, etc.

*IOL, intraocular lens

- Four times per day in 3rd week
- Three times per day in 4th week
- Four times per day in 5th week
- Two times per day in 6th week.

3. Non-steroidal eyedrops, such as flurbiprofen, ketorolac are prescribed four times per day for 6 weeks.
4. The patient is seen on the first postoperative day after 2 weeks and after 6 weeks. Visual rehabilitation in the form of spectacles is prescribed after 6 weeks.

Visual rehabilitation: Final spectacle correction is given after:
- 4 weeks after phacoemulsification.
- 6 weeks after SICS.
- 8 weeks after conventional ECCE after removal of sutures.

Postoperative Instructions
- Not to rub the operated eye.
- Avoid exposure of the operated eye to dust and smoke.
- To use protective eye goggles for 2 weeks.
- No head bath for 2 weeks.
- To use prescribed eyedrops as per the advice.
- To report immediately if the patient notices pain, redness and diminution of vision.

Timing of Surgery for Bilateral Mature Cataract or Significant Cataract in Both the Eyes

Normally only one eye is operated at a time and surgery for other eye is done after a gap of 1 week. The two eyes are not operated together to prevent risk of postoperative endophthalmitis, so that if it occurs at least one eye is spared.

Though the incidence of postoperative endophthalmitis has come down drastically with improvement in sterilization and surgical techniques, it still continues to be the single most dangerous complication, which may lead to painful blind eye if not treated early and effectively.

COMPLICATIONS OF CATARACT SURGERY***

With the advances in cataract surgery the complications have come down markedly and cataract surgery has become a day care surgery with very good visual prognosis.

The complications can be studied under three headings:
1. Preoperative complications.
2. Intraoperative complications.
3. Postoperative complications.

Preoperative Complications

Preoperative complications mainly include the complications during anesthesia, examples are given below.

Penetration or Perforation of Globe

Perforation of globe is seen in eyes with increased axial length as in pathological myopia, posterior staphyloma. It presents with sudden pain and hypotony. Perforation of the globe can lead to vitreous hemorrhage, retinal detachment, etc. which can lead to poor visual prognosis. The treatment is by sealing the perforation by laser or cryotherapy along with the treatment for the complications. The incidence of perforation of globe is less with peribulbar anesthesia compared to retrobulbar anesthesia.

Intravascular Injection

Intravascular injection is because of injection into the veins or arteries. Intra-arterial injection is very dangerous leading to central nervous system toxicity causing cardiopulmonary arrest.

Damage to Optic Nerve

Damage to optic nerve can occur either secondary to retrobulbar hemorrhage or because of direct injury to the optic nerve as in injection into the optic nerve sheath. The prognosis is usually poor with partial or total optic nerve atrophy being the end result. However this complication is of rare occurrence.

Brainstem Anesthesia

Brainstem anesthesia is a very rare complication occurring as a result of injection into the subdural or subarachnoid space around the optic nerve. Patient presents with symptoms of disorientation, unconsciousness and respiratory arrest. The treatment is by cardiopulmonary resuscitation.

Oculocardiac Reflex

Oculocardiac reflex is the reflex decrease in the heart rate as a result of manipulation of the extraocular muscle or because of pressure on the eye.

This is commonly seen in younger individuals and prior administration of intravenous atropine decreases the occurrence of oculocardiac reflex. However, the incidence is very less in elderly individuals who undergo cataract surgery in majority of cases.

Retrobulbar Hemorrhage

Retrobulbar hemorrhage is the most common anesthetic complication seen with retrobulbar anesthesia. The incidence is estimated to be about 2%. It presents as proptosis, subconjunctival hemorrhage with pain.

The management is by application of pressure to arrest bleeding. The next management depends on the IOP. If the IOP is elevated, surgery is postponed and central retinal artery pulsations are monitored as central retinal artery occlusion can occur. Such cases require lowering of IOP by lateral canthotomy, anterior chamber paracentesis and use of oral antiglaucoma drugs. Cataract surgery is performed after IOP is reduced.

As phacoemulsification has become the surgery of choice for cataract surgery, anesthesia-related complications have come down drastically as phacoemulsification is commonly performed on topical anesthesia.

Intraoperative Complications

Bridle Suture-related Complications

A bridle suture is applied for the purpose of fixation of globe in ECCE conventional and SICS. Perforation of the sclera and superior rectus muscle laceration and hematoma are the commonly seen complications. Since in phacoemulsification this step is not performed, these complications are rare.

Incision-related Complications

A well placed and constructed incision is very important for smooth conduct of surgery and stable wound in the postoperative period:

- Incision placed posteriorly on the sclera lead to troublesome bleeding
- Full thickness and deeper incisions lead to iris prolapse during surgery
- Superficial incisions lead to button holing especially during construction of tunnel
- Entry into the anterior chamber without construction of sclerocorneal tunnel called premature entry can lead to iris prolapse during surgery and following surgery.

Complications Because of Inadvertent Injury to the Intraocular Structures of the Eye

Detachment of Descemet's membrane: This can occur as a result of use of blunt keratome to enter the anterior chamber or because of entry of the instrument between the stroma and Descemet's membrane. This can lead to irreversible corneal edema and bullous keratopathy in the postoperative period. The treatment is by placing a large air bubble or by suturing the detached Descemet's membrane to the rest of the cornea.

Damage to endothelium: This can result from touching of instruments or nucleus against the endothelium. Damage to endothelium results in loss of endothelial cells resulting in corneal edema in the postoperative period. The normal endothelial cell count in adults is about 3,000 cells/mm^2. Reduction in the count below 500 cells/mm^2 leads to irreversible corneal edema.

Injury to iris: This occur in the form of injury to the sphincter pupillae resulting in postoperatively dilated pupil, iris prolapse during surgery, iridodialysis, constriction of pupil during surgery, etc. A large iridodialysis need to be sutured.

Injury to ciliary zonules: This can lead to zonular dialysis. A small zonular dialysis may not lead to much problems, but a large one can lead to nucleus drop.

Posterior capsular tear: This is one of the common intraoperative complications, which can lead to poor surgical outcome. It can occur during hydrodissection, nucleus removal or during irrigation and aspiration. In case of small posterior capsular tear posterior chamber IOL can be implanted, but a large one requires scleral fixated posterior chamber IOL (Figs 8.4.5A to C) or anterior chamber IOL (Fig. 8.4.6).

Vitreous Loss

Vitreous loss follows posterior capsule tear. It can lead to various complications such as vitreous touch syndrome, pupillary block glaucoma, increased incidence of cystoid macular edema, endophthalmitis and retinal detachment, incarceration into the operative wound resulting in epithelial ingrowth and fibrous downgrowth. If vitreous loss occurs during surgery, the first goal should be to clear it completely from the anterior segment by vitrectomy.

Retained Cortical Matter

Retained cortical matter can lead to phacogenic uveitis, phacoanaphylactic uveitis and increased incidence of postoperative after cataract.

Nucleus Drop

Nucleus drop is associated with posterior capsular tear, vitreous loss where nucleus fragments or whole of the nucleus can fall into the vitreous cavity. The treatment is by anterior vitrectomy in the initial stage and patient is referred to a posterior segment surgeon for vitrectomy and nucleus removal.

Intraocular Lens Drop

Intraocular lens drop results from implantation of posterior chamber IOL in presence of posterior capsule tear. An IOL in the periphery of the retina can be followed up as the IOL causes less inflammation compared to nucleus in the vitreous cavity. However an IOL, which is moving

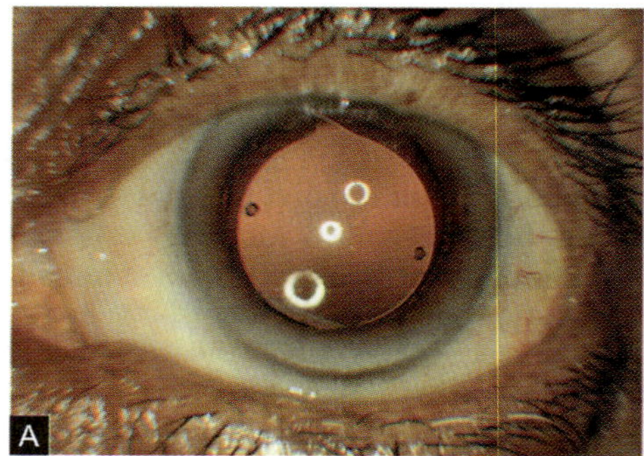

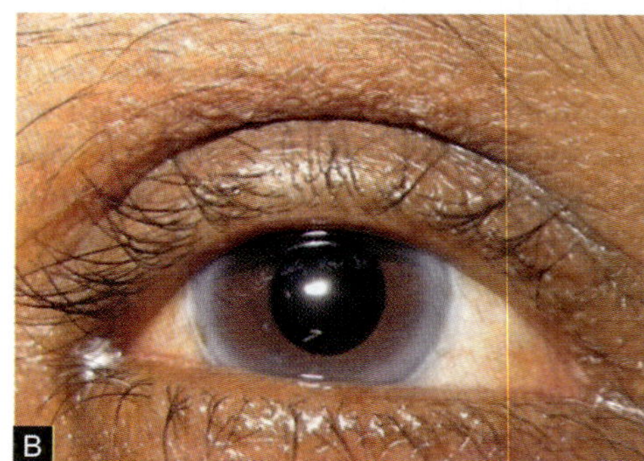

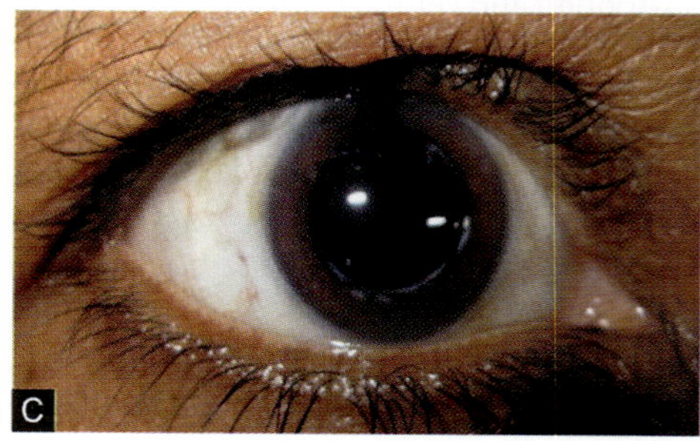

FIGS 8.4.5A to C: Pseudophakia with posterior chamber intraocular lens (Jet black pupil with shining reflexes).

with the movements of the eye or an IOL on the macula requires vitrectomy and repositioning of the IOL by scleral fixation.

Expulsive Choroidal Hemorrhage

Expulsive choroidal hemorrhage is rare, but blinding complication of cataract surgery and it is associated with complete loss of vision because of expulsion of the contents of the eye. It is seen in cases with increased IOP and uncontrolled hypertension. It manifests as increased vitreous pressure, posterior capsular rent, vitreous loss followed by expulsion of the intraocular contents of the eye including retina leading to complete loss of vision. The treatment is by immediate closure of the wound to prevent extrusion of the intraocular contents. This complication can be prevented by ensuring adequate control of hypertension before surgery and operating on a soft eye with adequate treatment of raised IOP.

Postoperative Complications

Complications can be early postoperative or late postoperative complications.

*Early Postoperative Complications (Within 3 Week)***

Iris prolapse: It is prolapse of iris through the surgical wound. It may result because of improper wound closure or because of associated iridodialysis. An iris prolapse, which is noticed within 48 hours duration is reposited back with wound closure, however an iris prolapse of more than 48 hours duration is excised because of risk of infection (Fig. 8.4.7).

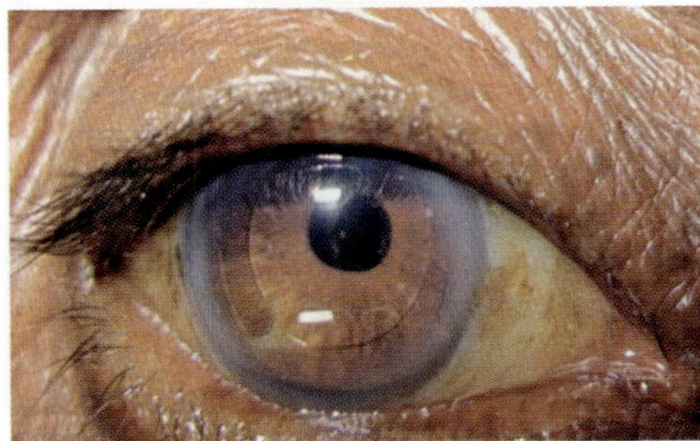

FIG. 8.4.6: Pseudophakia with anterior chamber intraocular lens (IOL)

*Shallow Anterior Chamber**

Shallow anterior chamber was one of the most common complications seen with ICCE and ECCE conventional type. The common causes for flat anterior chamber are wound leak, pupillary block glaucoma, ciliochoroidal detachment and malignant glaucoma:

1. Wound leak presents with hypotony and positive Seidel's test. The treatment is by reformation of the anterior chamber and suturing the wound.
2. Pupillary block glaucoma presents with raised IOP associated with shallow anterior chamber. It is caused by blockage of the pupil by either vitreous or lens matter or IOL thereby obstructing the flow of aqueous from posterior chamber to anterior chamber. The anterior chamber will be shallow in the periphery. The treatment is by using mydriatics to dilate the pupil to relieve the pupillary block. Cases not responding to medical treatment require laser peripheral iridotomy or surgical iridectomy to provide alternate pathway for aqueous.
3. Ciliochoroidal detachment is because of abnormal collection of fluid in the suprachoroidal space. It presents with shallow anterior chamber with or without leaking anterior chamber. Medical treatment is by mydriatics and cycloplegics. Surgical treatment is by suprachoroidal tap and reformation of anterior chamber.

Residual Lens Matter

The lens matter has to be removed because of the risk of phacogenic uveitis or phacoanaphylactic endophthalmitis and increased incidence after cataract. The residual lens matter is removed by anterior chamber wash by irrigation and aspiration (Fig. 8.4.8).

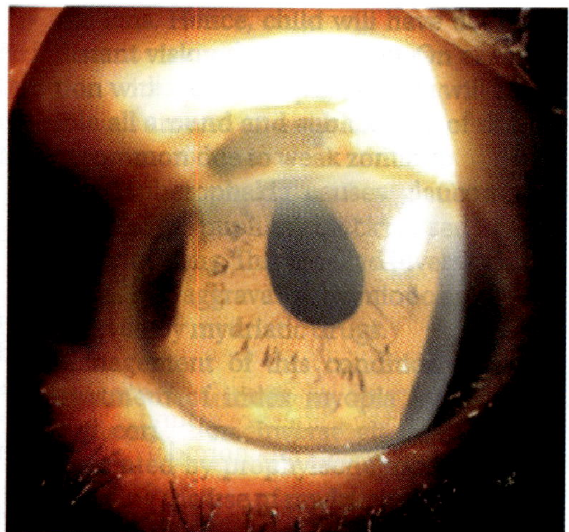

FIG. 8.4.7: Iris prolapse (pear-shaped pupil with iris in the scleral wound)

Severe Postoperative Inflammation

Severe postoperative inflammation may be in the form of postoperative iridocyclitis, phacotoxic uveitis or phacoanaphylactic endophthalmitis. The treatment is by intensive use of topical and systemic steroids to control the inflammation and by removal of residual lens matter if any.

*Endophthalmitis***

Endophthalmitis is the most dangerous complication of cataract surgery. This is described in detail under uvea.

Postoperative endophthalmitis is the most dangerous complication of cataract surgery. This requires early recognition and effective treatment failing, which it may lead to painful blind eye.

Hyphema

Hyphema is defined as collection of blood in the anterior chamber. Follow-up and observation is sufficient in small hyphema as it gets absorbed spontaneously. Hyphema associated with raised IOP is treated by antiglaucoma drugs. Hyphema not responding to treatment and associated with persistent raised IOP is treated by paracentesis and anterior chamber wash to drain the blood.

Striate Keratopathy

Striate keratopathy is because of corneal edema as a result of intraoperative damage to the corneal endothelium. This is treated by hyperosmotic agent, e.g. hypertonic saline. Marked loss of endothelium or total Descemet's detachment can result in irreversible corneal edema leading to bullous keratopathy.

Late Postoperative Complications**

Posterior Capsular Calcification or After Cataract

Posterior capsular calcification is the most common late postoperative complication leading to decrease in the visual acuity in the late postoperative period. It is described in detail later in the chapter.

Cystoid Macular Edema

Cystoid macular edema (CME) was first described by Irvine hence called Irvine-Gass syndrome. It is because of release of inflammatory

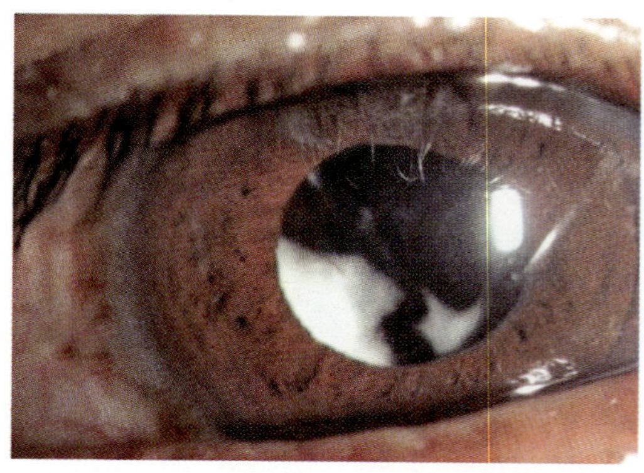

FIG. 8.4.8: Retained lens matter (white lens matter in the inferonasal quadrant with pseudophakia)

mediators (prostaglandins) as a result of postoperative inflammation because of iridocyclitis. Increased incidence is seen in cases associated with systemic diseases such as uncontrolled diabetes and hypertension and vitreous disturbances during surgery such as vitreous loss, vitreous incarceration in the wound.

Cystoid macular edema can be prevented by pre- and post-operative use of antiprostaglandin, e.g. flurbiprofen and by control of systemic diseases such as diabetes mellitus. Treatment is by control of inflammation with steroids and antiprostaglandins. In cases of CME associated with vitreous disturbances, treatment is by anterior vitrectomy and steroids.

After cataract and CME are the most common late postoperative complications responsible for diminution of vision in the late postoperative period.

Postoperative Astigmatism

Surgically-induced astigmatism is directly proportional to the cube of the length of the incision and hence larger the incision more is the postoperative astigmatism.

Average astigmatism following phakoemulsification is about 0.5 D, following SICS it is between 0.5 D and 1.0 D and following ECCE it is 1.0–2.0 D.

Chronic Postoperative Endophthalmitis

Chronic postoperative endophthalmitis is a rare complication of cataract surgery presenting as intraocular inflammation after 6 weeks of cataract surgery. The causative organisms are *Propionibacterium acnes* and fungi.

Retinal Detachment

The incidence of retinal detachment is more common in pseudophakics as compared to phakic and in aphakic than pseudophakic. The incidence is more in cases associated with vitreous loss and other vitreous disturbances.

Corneal Endothelial Decompensation

Corneal endothelial decompensation is seen in cases with pre-existing corneal endothelial diseases such as corneal dystrophies or in cases with extensive damage to corneal endothelial cells. Bullous keratopathy is the end result of corneal endothelial decompensation.

Bullous keratopathy is further classified into pseudophakic and aphakic bullous keratopathy depending on phakic status of the eye. Aphakic bullous keratopathy is more common than pseudophakic bullous keratopathy. Treatment is by keratoplasty.

Anterior Capsular Contraction Syndrome and Capsular Bag Distension Syndrome

Anterior capsular contraction syndrome and capsular bag distension syndrome is seen rarely as a complication of capsulorhexis. The treatment is by yttrium-aluminum-garnet (YAG) laser radial anterior relaxing capsulotomy.

Epithelial Ingrowth and Fibrous Downgrowth

Epithelial ingrowth and fibrous downgrowth are relatively rare complications seen because of defective wound apposition or closure, hence were common with ICCE and ECCE conventional surgeries.

Most Dangerous Complications

Intraoperative: Expulsive choroidal hemorrhage.
Postoperative: The postoperative endophthalmitis.

Most Common Postoperative Complication

Cystoid macular edema and after cataract.

Intraocular Lens-related Complications

They are described below under IOL.

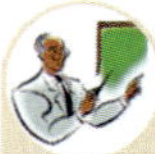

Complications of Untreated Cataracts*

Cataract if not operated even after maturity and hypermaturity, can lead to complications such as:
- *Lens-induced glaucoma:* Described in detail under lens-induced glaucoma.
- *Subluxation and dislocation of the lens:* It is because of degeneration of ciliary zonules.
- *Phacoanaphylactic uveitis:* It is because of leakage of lens proteins, which initiate antigen-antibody reaction leading to uveitis.

INTRAOCULAR LENSES**

The use of IOLs in cataract surgery was the major breakthrough, which was responsible for rapid visual rehabilitation. Sir Harold Ridley, a British ophthalmologist was the first to use IOLs in cataract surgery in the year 1949.

The IOLs have undergone rapid changes since then, and the various IOLs can be studied under six generations:
1. First generation: Posterior chamber IOL (Ridley's posterior chamber IOL).
2. Second generation: Anterior chamber angle fixated lenses.
3. Third generation: Iris supported lenses.
4. Fourth generation: Anterior chamber one piece.
5. Fifth generation: Posterior chamber lenses.
6. Sixth generation: Modern capsular posterior chamber IOL and modern anterior chamber IOL.

Multifocal IOL, foldable IOL, toric IOL, rollable IOL are the recent advancements in IOL and can be called modern generation IOLs.

Parts of Intraocular Lens

Intraocular lens has got two parts, optic and haptic. Optic is the central part of the IOL required for the vision and it measures about 5.5–6.5 mm. Haptic is the peripheral part of the IOL, which supports the optic. The overall diameter of the IOL is 12.5–13.5 mm. Optic of IOLs are made of:*
- Polymethyl methacrylate (PMMA)
- Silicone
- Acrylic
- Hydrogels.

Haptics of IOLs are made of:
- Polypropylene
- Polyamides
- Polymethyl methacrylate.

Types of Intraocular Lenses (Fig. 8.4.9)*

They are classified as:
- Depending on the site where they are placed:
  - Anterior chamber IOL
  - Iris fixated IOL
  - Posterior chamber IOL.
- Depending on nature:
  - Rigid IOL
  - Foldable IOL.

Sterilization of Intraocular Lens*

1. *Chemical sterilization:* It is done by soaking the lens in 10% sodium hydroxide solution.
2. *Gas sterilization:* It is done by exposing the lens to ethylene oxide.
3. *Radiation sterilization:* It is done by exposing to gamma (γ) rays up to 2.5 mrad.

Complications of Intraocular Lens Implantation**

1. Malposition of IOLs (Fig. 8.4.10):
   a. Decenteration.
   b. *Subluxation:* Sunset syndrome—inferior subluxation and sunrise syndrome—superior subluxation.
   c. *Dislocation:* Lost lens syndrome dislocation of IOL into vitreous chamber.
   d. *Windshield wiper syndrome:* Movement of the IOL with movements of the eye as a result of small IOL placed in the ciliary sulcus.
2. *Pupillary capture:* The presence of IOL in the pupillary plane blocking the pupil partly or completely because of synechiae

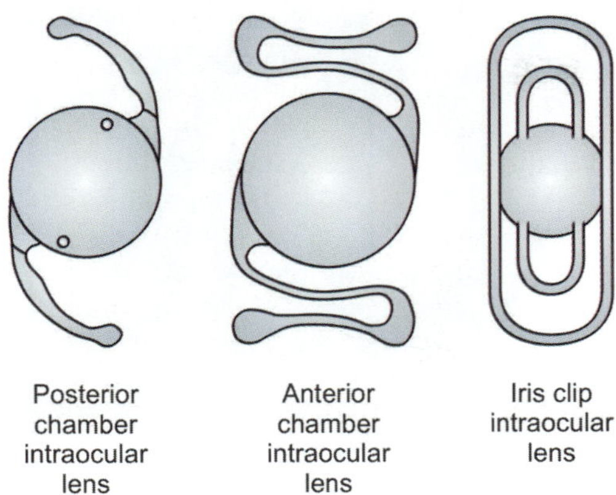

FIG. 8.4.9: Different types of intraocular lenses

between the posterior surface of the optic and the underlying iris. Pupillary capture is commonly in pediatric cataract surgeries.

3. *Iris tuck:* It is the entrapment of peripheral iris in between the IOL haptic resulting in distortion of the shape of the pupil.
4. *Uveitis-glaucoma-hyphema syndrome:* The uveitis-glaucoma-hyphema is because of mechanical rubbing of the iris by the IOL. It was seen usually with anterior chamber IOLs and iris fixated IOLs.
5. *Corneal retinal inflammatory syndrome (CRIS):* It is the chronic inflammation seen because of chronic rubbing of IOL against the iris releasing iris pigments.
6. *Posterior capsular opacification:* This is described in detail under 'After Cataract'.
7. *Toxic lens syndrome:* Uveitis caused by toxins associated with lens-like ethylene gas used for sterilizing lens.

AFTER CATARACT**

Definition

After cataract is also called posterior capsule opacification (PCO). After cataract is opacification of posterior capsule of the lens following ECCE (Figs 8.4.11A and B). The incidence of after cataract is 10–50% following ECCE.

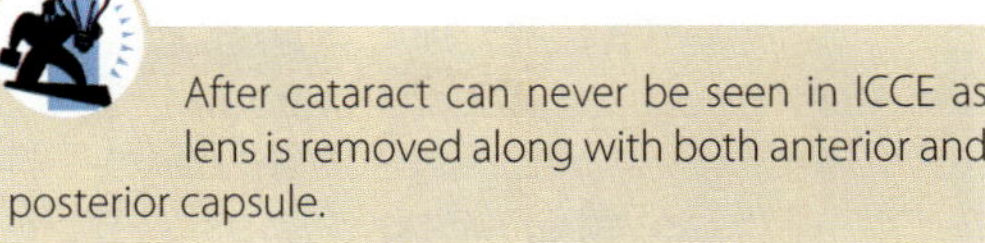

After cataract can never be seen in ICCE as lens is removed along with both anterior and posterior capsule.

Pathogenesis

The equatorial epithelium, which remains active throughout life, is the primary source of after cataract, especially for Elschnig's pearl and Soemmering's ring. The membranous type is because of posterior proliferation of anterior epithelium cells.

The time of onset, incidence and severity depend on various factors such as surgical technique and IOL.

Clinical Features

1. Diminution of vision gradual in onset and progressive in nature following cataract surgery by ECCE method is the presenting feature.
2. On examination, opacity of the posterior capsule behind the IOL can be made out; depending on the appearance of the opacity.

Types*

1. Membranous after cataract: Cells proliferate such as membrane.
2. Elschnig's pearl: Cells proliferate and distend to form spherical cells.

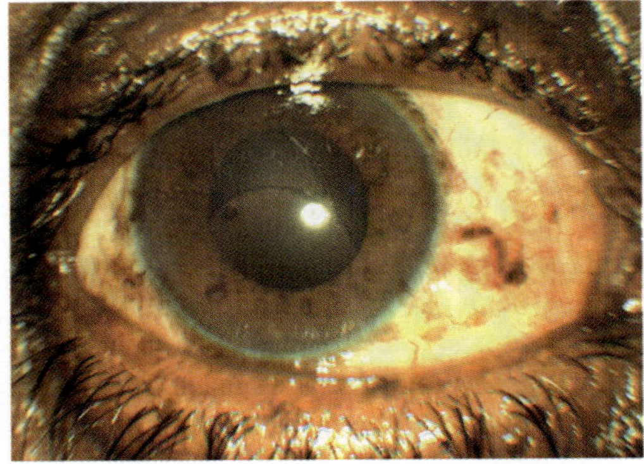

FIG. 8.4.10: Malposition of intraocular lens (IOL)

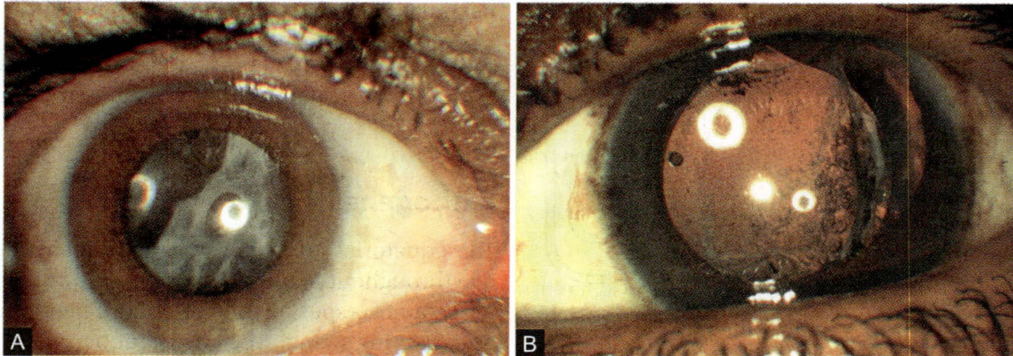

FIGS 8.4.11A and B: After cataract (the opacification of the posterior capsule behind the intraocular lens)

3. Soemmering's ring: Cells proliferate and get enclosed between two layers of lens capsule and appear like ring. It is seen in the periphery hence it will not affect vision.

Treatment*

1. After cataract is treated by neodymium yttrium-aluminum-garnet (Nd-YAG) capsulotomy—central part of the posterior capsule is removed by laser energy.
2. Dense membranous after cataract, which cannot be removed by laser, has to be treated by surgical posterior capsulotomy.

Prevention

- By reducing the source for after cataract by:
  - Complete removal of cortical matter
  - Polishing of the posterior capsule
  - Polishing of the under surface of the remaining anterior capsule to remove the anterior and equatorial epithelial cells.
- Reduce the stimulus for after cataract by:
  - Using biocompatible IOL to reduce stimulation of cellular proliferation.
- Prevent the after cataract from reaching posterior capsule by:
  - Using IOL with square truncated edges, which prevent migration of anterior epithelial cells posteriorly
  - Using biconvex IOL or planoconvex IOL with convexity toward the posterior capsule and placing it in the capsular bag, so that it obliterates the space between IOL and posterior capsule.

GIST BOX 8.4

- Cataract surgery is the most commonly performed eye surgery and it is one of the most commonly performed surgeries worldwide.
- The techniques for cataract surgery have undergone evolution starting from couching, which was practiced in the ancient times to the modern cataract surgery by phacoemulsification.
- Extracapsular cataract extraction (ECCE) is a surgical procedure for cataract where cataractous lens is removed leaving behind intact posterior capsule. Conventional ECCE, small incision cataract surgery (SICS) and phacoemulsification are the different types of ECCE.
- After cataract is also called posterior capsule opacification (PCO). After cataract is opacification of posterior capsule of the lens following ECCE.

CHAPTER

8.5 Lens-induced Glaucoma

DEFINITION***

Lens-induced glaucoma is a group of secondary glaucoma caused by the lens pathology (Figs 8.5.1A and B).

ETIOPATHOGENESIS

Lens-induced glaucoma can be either open-angle glaucoma or narrow-angle glaucoma, or combination of both mechanisms:

1. Open-angle glaucoma is caused by blockage of aqueous drainage system:
   a. Obstruction of trabecular meshwork by lens material and inflammatory cells as in phacolytic glaucoma, phacoanaphylactic glaucoma and lens particle glaucoma.
   b. Pupillary block caused by subluxated or dislocated lens.
2. Narrow-angle glaucoma is caused by direct mechanical closure of the angle of the anterior chamber as in phacomorphic glaucoma and dislocation of lens into anterior chamber.
3. Conditions causing glaucoma by open-angle mechanism will secondarily cause angle closure because of formation of synechiae due to inflammation resulting in synechial angle closure. Thus, resulting in combined mechanism glaucoma.

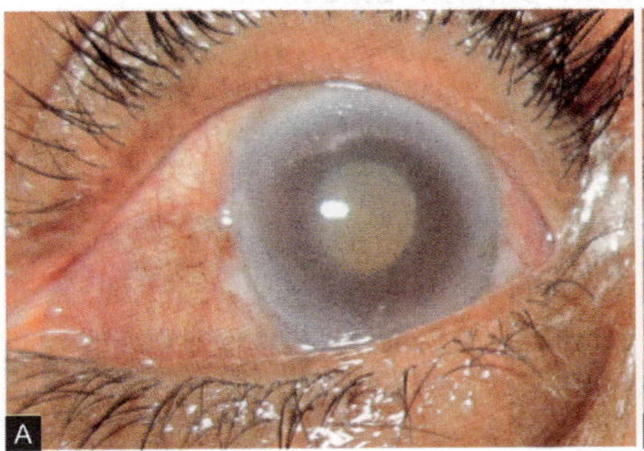

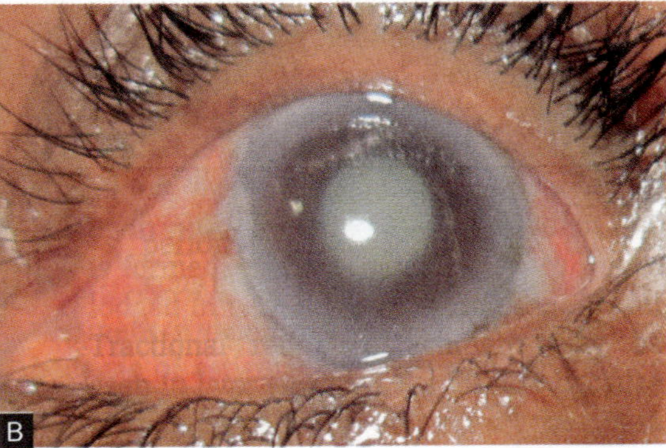

FIGS 8.5.1A and B: Lens-induced glaucoma

CLINICAL TYPES

Phacomorphic Glaucoma**

Phacomorphic glaucoma is a type of angle-closure lens-induced glaucoma caused by swollen or intumescent lens resulting in mechanical closure of the angle of the anterior chamber.

Clinical Features

1. Acute onset pain, redness superimposed on symptoms of cataract or dislocation of lens as in diminution of vision.
2. Examination reveals circumcorneal congestion, raised intraocular pressure (IOP), variable degrees of corneal edema, shallow anterior chamber and presence of intumescent cataractous lens or dislocated lens in anterior chamber.

Phacomorphic glaucoma has to be differentiated from pupillary block glaucoma, which can be caused by intumescent lens or dislocated lens. Peripheral iridotomy will relieve pupillary block and can distinguish it from phacomorphic glaucoma.

Treatment

1. Initial treatment is by reduction of raised IOP by medical management by using hyperosmotics such as mannitol, oral carbonic anhydrase inhibitors, e.g. acetazolamide and topical antiglaucoma drugs, beta blockers such as timolol 0.5% eyedrops.
2. Once raised IOP is controlled by medical management cataract surgery is done.
3. Long-standing cases, which may have led to secondary synechial angle closure may require filtration surgeries such as trabeculectomy depending on the amount of synechial angle closure.

Phacolytic Glaucoma**

Phacolytic glaucoma is a type of open-angle lens-induced glaucoma caused by obstruction of aqueous outflow in the trabecular meshwork by high-molecular weight lens proteins, which leak from microscopic defects in the intact capsule of mature or hypermature cataract. It is also called lens protein glaucoma.

Clinical Features

1. Acute onset pain, redness superimposed on symptoms of cataract, i.e. gradual progressive painless diminution of vision.
2. Examination reveals circumcorneal congestion, raised IOP, variable degrees of corneal edema, deep anterior chamber and presence of severe flare and cells in the anterior chamber.

Treatment

1. Initial treatment is by reduction of raised IOP and control of inflammation of eye. IOP is reduced by hyperosmotics—mannitol, oral carbonic anhydrase inhibitors such as acetazolamide and topical antiglaucoma drugs, beta blockers, e.g. timolol 0.5% eyedrops. Inflammation of the eye is treated by topical steroid eyedrops and oral steroids.
2. Once raised IOP is controlled by medical management, cataract surgery is done.

Lens-particle Glaucoma

Lens-particle glaucoma is a type of open-angle lens-induced glaucoma caused by obstruction of aqueous outflow in the trabecular meshwork by lens particles liberated into the anterior chamber following disruption of the lens capsule after cataract surgery or following trauma.

Clinical Features

Lens-particle glaucoma usually follows cataract surgery or history of trauma. Examination reveals circumcorneal congestion, raised IOP, variable degrees of corneal edema and presence of lens matter in the anterior chamber.

Treatment

Treatment is by the reduction of IOP with antiglaucoma drugs and removal of lens particles from anterior chamber by irrigation and aspiration.

Phacoanaphylactic Glaucoma

Phacoanaphylactic glaucoma is a type of open-angle lens-induced glaucoma caused by obstruction of aqueous outflow in the trabecular meshwork by lens particles liberated into the anterior chamber following disruption of the lens capsule and inflammatory cells in response to inflammatory reaction elicited by lens antigen.

> Lens antigen is sequestered antigen not exposed to the immune system, when lens antigen is liberated into anterior chamber following disruption of lens capsule induces granulomatous inflammation.

Clinical Features

1. It usually follows a latent period after cataract surgery or history of trauma during which sensitization to the liberated lens particles occur.
2. Examination shows circumcorneal congestion, raised IOP, variable degrees of corneal edema and signs of uveitis such as presence of keratic precipitates, hypopyon, posterior synechiae, cells and flare in the anterior chamber.

Treatment

Phacoanaphylactic glaucoma is similar to phacolytic glaucoma except that it requires more aggressive use of steroids to control granulomatous inflammation.

GLAUCOMA ASSOCIATED WITH ECTOPIA LENTIS

Glaucoma associated with ectopia lentis is the glaucoma resulting from subluxation or dislocation of lens. Glaucoma results from various mechanisms depending on the cause for ectopia lentis.

Pupillary Block Glaucoma

Pupillary block glaucoma is because of obstruction of the aqueous outflow from posterior chamber to anterior chamber through pupil because of pupillary block. It is commonly seen in cases of Weill-Marchesani syndrome because of microspherophakia or because of subluxation or dislocation of lens into pupil.

Abnormalities of the Angle of the Anterior Chamber

Abnormalities of the angle of the anterior chamber are associated with underlying causative diseases of ectopia lentis. Marfan's syndrome, one of the common causes of ectopia lentis, is usually associated with abnormalities of the angle of the anterior chamber like broad trabecular meshwork, dense iris processes.

Phacolytic Glaucoma

Dislocated lens into the anterior chamber may undergo degeneration resulting in liberation of lens proteins into anterior chamber, thus causing phacolytic glaucoma.

Traumatic Glaucoma

In cases of traumatic ectopia lentis, other associated factors seen along with trauma may be responsible for glaucoma as described in Chapter 9.6 'Secondary Glaucoma'.

DIFFERENCES BETWEEN VARIOUS TYPES OF LENS-INDUCED GLAUCOMA

The differences between various types of lens-induced glaucoma are discussed in Table 8.5.1.

TABLE 8.5.1: Differences between various types of lens-induced glaucoma

Features	*Phacomorphic glaucoma*	*Phacolytic glaucoma*	*Lens-particle glaucoma*	*Phacoanaphylactic glaucoma*
Type of glaucoma	Angle-closure glaucoma	Open-angle glaucoma	Open-angle glaucoma	Open-angle glaucoma
Mechanism	Mechanical closure of the angle of the anterior chamber by swollen lens	Obstruction of trabecular meshwork by lens proteins, which leak from microscopic defects in the intact capsule of mature or hypermature cataract	Obstruction of trabecular meshwork by lens particles liberated into the anterior chamber following disruption of the lens capsule after cataract surgery or following trauma	Obstruction of trabecular meshwork by lens particles liberated into the anterior chamber following disruption of the lens capsule and inflammatory cells in response to inflammatory reaction elicited by lens antigen
Symptoms	Pain, redness in a patient with history of cataract	Pain, redness in a patient with history of cataract	Pain, redness following cataract surgery or following trauma	Pain, redness following cataract surgery or following trauma and presence of latent period
Anterior chamber signs	Shallow anterior chamber	Deep anterior chamber with presence of cells and flare	Presence of lens particle in anterior chamber	Presence of lens particle in anterior chamber and signs of uveitis such as keratic precipitates, cells and flare, synechiae, hypopyon, etc.
Treatment	Reduction of raised intraocular pressure (IOP) followed by extraction of cataractous lens	Reduction of raised IOP and control of ocular inflammation followed by extraction of cataractous lens	Reduction of raised IOP followed by removal of lens particles from anterior chamber	Reduction of raised IOP and control of ocular inflammation followed by extraction of cataractous lens

GIST BOX 8.5

- Lens-induced glaucoma is a group of secondary glaucoma caused by lens pathology.
- Phacomorphic glaucoma is a type of angle-closure lens-induced glaucoma caused by swollen or intumescent lens resulting in mechanical closure of the angle of the anterior chamber.
- Phacolytic glaucoma is a type of open-angle lens-induced glaucoma caused by obstruction of aqueous outflow in the trabecular meshwork by high-molecular weight lens proteins, which leak from microscopic defects in the intact capsule of mature or hypermature cataract.
- Lens particle glaucoma is a type of open-angle lens-induced glaucoma caused by obstruction of aqueous outflow in the trabecular meshwork by lens particles liberated into the anterior chamber following disruption of the lens capsule after cataract surgery or following trauma.
- Phacoanaphylactic glaucoma is a type of open-angle lens-induced glaucoma caused by obstruction of aqueous outflow in the trabecular meshwork by lens particles liberated into the anterior chamber following disruption of the lens capsule and inflammatory cells in response to inflammatory reaction elicited by lens antigen.

CHAPTER

8.6 Ectopia Lentis

DEFINITION**

Displacement of lens from its normal position is called ectopia lentis. The causes include congenital and acquired. Congenital ectopia lentis is usually bilaterally symmetrical in both the eyes.

Ectopia lentis can be either subluxation or dislocation. Partial displacement of the lens due to partial zonular defect is called subluxation. In subluxation, lens is displaced sideways, but stays within the patellar fossa.

Complete displacement of the lens due to complete loss of zonular support is called dislocation or luxation. In dislocation lens is completely displaced out of the patellar fossa and lies either in the anterior chamber or in the vitreous chamber (Figs 8.6.1A to C, 8.6.2A and B).

ETIOLOGY

Simple Ectopia Lentis

Ectopia lentis without any ocular or systemic diseases is called simple ectopia lentis. It is transmitted as autosomal dominant inherited condition.

Ectopia Lentis et Pupillae

Ectopia lentis associated with abnormality of pupil, normal round pupil being replaced by slit-shaped pupil or oval-shaped pupil. Pupil is displaced in the direction opposite to that of lens. It is transmitted as autosomal recessive inherited condition.

ECTOPIA LENTIS ASSOCIATED WITH SYSTEMIC CONDITIONS

Ectopia lentis is associated with systemic conditions as follows:

- Marfan's syndrome
- Homocystinuria
- Weill-Marchesani syndrome
- Hyperlysinemia
- Ehlers-Danlos syndrome
- Sulfite oxidase deficiency
- Crouzon's syndrome
- Refsum's syndrome.

Marfan's Syndrome*

Autosomal dominant disorder characterized by skeletal, cardiovascular and ocular features:

- Skeletal abnormalities include long thin extremities, hyperextensibility of joints, arachnodactyly and scoliosis of spine
- Cardiovascular abnormalities include dissecting aortic aneurysm and dilatation of the aortic valve
- Ocular abnormalities include bilateral down and out subluxation of lens. Subluxation is usually stable and nonprogressive (Fig. 8.6.3).

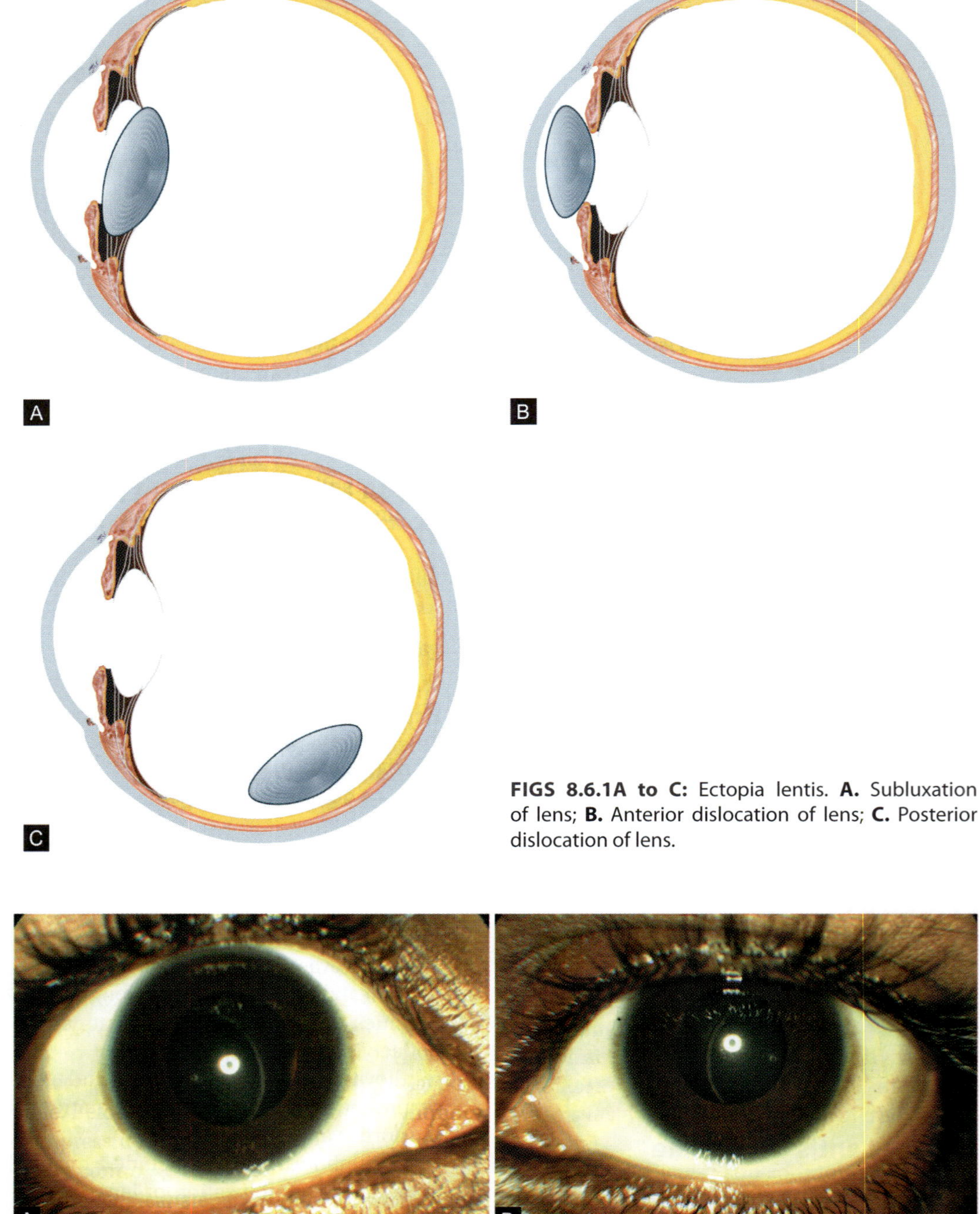

FIGS 8.6.1A to C: Ectopia lentis. **A.** Subluxation of lens; **B.** Anterior dislocation of lens; **C.** Posterior dislocation of lens.

FIGS 8.6.2A and B: Bilateral subluxation of lens

Homocystinuria*

Homocystinuria is an autosomal recessive disorder due to deficiency of enzyme cystathione synthetase affecting the metabolism of sulfur containing amino acids, e.g. methionine resulting in increased urinary excretion of homocystine. Since the zonules of lens have a high concentration of cysteine normally, deficiency of cysteine makes the zonules weak resulting in subluxation of the lens:

1. *Ocular features:* It include subluxation of lens downward and nasally. It is usually progressive resulting in the complete dislocation of lens later (Fig. 8.6.4).
2. *Systemic features:* It include mental retardation, skin abnormalities such as malar flush, increased thromboembolic phenomenon due to increased platelet stickiness, skeletal abnormalities similar to Marfan's syndrome such as arachnodactyly.

Weill-Marchesani Syndrome

Autosomal recessive disorder characterized by:

1. *Systemic features:* It like short stature, stubby fingers, short broad extremities, stiff joints, mental retardation.
2. *Ocular features:* It include microspherophakia and forward subluxation of lens causing pupillary block glaucoma.

Ehlers-Danlos Syndrome

Ehlers-Danlos syndrome is a rare inherited syndrome characterized by:

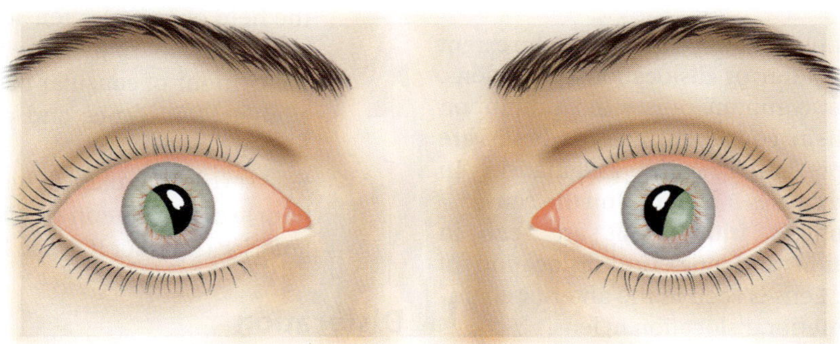

FIG. 8.6.3: Bilateral down and out subluxation of lens

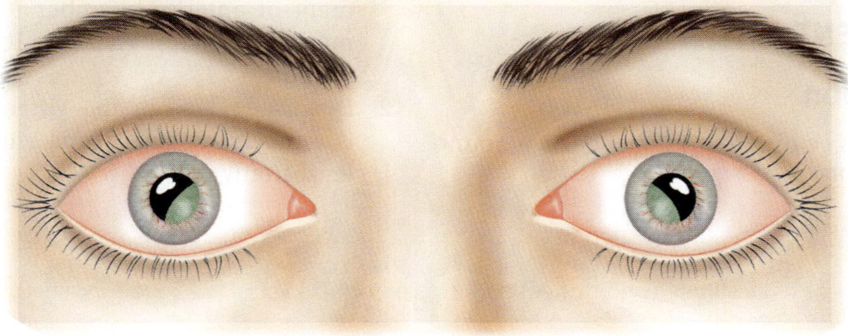

FIG. 8.6.4: Bilateral down and in subluxation of lens

1. *Ocular features:* Subluxation of lens, blue sclera (sclera thinning), keratoconus.
2. *Systemic features:* It include hyperextensibility of joints and hyperstretchability of skin.

Acquired Causes for Subluxation or Dislocation of Lens*

- Trauma (most common cause).
- Spontaneous lens dislocation because of stretching of the zonules or degeneration of zonules as in:
  - Hypermature cataract.
  - High myopia.
  - Buphthalmos.
  - Chronic uveitis.
  - Keratoglobus.
  - Intraocular tumors.
  - Aniridia.
  - Coloboma of iris and ciliary body.

CLINICAL FEATURES

1. Diminution of vision depends on the extent of subluxation or dislocation of the lens. The most common causes for diminution of vision in congenital ectopia lentis are amblyopia and irregular astigmatism. In acquired causes it depends on the cause.
2. Phacodonesis, iridodonesis are seen in subluxation and posterior dislocation of the lens. Lens is seen in the anterior chamber in anterior dislocation of lens.
3. Examination for associated ocular features and systemic features should be done in all the cases for the congenital and acquired causes.

TREATMENT

Subluxation

Treatment of ectopia lentis depends on amount of subluxation:

1. Minimal subluxation of lens is managed by periodic follow-up in cases of progressive ectopia lentis.
2. Subluxation of lens causing visual disturbances due to astigmatism is managed by refraction and correction.
3. Subluxation of lens causing visual disturbance and diplopia because of partly aphakic zone and partly phakic zone is treated by Nd-YAG laser iridoplasty to enlarge the aphakic zone and treatment of aphakia by aphakic correction.
4. Subluxated cataractous lens is treated by extracapsular cataract extraction and intraocular lens (IOL) placement:
   a. For minimal zonular dehiscence (< 3 hour) placement of IOL in ciliary sulcus for minimal subluxation is advised.
   b. For moderate zonular dehiscence (3–5 hour) placement of IOL is done with the help of capsular tension ring (capsular tension ring helps to maintain the contour of capsular bag in cases of zonular dehiscence and prevents IOL decentration).
   c. For severe zonular dehiscence (> 5 hour) scleral fixation of IOL is done or anterior chamber IOL can be used.

Dislocation

Dislocated lens should always be removed by appropriate surgical technique:

1. Dislocated lens in anterior chamber is removed by extraction of the lens and placement of anterior chamber IOL or placement of posterior chamber IOL by scleral fixation.
2. Dislocated lens in the vitreous chamber is removed by pars plana vitrectomy and lensectomy.

GIST BOX 8.6

- Displacement of lens from its normal position is called ectopia lentis. The causes include congenital and acquired.
- Ectopia lentis can be either subluxation or dislocation.
- Trauma is the commonest acquired cause for ectopia lentis.

FREQUENTLY ASKED QUESTIONS (FAQs)

*Short Answers

1. Histology of lens.
2. Metabolism of lens.
3. Embryology of lens.
4. Microspherophakia.
5. Coloboma of lens.
6. Zonular cataract.
7. Drug-induced cataract.
8. Heat cataract.
9. Hypermature cataract.
10. Intumescent cataract.
11. Mention the methods of nucleus removal in small incision cataract surgery.
12. Mention the causes for postoperative shallow anterior chamber after cataract surgery.
13. Mention the complications of hypermature cataract.
14. Classify intraocular lenses (IOLs).
15. Mention the different types of IOL.
16. Sterilization of intraocular lens.
17. Mention the materials used for manufacturing IOL.
18. Mention the types of after cataract.
19. Treatment of after cataract.
20. Mention the ocular manifestations of Marfan's syndrome.
21. Mention the causes for acquired ectopia lentis.
22. Mention the advantages and disadvantages of phacoemulsification.
23. Mention the different types of anesthesia used for different techniques of cataract surgery.

**Short Essays

1. Mention the classification of cataract.
2. Describe the management of congenital and developmental cataract.
3. Describe the clinical types of congenital and developmental cataract.
4. Nuclear cataract.
5. Presenile cataract.
6. Complicated cataract.
7. Diabetic cataract.
8. Metabolic cataract.
9. Retinal and macular function tests.
10. IOL power calculation.
11. Couching.
12. Intracapsular cataract extraction (ICCE).
13. Recent advances in cataract surgery.
14. Postoperative management after cataract surgery.
15. Early postoperative complications of cataract surgery.
16. Late postoperative complications of cataract surgery.
17. Postoperative endophthalmitis.
18. IOL.
19. Describe the IOL-related complications after cataract surgery.
20. After cataract.
21. Phacomorphic glaucoma.
22. Phacolytic glaucoma.
23. Ectopia lentis.

***Long Essays

1. Define cataract. Describe etiology, pathogenesis and clinical features of senile cataract.
2. Describe the etiology, clinical features and treatment of congenital, and developmental cataract.
3. Define senile cataract. Describe the etiology, clinical features and management of senile cataract.
4. Describe the preoperative investigations of cataract surgery and methods of calculation of IOL power.
5. Mention the different techniques of cataract surgery. Describe the steps of small incision cataract surgery.
6. Define and classify extracapsular cataract extraction (ECCE). Describe the steps of phacoemulsification.
7. Describe the postoperative complications of cataract surgery.
8. Define lens-induced glaucoma. Describe the etiopathogenesis, clinical features and treatment of lens-induced glaucoma.

BIBLIOGRAPHY

1. Angra SK, Gupta S, Dada VK, et al. Coloboma of lens. Indian J Ophthalmol. 1984;32(1):21-2.
2. Bavbek T, Ogüt MS, Kazokoglu H. Congenital lens coloboma and associated pathologies. Doc Ophthalmol. 1993;83(4):313-22.
3. Bhattacharjee H, Bhattacharjee K, Medhi J, et al. Clear lens extraction and intraocular lens implantation in a case of microspherophakia with secondary angle closure glaucoma. Indian J Ophthalmol. 2010;58(1):67-70.
4. Bhattacharjee K, Bhattacharjee H, Bhattacharjee P. Lens subluxation and its management. In: Dutta LC (Ed). Modern Ophthalmology, vol. 2, 3rd edition. New Delhi: Jaypee Brothers Medical Publishers (P) Ltd; 2005.
5. Damji KF, Freedman SF, Moroi SE, et al. Shields' Textbook of Glaucoma, 5th edition. China: Lippincott Williams & Wilkins; 2011.
6. Durcan JF. Lens induced glaucoma. In: Morrison JC, Pollack IP (Eds). Glaucoma: Science and Practice. Hong Kong: Thieme Medical Publishers, Inc; 2002.
7. Dutta LC. Modern Ophthalmology, vol. 1, 3rd edition. New Delhi: Jaypee Brothers Medical Publishers (P) Ltd; 2005.
8. Goyal M, Hogeweg M. Couching and cataract extraction a clinic based study in northern Nigeria. Comm Eye Health. 1997;10(21):6-7.
9. John SR, Chakrabarti M, Chakraborty A. Management of subluxated lenses. Kerala Journal of Ophthalmology. 2009;21(2);163-70.
10. Khurana AK, Indu khurana. Anatomy & Physiology of Eye, 2nd edition. New Delhi: CBS Publishers and Distributors; 2007.
11. Mukherjee PK. Pediatric Ophthalmology. New Delhi: New Age International Publishers Private Limited; 2005. pp. 303-46.
12. Ravishankar K, Garg D. Phacoemulsification in difficult situations. In: LC Dutta (Ed). Modern Ophthalmology, vol. 1, 3rd edition. New Delhi: Jaypee Brothers Medical Publishers; 2005.
13. Yanoff M, Duker JS. Ophthalmology, 3rd edition. China: Mosby Elsevier Inc; 2006.

SECTION 9

Glaucoma

CHAPTER

9.1 Anatomy and Physiology of Glaucoma

Glaucoma is a heterogeneous group of diseases characterized by damage to retinal ganglion cells and axons. Multiple factors are responsible for glaucomatous damage of which raised intraocular pressure (IOP) is considered as prime factor.

The pathophysiology of glaucoma is unique when compared to other ophthalmic diseases, as it involves the structures in both anterior and posterior segment of the eye. The pathophysiology of glaucoma involves aqueous humor production and aqueous outflow system in anterior segment, and it involves retinal ganglion cells and axons in the posterior segment, the damage to which leads to the characteristic optic disk changes and visual field defects.

AQUEOUS HUMOR

Aqueous humor is a transparent, colorless fluid present in the anterior and posterior chamber of the eye.

Functions*

1. Aqueous humor maintains IOP.
2. Being clear and transparent it forms part of optical medium of eye.
3. It provides essential nutrition and oxygen, and washes away metabolic waste products from avascular structures of the eye such as cornea, lens and anterior vitreous.
4. Because of presence of immunoglobulins aqueous humor plays a defensive or protective role.

Production of Aqueous Humor*

Aqueous humor is produced from ciliary body. Aqueous is derived from plasma within the capillary network of the ciliary processes and it is secreted into posterior chamber of the eye. Aqueous humor is produced from plasma by:

- Diffusion
- Ultrafiltration
- Active transport or secretion.

Diffusion

Diffusion is a passive mechanism in which lipid-soluble substances are transported across the cell membrane.

Ultrafiltration

Ultrafiltration is a passive mechanism in which water and water-soluble substances are transported across the cell membrane through micropores in the cell membrane in response to an osmotic gradient.

Active Transport

Active transport is active secretion of substances across the cell membrane.

The rate of formation of aqueous humor is 2.4 μL/min. The volume of aqueous humor is 310 μL (0.31 mL) with 250 μL (0.25 mL) in anterior chamber and 60 μL (0.6 mL) in posterior chamber.

Drainage of Aqueous Humor*

The aqueous humor is secreted into the posterior chamber and from posterior chamber it enters the anterior chamber through the pupil (through the space between iris and lens). From anterior chamber of the eye, aqueous humor flows out of the eye by two routes (Fig. 9.1.1).

Conventional Outflow

Conventional outflow is via trabecular meshwork present in the angle of the anterior chamber. It is the major drainage route for aqueous humor accounting for 80–90% of aqueous outflow.

Trabecular meshwork is a layer of connective tissue present in the angle of the anterior chamber. Trabecular meshwork consists of uveal meshwork, corneoscleral meshwork and juxtacanalicular meshwork:

1. Uveal meshwork is the innermost part of the trabecular meshwork. It consists of trabecular bands with irregular pores measuring about 25–75 μm extending from the iris root and ciliary body to Schwalbe's line.
2. Corneoscleral meshwork is the middle part of the trabecular meshwork. It consists of trabecular bands with elliptical openings measuring about 5–50 μm extending from the scleral spur to the scleral sulcus.
3. Juxtacanalicular meshwork is the outermost part of the trabecular meshwork. It is composed of a connective tissue core lined on either side by endothelium. The outer endothelial layer is continuous with the inner wall of Schlemm's canal. It is the site, which accounts for major resistance to aqueous outflow.

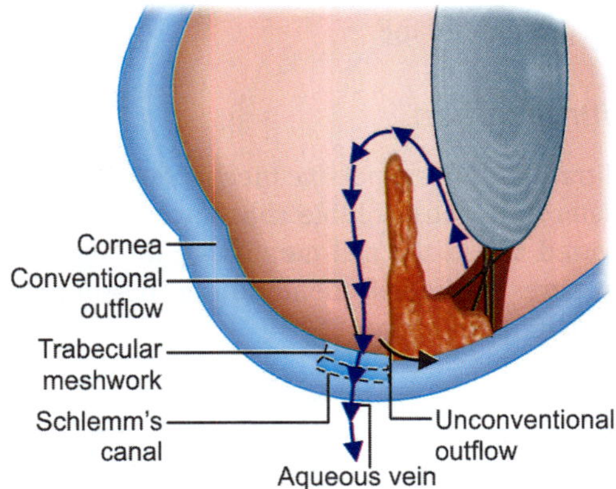

FIG. 9.1.1: Drainage of aqueous humor

From trabecular meshwork, aqueous enters into Schlemm's canal. Schlemm's canal is an endothelium lined collecting duct present in the scleral sulcus. Aqueous is drained from Schlemm's canal into episcleral veins via collector channels. Episcleral veins drain into anterior ciliary and superior ophthalmic veins, which ultimately drain aqueous humor into cavernous sinus.

Unconventional Outflow

Unconventional outflow is also called uveoscleral outflow and it accounts for 10–20% of aqueous outflow. Aqueous drainage occurs through ciliary body to suprachoroidal space and supraciliary space. From suprachoroidal and supraciliary spaces aqueous is drained by the veins in the ciliary body and choroid.

ANATOMY OF ANGLE OF ANTERIOR CHAMBER

The space between the root of the iris and peripheral cornea is called angle of the anterior chamber. Trabecular meshwork and Schlemm's canal lie in the angle of the anterior chamber, which is responsible for conventional drainage of aqueous humor. Hence, it is also called filtration angle.

The structures of the angle of the anterior chamber are not visible to naked eye during examination because of overhanging scleral shelf, which obscures the view of the angle of anterior chamber and total internal reflection that occurs as the angle of incidence of the rays from the angle of the anterior chamber is more than the critical angle.

Angle of the anterior chamber is examined by gonioscopy.

Structures of the Angle of Anterior Chamber*

The structures of the angle of the anterior chamber from anterior to posterior are (Fig. 9.1.2):

1. *Schwalbe's line:* It represents the termination of Descemet's membrane of cornea.
2. *Trabecular meshwork:* It is the layer of connective tissue, which consists of pores for the drainage of aqueous.
3. *Scleral spur:* It is the posterior lip of the scleral spur. It provides attachment to meridional fibers of ciliary body.
4. *Ciliary body band:* It is the part of ciliary body, which is visible anterior to the insertion of iris.
5. *Root of the iris:* It is the outer margin of the iris, which is attached to the ciliary body.

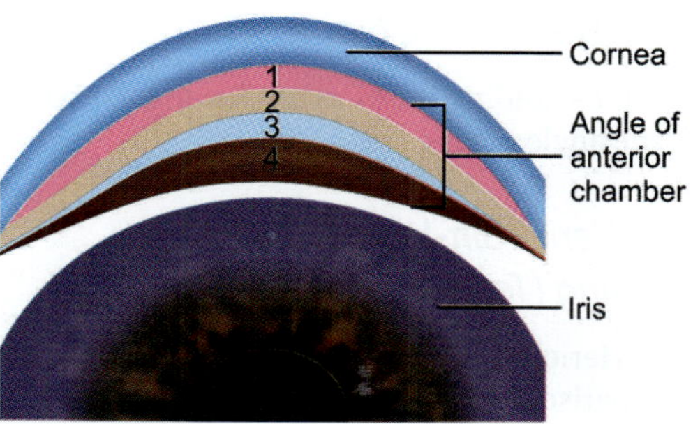

FIG. 9.1.2: Structures of the angle of anterior chamber. 1. Schwalbe's line; 2. Trabecular meshwork; 3. Scleral spur; 4. Ciliary body.

Grading of the Angle of Anterior Chamber (Fig. 9.1.3)*

Scheie's Grading (Table 9.1.1)

Scheie's grading is based on the structures visualized on gonioscopy.

TABLE 9.1.1: Scheie's grading

Grade	*Findings*	*Remarks*
Grade 0	All structures visible	Wide open angle
Grade 1	Root of the iris not visible	Open angle
Grade 2	Ciliary body band not visible	Narrow angle
Grade 3	Posterior trabecular meshwork not visible	Extremely narrow angle
Grade 4	Only Schwalbe's line visible	Closed angle

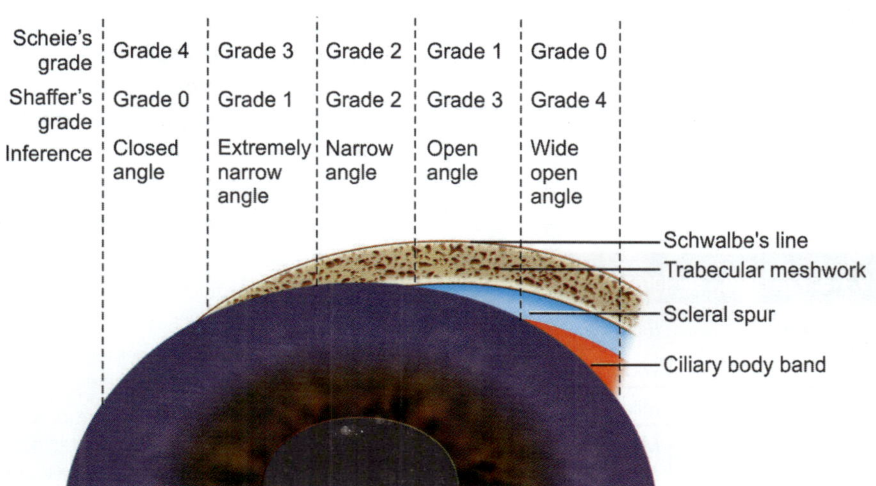

FIG. 9.1.3: Grading of the angle of anterior chamber

Shaffer's Grading (Table 9.1.2)

Shaffer's grading is based on the angular width of the angle recess.

Van Herick Slit-lamp Grading (Table 9.1.3)

Van Herick slit-lamp grading is based on the comparison between the peripheral anterior chamber (PAC) depth and corneal thickness (CT). It is done by focusing a narrow slit beam at a 60° angle across the peripheral part of the cornea and by comparing the peripheral anterior chamber depth to the corneal thickness.

INTRAOCULAR PRESSURE**

Definition

Intraocular pressure is defined as pressure exerted by fluids inside the eyeball.

Elevated IOP is considered as the most important factor in pathogenesis of glaucoma. Reduction of IOP is the only effective known treatment available to prevent the progression of the disease.

TABLE 9.1.2: Shaffer's grading

Grade	*Findings*	*Remarks*
Grade 4	35°–45° angle	Wide open angle
Grade 3	20°–35° angle	Open angle
Grade 2	20° angle	Narrow angle
Grade 1	10° angle	Extremely narrow angle
Grade 0	0° angle	Angle closed

TABLE 9.1.3: Van Herick slit-lamp grading

Grade	*Findings*	*Remarks*
Grade 4	PAC* > ½ CT†	Wide open angle
Grade 3	PAC = ¼–½ CT	Mild narrow angle
Grade 2	PAC = ¼ CT	Moderately narrow angle
Grade 1	PAC < CT	Severely narrow angle

*PAC, peripheral anterior chamber; †CT, corneal thickness.

The IOP is determined by the equilibrium between the production and drainage of aqueous humor. An IOP between 10 and 21 mm Hg with a mean IOP of 16 mm Hg with standard deviation of 3 mm Hg is considered as normal IOP.

Factors Influencing IOP

1. *Age:* Intraocular pressure increases with increasing age.
2. *Gender:* The IOP is higher in females compared to males, more so in the elderly age group.
3. *Diurnal variation:* Normally, the IOP is elevated early in the morning and decreases as the day progresses, and it is usually at its lowest level during night. In normal individuals, the diurnal variation is within 5 mm Hg. This will be in the range of 5–10 mm Hg in patients with glaucoma.
4. *Blood pressure:* Increased IOP is found in hypertensives compared to normotensives.
5. *Anesthetics:* Most anesthetic agents lowers IOP except ketamine, a dissociative anesthetic agent causes transient rise in IOP when administered by intravenous (IV) route.
6. *Exercise:* Regular exercise tends to lower the IOP.
7. *Drugs:* Corticosteroids tends to increase IOP and antiglaucoma drugs lowers the IOP.
8. *Fluid intake:* This decreases osmolarity of plasma and increases IOP.
9. *Alcohol:* Consumption of alcohol decreases IOP.

Methods of Measurement of IOP/Tonometry**

Digital tonometry: A crude method of measuring the IOP is by feeling the fluctuation produced by indentation of the globe by finger.

Indentation tonometry: Measurement of IOP by indentation tonometer, Schiotz tonometer.

Applanation tonometry: Measurement of IOP by applanation tonometer, Goldmann tonometer (gold standard and the most accurate method), Perkin's tonometer.

Non-contact tonometry: Measurement of IOP by non-contact method by using air puff tonometers.

Indentation Tonometry**

Indentation tonometry is done by using Schiotz tonometer.

Principle

Indentation tonometry works on the principle of indentation. A fluid-filled sphere when indented by a plunger, the plunger will indent the sphere till the pressure of the plunger equals the pressure inside the sphere.

Technique of Schiotz Indentation Tonometry

1. Schiotz indentation tonometry is done under topical anesthesia with 4% lignocaine eyedrops with patient lying in supine position.
2. The foot plate of the Schiotz tonometer is placed gently over the cornea and the deflection of the indicator on the scale is noted.
3. Procedure is started with the fixed 5.5 g weight, if the deflection is less than 3 on the scale, 7.5 g, 10 g, 15 g weights one after the other are used and the average of the three readings is taken as mean IOP.
4. The IOP in mm Hg is derived by comparing the scale reading and plunger weight using Friedenwald nomogram, a conversion table.

Disadvantages

Indentation is influenced by scleral rigidity; hence, it is not an accurate method. Scleral rigidity is influenced by several factors. It is decreased in high myopia and following intraocular surgeries. It is increased in hypermetropia.

Advantages

As it is cheaper and easy to use, it continues to be in use in spite of the drawbacks.

Applanation Tonometry**

Goldmann Applanation Tonometer

Principle

Goldmann applanation tonometer is based on Imbert-Fick law. It states that the pressure inside the sphere (P) is equal to the force necessary to flatten the surface (F) divided by the area of flattening (A). It can be expressed as:

$$P = F/A$$

Technique

1. Goldmann applanation tonometer is done under topical anesthesia with 4% lignocaine eyedrops; it requires the tear film to be stained with fluorescein and it is done using slit lamp.
2. Topical anesthesia is achieved by 4% lignocaine and the tear film is stained with fluorescein.
3. Patient is seated in front of the slit lamp and asked to look straight ahead with both eyes kept wide open.
4. Biprisms are illuminated from slit lamp with light intensity kept to maximum with cobalt blue filter.
5. Slit lamp is moved forward till the biprism touches the cornea in the center.
6. When the prisms touch the cornea, two semicircles are seen through the eye piece of slit lamp and the applanation force is adjusted till the inner edges of the semicircles touch.
7. The IOP is derived by multiplying the reading on the dial by 10.

Advantages

Goldmann applanation tonometer is the most accurate method considered as gold standard for measurement of IOP because it is not affected by scleral rigidity.

Other Applanation Tonometers

- Perkins hand-held applanation tonometer
- Air-puff tonometer
- Tono-Pen
- Non-contact tonometer.

OPTIC DISK

Glaucoma is characterized by optic neuropathy and irreversible visual field defects because of damage to the retinal ganglion cells. Examination of optic disk forms a vital part of examination in glaucoma to diagnose the disease as well as to study the progression of the disease and response to treatment.

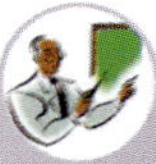

Examination of Optic Disk

It is done by:
- Direct ophthalmoscope.
- Indirect ophthalmoscope.
- Slit-lamp biomicroscopic examination of optic disk by using 78 D lens, 90 D lens, Hruby lens, Goldmann lens and Zeis lens.

Features of Normal Optic Disk (Fig. 9.1.4)

1. Shape and color: Normal optic disk is vertically oval in shape and normally it is orange to pink in color.
2. Size: Normal size of optic disk varies from individual to individuals with average horizontal dimension of 1.75 mm and vertical dimension of 1.90 mm.

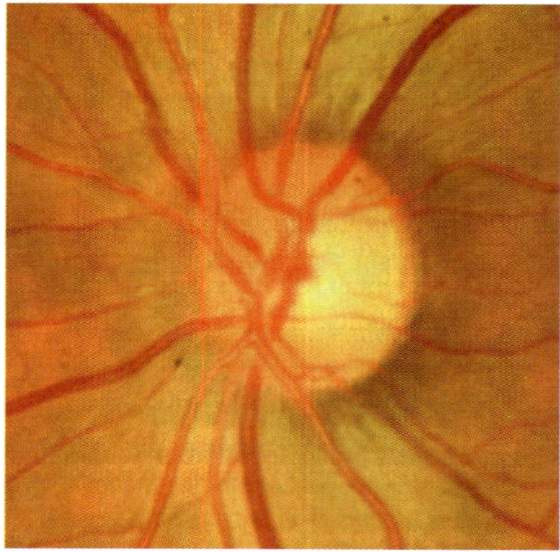

FIG. 9.1.4: Normal optic disk

3. Cup: Normal depression present in the center of the disk is called cup. The size of the cup depends on the size of scleral canal and the number of retinal nerve fibers passing through it.
4. Neuroretinal rim: It is the area between the margin of the cup and the margin of the disk. It represents the retinal nerve fibers. Normally, the rim is widest **I**nferiorly followed by **S**uperior, **N**asal and **T**emporal zone (ISNT rule). Normally, the neuroretinal rim will not show any thinning, notching or hemorrhages.
5. Cup-to-disk ratio (CD ratio): Normal CD ratio is 0.3 or less. It depends on the width of scleral canal and the width of neuroretinal rim.
6. Normally, the size of the disk, size of the cup, CD ratio and neuroretinal rim will be symmetrical in both eyes.

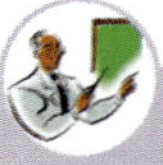

Pathogenesis of Optic Nerve Damage in Glaucoma**

It is characterized by retinal ganglion cell death, occurs by apoptosis as a result of increase in intracellular nitric oxide and glutamate. This is initiated by mechanical factors, vascular factors and cellular factors.

Mechanical factors: Misalignment of the pores of the lamina cribrosa because of posterior bowing of lamina cribrosa in response to raised IOP. The axons of the optic nerve are damaged as they pass through the misaligned pores of lamina cribrosa by direct mechanical compression or by blockage of retrograde axoplasmic flow resulting in deposition of extracellular materials such as glutamate causing death of retinal ganglion cells.

Vascular factors: Ischemia of the optic nerve head and decreased optic nerve head perfusion because of compression of blood vessels supplying the optic nerve head leading to interference with the delivery of nutrients or removal of metabolic products.

Cellular factors: Astrocytes are found along with axons in the optic nerve and are essential for survival of retinal ganglion cells. Loss of astrocytes or dysfunction of the astrocytes in response to mechanical and vascular factors results in damage of the optic nerve by increasing levels of neurotoxic nitric oxide.

VISUAL FIELD

Normal visual field is defined by Traquair as 'island of vision in a sea of blindness'. The peak of the island, which represents the highest visual acuity is because of fovea and the bottomless pit with no vision is because of optic disk, called blind spot.

The normal visual field extends 60° superiorly and nasally, 70° inferiorly and 90° temporally. The area of maximum visual acuity is the point of fixation and is represented by fovea. Blind spot is the nonseeing or blind area within the visual field corresponding to optic disk. Blind spot is located 15° temporal to the point of fixation.

Visual field and retina have got inverted and reversed relationship. Inferior retina is represented by superior visual field and vice versa. Similarly, nasal retina is represented by temporal visual field and vice versa. This also explains the relation of blind spot in relation to fovea (though optic disk lies nasal to fovea on visual field it lies temporal to fovea).

Measurement of visual field is helpful in diagnosing glaucoma, staging the severity of glaucoma and knowing the response to treatment and progression of glaucoma.

Measurement of Visual Field

Visual field is measured by:
- Confrontation method.
- Perimetry.

Standard automated perimetry is the standard method used to measure visual field in glaucoma. Humphery Field Analyzer and Octopus are the two types of automated perimeters available. Short-wavelength automated perimetry (SWAP) using blue stimulus on yellow background and frequency doubling technology (FDT) are the recent testing methods employed.

Anatomical Basis of Glaucomatous Visual Field Defects*

1. *Arrangement of retinal nerve fibers explain the anatomical basis of visual field defects (Fig. 9.1.5)*:
   a. Retinal nerve fibers from the macula reach the optic disk through a horizontal path called papillomacular bundle.
   b. Retinal nerve fibers from the temporal part of the retina reach the optic disk by arching above and below the papillomacular bundle called superior and inferior arcuate fibers.

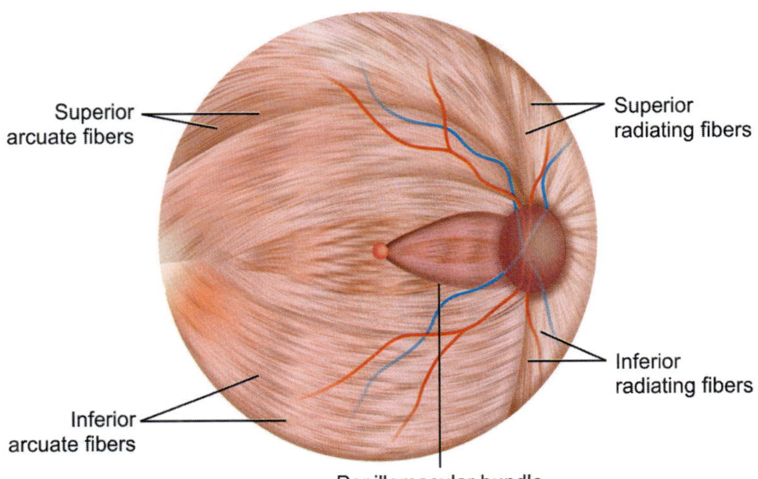

FIG. 9.1.5: Arrangement of retinal nerve fibers

c. Retinal nerve fibers from the nasal part of the retina reach the optic disk directly as superior radiating fibers and inferior radiating fibers.

2. *Susceptibility of retinal nerve fibers to glaucomatous damage:*
   a. The arcuate fibers are most susceptible to glaucomatous damage explaining the paracentral scotoma, Seidel's scotoma and Bjerrum's scotoma early in the disease.
   b. The macular fibers are most resistant to glaucomatous damage explaining the persistence of central vision till the late advanced stages of glaucoma.

RETINAL NERVE FIBER LAYER ANALYSIS

Retinal nerve fiber layer analysis helps in early detection of glaucoma as retinal nerve fiber layer damage is the earliest event to occur preceding the irreversible changes in optic disk and visual field. In fact, the detectable visual field loss is seen only after 30–40% of retinal nerve fiber layer is damaged. It is done by:

- Optical coherence tomography (OCT)
- Scanning laser polarimetry: GDx analyzer
- Confocal scanning laser ophthalmoscopy: Heidelberg retinal tomograph (HRT).

GIST BOX 9.1

- Glaucoma is a heterogeneous group of diseases characterized by damage to retinal ganglion cells and axons.
- Aqueous humor is transparent, colorless fluid present in the anterior and posterior chamber of the eye. Aqueous humor maintains intraocular pressure (IOP).
- Aqueous humor is produced from plasma by ciliary processes by diffusion, ultrafiltration and active transport or secretion.
- The aqueous humor is secreted into the posterior chamber; from posterior chamber it enters the anterior chamber through the pupil (through the space between iris and lens). From anterior chamber of the eye, aqueous humor flows out of the eye by two routes, conventional outflow via trabecular meshwork accounting for 80–90% of outflow and uveoscleral outflow accounting for 10% of outflow.
- The space between the root of the iris and peripheral cornea is called angle of the anterior chamber. The structures of the angle of the anterior chamber from anterior to posterior are Schwalbe's line, trabecular meshwork, scleral spur, ciliary body band and root of the iris.
- Intraocular pressure is defined as pressure exerted by fluids inside the eyeball. Elevated intraocular pressure is considered as the most important factor in pathogenesis of glaucoma. Reduction of IOP is the only known effective treatment available to prevent the progression of the disease.

CHAPTER

9.2 Introduction and Classification of Glaucoma

DEFINITIONS

Glaucoma**

Glaucoma indicates group of diseases characterized by characteristic optic nerve damage and irreversible visual field defects caused by either raised or normal intraocular pressure (IOP).

Ocular Hypertension

Presence of raised IOP along with absence of the characteristic optic nerve damage and visual field defects seen in glaucoma is called ocular hypertension.

Normal Intraocular Pressure

Intraocular pressure in the range of 10–21 mm Hg is considered as normal IOP.

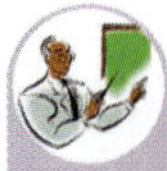

Magnitude of Glaucoma

Glaucoma is the second commonest cause of blindness and leading cause of irreversible blindness worldwide. It affects about 70 million people worldwide.

Glaucoma is called silent thief of sight as in most cases it will cause painless, gradually progressive irreversible loss of vision.

CLASSIFICATION OF GLAUCOMA**

Glaucoma is classified on the basis of etiology and pathogenesis/mechanism of glaucoma.

Etiological Classification of Glaucoma

Based on the etiology, glaucoma is classified into:

1. *Childhood glaucoma:*
   a. Primary congenital glaucoma.
   b. Developmental glaucoma.
   c. Secondary glaucoma.
2. *Adult glaucoma:*
   a. Primary open-angle glaucoma.
   b. Primary angle-closure glaucoma.
   c. Secondary glaucoma.

Classification of Glaucoma Based on the Mechanism

Open-angle Glaucoma

Open-angle glaucoma is associated with open angle and the cause for rise in IOP is assumed to be because of increased resistance to aqueous outflow in the trabecular meshwork. Open-angle glaucoma can be primary or secondary.

Primary open-angle glaucoma: It is open-angle glaucoma, which is not associated with any known ocular or systemic disorder that causes increased resistance to aqueous outflow.

Secondary open-angle glaucoma: It is open-angle glaucoma, which is associated with known ocular or systemic disorder that causes increased resistance to aqueous outflow.

Pigmentary glaucoma, pseudoexfoliation glaucoma, phacolytic glaucoma, steroid-induced glaucoma, etc. are examples for secondary open-angle glaucoma because of associated with ocular disease.

Angle-closure Glaucoma

Angle-closure glaucoma is associated with either shallow/closed angle or pupillary block causing gradual shallowing of the anterior chamber leading to aqueous outflow obstruction. Angle-closure glaucoma can be primary or secondary.

Primary angle-closure glaucoma: It is angle-closure glaucoma, which is not associated with any known ocular or systemic disorders.

Secondary angle-closure glaucoma: It is angle-closure glaucoma, which is associated with known ocular or systemic disorder that causes shallowing of the anterior chamber (e.g. phacomorphic glaucoma, glaucoma caused by microspherophakia) or closure of the angle of the anterior chamber (e.g. neovascular glaucoma).

Combined-mechanism Glaucoma

Combined-mechanism glaucoma is a type of glaucoma, which results from both because of increased resistance to aqueous outflow in the trabecular meshwork as in open-angle glaucoma and closure of the angle of the anterior chamber as in angle-closure glaucoma.

GIST BOX 9.2

- Glaucoma indicates group of diseases characterized by characteristic optic nerve damage and irreversible visual field defects caused by either raised or normal intraocular pressure (IOP).
- Presence of raised IOP along with absence of the characteristic optic nerve damage and visual field defects seen in glaucoma is called ocular hypertension.

CHAPTER

9.3 Childhood Glaucoma

Childhood glaucoma include:

- Primary congenital glaucoma
- Developmental glaucoma
- Secondary glaucoma.

PRIMARY CONGENITAL GLAUCOMA***

Definition

Primary congenital glaucoma is defined as a glaucoma caused by aqueous outflow obstruction due to maldevelopment of the angle of the anterior chamber without other ocular and systemic abnormalities.

Etiology

- The incidence of congenital glaucoma is 1 in 10,000
- More common in males than females with 65% being seen in boys
- About 70% of the cases are bilateral
- Most cases are sporadic in occurrence and about 10% of the cases are familial showing autosomal recessive pattern with incomplete or variable penetrance
- Loci GLC3A and GLC3B on chromosomes 1 and 2, which are associated with *cytochrome P450* gene responsible for development of the angle of the anterior chamber have been identified as the genetic loci of congenital glaucoma.

Classification of Congenital Glaucoma

True congenital glaucoma: Glaucoma is present at birth. It accounts for 40% of congenital glaucoma.

Infantile glaucoma: Glaucoma manifests within first 3 years of life. It accounts for 55% of congenital glaucoma.

Juvenile glaucoma: Glaucoma manifests between 3 and 16 years. It accounts for 5% of congenital glaucoma.

Buphthalmos*

Buphthalmos refers to marked enlargement of the eyeball seen in congenital and infantile glaucoma (in childhood glaucoma manifesting before 3 years of age).

The word buphthalmos is derived from Greek word 'bous' meaning ox and 'ophthalmos' meaning eyes (buphthalmos literally means ox-like eyes).

Hydrophthalmos: It refers to high-fluid content of the eyeball as a result of obstruction to aqueous outflow seen in congenital and infantile glaucoma.

Pathogenesis

1. Congenital glaucoma is because of maldevelopment of the angle of the anterior chamber. It is usually because of isolated trabeculodysgenesis, which is not associated with other congenital anomalies of the eye.
2. Presence of anomalous impermeable trabecular meshwork or presence of a membrane covering the trabecular meshwork (called Barkan's membrane, described by Barkan) has been proposed to be the cause for aqueous obstruction.
3. Aqueous obstruction leads to rise in intraocular pressure (IOP) resulting in the development of glaucoma.

Clinical Features*

Symptoms

Epiphora, photophobia and blepharospasm in a newborn are described as classical triad of the congenital glaucoma. The classical triad is because of the corneal edema causing irritation of the corneal nerves.

Signs

1. *Eyeball:*
   a. Enlargement of the eyeball resulting in buphthalmos (Fig. 9.3.1) is seen in children below 3 years of age because of stretching of collagen in cornea and sclera in response to raised IOP.
   b. Axial length of the eyeball is increased and it can be diagnosed by ultrasound.
2. *Cornea:*
   a. Corneal edema secondary to raised IOP. Initially, the corneal edema involves epithelium of cornea, later involves stroma of the cornea. Long-standing edema of the cornea leads to stromal scarring.
   b. Corneal enlargement along with the enlargement of the eyeball, because of stretching of the immature collagen in children aged less than 3 years. Horizontal diameter of more than 12 mm indicates corneal enlargement.
   c. Breaks in the Descemet's membrane called Haab's striae. They appear as linear curvilinear lines (Fig. 9.3.2).
3. *Sclera:* It is thinned out because of stretching and shows bluish discoloration.
4. *Anterior chamber:* It is deep because of enlargement of the eyeball.
5. *Iris:* It shows atrophic patches and may show tremulousness.
6. *Lens:* It may show subluxation because of stretching of the zonules as a result of enlargement of the eyeball.

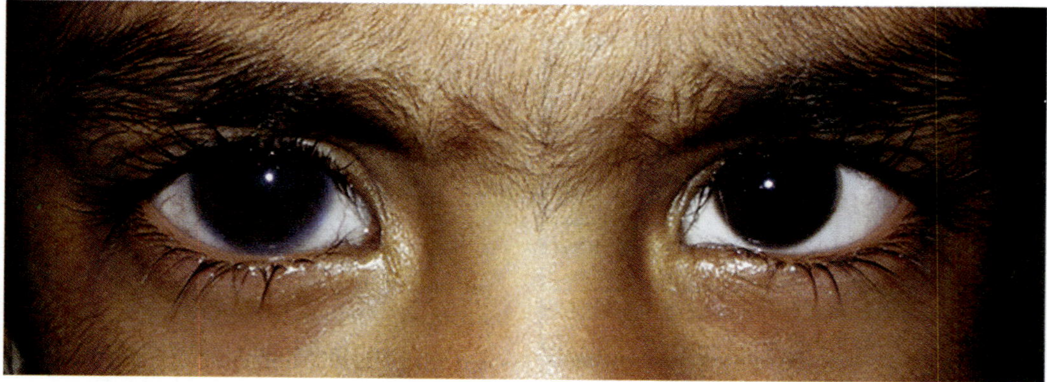

FIG. 9.3.1: A child with unilateral congenital glaucoma of right eye presenting as buphthalmos

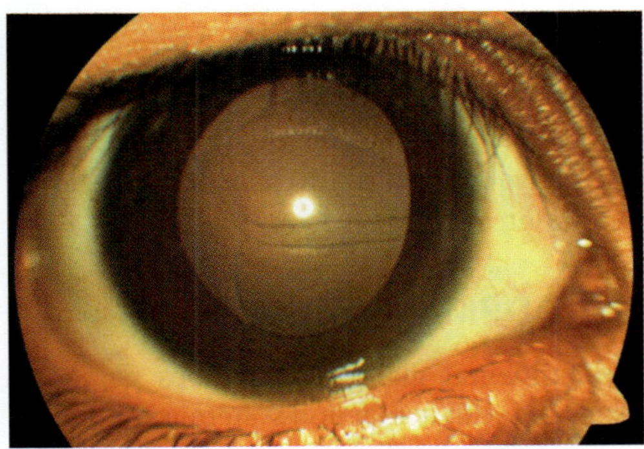

FIG. 9.3.2: Breaks in the Descemet's membrane—Haab's striae

7. *Optic disk:*
   a. Optic disk shows variable amount of cupping. It differs from that of adults from the fact that cupping in children less than 3 years is reversible.
   b. In response to increased IOP the immature connective tissue in lamina cribrosa of sclera allows posterior movement. This returns back to normal position once the IOP is decreased.
   c. The cup tends to enlarge circumferentially compared to oval in adults. It is because of stretching of sclera in children.
8. *Intraocular pressure:* Measurement of IOP shows raised IOP.

EXAMINATION OF CHILDREN WITH SUSPICION OF CONGENITAL GLAUCOMA

Examination is done under general anesthesia. This includes:

1. *Measurement of corneal diameter:* It is done by calipers. Horizontal diameter more than 12 mm in 1st year of life is pathological and indicates congenital or infantile glaucoma.
2. *Measurement of IOP:* Since most of the anesthetic agents alter the IOP, it has to be recorded immediately after intubation. Applanation tonometer such as Perkins handheld tonometer or Tono-Pen are preferred for measurement of IOP as indentation tonometry is not accurate because of low-sclera rigidity in children. An IOP of more than 21 mm Hg is pathological.
3. *Gonioscopy:* It is done by Koeppe's lens with handheld slit lamp. In congenital glaucoma, the angle is open with flat iris insertion most commonly and iris is inserted anteriorly into the trabecular meshwork.

Normal Gonioscopy in Children

It shows iris insertion at or posterior to scleral spur. Vessels from major arterial circle are seen on the iris called Loch Ness Monster phenomenon and peripheral part of iris is covered by fluffy tissue called Lister's morning mist.

4. *Ophthalmoscopy:* It is done by direct ophthalmoscope for examination of the optic disk.
5. *Retinoscopy:* It is done by streak retinoscope and usually shows axial myopia.

Differential Diagnosis

Major symptoms and signs of congenital glaucoma such as corneal edema, corneal enlargement, watering, photophobia and raised IOP have to be differentiated from other causes, which cause similar findings:

1. Corneal enlargement and cloudy cornea has to be differentiated from other causes of congenital corneal opacity such as **STUMPED** (**S**—sclerocornea, **T**—trauma, **U**—ulcer, **M**—metabolic conditions, **P**—posterior corneal defect, **E**—endothelial dystrophies and **D**—dermoid).
2. Corneal enlargement has to be differentiated from megalocornea and axial myopia.
3. Watering has to be differentiated from neonatal conjunctivitis and congenital nasolacrimal duct obstruction.
4. Photophobia has to be differentiated from that caused by iridocyclitis and keratitis.
5. Raised IOP has to be differentiated from primary diseases of the eye causing secondary rise in IOP such as retinoblastoma, retinopathy of prematurity, persistent hyperplastic primary vitreous, etc.

Treatment*

Surgical treatment is the treatment of choice for congenital glaucoma. Medical treatment is indicated to control increased IOP before surgical treatment.

Medical Treatment

Beta blockers such as timolol, carbonic anhydrase; inhibitors such as acetazolamide, dorzolamide; prostaglandin analogues such as latanoprost; and α agonists such as brimonidine are used to reduce IOP.

Surgical Treatment

1. Goniotomy: It involves incising the angle of anterior chamber by visualizing the angle with goniolens. The principle of surgery is to increase the aqueous outflow through the angle of the anterior chamber.
2. Trabeculotomy: It involves incising the trabecular meshwork by passing a probe through Schlemm's canal. It is done in cases in which corneal clouding is preventing the visualization of the angle of the anterior chamber.
3. Trabeculectomy.
4. Combined trabeculotomy and trabeculectomy.
5. Refractory cases may require trabeculectomy with antimetabolite drugs, glaucoma drainage implants.
6. Non-responding cases may require cyclodestructive procedures such as cyclocryotherapy and cyclophotocoagulation for reducing IOP and pain management.

Follow-up

Children with congenital or infantile glaucoma require regular follow-up with recording of IOP and corneal diameter at each visit. Progressive enlargement in corneal diameter indicates progression of glaucoma.

Complications

Corneal scarring, progressive optic nerve damage and anisometric amblyopia because of progressive myopia are the common causes for diminution of vision.

DEVELOPMENTAL GLAUCOMA

Developmental glaucoma includes glaucoma associated with ocular and systemic anomalies.

Glaucoma Associated with Iridotrabeculodysgenesis

Axenfeld-Rieger Syndrome

- It is a group of congenital anomalies due to iridotrabeculodysgenesis characterized by abnormal development of the angle of the anterior chamber, iris and trabecular meshwork. It is inherited as autosomal dominant trait with 50% of the cases being associated with glaucoma.
- It compromises of Axenfeld anomaly, Rieger anomaly and Rieger syndrome.
- *Axenfeld anomaly:* It is characterized by posterior embryotoxon (prominent and anteriorly displaced Schwalbe's line) with attachment of peripheral iris strands to it.
- *Rieger anomaly:* It is characterized by Axenfeld anomaly plus hypoplasia of iris and corectopia of pupil (Fig. 9.3.3).
- *Rieger syndrome:* It is characterized by Rieger anomaly plus presence of extraocular features such as dental anomalies (hypodontia, microdontia), facial anomalies (maxillary hypoplasia, hypertelorism, broad nasal bridge and telecanthus), redundant paraumbilical skin and hypospadias (Fig. 9.3.4).
- Axenfeld-Rieger syndrome has to be differentiated from iridocorneal endothelial (ICE) syndrome. Axenfeld-Rieger syndrome is a bilateral condition occurring in newborns as a congenital anomaly, whereas ICE syndrome is a unilateral condition occurring in middle-aged individuals as a degenerative condition.

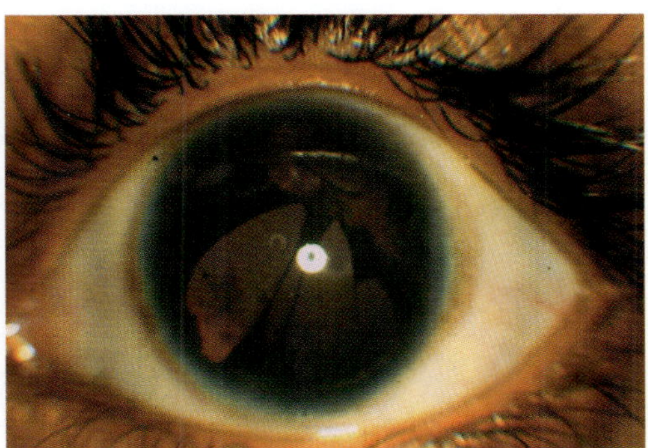

FIG. 9.3.3: Ocular features of Axenfeld-Rieger syndrome (*Note:* Hypoplasia of iris and corectopia of pupil).

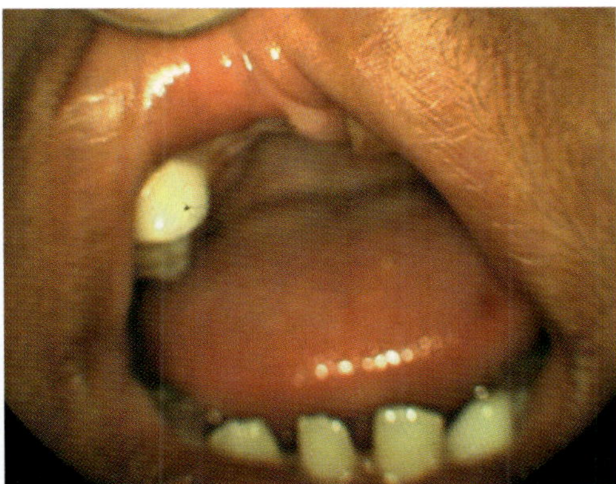

FIG. 9.3.4: Extraocular features of Axenfeld-Rieger syndrome (*Note:* Hypodontia).

Glaucoma Associated with Irido Corneal Trabeculodysgenesis

Peter's Anomaly

- Peter's anomaly is a rare congenital ocular anomaly characterized by central leukomatous corneal opacity with underlying defect in the posterior cornea with iridocorneal or lenticulocorneal adhesions.
- It is because of irido corneal trabeculodysgenesis.
- About 50% of the cases are associated with glaucoma because of associated maldevelopment of the angle of the anterior chamber.

Glaucoma Associated with Aniridia

Aniridia is a rare hereditary disorder characterized by hypoplasia of iris. Glaucoma develops in more than 50% of patients with aniridia in late childhood because of synechial angle closure by contraction or anterior rotation of the rudimentary/hypoplastic iris tissue.

Glaucoma Associated with Systemic Syndromes

Glaucoma is associated with systemic syndromes like:

- Marfan's syndrome
- Weill-Marchesani syndrome
- Sturge-Weber syndrome
- Neurofibromatosis or von Recklinghausen syndrome.

Glaucoma Associated with Chromosomal Syndromes

Glaucoma is associated with chromosomal syndromes such as:

- Down syndrome
- Turner's syndrome.

The treatment for developmental glaucoma is in similar lines as that of primary congenital glaucoma. However, the prognosis is poor because of associated ocular anomalies.

SECONDARY GLAUCOMA

Secondary glaucoma is similar to that developing in adults. It is defined as rise in IOP as a complication of primary intraocular disease resulting in development of glaucoma. The common causes in children include:

- Retinoblastoma
- Retinopathy of prematurity
- Persistent hyperplastic primary vitreous
- Juvenile xanthogranuloma.

GIST BOX 9.3

- Childhood glaucoma includes primary congenital glaucoma, developmental glaucoma and secondary glaucoma.
- Primary congenital glaucoma is defined as glaucoma caused by aqueous outflow obstruction due to maldevelopment of the angle of the anterior chamber without other ocular and systemic abnormalities.
- The incidence of congenital glaucoma is 1 in 10,000. It is because of maldevelopment of the angle of the anterior chamber. It is usually because of isolated trabeculodysgenesis, which is not associated with other congenital anomalies of the eye. Epiphora, photophobia and blepharospasm in a newborn are described as classical triad of congenital glaucoma. Surgical treatment is the treatment of choice for congenital glaucoma. Medical treatment is indicated to control raised intraocular pressure before surgical treatment.
- Developmental glaucoma includes glaucoma associated with ocular and systemic anomalies.

CHAPTER

9.4 Primary Open-angle Glaucoma

DEFINITION

Primary open-angle glaucoma (POAG)*** is also called chronic simple glaucoma. It is characterized by triad of raised intraocular pressure (IOP), optic nerve head damage and visual field defects with an open angle of the anterior chamber.

Primary open-angle glaucoma is defined as chronic progressive optic neuropathy characterized by:

- Open and normal appearing angle of the anterior chamber
- Characteristic retinal nerve fiber layer or optic nerve head damage with or without visual field defects
- Raised IOP consistently above 21 mm Hg
- Absence of secondary causes of open-angle glaucoma.

ETIOLOGY*

The risk factors for POAG can be divided into ocular and nonocular.

Ocular Risk Factors

- Intraocular pressure.
- Optic nerve head cupping.
- Central corneal thickness.
- Myopia.

Non-ocular Risk Factors

- Age.
- Race.
- Family history.
- Diabetes.
- Hypertension.
- Migraine.
- Cardiovascular disease.
- Smoking.

Ocular

Intraocular Pressure

Increase in IOP results in increased incidence of POAG. Increased IOP causes glaucomatous optic nerve damage by causing vascular ischemia and decreased perfusion of optic nerve head.

Intraocular pressure is the only reversible ocular risk factor. The progression of glaucoma can be controlled by reduction in the IOP.

Optic Nerve Head Cupping

Increased optic disk cup ratio as in physiological cupping is associated with increased risk of developing POAG.

Central Corneal Thickness

Central corneal thickness (CCT) affects the measurement of IOP. Patients with decreased

CCT are more likely to be underdiagnosed or misdiagnosed because of false decrease in the measurement of IOP.

Central Corneal Thickness

Normal CCT is 540 μm. CCT is measured by pachymetry.

Effect of CCT on IOP

Intraocular pressure increases by about 5 mm Hg for every 100 μm increase in corneal thickness:

- Increased CCT results in artificially raised IOP as thicker corneas resist indentation.
- Decreased CCT results in artificially decreased IOP.

Myopia

Myopia is associated with more incidence of POAG probably because of increased susceptibility of the optic disk in myopic eyes to sustain glaucomatous damage as thinned parapapillary sclera in myopic eyes exert high tension on the lamina cribrosa.

Nonocular

Age

The risk of POAG increases with increasing age. This may be explained by the fact that ageing optic nerve becomes increasing susceptible to IOP.

Race

The highest prevalence of open-angle glaucoma occurs in Africans. It is more common in black races compared to white may be because of presence of thinner corneas and large optic disk and cup in blacks.

Family History

The risk of POAG increases with positive family history. An individual is three to four times at risk if a sibling has glaucoma, two times at risk if a parent is having glaucoma. It is explained by the presence of susceptibility genes, which are inherited mainly in autosomal dominant pattern and the interaction between the genetic and environmental factors may lead to development of glaucoma.

Systemic diseases such as diabetes, hypertension, cardiovascular disease, migraine and systemic factors such as smoking and their role as risk factor for development of POAG is not well established, but it has been observed in few studies. This may be explained by the fact that abnormalities in the vascular component (retinal microcirculation) and vasospasm, which is seen in all these conditions as a possible pathway for development of glaucoma.

PATHOGENESIS

Pathogenesis of POAG is characterized by rise in IOP and progressive optic nerve damage (Fig. 9.4.1).

CLINICAL FEATURES

The disease is generally bilateral, but asymmetrical in nature.

Symptoms

1. Initially, the patient is asymptomatic without any symptoms.
2. Diminution of vision insidious in onset, gradually progressive and painless in nature, bilateral, but often asymmetrical.

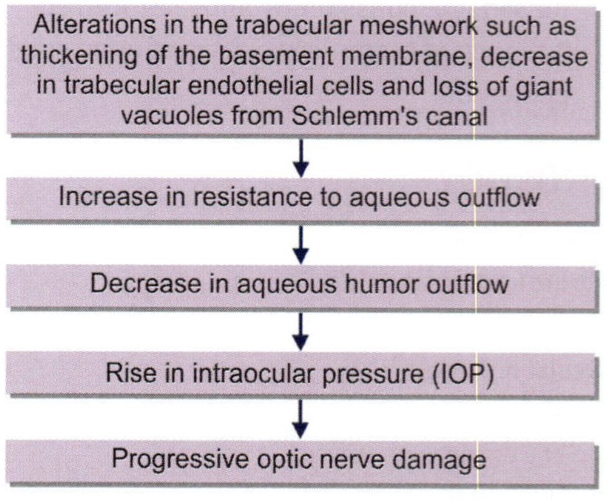

FIG. 9.4.1: Pathogenesis of primary open-angle glaucoma

3. Defect or loss of visual field.
4. Mild headache or eye ache.
5. Frequent changes in presbyopic glasses, because of failure in accommodation as a result of pressure on the ciliary muscle.

Signs

1. Visual acuity is normal in the initial stages; it will be decreased in the later stages.
2. Anterior segment examination is normal with normal anterior chamber depth and open angle of the anterior chamber.
3. Pupils are normal in reaction; in advanced stages changes such as sluggishly reactive pupil, relative afferent pupillary pathway defect are seen.
4. Intraocular pressure is usually increased and it shows large diurnal variation.
5. Optic disk (Fig. 9.4.2) shows varying degrees of glaucomatous disk changes.

Variation in Intraocular Pressure

1. *Elevated IOP:* An IOP of more than 21 mm Hg is considered as abnormal.
2. *Wider diurnal variation in IOP:* Since IOP has got diurnal variation, a single measurement of IOP less than 21 mm Hg does not rule out glaucoma. Normally, the IOP is elevated early in the morning and decreases as the day progresses and it is usually at its lowest level during night. In normal individuals, the diurnal variation is within 5 mm Hg. This will be in the range of 5–10 mm Hg in patients with glaucoma.

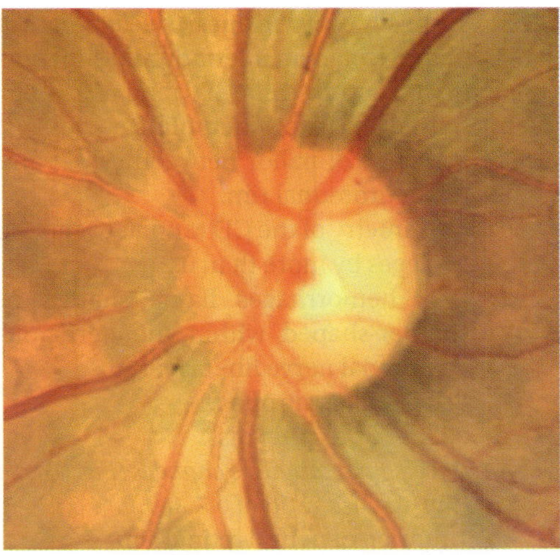

FIG. 9.4.2: Normal optic disk

*Glaucomatous Optic Disk Changes***

1. *Early glaucomatous changes (Figs 9.4.3A and B):*

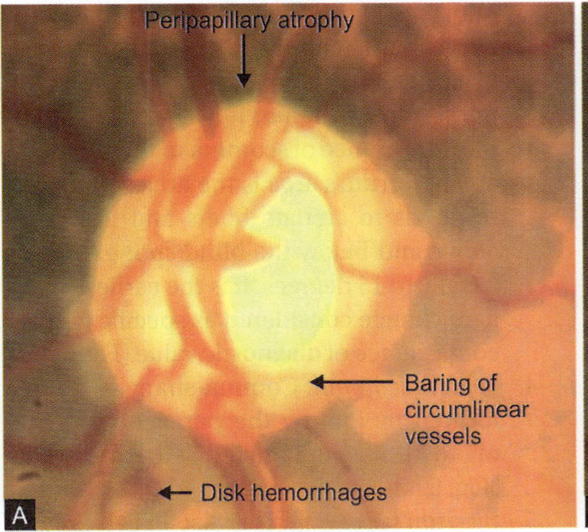

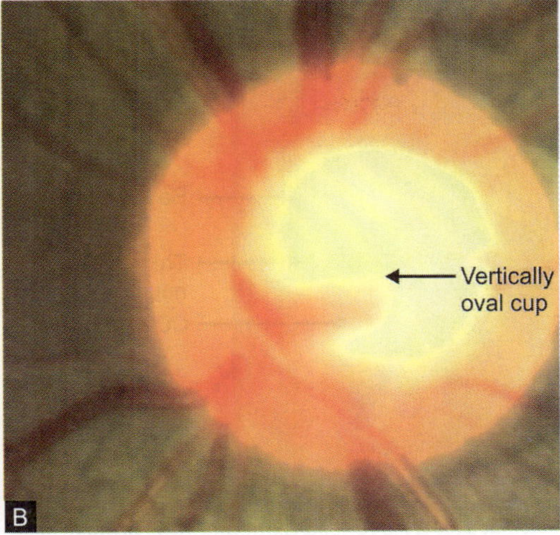

FIGS 9.4.3A and B: Early glaucomatous optic disk changes

a. Vertically oval cup due to selective loss of neuroretinal rim inferiorly and superiorly with cup-to-disk (CD) ratio of 0.4–0.6.
b. Baring of the circumlinear vessels: Presence of pallor between vessel and the neuroretinal rim.
c. Asymmetry of the CD ratio between the two eyes by more than 0.2.
d. Disk hemorrhages flame shaped or splinter-shaped within the peripapillary retinal nerve fiber layer.
e. Peripapillary atrophy.
f. Pallor of the optic disk.

2. *Advanced glaucomatous changes (Fig. 9.4.4):*
   a. Cup-to-disk ratio of 0.7–0.9.
   b. Thinning of neural retinal rim.
   c. Nasal shifting of blood vessels.
   d. *Bayoneting sign:* Double angulation of the retinal blood vessels giving the appearance of being broken at the disk margin is called bayoneting sign (Fig. 9.4.5).
   e. *Lamellar dot sign:* Visibility of the pores of the lamina cribrosa because of loss of retinal ganglion cells is called lamellar dot sign.
3. *Glaucomatous optic atrophy (Figs 9.4.6A and B, Fig. 9.4.7):*
   a. Total cupping of the optic disk with CD ratio of 1.0.
   b. Total pallor of the optic disk.
   c. Complete loss of neuroretinal rim.

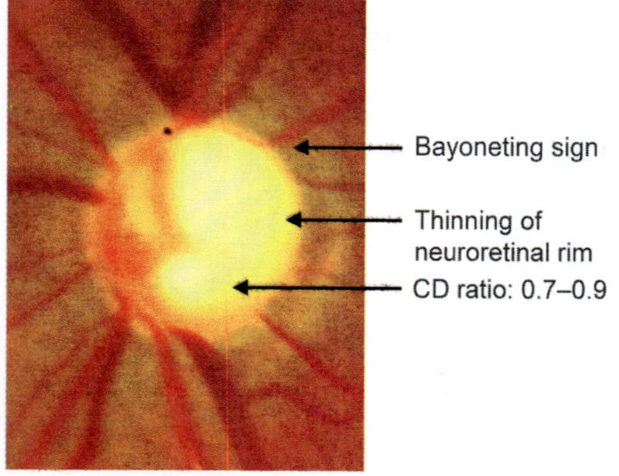

FIG. 9.4.4: Advanced glaucomatous optic disk changes (CD, cup-to-disk)

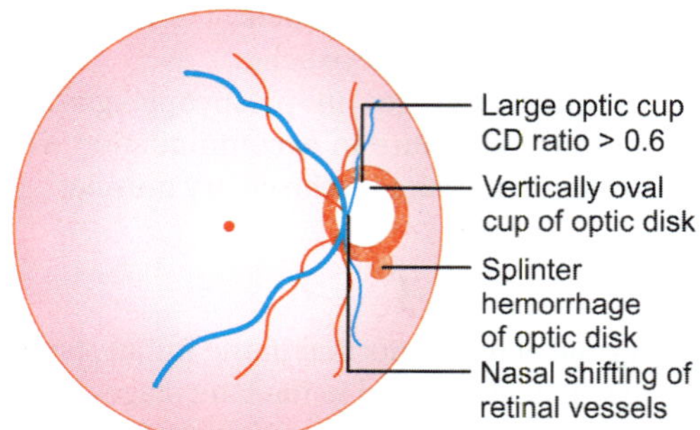

FIG. 9.4.5: Optic disk changes in glaucoma (vertically oval cup of optic disk, nasal shift of retinal vessels, bayoneting, splinter hemorrhage of optic disk; CD, cup-to-disk).

   d. Optic disk appears deeply excavated with bending of all the retinal vessels at the margin of the optic disk.

*Glaucomatous Visual Field Changes***

The glaucomatous visual field defects are:

1. *Isopter contraction:* It is the earliest visual field defect of glaucoma characterized by generalized constriction of peripheral field.
2. *Baring of the blind spot:* It is one of the early defects seen in glaucoma characterized by exclusion of blind spot from the visual field.

   Isopter contraction and baring of the blind spot are not diagnostic of glaucoma as they are seen in other ocular diseases like cataract, etc.
3. *Paracentral scotoma:* It is characterized by the appearance of scotoma in the Bjerrum's area. Bjerrum's area is the area, which corresponds to arcuate fibers and it extends above and below the blind spot extending nasally to 15 degrees. It is the earliest visual field change considered as specific to glaucoma, hence of diagnostic value (Fig. 9.4.8).
4. *Seidel's scotoma:* Comma-shaped scotoma formed by joining the paracentral scotoma to blind spot is called Seidel's scotoma (Fig. 9.4.9).
5. *Bjerrum's scotoma:* It is also called arcuate scotoma. Scotoma involving whole of the

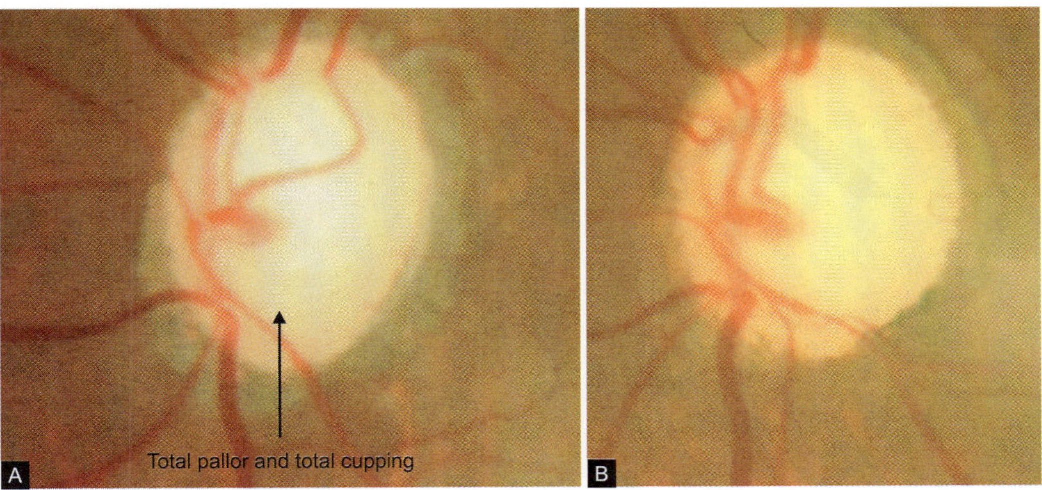

FIGS 9.4.6A and B: Glaucomatous optic atrophy

Bjerrum's area is called Bjerrum's scotoma. It is formed by extension of the Seidel's scotoma to the horizontal line (Fig. 9.4.10).

6. *Double arcuate scotoma:* It is also called ring scotoma. Joining of the superior and inferior arcuate scotomas result in the formation of double arcuate scotoma.
7. *Roenne's nasal step:* Step-like defect seen at the meeting point of the superior and inferior arcuate scotomas is called Roenne's nasal step. It is because of the fact that the scotomas usually involve different arcs (Fig. 9.4.11).
8. *Tubular vision/temporal island of vision:* It refers to presence of central tunnel vision or tubular vision seen in advanced glaucoma. Retention of central vision (tubular vision and temporal island of vision) till late in advanced glaucoma is because of the fact that the macular fibers are most resistant to glaucomatous damage (Fig. 9.4.12).
9. Complete loss of vision with perception of light negative end result of glaucomatous optic atrophy (Fig. 9.4.13).

INVESTIGATIONS

Retinal Nerve Fiber Layer Analysis

Retinal nerve fiber layer analysis is done to diagnose early changes of glaucoma in the form of retinal nerve fiber layer damage before the development of visual defects. It is done by:

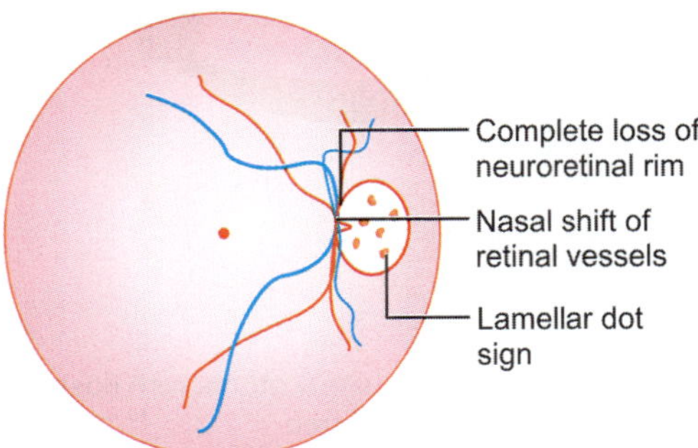

FIG. 9.4.7: Glaucomatous optic atrophy

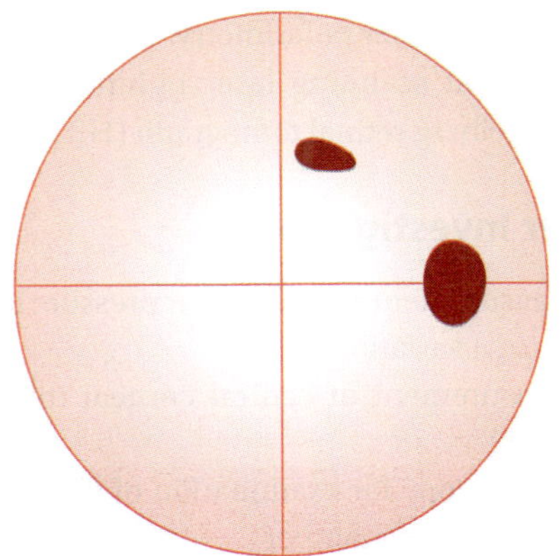

FIG. 9.4.8: Paracentral scotoma

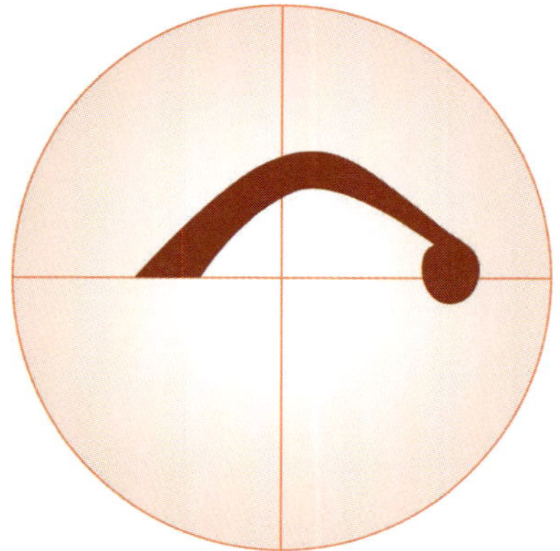

FIG. 9.4.9: Seidel's scotoma

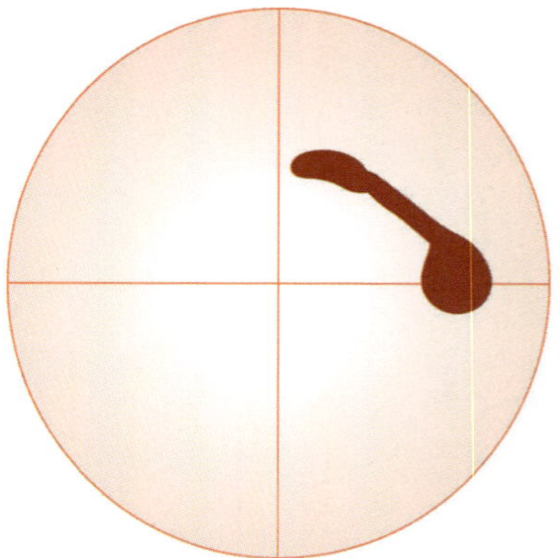

FIG. 9.4.10: Bjerrum's scotoma

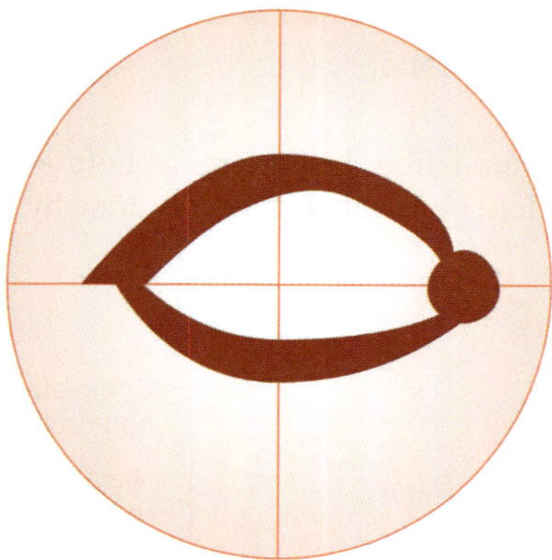

FIG. 9.4.11: Double arcuate scotoma with Roenne's nasal step

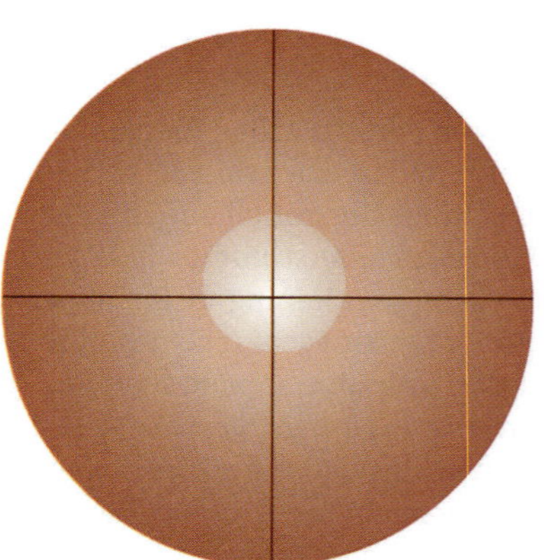

FIG. 9.4.12: Tubular vision

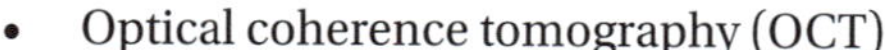

- Optical coherence tomography (OCT)
- Scanning laser polarimetry: GDx analyzer
- Confocal scanning laser ophthalmoscopy: Heidelberg retinal tomograph (HRT).

Other Investigations

- Measurement of intraocular pressure and its diurnal variation
- Measurement of central corneal thickness (CCT)
- Gonioscopy for examination of the angle of the anterior chamber

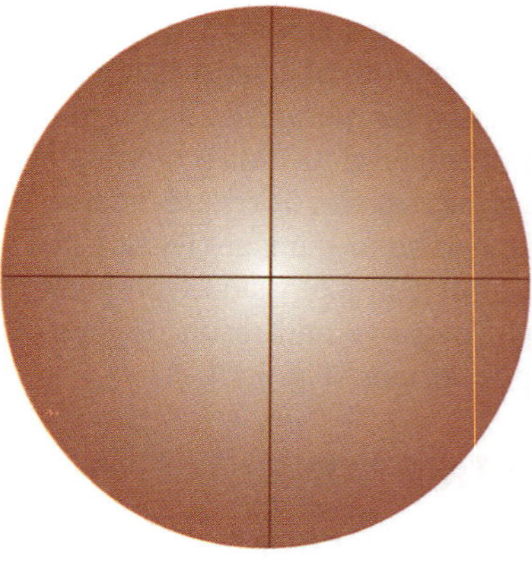

FIG. 9.4.13: Complete loss of vision

- Retinal nerve fiber analysis to look for nerve fiber damage
- Evaluation of optic disk
- Measurement of visual fields by perimetry
- Provocative test.

Provocative Test for Open-angle Glaucoma

It is done in glaucoma suspect cases with IOP in the borderline range. It is done by water drinking test. It is done by asking the patient to report in the morning with empty stomach. Initially, baseline IOP is measured. Patient is asked to drink 1 liter of water. IOP is measured at every 15-minute intervals for 1 hour. A raise of IOP by more than 8 mm Hg is taken as positive provocative test. However, it is not done commonly nowadays because of availability of recent diagnostic tools like OCT, HRT, GDx for retinal nerve fiber analysis, the defect of which is more significant compared to rise in IOP.

DIFFERENTIAL DIAGNOSIS

Primary open-angle glaucoma has to be differentiated from:

1. *Ocular hypertension:* It can be differentiated from the absence of glaucomatous optic disk changes and glaucomatous visual field loss. It is associated only with raised IOP above 21 mm Hg and open angles on gonioscopy similar to POAG.
2. *Normal tension glaucoma:* It can be differentiated from the presence of normal IOP. It is associated with glaucomatous optic disk and visual field changes, and open angles on gonioscopy similar to POAG.
3. *Primary angle-closure glaucoma:* Presence of narrow angle of anterior chamber on gonioscopy differentiates it from POAG.
4. Secondary open-angle glaucoma, e.g. pseudoexfoliation glaucoma, pigmentary glaucoma, steroid-induced glaucoma, etc. They can be differentiated from POAG from the presence of secondary factors responsible for glaucoma, e.g. pseudoexfoliative material, pigment dispersion, history of using steroid drugs, etc.

TREATMENT

The aims of treatment are:

1. Glaucoma leads to irreversible visual loss, because of progressive damage of the optic nerve. Reduction of IOP is the only effective known treatment available to prevent the progression of the disease.
2. The aim of treatment is to reduce the IOP and monitor the changes in optic disk and visual fields at regular intervals to prevent the progression of the disease.
3. To find out the target IOP and to maintain it below the target pressure by medical, laser, surgical or combined treatment approach.

Target Intraocular Pressure

- It is defined as level of IOP below which the glaucomatous optic nerve damage is usually not seen.
- It depends on the pretreatment IOP and the stage of disease. An advanced stage of glaucoma needs lower IOP as target pressure. Routinely accepted target pressures are:
  - *Early glaucoma:* Below 15 mm Hg
  - *Moderate glaucoma:* Below 12 mm Hg
  - *Advanced glaucoma:* Below 10 mm Hg.

Target pressure individual varies from individual and it has to be closely monitored and adjusted according to the progression of the disease.

The treatment options for POAG include:

- Medical treatment
- Laser treatment
- Surgical treatment.

Medical Treatment

Medical treatment is by antiglaucoma drugs.

Antiglaucoma drugs: These are the drugs, which reduce the IOP by either decreasing the production of aqueous humor or by increasing the outflow of aqueous humor. The available antiglaucoma drugs are:**

1. *Prostaglandin analogues:* Latanoprost 0.005%, travoprost 0.004%, bimatoprost 0.03%.
2. *Adrenergic antagonists:* Timolol 0.25%, 0.5%, betaxolol 0.25%, 0.5%.

3. *Adrenergic agonists:* Apraclonidine 1%, brimonidine 0.5%, 1%.
4. *Parasympathomimetics:* Pilocarpine 1%, 2%, 4%.
5. *Carbonic anhydrase inhibitors:* For oral use like acetazolamide, topical like dorzolamide, prostaglandin analogue such as latanoprost 0.005% eyedrops once daily or beta blocker like timolol 0.5% eyedrops twice daily is the drug used initially as first-line drug.

To begin with one drug is used, if it is not able to achieve the target IOP, it is either replaced by a more efficient drug or a combination of two drugs are used. Most commonly used drug combinations are latanoprost with timolol, latanoprost with carbonic anhydrase inhibitors, e.g. dorzolamide.

Oral drug, e.g. acetazolamide is used only for few days and they are not recommended for long-term usage.

Laser Treatment

Indications

- Failure of medical treatment to reduce the IOP below the target pressure
- Non-compliant patient.

The treatment options available are:

- Argon laser trabeculoplasty (ALT)
- Selective laser trabeculoplasty (SLT).

Laser Trabeculoplasty

- Trabeculoplasty is done by application of laser burns to trabecular meshwork. It acts by increasing the aqueous outflow, because of shrinkage of collagen and opening of intertrabecular spaces.
- Argon laser trabeculoplasty is done by application of argon laser burns at the junction of the pigmented and non-pigmented trabecular meshwork.
- Selective laser trabeculoplasty is done by application of frequency doubled neodymium-yattrium-aluminum-garnet (Nd-YAG) laser. It selectively affects the pigmented cells; hence, it is called selective laser trabeculoplasty. Since it selectively affects the cells, it is safer than ALT.

Surgical Treatment

Indications

- Failure of medical treatment to reduce the IOP below the target pressure
- Non-compliant patient
- As a primary procedure in patients with advanced glaucoma, who requires lower target pressure.

The treatment options available are:

- Partial thickness filtration surgery, e.g. trabeculectomy
- Aqueous drainage devices (e.g. Ahmed valve implants): Usually reserved for patients in whom the trabeculectomy is failed.

RECENT ADVANCES IN TREATMENT OF GLAUCOMA

Neuroprotection in Glaucoma*

Glaucoma is considered as a neurodegenerative disease characterized by progressive damage to retinal ganglion cells. This is supported by the fact that in spite control of IOP, the disease progresses in few individuals. Neuroprotection in glaucoma is aimed at protecting the retinal ganglion cells from progressive damage.

Calcium Channel Blockers

1. Calcium channel blockers act directly by decreasing the influx of calcium, thereby preventing the calcium-induced apoptosis and indirectly by increasing the blood supply to retinal ganglion cells.
2. Calcium channel blockers such as nifedipine, verapamil and flunarizine have been known to have neuroprotection effect.

N-methyl-D-aspartate Receptor Antagonists

1. Increased glutamate leads to N-methyl-D-aspartate (NMDA) receptor overactivation

and excitotoxicity. NMDA receptor antagonist would be able to prevent excitotoxic damage to retinal ganglion cells.
2. Memantine, a NMDA receptor antagonist is in clinical trial phase and may be available as neuroprotective drug.

Nitric Oxide Synthetase Inhibitors

1. Increased levels of nitric oxide are known to be neurotoxic and nitric oxide synthetase inhibitors act by preventing the synthesis of nitric oxide.
2. Aminoguanidine is a nitric oxide synthetase inhibitor, but its effectiveness is not proven yet.

Antioxidants

Antioxidants such as vitamin C and E are known to reduce damage to retinal ganglion cells by reducing the NMDA-induced toxicity.

Neurotrophins

Brain-derived neurotrophic factor (BDNF) has shown to reduce the retinal ganglion cell death in animal models.

Immunomodulation and Glaucoma Vaccine

Immunization against the myelin basic protein to prevent the death of retinal ganglion cells is seen as a possible way of developing a glaucoma vaccine.

Neuroprotective Action of the Presently Used Antiglaucoma Drugs

Presently used antiglaucoma drugs such as brimonidine, betaxolol, prostaglandins and carbonic anhydrase inhibitors are known to have neuroprotective action. Further studies are underway to get conclusive evidence regarding the neuroprotective action.

NORMAL-TENSION GLAUCOMA**

Definition

Normal-tension glaucoma (NTG) is also called low-tension glaucoma. It is defined as a type of primary open-angle glaucoma characterized by all the features of open-angle glaucoma (i.e. open and normal appearing angle of the anterior chamber, characteristic retinal nerve fiber layer or optic nerve head damage with or without visual field defects, absence of secondary causes of open-angle glaucoma) other than the raised IOP.

Etiopathogenesis

Normal-tension glaucoma is more often seen in elderly aged people with incidence being more in females. Local vascular factors, which reduce the blood supply to optic nerve head play a significant role in the development of NTG. Higher prevalence of NTG is seen in people, who are suffering from vasospastic diseases such as ischemic vascular disease, Raynaud's disease, migraine, etc.

Clinical Features

Clinical features are similar to that of POAG with all features being present except raised IOP. Optic disk in NTG shows more often disk hemorrhages and focal notching of the disk. Visual field defects in NTG occur more often close to fixation as compared to POAG.

Investigations

Normal-tension glaucoma is usually diagnosis of exclusion and all other causes of optic nerve damage should be ruled out. The causes include:

1. Undetected raised IOP as in:
   a. Primary open-angle glaucoma with diurnal variation.
   b. Secondary glaucoma, e.g. like steroid-induced glaucoma in remission.

   c. Patient on systemic drugs as a treatment of some other systemic disease, which is lowering IOP (e.g. beta blockers used for treatment of hypertension may reduce IOP also).
2. Diseases other than glaucoma causing optic nerve damage as in:
   a. Compressive lesions of optic nerve.
   b. Ischemic optic neuropathy.
   c. Hereditary optic atrophy.
   d. Systemic diseases such as multiple sclerosis, syphilis and tuberculosis, which produce optic neuropathies.

Treatment

- Treatment is indicated in patients with progressive disease
- Treatment is guided by NTG study; the observations of the study suggest a reduction of IOP by 30% to reduce the progression of the disease
- Treatment is done by:
  - Antiglaucoma drugs to lower the IOP by 30%
  - Improving the vascular supply to optic nerve head by treating the vasospasm by drugs such as calcium channel blockers
  - Treatment of any underlying vasospastic diseases such as ischemic vascular diseases, migraine, etc.
  - Neuroprotection may play a significant role in the treatment of glaucoma.

OCULAR HYPERTENSION*

Presence of raised IOP alone with absence of the characteristic optic nerve damage and visual field defects seen in glaucoma is called ocular hypertension.

The treatment for ocular hypertension is guided by Ocular Hypertension Treatment Study. The observations of the study suggest a reduction of IOP by 20% to reduce the risk of developing glaucoma.

GIST BOX 9.4

- Primary open-angle glaucoma (POAG) is also called chronic simple glaucoma. It is characterized by triad of raised intraocular pressure (IOP), optic nerve head damage and visual field defects with an open angle of the anterior chamber.
- Pathogenesis of POAG is characterized by rise in IOP and progressive optic nerve damage.
- The IOP is usually increased and it shows large diurnal variation and optic disk shows varying degrees of glaucomatous disk changes.
- The treatment options for POAG include medical treatment, laser treatment and surgical treatment.

CHAPTER

9.5 Primary Angle-closure Glaucoma

DEFINITION

Primary angle-closure glaucoma (PACG)*** is a type of glaucoma caused by closure of the angle by the peripheral iris, obstructing the aqueous outflow.

ETIOLOGY*

The risk factors for PACG can be divided into ocular factors and non-ocular factors.

Ocular Risk Factors

- Eyes, which are predisposed to development of angle closure show the following anatomical features:
  - Shorter axial length
  - Shallow anterior chamber
  - Increased lens thickness
  - Anterior placement of lens iris diaphragm
  - Plateau iris configuration
  - Smaller corneal diameter.
- Primary angle-closure glaucoma is more common in hypermetropic eyes as these eyes are smaller with shorter axial length, shallow anterior chamber.

Non-ocular Risk Factors

- *Age:* The incidence of PACG increases with age, probably because of increasing lens thickness with increasing age. PACG is more common in fifth to sixth decade of age.
- *Gender:* The incidence is two to four times more common in females, probably because females tend to have smaller eye dimensions compared to males.
- *Race:* PACG is more common in Chinese and East Asian population, probably because of smaller eye dimensions.
- *Family history:* PACG is more common in first-degree relatives of patients with PACG, probably because of inherited anatomical features of eye.
- *Personality:* PACG is more common in emotional nervous individuals. This is explained by the fact that increased sympathetic tone in emotional stress causing mydriasis of pupil may act as precipitating factor.

Precipitating Factors

In individuals, who are prone to angle closure because of the presence of ocular and non-ocular risk factors, the precipitating factors, which can cause mydriasis of pupil can precipitate angle closure. The precipitating factors are:

- *Physiological factors:* Mydriasis caused by factors such as dim illumination.
- *Pharmacological factors:* Drugs causing mydriasis such as parasympatholytics (e.g. atropine, etc.), sympathomimetics (e.g. adrenaline, etc.).
- *Psychological factors:* Emotional stress, anxiety, etc.

PATHOGENESIS**

The pathogenesis of PACG is explained by the following mechanisms:

- Pupillary block mechanism
- Plateau iris mechanism
- Lens mechanism.

Pupillary Block Mechanism

Resistance to the flow of aqueous humor from posterior chamber to anterior chamber because of small dimensions of eyeball results in pressure difference between anterior and posterior chamber with higher pressure in posterior chamber. This resistance to the flow of aqueous becomes maximum in mid-dilated pupillary position resulting in relative pupillary block. The relative pupillary block becomes absolute pupillary block causing forward pushing of the iris resulting in closure of the angle of the anterior chamber. Initially, the angle is closed by appositional closure; later, it becomes synechial closure. Closure of the angle of the anterior chamber results in elevation of IOP. Peripheral iridotomy can break the pupillary block, which is helpful in reducing the IOP.

Plateau Iris Mechanism

Plateau iris is an abnormal anatomical configuration caused by anteriorly positioned ciliary processes leading to narrow angle of the anterior chamber by pushing the peripheral iris forward. The angle of the anterior chamber is closed here because of abnormal configuration of the iris without significant pupillary block; hence, peripheral iridotomy will not help to reduce IOP.

Lens Mechanism

Lens-related factors such as thicker lens and anterior lens movement lead to relative pupillary block resulting in closure of the angle of the anterior chamber. In these cases, angle closure persists even after peripheral iridotomy. Lens extraction plays a significant role in the management of these cases.

CLASSIFICATION (International Society of Geographical and Epidemiological Ophthalmology Classification)*

Primary angle-closure glaucoma is classified into three types.

Primary Angle-closure Suspect

Appositional angle closure of more than 270° or more than three quadrants with absence of peripheral anterior synechiae and normal IOP, optic disk and visual fields (Table 9.5.1).

Primary Angle Closure

Appositional and/or synechial angle closure of more than 270° with presence or absence of peripheral anterior synechiae and raised IOP, and normal optic disk and visual fields (Table 9.5.2).

Primary Angle-closure Glaucoma

Appositional and synechial angle closure of more than 270° with presence of peripheral anterior synechiae and raised IOP, and glaucomatous optic disk and visual field changes (Table 9.5.3).

TABLE 9.5.1: Primary angle-closure suspect

Gonioscopy	Appositional angle closure > 270° and absence of peripheral anterior synechiae
IOP*	Normal
Optic disk	Normal
Visual fields	Normal

*IOP, intraocular pressure

TABLE 9.5.2: Primary angle closure

Gonioscopy	Appositional and/or synechial angle closure of 270° and +/- peripheral anterior synechiae
IOP*	Raised
Optic disk	Normal
Visual fields	Normal

*IOP, intraocular pressure

TABLE 9.5.3: Primary angle-closure glaucoma

Gonioscopy	Appositional and synechial angle closure with presence of peripheral anterior synechiae
IOP*	Raised
Optic disk	Glaucomatous changes
Visual fields	Glaucomatous field defects

*IOP, introcular pressure

CLINICAL STAGES OF ANGLE-CLOSURE GLAUCOMA*

- Prodromal stage or latent glaucoma
- Stage of constant instability or intermittent glaucoma
- Acute congestive stage or acute angle-closure glaucoma
- Chronic congestive stage or chronic congestive glaucoma
- Absolute glaucoma.

Prodromal Stage or Latent Glaucoma

Latent glaucoma is seen in eyes, which come under angle-closure suspect and show shallow anterior chamber, narrow angle of the anterior chamber. In the eyes, which are prone to develop angle closure, intermittent attacks of transient rise in IOP lasting for few seconds are seen because of intermittent closure of the angle precipitated by the precipitating factors.

Symptoms

- Patient is usually asymptomatic
- Patient may complain of occasional headache, blurring of vision and colored halos.

Signs

Eye shows features of angle-closure suspects such as shallow anterior chamber, narrow angle of the anterior chamber with IOP, optic disk and visual fields being normal.

Stage of Constant Instability or Intermittent Glaucoma

The transient rise in IOP, which is seen in the prodromal phase are seen in this stage repeatedly and regularly with each attack lasting for few minutes to few hours. The attacks are generally milder and spontaneously without any treatment. A typical patient complains of headache, colored halos and blurring of vision on exposure to any of the precipitating factors such as dim illumination, drugs, anxiety, etc. Patient becomes normal once the exposure to precipitating factors are removed or after sleeping (miosis during sleep may break the pupillary block).

Symptoms

Patient complains of headache, blurring of vision and colored halos during attack of angle closure.

Signs

1. During the attack, the eye shows circumcorneal congestion, corneal edema, shallow anterior chamber, mid-dilated pupil and raised IOP.
2. Eye shows features of angle closure such as shallow anterior chamber, narrow angle of the anterior chamber with or without peripheral synechiae, raised IOP during the attack and normal IOP in between the attacks, normal optic disk and normal visual fields.

Acute Congestive Stage or Acute Angle-closure Glaucoma***

Acute angle-closure glaucoma results from total closure of the angle of the anterior chamber resulting in acute raise of IOP.

Pathogenesis

Pathogenesis of acute congestive stage is given in Figure 9.5.1.

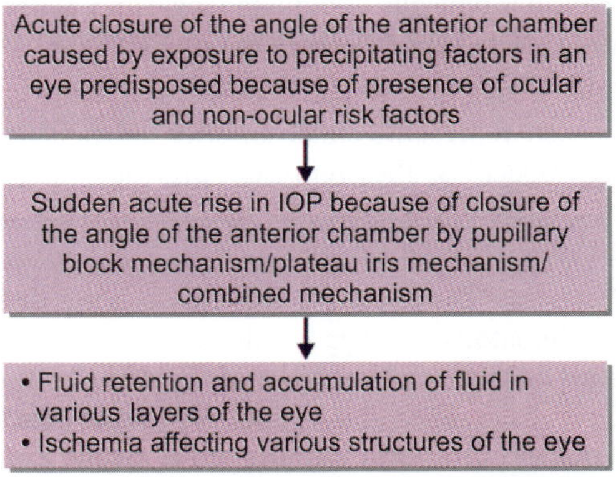

Acute closure of the angle of the anterior chamber caused by exposure to precipitating factors in an eye predisposed because of presence of ocular and non-ocular risk factors

↓

Sudden acute rise in IOP because of closure of the angle of the anterior chamber by pupillary block mechanism/plateau iris mechanism/ combined mechanism

↓

- Fluid retention and accumulation of fluid in various layers of the eye
- Ischemia affecting various structures of the eye

FIG. 9.5.1: Pathogenesis (IOP, intraocular pressure)

Symptoms

- Acute onset of severe eye pain radiating along the distribution of the trigeminal nerve
- Marked diminution of vision associated with redness, watering and photophobia
- Severe headache associated with vomiting.

Signs

Visual acuity: Gross diminution of vision. Visual acuity is reduced to counting fingers close to face or hand movements. Diminution of vision is because of corneal edema and because of ischemia of the optic nerve head and depressed retinal function.

Lids: It shows variable amount of lid edema depending on the amount of inflammation.

Conjunctiva: It shows circumcorneal congestion and chemosis.

Cornea: It shows variable amount of edema of the cornea because of accumulation of fluid as a result of endothelial dysfunction caused by sudden rise in IOP.

Anterior chamber: Depth of anterior chamber is shallow. Anterior chamber shows variable amount of cells and flare because of inflammation caused by ischemia.

Iris: It is edematous initially and later it shows atrophic patches typically in the sphincter papillae area as a result of ischemia.

Pupil: It is typically mid dilated, oval and nonresponsive to light as a result of pupillary block.

Lens: This may show glaucomflecken. Glaucomflecken represents small anterior subcapsular lens opacities. They represent previous attacks of angle closure glaucoma and are because of atrophy of the lens fibers.

Optic disk: During the acute attack, optic disk is edematous and hyperemic, because of ischemia of the optic nerve head. Cupping of the optic disk sets in after 2–4 weeks of acute attack because of ischemic damage to the retinal ganglion cells.

Gonioscopy: It shows appositional closure with or without peripheral anterior synechiae initially, later or following repeated attacks synechial closure of the angle.

Intraocular pressure: It is markedly increased, usually more than 40 mm Hg.

Examination of other eye: Examination of other eye shows the presence of ocular risk factors such as shallow anterior chamber, etc. (Fig. 9.5.2).

> Examination of optic disk and gonioscopy may be difficult in the acute congestive stage because of corneal edema and inflammation of the eye. Glycerine or hypertonic saline eyedrops may be used to reduce corneal edema and to proceed with fundoscopy for examination of optic disk and gonioscopy for examination of the angle of the anterior chamber.

Chronic Congestive Stage or Chronic Congestive Glaucoma

Chronic congestive stage can follow an acute attack of acute congestive glaucoma or repeated attacks of intermittent glaucoma, or as a chronic closure of the angle because of gradual closure of the angle of the anterior chamber by synechiae.

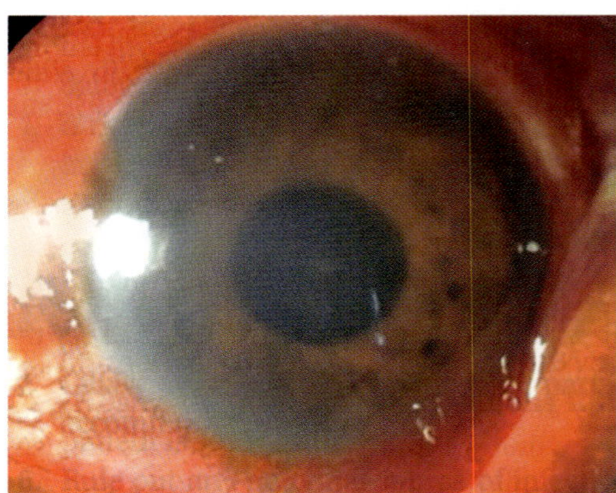

FIG. 9.5.2: Acute angle-closure glaucoma (*Note:* Circumcorneal congestion, corneal edema, mid-dilated pupil and shallow anterior chamber).

Symptoms

Symptoms depend on the nature of onset of chronic congestive glaucoma:

1. If it follows acute congestive glaucoma, patient gives history of a previous acute attack, in cases following intermittent glaucoma history of repeated attacks of glaucoma such as transient diminution of vision, colored halos and headache is available.
2. In cases of chronic angle-closure glaucoma, symptoms are usually minimal.

Signs

On examination, visual acuity is decreased because of glaucomatous damage to the optic nerve, anterior chamber is shallow, IOP shows moderate elevation, gonioscopy shows angle closure and presence of synechiae, optic disk and visual fields show glaucomatous changes similar to those seen in open-angle glaucoma.

Stage of Absolute Glaucoma**

Absolute glaucoma (Fig. 9.5.3) is the end result of angle-closure glaucoma. Increased IOP leads to irreversible damage to the structures of the eye resulting in painful blind eye.

Symptoms

Patient complains of chronic pain and complete loss of vision with perception of light negative.

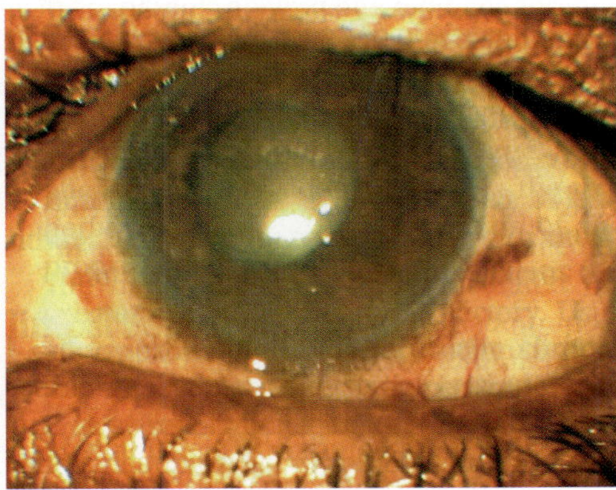

FIG. 9.5.3: Absolute glaucoma

Signs

Visual acuity: Eye is totally blind with perception of light being negative.

Cornea: It is edematous and may show bullous keratopathy.

Anterior chamber: It is shallow and angle of the anterior chamber shows synechial closure.

Iris: It shows atrophic patches.

Pupil: It is fixed, dilated and absence of reaction to light and accommodation.

Optic disk: It shows glaucomatous optic atrophy.

Intraocular pressure: It remains elevated.

Complications of Absolute Glaucoma

Staphyloma: High IOP leads to thinning of sclera and ectasia resulting in the formation of staphyloma.

Atrophic bulbi: Constantly elevated IOP leads to atrophy of ciliary body resulting in decreased aqueous production leading to soft, shrunken, sightless eye called atrophic bulbi.

DIFFERENTIAL DIAGNOSIS

1. Diagnosis of glaucoma is usually obvious in acute congestive glaucoma, chronic congestive glaucoma and in absolute glaucoma.
2. Acute congestive glaucoma has to be differentiated from the other causes of acute red eye such as acute conjunctivitis and acute iridocyclitis.
3. Investigations are required in prodromal stage and stage of intermittent glaucoma.

INVESTIGATIONS

Provocative Tests

Provocative tests are tests, which provoke angle closure in individuals, who come under the classification of primary angle-closure suspect. They act as precipitating factors to cause an attack of angle closure under supervision of an ophthalmologist, so that effective treatment can be planned. Patients with positive provocative test should undergo prophylactic treatment.

Dark-room test: After baseline measurement of IOP, patient is asked to stay in a darkroom for 1 hour. An increase in IOP by more than 8 mm Hg is taken as positive. It is based on the principle that physiological mydriasis, which occurs in darkness may act as precipitating factor to provoke angle closure.

Prone test: After baseline measurement of IOP, patient is asked to stay in prone position or place his/her head in face-down position for 1 hour. An increase in the IOP by more than 8 mm Hg is taken as positive. It is based on the principle that forward movement of iris lens diaphragm during prone position or face-down position may act as precipitating factor to provoke angle closure.

Dark-room prone-position test: It is combination of dark-room test and prone test. Here, patient is asked to stay in a darkroom in prone position or face-down position for 1 hour. An increase in the IOP by more than 8 mm Hg is taken as positive.

During the above mentioned provocative tests, patient is asked to remain awake. If the patient sleeps off during the tests, physiological miosis during sleep may lead to false negative interpretation.

Mydriatic provocative test: After baseline measurement of IOP, mydriatic drugs such as phenylephrine, tropicamide, etc. are instilled. IOP is measured at 15-minute intervals. An increase in the IOP by more than 8 mm Hg is taken as positive. It is based on the principle that mydriasis may act as precipitating factor to provoke angle closure.

Mapstone test: After baseline measurement of IOP, phenylephrine (mydriatic drug) and pilocarpine (miotic drug) are instilled to achieve mid-dilated pupil. IOP is measured after 1 hour. An increase in the IOP by more than 8 mm Hg is taken as positive. It is based on the principle that pupillary block is maximum in mid-dilated pupil.

Role of Provocative Tests in Today's Practice

Provocative tests are rarely used today, because of drawbacks, e.g. negative test does not rule out the possibility of angle closure. They were practiced in olden days when laser iridotomy was not available and the prophylactic treatment done was surgical iridectomy.

Availability of safe prophylactic treatment such as laser iridotomy, which can be used in primary angle-closure glaucoma suspects has almost made provocative tests only of historical significance.

Evaluation of the Angle of the Anterior Chamber

Gonioscopy: It differentiates glaucoma broadly into two categories, namely open-angle glaucoma and angel-closure glaucoma. Gonioscopy in primary angle-closure glaucoma suspects show appositional closure of the angle for more than 270° with absence of peripheral anterior synechiae. In primary angle closure, gonioscopy shows angle closure with or without peripheral synechiae. In primary angle-closure glaucoma, gonioscopy shows angle closure with peripheral synechiae

Indentation gonioscopy is done to differentiate appositional angle closure by synechial closure.

Ultrasound biomicroscopy (UBM) and anterior segment optical coherence topography (OCT): These methods provide view of the angle of the anterior chamber and provide clues to the diagnosis of various types of glaucoma.

Colored Halos in Glaucoma**

- A condition in which patient perceives colored rings around light source is called colored halos. They are seen because of prismatic dispersion of light because of abnormal collection of fluid in the cornea or lens.
- In glaucoma, colored halos are because of corneal edema. Colored halos are one of the earliest symptoms seen in the early stages of glaucoma and patients complaining of colored halos should be examined to rule out glaucoma.

Contd...

Contd...

- The other causes for colored halos include conjunctivitis, because of collection of mucus on corneal surface and early stages of immature cataract.
- Colored halos in glaucoma can be differentiated from those due to other causes by following methods:
  - Colored halos in conjunctivitis disappear on removal of the collected mucus over the corneal surface either by eye wash or by manual removal
  - Colored halos due to corneal edema and because of immature cataract can be differentiated by Fincham stenopeic slit test.

Fincham Stenopic Slit Test

The test is done by passing a stenopic slit in front of the eye, while the patient is looking at a bright source of light. The colored halos because of cataract are broken into segments whereas the colored halos because of corneal edema as in case of glaucoma remain intact. The colored halos in immature cataract are broken into segments, because of diffraction of light caused by regularly arranged lens fibers.

TREATMENT

The treatment depends on the stage of the disease.

Treatment of Latent Glaucoma and Intermittent Glaucoma

Primary angle-closure glaucoma suspect and primary angle closure:

- This stage involves patients, who are at risk of angle closure; these patients are treated by prophylactic laser iridotomy
- Medical treatment in the form of pilocarpine eyedrops four times per day is advised as a temporary measure to induce miosis of pupil and to prevent angle closure till laser iridotomy is performed.

Treatment of Acute Angle-closure Glaucoma**

Acute angle-closure glaucoma is an ophthalmological emergency; hence, treatment should be started immediately. The principles of treatment of acute angle-closure glaucoma are:

1. To reduce IOP and control of inflammation.
2. To open of angle of the anterior chamber to increase aqueous outflow.
3. To prevent angle closure in future.
4. Prophylactic treatment of other eye by laser iridotomy.
5. Reduction of IOP and control of inflammation is done by:
   a. Intravenous (IV) mannitol 20%, 1.5–2 g/kg body weight given over period of 45 minutes to 1 hour or oral glycerol in cases in which IV mannitol is contraindicated.
   b. Oral acetazolamide 250 mg one or two tablets stat.
   c. Topical timolol 0.5% eyedrops.
   d. Topical steroid eyedrops to control inflammation.
   e. Oral and systemic analgesic drugs to relieve pain.
6. Treatments aimed at opening of angle of the anterior chamber to increase aqueous outflow:
   a. Patient is asked to lie in supine position, so that the iris lens diaphragm falls back, thereby increasing the anterior chamber depth.

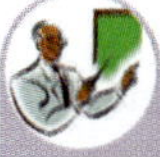

Role of Pilocarpine in Acute Angle-closure Glaucoma

Pilocarpine acts in angle-closure glaucoma by breaking the pupillary block. It acts by causing miosis, thereby pulling the peripheral iris away from the trabecular meshwork, thus preventing the crowding of iris at the angle of the anterior chamber.

If the angle closure is caused by anterior lens movement or intumescent lens, which may occur in few cases, pilocarpine increases the angle closure because of ciliary spasm leading to further anterior movement of the iris lens diaphragm.

Hence, use of pilocarpine should be followed with close monitoring of IOP to find out the cases in which angle closure is caused by lens mechanism. In these cases, pilocarpine eyedrops are contraindicated.

   b. After the IOP is controlled by the above measures, pilocarpine 2–4% eyedrops four times per day are started. Once the

IOP is controlled, the corneal edema is subsided and anterior chamber inflammation is controlled laser iridotomy or surgical iridectomy is done to eliminate pupillary block.

c. If the IOP increases on treatment with pilocarpine as in case of lens-related angle closure, pilocarpine eyedrops are stopped and argon laser iridoplasty is done.

7. Treatment to prevent angle closure in future: After laser iridotomy, surgical iridectomy or iridoplasty is performed and the patient is examined repeatedly at frequent intervals; at each visit IOP recording and gonioscopy are done and depending on the examination findings the following treatment is followed:
   a. If the IOP is under control with open angle, patient is examined frequently and followed up with optic disk changes, visual field defects as done for open-angle glaucoma.
   b. If the IOP is elevated with open angle, medical treatment similar to open angle-glaucoma is continued.
   c. If the IOP is elevated with synechial angle closure less than 180°, argon laser trabeculoplasty is carried out.
   d. If the IOP is elevated with synechial angle closure more than 180°, trabeculectomy is indicated.
   f. If the IOP is still elevated, more complex surgeries such as glaucoma artificial drainage devices are indicated.

Treatment of other eye is very important in every patient with acute congestive glaucoma. Other eye should be examined and if the anterior chamber is shallow and angle of the anterior chamber is narrow prophylactic laser iridotomy has to be done.

Treatment of Chronic Angle-closure Glaucoma

1. Initial treatment in chronic angle-closure glaucoma is aimed at controlling the elevated IOP and performing laser iridotomy to prevent pupillary block.
2. After iridotomy surgical treatment in the form of trabeculectomy is indicated depending on the amount of synechial angle closure.
3. Patients with elevated IOP after trabeculectomy surgery are candidates for glaucoma surgery with artificial drainage devices or cyclophotocoagulation.

Treatment of Absolute Glaucoma*

The treatment of absolute glaucoma is mainly aimed at pain management. It is done by destructive procedures targeted at ciliary body to shut down the production of aqueous humor.

The treatment options available are:

1. *Cyclocryotherapy:* Destruction of ciliary body by cryoprobe.
2. *Cyclophotocoagulation:* Destruction of ciliary body by laser photocoagulation.
3. *Retrobulbar injection of absolute alcohol:* 96% absolute alcohol is injected by retrobulbar injection; alcohol provides pain relief by causing coagulation of proteins of sensory nerve fibers.

If the patient is not responsive and presents with painful blind eye, destructive surgeries of the eye such as enucleation and evisceration are considered.

GIST BOX 9.5

- Primary angle-closure glaucoma (PACG) is a type of glaucoma caused by closure of the angle by the peripheral iris, obstructing the aqueous outflow.
- The PACG is more common in hypermetropic eyes as these eyes are smaller with shorter axial length, shallow anterior chamber.
- Clinical stages of angle-closure glaucoma are prodromal stage or latent glaucoma, stage of constant instability or intermittent glaucoma, acute congestive stage or acute angle-closure glaucoma, chronic congestive stage or chronic congestive glaucoma and absolute glaucoma.
- Acute angle-closure glaucoma is an ophthalmological emergency; hence, treatment should be started immediately. The principles of treatment of acute angle-closure glaucoma are:
  - To reduce the intraocular pressure and control of inflammation
  - To open the angle of the anterior chamber to increase aqueous outflow
  - To prevent angle closure in future
  - Prophylactic treatment of other eye by laser iridotomy.

CHAPTER

9.6 Secondary Glaucoma

DEFINITION**

Secondary glaucoma is defined as rise in intraocular pressure (IOP) as a complication of primary intraocular disease, systemic disease resulting in development of glaucoma.

Secondary glaucoma can be open-angle, angle-closure or mixed-mechanism glaucoma. Secondary glaucoma accounts for about 10% of all the varieties of glaucoma with about 10 million people suffering from secondary glaucoma worldwide. The causes for secondary glaucoma* are of diverse etiology and can be:

- Pigmentary glaucoma
- Pseudoexfoliation glaucoma
- Steroid-induced glaucoma
- Inflammatory glaucoma
- Lens-induced glaucoma
- Traumatic glaucoma
- Neovascular glaucoma
- Glaucoma following ocular surgeries
- Glaucoma associated with intraocular tumors
- Glaucoma associated with intraocular hemorrhage
- Glaucoma associated with elevated episcleral venous pressure
- Glaucoma associated with iridocorneal endothelial (ICE) syndrome
- Glaucoma associated with rhegmatogenous retinal detachment.

PIGMENTARY GLAUCOMA**

Definition

Pigmentary glaucoma is a secondary open-angle glaucoma characterized by deposition of iris pigments in the trabecular meshwork causing resistance to aqueous outflow resulting in glaucoma.

Etiopathogenesis

Pigmentary glaucoma is seen in association with pigment dispersion syndrome. The risk factors for development of pigmentary glaucoma are pigment dispersion syndrome with young age, myopia and white race. It is seen more often in males with male to female ratio of 2:1.

Pigment Dispersion Syndrome

Pigment dispersion syndrome is a clinical syndrome characterized by presence of pigmented trabecular meshwork, iris transillumination defects and Krukenberg's spindle (spindle-shaped deposition of pigment over the posterior surface of cornea).

The risk of development of glaucoma is about 15% after 15 years. The overall incidence of development of glaucoma in pigment dispersion syndrome is about 25–50%.

The eyes with pigment dispersion syndrome typically show deep anterior chamber with concave configuration of the iris. This leads to development of reverse pupillary block (in pupillary block, the pupil gets blocked whereas here iris gets blocked). Because of the repeated rubbing of the iris against the zonules of the lens leads to liberation of pigments. The liberated pigments get deposited throughout the anterior chamber, posterior surface of cornea and in the trabecular meshwork. The pigments deposited in the trabecular meshwork cause resistance to flow of aqueous humor resulting in elevation of IOP and glaucoma.

Clinical Features

1. The classic clinical features are triad of presence of pigmented trabecular meshwork on gonioscopy, iris transillumination defects and Krukenberg's spindle along with raised IOP, visual field and optic disk changes.
2. Along with the triad, the structures in the anterior segment show pigmentation.

Treatment

1. Prophylactic treatment is by laser iridotomy, which treats the reverse pupillary block; laser iridotomy acts by flattening the concave contour of the iris.
2. Treatment of pigmentary glaucoma is on similar lines as primary open-angle glaucoma with antiglaucoma drugs. The prognosis is poorer compared to primary open-angle glaucoma. Cases not responding to medical treatment are managed by argon laser trabeculoplasty and trabeculectomy.

PSEUDOEXFOLIATION GLAUCOMA**

Definition

1. Pseudoexfoliation glaucoma is secondary open-angle glaucoma characterized by deposition of exfoliation material in the trabecular meshwork causing resistance to aqueous outflow resulting in glaucoma.
2. It is also called glaucoma capsulare because of visible deposition of exfoliation material over the lens capsule.
3. It is the commonest cause of secondary open-angle glaucoma.

Etiopathogenesis

Pseudoexfoliation glaucoma is seen in association with pseudoexfoliation syndrome.

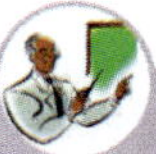

Pseudoexfoliation Syndrome

It is a clinical syndrome characterized by deposition of pseudoexfoliation material on the anterior capsule of the lens, zonules of lens, pupillary margin of the iris, endothelium of cornea, trabecular meshwork and other structures of the anterior segment of the eye.

It is a systemic syndrome with clinical manifestations predominantly limited to eye. Though pseudoexfoliation material is also seen in other organs such as kidneys, liver, lung, myocardium, etc. Systemic manifestations of the disease are not well known clinically.

The risk of development of glaucoma in pseudexfoliation syndrome is about 50%. Hence, all patients with pseudoexfoliation syndrome should be examined at regular intervals once in 1–2 years for development of glaucoma.

Pseudoexfoliation syndrome should be differentiated from true exfoliation seen following exposure to heat, radiation (true exfoliation was seen in the past in glass blowers because of constant exposure to heat).

Pseudoexfoliation glaucoma is seen in more commonly in elderly individuals in fifth or sixth decade of age; in females it is more than males. Pseudoexfoliation glaucoma is characterized by presence of dandruff-like flaky white material distributed in the structures of the anterior segment. The deposition of exfoliation material in the trabecular meshwork leads to increase in resistance to the aqueous outflow resulting in increased IOP.

Clinical Features

1. The clinical features of pseudoexfoliation syndrome are presence of exfoliation material on the pupillary margin of the iris, anterior capsule of lens and gonioscopy shows deposition of exfoliation material and excessive pigmentation of the trabecular meshwork.
2. The other associated features are poor pupillary dilatation, transillumination defects in the iris and weakness of zonules. Poor pupillary dilatation and weakness of zonules leads to high risk for intraoperative complications such as posterior capsular rent, posterior dislocation of nucleus of lens during cataract surgery on eyes with pseudoexfoliation syndrome.
3. Pseudoexfoliation glaucoma usually presents as unilateral glaucoma or bilateral with asymmetrical in nature. Pseudoexfoliation glaucoma is usually open-angle glaucoma; however, secondary angle-closure glaucoma is also known to occur in few eyes.

Differential Diagnosis

Pseudoexfoliation glaucoma has to be differentiated from:

1. *Pigmentary glaucoma:* It is seen basically in young myopic males with presence of pigments distributed throughout the anterior segment.
2. *Primary open-angle glaucoma:* Absence of pseudoexfoliation material differentiates it from pseudoexfoliation glaucoma.
3. *Amyloidosis:* It is a systemic disease characterized by deposition of whitish material similar to pseudoexfoliation, but presence of systemic features involving renal system, liver, skin, neuropathies, etc. differentiates it from pseudoexfoliation glaucoma.

Treatment

Treatment of pseudoexfoliation glaucoma is on similar lines as primary open-angle glaucoma with antiglaucoma drugs. The prognosis is poorer compared to primary open-angle glaucoma. Cases not responding to medical treatment are managed by argon laser trabeculoplasty and trabeculectomy.

STEROID-INDUCED GLAUCOMA**

Definition

Steroid-induced glaucoma is secondary open-angle glaucoma characterized by elevated IOP following administration of steroids.

Etiopathogenesis

Steroid-induced glaucoma can occur following any route of administration of steroids—topical, periocular or systemic steroids. Topical and intravitreal routes of administration of steroids are most commonly associated with elevation of IOP.

Elevation of the IOP as high as more than 15 mm Hg as a response to steroid use for more than 4 weeks is seen in 5% of general population. They are known as high steroid-responders. Steroid responders are more prone for development of glaucoma, when steroids are administered.

Accumulation of polymerized glycosaminoglycans in the trabecular meshwork as a result of lysosomal membrane stabilization caused by steroids, thus preventing their degradation. Glycosaminoglycans normally undergo depolymerization and undergo degradation caused by hyaluronidase enzymes present in the lysosomes and hence lysosomal membrane stabilization leads to accumulation of glycosaminoglycans in the trabecular meshwork, which leads to increased resistance to aqueous outflow in the trabecular meshwork resulting in elevation of IOP.

Other proposed mechanisms of steroid-induced glaucoma are:

1. Accumulation of debris in the trabecular meshwork causing increased resistance to aqueous outflow as a result of inhibition of phagocytosis by endothelial cells lining the trabecular meshwork.

2. Inhibition in the synthesis of prostaglandins by steroids, which increase the aqueous outflow.
3. Increased expression of myocilin, glaucoma gene.

Clinical Features

The clinical features are similar to primary open-angle glaucoma, the only differentiating feature being history of use of steroids.

Treatment

1. The basic principle of treatment is to stop steroids and use of antiglaucoma drugs to reduce the raised IOP. Usually, IOP decreases on withdrawal of steroids. Rarely other treatment options such as laser trabeculoplasty or filtration surgery are required.
2. Steroid-induced glaucoma can be reduced by optimal use of steroids and regular follow-up of those, who require steroids to find out steroid responders and by use of steroid sparing drugs in steroid responders.

INFLAMMATORY GLAUCOMA**

Definition

Inflammatory glaucoma is a secondary glaucoma caused by alterations in the aqueous humor dynamics as a result of ocular inflammation.

Etiopathogenesis

Uveitis is the most common ocular inflammation associated with inflammatory glaucoma. Keratitis, episcleritis, scleritis and other inflammatory conditions are also associated with inflammatory glaucoma.

The mechanism of inflammatory glaucoma caused by uveitis is well understood and inflammatory glaucoma is seen in about 15–20% of uveitis patients.

Inflammatory glaucoma in uveitis can be caused by open angle or angle closure, or combined mechanism:

1. Obstruction of the trabecular meshwork by inflammatory cells, hypersecretion of the aqueous humor caused by prostaglandins and other inflammatory mediators, steroid-induced glaucoma caused by steroids used in the treatment of glaucoma are some of the mechanisms involved in causing open-angle inflammatory glaucoma.
2. Synechial closure of the angle of anterior chamber, posterior synechiae causing pupillary block glaucoma, neovascularization and formation of fibrovascular membrane involving the angle of anterior chamber are some of the mechanisms involved in causing angle-closure inflammatory glaucoma.
3. Combined mechanism is because of presence of both the above causes together.

The mechanism of inflammatory glaucoma in keratitis may be because of associated uveitis. The mechanism of inflammatory glaucoma in scleritis and episcleritis is not well understood; it may be because of associated uveitis or elevated episcleral venous pressure.

Clinical Features

Inflammatory glaucoma presents with the clinical features of the primary ocular disease and elevated IOP with open or closed angle depending on the mechanism of glaucoma (Figs 9.6.1A and B).

Glaucomatocyclitic crisis, Fuchs' heterochromic iridocyclitis, intermediate uveitis, phacogenic uveitis, uveitis associated with systemic diseases such as juvenile rheumatoid arthritis, sarcoidosis, ankylosing spondylitis, Behcet's disease, psoriatic arthritis, etc. are some of the common uveitic conditions associated with inflammatory glaucoma.

Treatment

The treatment of inflammatory glaucoma is by treatment of ocular inflammation by use of steroids, cycloplegic agents, etc. and reduction of elevated IOP by use of antiglaucoma drugs. Cases not responding to medical line of management are treated by glaucoma surgery.

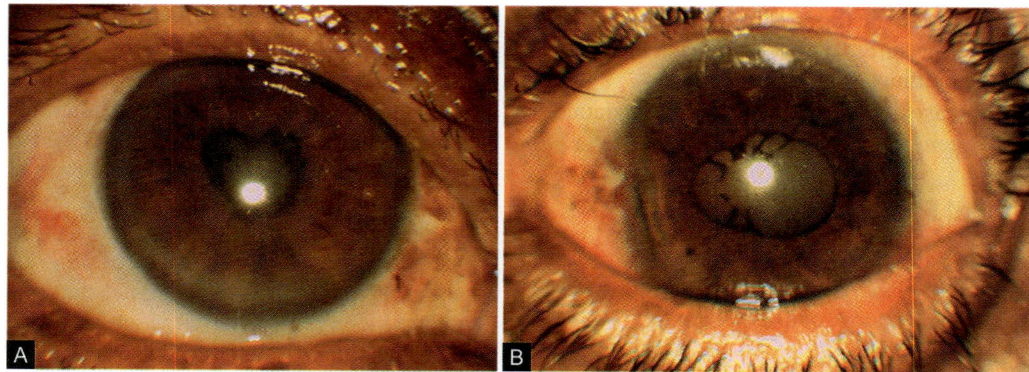

FIGS 9.6.1A and B: Inflammatory glaucoma

LENS-INDUCED GLAUCOMA

Lens-induced glaucoma is described in detail under Section 8, Chapter 8.5 'Lens-induced Glucoma'.

TRAUMATIC GLAUCOMA**

Definition

Traumatic glaucoma is a type of secondary glaucoma following ocular trauma.

Etiopathogenesis

Glaucoma can result from blunt injury or penetrating injury:

- Traumatic glaucoma is more common following blunt injury
- Traumatic glaucoma can be caused by either open-angle or angle-closure or combined mechanism
- Traumatic glaucoma can follow either immediately following injury or can have late onset.

Causes for Traumatic Glaucoma Following Blunt Injury

Inflammation: It leads to obstruction of the trabecular meshwork by inflammatory cells and causes glaucoma in the early period following injury with open-angle mechanism.

Hemorrhage: This in the form of hyphema leads to glaucoma in the early period following injury. Vitreous hemorrhage can lead to glaucoma in the late period because of ghost cells called ghost-cell glaucoma.

Subluxation or dislocation of the lens: It can lead to glaucoma in the early period following injury because of pupillary block or angle-closure mechanism.

Angle recession: It is caused by trauma leads to hypotony, but as the angle structures heal, it leads to fibrosis and formation of synechial closure causing glaucoma by angle-closure glaucoma.

Causes for Traumatic Glaucoma Following Penetrating Injury

In addition to the above explained mechanisms other mechanisms specific to penetrating injuries are:

- Epithelial downgrowth or fibrous in growth
- Adherent leukoma
- Toxic effect of retained intraocular foreign body.

Clinical Features

Initially following injury, hypotony may be seen, but later glaucoma sets in because of one of the mechanisms as described previously.

Hence, patients presenting with trauma of the eye should be evaluated to rule out glaucoma.

Patients with high risk of developing traumatic glaucoma are those who present initially with:

- Hyphema
- Vitreous hemorrhage
- Angle recession
- Lens subluxation or dislocation.

Treatment

Treatment depends on the underlying cause. Initially, IOP is reduced by antiglaucoma drugs.

Angle-recession Glaucoma**

Angle recession is a secondary chronic open-angle glaucoma seen in eyes with angle recession.

Angle recession is defined as separation of circular and longitudinal fibers of the ciliary muscle as a result of blunt trauma to the eye.

The risk of secondary glaucoma following angle recession is about 10%. Eyes with angle recession of less than 180° usually will not develop glaucoma. Glaucoma is more commonly seen in eyes with more than 180° of angle recession.

The exact mechanism of development of angle-recession glaucoma is poorly understood. The degenerative changes in the trabecular meshwork following trauma leading to formation of membrane covering the trabecular meshwork may be the cause for angle-recession glaucoma.

Angle-recession glaucoma is secondary open-angle glaucoma, which usually presents late after injury. About 50% of those who develop angle-recession glaucoma, have a tendency to develop primary open-angle glaucoma in the normal fellow eye. Angle-recession glaucoma typically presents as unilateral glaucoma. Angle recession is diagnosed by presence of deep anterior chamber and irregular, and wide ciliary body band as seen on gonioscopy. Ultrasound biomicroscopy can show angle recession.

Treatment of angle-recession glaucoma is on similar lines as for primary open-angle glaucoma.

NEOVASCULAR GLAUCOMA**

Definition

Neovascular glaucoma is a severe type of secondary glaucoma caused by proliferation of new vessels over iris and trabecular meshwork resulting in formation of fibrovascular membrane involving the angle of the anterior chamber obstructing the flow of aqueous humor.

It is called by various names such as rubeotic glaucoma, hemorrhagic glaucoma, 100-days' glaucoma and thrombotic glaucoma.

Neovascular glaucoma is one of the severe types of secondary glaucoma, which is difficult to treat and it often results in blindness.

Etiopathogenesis

Hypoxia resulting from ischemia of retina is the initiating event in the development of neovascularization. The angiogenic factor vascular endothelial growth factor (VEGF) and other inflammatory mediators are responsible for neovascularization.

The mechanism of glaucoma in the early stages is by open-angle mechanism by the obstruction of the trabecular meshwork caused by fibrovascular membrane. In the later stages, angle closure caused by contraction of the fibrovascular membrane leads to glaucoma.

Diabetic retinopathy and central retinal vein occlusion are the commonest causes associated with neovascularization and neovascular glaucoma.

*Causes for Neovascularization and Neovascular Glaucoma**

The causes for neovascularization and neovascular glaucoma are:

1. *Diseases of retina associated with retinal ischemia* such as:
   - Diabetic retinopathy
   - Retinal vascular occlusive diseases such as central retinal vein occlusion, hemicentral retinal vein occlusion
   - Ocular ischemic syndrome
   - Sickle cell retinopathy.
2. *Inflammatory diseases of the eye*:
   - Chronic uveitis
   - Retinal vasculitis associated with diseases, e.g. Eale's disease, Behcet's disease, etc.

3. *Tumors of the eye*:
   - Retinoblastoma
   - Melanoma of iris, ciliary body, choroid
   - Metastatic tumors.

Central retinal artery occlusion is not commonly associated with neovascular glaucoma as it causes rapid necrosis of retina, whereas central retinal vein occlusion results in chronic hypoxia resulting in production of vasoproliferative factors.

Branch retinal vein occlusion is not commonly associated with neovascular glaucoma as it involves less than half of the retina; production of adequate neovascular stimulus requires involvement of half or more than of retina to be involved by hypoxic stimulus. Hence, neovascular glaucoma is commonly seen in central retinal vein occlusion and hemicentral retinal vein occlusion.

Clinical Features

The disease can be classified into three stages:

1. *Rubeosis stage:* This stage is asymptomatic with presence of symptoms of the underlying disease only. On examination, presence of new vessels along the pupillary margin extending toward the angle of the anterior chamber is seen.
2. *Open-angle glaucoma stage:* It is characterized by mild-to-moderate rise of IOP. On examination, gonioscopy shows open angle with absence of synechiae. It is because of formation of fibrovascular membrane involving the angle of the anterior chamber.
3. *Angle-closure glaucoma stage:* It is characterized by very high IOP presenting as acute red eye. It is because of contraction of fibrovascular membrane resulting in synechial closure of the angle of the anterior chamber. This stage is characterized by inflammation of the anterior chamber, corneal edema with high IOP.

Treatment

1. Prophylactic treatment is by panretinal photocoagulation to prevent the production of neovascular stimulus from hypoxic retina.
2. Panretinal cryotherapy is done in cases in which panretinal photocoagulation cannot be done because of opacities in the media.
3. Once glaucoma is developed, treatment is by control of IOP; it is done by antiglaucoma drugs.
4. Cases presenting late with angle-closure glaucoma require steroids and cycloplegic drugs to control associated inflammation.
5. Most of the cases of neovascular glaucoma develop blindness because of neovascular glaucoma itself and because of the underlying disease causing glaucoma. The response to medical line of treatment for neovascular glaucoma is unsatisfactory, and most cases may require surgical treatment such as trabeculectomy or artificial drainage devices.

GLAUCOMA FOLLOWING OCULAR SURGERIES

Glaucoma is seen as a complication of ocular surgery. The most common surgeries associated with development of glaucoma are:

- Cataract surgery
- Penetrating keratoplasty
- Vitrectomy.

The mechanisms of development of glaucoma are:

- Early complications related to surgery in case of hyphema, postoperative inflammation, retained viscoelastic material, pupillary block glaucoma, malignant glaucoma, etc.
- Late complications such as epithelial ingrowth and fibrous downgrowth
- Steroid-induced glaucoma caused by use of steroids in the postoperative period.

Malignant Glaucoma**

Malignant glaucoma is a rare, but aggressive type of postoperative glaucoma. It is also known as aqueous misdirection glaucoma or ciliary block glaucoma.

It is seen typically following surgery on eyes with narrow angles or angle closure. It is called malignant glaucoma because of aggressive nature of the disease, which responds poorly to treatment with rapid progression to glaucomatous optic atrophy.

The mechanism of malignant glaucoma is explained by misdirection of the aqueous posteriorly resulting in increase in the vitreous volume, which leads to shallowing of the anterior chamber, angle closure and elevation of IOP. Abnormal and thickened anterior hyaloid is known to play a vital role in the pathogenesis of malignant glaucoma (Figs 9.6.2A and B).

Malignant glaucoma presents as painful, acute red eye following surgery with shallow anterior chamber and elevated IOP.

Malignant glaucoma has to be differentiated from pupillary block glaucoma. Pupillary block glaucoma is because of pupillary block caused by intraocular lens in pseudophakia, vitreous in cases of aphakia and other materials such as lens matter, fibrinous membrane, etc. It is characterized by peripheral shallow and central deep anterior chamber and it responds to peripheral iridectomy or iridotomy, thus differentiating it from malignant glaucoma in which the anterior chamber is uniformly shallow and it will not respond to peripheral iridectomy or iridotomy.

The treatment of malignant glaucoma is by use of:

- Antiglaucoma drugs, including hyperosmotic agents to decrease IOP
- Cycloplegic agents, which cause contraction of the zonules, backward movement of the lens and thus help in formation of anterior chamber
- Laser treatment for disruption of anterior hyaloid face
- Laser treatment to ciliary processes to cause shrinkage of the ciliary processes
- Surgical treatment in the form of vitreous aspiration or anterior vitrectomy is indicated in non-responding cases.

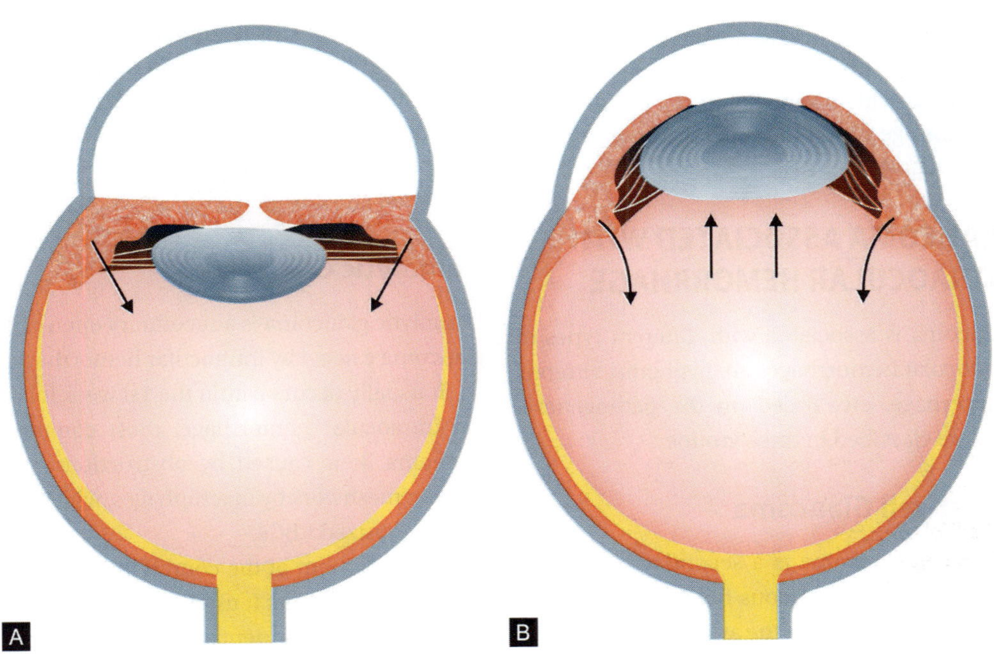

FIGS 9.6.2A and B: Mechanism of malignant glaucoma

GLAUCOMA ASSOCIATED WITH INTRAOCULAR TUMORS

Glaucoma is seen in benign and malignant tumors of the eye. The mechanisms involved in development of glaucoma because of intraocular tumors are:

1. Tumors of the anterior segment such as tumors of iris and ciliary body result in glaucoma by:
   a. Infiltration of the trabecular meshwork by tumor cells.
   b. Extension of tumor to involve the trabecular meshwork.
2. Tumors of the posterior segment such as tumors of choroid and retina result in glaucoma by:
   a. Neovascularization of the angle of the anterior chamber resulting in neovascular glaucoma.
   b. Anterior displacement of iris lens diaphragm resulting in angle closure.

The treatment of glaucoma is by treatment of the underlying tumor along with antiglaucoma treatment. Presence of secondary glaucoma in a patient with intraocular tumor indicates advanced stage of the intraocular tumor and is a bad prognostic sign.

GLAUCOMA ASSOCIATED WITH INTRAOCULAR HEMORRHAGE

Glaucoma is associated with different types of intraocular hemorrhages are hyphema, vitreous hemorrhage, etc. Based on the pathogenesis they are classified in three groups.

Ghost-cell Glaucoma*

Ghost-cell glaucoma is a secondary glaucoma seen in eyes with vitreous hemorrhage associated with disruption of the anterior hyaloid face. It is also called khaki-cell glaucoma.

Ghost Cells

The degenerated red blood cells (RBC) after vitreous hemorrhage are called ghost cells. They usually develop 2–4 weeks after vitreous hemorrhage. The RBC lose hemoglobin, undergo degeneration and appear as khaki-colored cells. The ghost cells are rigid and less flexible compared to RBC.

These ghost cells gain access into anterior chamber in cases of disruption of the anterior hyaloid face. Since, these ghost cells are less flexible and they cannot pass through the trabecular meshwork, they get accumulated in the trabecular meshwork and cause elevation of IOP.

It presents in patients with vitreous hemorrhage with symptoms of sudden increase of IOP. On examination, khaki-colored ghost cells are seen in the anterior chamber and on gonioscopy, the ghost cells are seen over the trabecular meshwork.

The treatment is by antiglaucoma drugs to control IOP. Cases not responding to medical line of treatment require anterior chamber wash to remove the ghost cells followed by vitrectomy to clear vitreous hemorrhage, the source of degenerated ghost cells.

Hemolytic Glaucoma

Hemolytic glaucoma is a secondary open-angle glaucoma caused by intraocular hemorrhage.

It usually occurs within the 1st week following intraocular hemorrhage, most commonly hyphema. It is caused by obstruction of trabecular meshwork by macrophages, which have phagocytosized RBCs.

The treatment of the condition is similar to ghost-cell glaucoma. It usually responds well to medical line of treatment and surgical intervention is rarely required.

Hemosiderotic Glaucoma

Hemosiderotic glaucoma is a secondary open-angle glaucoma caused by siderosis of the trabecular meshwork. It is a relatively rare condition seen in long-standing intraocular hemorrhage.

The endothelial cells of the trabecular meshwork phagocytose the hemoglobin released from degenerated RBCs. The iron released from the hemoglobin causes siderosis of trabecular meshwork leading to sclerotic changes, which causes increased resistance to flow of aqueous humor.

GLAUCOMA ASSOCIATED WITH ELEVATED EPISCLERAL VENOUS PRESSURE

Glaucoma associated with elevated episcleral venous pressure include a group of conditions characterized by elevated IOP associated with elevated episcleral venous pressure.

Aqueous outflow depends on pressure gradient between the episcleral venous pressure and IOP. The normal episcleral venous pressure is about 10 mm Hg. An increase in episcleral venous pressure leads to decreased aqueous outflow, which results in increased IOP.

The causes for elevated episcleral venous pressure are:

- Arteriovenous anomalies, e.g. carotid- cavernous fistula, Sturge-Weber syndrome
- Venous obstruction caused by a variety of causes such as cavernous sinus thrombosis, superior vena cava syndrome and thyroid ophthalmopathy.

Glaucoma associated with elevated episcleral venous pressure along with increased IOP present with clinical features of dilated and tortuous episcleral veins and chemosis of conjunctiva. Gonioscopy shows open angles with presence of blood in the Schlemm's canal.

Treatment of the condition is by treatment of the underlying cause along with treatment of the raised IOP by antiglaucoma drugs.

GLAUCOMA ASSOCIATED WITH IRIDOCORNEAL ENDOTHELIAL SYNDROME

Secondary glaucoma is seen in ICE syndrome, a degenerative disease involving the uveal tract. It is described in Chapter 7.8 'Dystrophies and Degenerations of Uveal Tract'.

GLAUCOMA ASSOCIATED WITH RHEGMATOGENOUS RETINAL DETACHMENT

Schwartz's Syndrome*

Schwartz syndrome is characterized by secondary chronic open-angle glaucoma following retinal detachment. It is named after Schwartz, who first described the disease.

Rhegmatogenous retinal detachment usually results in hypotony because of increased uveoscleral outflow through the retinal break. Rarely few patients present with elevated IOP because of chronic secondary open-angle glaucoma.

The mechanism of secondary glaucoma is not well known. It is supposed to be because of:

- Associated iridocyclitis resulting in trabeculitis leading to decreased aqueous outflow
- Obstruction of the trabecular meshwork by outer segments of the photoreceptors.

The treatment of the condition is by using antiglaucoma drugs to decrease the raised IOP and surgery for retinal detachment.

GIST BOX 9.6

- Secondary glaucoma is defined as rise in intraocular pressure as a complication of primary intraocular disease—systemic disease resulting in development of glaucoma.
- Secondary glaucoma can be open-angle, angle-closure or mixed-mechanism glaucoma. Secondary glaucoma accounts for about 10% of all the varieties of glaucoma with about 10 million people suffering from secondary glaucoma worldwide.

The causes for secondary glaucoma can be:

- Pigmentary glaucoma
- Pseudoexfoliation glaucoma
- Steroid-induced glaucoma
- Inflammatory glaucoma
- Lens-induced glaucoma
- Traumatic glaucoma
- Neovascular glaucoma
- Glaucoma following ocular surgeries
- Glaucoma associated with intraocular tumors
- Glaucoma associated with intraocular hemorrhage
- Glaucoma associated with elevated episcleral venous pressure
- Glaucoma associated with iridocorneal endothelial (ICE) syndrome
- Glaucoma associated with rhegmatogenous retinal detachment.

CHAPTER

9.7 Treatment Modalities of Glaucoma

Glaucoma leads to irreversible visual loss because of progressive damage of the optic nerve. Reduction of intraocular pressure (IOP) is the only effective known treatment available to prevent the progression of the disease.

The aim of treatment is to reduce the IOP and monitor the changes in optic disk and visual fields at regular intervals to prevent the progression of the disease.

The decision to start treatment in glaucoma is taken depending on the patient's IOP, amount of damage to the optic nerve and rate of progression of glaucoma. Once started treatment is required for rest of the life of the patient.

The treatment options available are medical treatment by using antiglaucoma drugs, laser treatment and glaucoma surgeries. Generally, antiglaucoma drugs are the first line of management. The treatment is modified depending on the patient's response to antiglaucoma drugs, compliance of the patient, adverse effects of antiglaucoma drugs, coexisting systemic diseases, etc.

Antiglaucoma drugs are described in detail under Chapter 8 'Drugs Used in Ophthalmology' in Author's textbook *Clinical Methods in Ophthalmology*.

LASER TREATMENT MODALITIES FOR GLAUCOMA

Laser Peripheral Iridotomy

Laser peripheral iridotomy involves creation of a full-thickness hole in the periphery of iris to create an alternate pathway for flow of aqueous from posterior to anterior chamber by using laser energy.

Laser iridotomy has almost replaced surgical iridectomy, which was done before laser was available.

*Indications**

- Acute angle-closure glaucoma
- Chronic angle-closure glaucoma
- As a prophylaxis against development of angle closure in fellow eye in a patient with acute angle-closure glaucoma
- Aphakic or pseudophakic pupillary block
- As a prophylaxis to prevent pigmentary glaucoma in a patient with pigment dispersion syndrome.

Procedure

Topical pilocarpine 1% eyedrops are applied to the eye before 1 hour of the procedure. Pilocarpine helps by stretching the peripheral iris and making it thin, which helps in easy penetration of the laser energy. One drop of 0.5% apraclonidine or 0.2% brimonidine is applied to prevent postoperative elevation of the IOP.

The procedure is done under topical anesthesia. The laser commonly used is neodymium-yttrium-aluminum-garnet (Nd-YAG) laser, which acts by photodisruption. Though it can be done by argon laser, which acts by photocoagulation, it is not preferred as it requires the laser energy to be absorbed by the pigments in the iris; it may not act on light-colored iris.

Usually, iridotomy is done in the periphery of the iris, which is covered by upper eyelid to prevent postoperative glare or diplopia. It is done as an office procedure in sitting position by a slit lamp fitted with laser. Though it can be done without using contact lens Abraham iridotomy lens or wise iridotomy lens is used as the contact lenses minimize the eye movements and concentrate the laser energy.

Topical steroids are used in the postoperative period to treat the inflammation induced by laser for 1 week.

Laser Trabeculoplasty

Laser trabeculoplasty involves application of laser burns to trabecular meshwork to increase the aqueous outflow as a result of shrinkage of collagen and opening of intratrabecular spaces.

Indications

- Primary open-angle glaucoma with failure of medical treatment to reduce the IOP below the target pressure
- Pseudoexfoliation glaucoma and pigmentary glaucoma not responding to medical treatment.

Procedure

Laser trabeculoplasty is done under topical anesthesia with patient seated with slit lamp fitted with laser. One drop of 0.5% apraclonidine or 0.2% brimonidine is applied before the procedure to prevent postoperative elevation of the IOP. It is done by using gonioprism or four mirror gonioscopic lens.

Laser trabeculoplasty can be of various types depending on the lasers used:

- Argon laser trabeculoplasty (ALT)
- Selective laser trabeculoplasty (SLT)
- Diode laser trabeculoplasty (DLT).

Argon laser trabeculoplasty is done by application of argon laser burns at the junction of the pigmented and non-pigmented trabecular meshwork. The SLT is done by application of frequency doubled Nd-YAG laser. It selectively affects the pigmented cells; hence, it is called selective laser trabeculoplasty. Since, it selectively affects the cells, it is safer than ALT. DLT is similar to ALT except that the laser used is diode laser. Laser trabeculoplasty requires presence of open angle in more than 180° for visibility and success of the procedure.

Topical steroids are used in the postoperative period to treat the inflammation induced by laser for 1 week.

Laser Iridoplasty

Laser iridoplasty involves application of partial thickness laser burns to the periphery of the iris to cause contraction of stroma of iris to widen the angle.

Indications

- Plateau iris syndrome
- Before doing trabeculoplasty in patients with narrow angles to increase the visibility of the angle of the anterior chamber.

It is done by argon green laser by using Abraham iridotomy lens.

SURGICAL TREATMENT MODALITIES FOR GLAUCOMA

Iridectomy*

Iridectomy involves creation of a full thickness hole in the periphery of iris to create an alternate pathway for flow of aqueous from posterior to anterior chamber. The indications are similar to laser iridotomy.

With the advent of laser iridotomy, surgical iridectomy is not popular because of the involvement of the risks of the intraocular surgery.

Filtration Surgeries

The surgical treatment modalities consist of making a channel or fistula for filtration of the aqueous from the eye and are called filtration surgeries. Depending on the thickness of the tissue removed, the filtration surgeries are classified are as follows.

Full-thickness Filtration Surgery

Full-thickness filtration surgery includes removal of full thickness of sclera by punch forceps or trephination or thermosclerostomy by using thermal energy under a conjunctival flap. Because of the high rate of complications, they are no longer done.

Partial-thickness Filtration Surgery

Partial-thickness surgery includes removal of partial thickness of sclera including a part of trabecular meshwork under a scleral flap and it is called trabeculectomy.

Trabeculectomy**

Trabeculectomy is the most common form of glaucoma surgery performed in clinical practice.

Trabeculectomy is described in detail in Chapter 9 'Common Ophthalmic Surgeries' in Author's textbook *'Clinical Methods in Ophthalmology'*.

*Non-penetrating Glaucoma Surgery**

Non-penetrating glaucoma surgery are relatively new surgical techniques and are safer than trabeculectomy with similar efficacy.

Deep sclerectomy, viscocanalostomy and canaloplasty are the recent non-penetrating glaucoma surgeries with promising results for control of IOP.

Deep sclerectomy

Deep sclerectomy involves making superficial and deep partial-thickness scleral flaps, removing the deep scleral flap and unroofing the Schlemm's canal, leaving behind the Descemet's membrane. The superficial flap is sutured. It differs from trabeculectomy by the fact here Descemet's membrane is left behind and this acts as semipermeable tissue to allow the aqueous to flow through it.

Viscocanalostomy

Viscocanalostomy is done in a similar fashion as deep sclerectomy after exposing the Schlemm's canal; it is expanded by injecting viscoelastic material.

Canaloplasty

Canaloplasty is done in similar fashion as viscocanalostomy; here after exposing the Schlemm's canal, it is enlarged by inserting a microcatheter.

Surgeries for Congenital and Developmental Glaucoma

They are described under Section 9, Chapter 9.3 'Childhood Glaucoma'.

Antimetabolites/Antifibrotic Agents in Trabeculectomy*

Antimetabolites are used in trabeculectomy surgery to prevent scarring by inhibition of fibroblasts and modulation of wound healing.

Mitomycin-C and 5-fluorouracil are the most antimetabolites used as an adjuvant in trabeculectomy surgery.

Indications

- Previously failed trabeculectomy
- Secondary glaucoma such as neovascular glaucoma, inflammatory glaucoma, etc. which have high risk for failure with only trabeculectomy
- Previous conjunctival scarring as a result of previous surgeries involving the site of trabeculectomy.

Mitomycin-C is used intraoperatively by applying over the scleral bed in a concentration of 0.2–0.5 mg/mL applied for 1–5 minutes after taking all precautions to avoid entry of the drug into anterior chamber.

The drug 5-fluorouracil is used either intraoperatively in a concentration of 50 mg/mL or postoperatively as subconjunctival injection of 0.5 mL daily for 1 week.

Artificial Drainage Devices

Artificial drainage devices are used in glaucoma cases, which are refractory to treatment. They act by providing an alternative pathway for drainage of aqueous through the tube implant from anterior chamber to subconjunctival space.

Indications

- Glaucoma cases not responding to conventional glaucoma surgeries
- Inflammatory glaucoma, neovascular glaucoma, glaucoma associated with penetrating keratoplasty, developmental glaucoma, etc.

Types

Artificial drainage devices are of two types:

1. Non-valved implants: Molteno implant, Baerveldt implant, Schocket implant, etc.
2. Valved implants: Ahmed implant, Krupin implant, etc.

Artificial drainage devices are associated with potential intraoperative complications such as hyphema, expulsive choroidal hemorrhage, vitreous hemorrhage, etc. and postoperative complications such as hypotony, closure of the implant, expulsion of the implant, endophthalmitis, etc. Hence, artificial drainage devices are used as last resort in treatment of glaucoma, which are refractory to all modalities of treatment and patients implanted with artificial drainage devices require regular monitoring.

Cyclodestructive Procedures

Definition

The procedures aimed at destroying the ciliary body to decrease IOP by decreasing the production of aqueous by ciliary body are called cyclodestructive procedures.

Cyclodestructive procedures lead to irreversible loss of function of ciliary epithelium to secrete aqueous; they are associated with complications such as hypotony, phthisis bulbi with no scope for improvement of vision.

Indications

Cyclodestructive procedures are indicated in eyes with poor vision where all other modalities of treatment have failed for pain relief.

Types

Cyclodestructive procedures include:

1. *Cyclocryotherapy:* It includes use of cryo probe with temperature of –80°C at the sclera produce a temperature of –10°C in the ciliary processes to cause necrosis of ciliary body. It is done by placing the cryo probe 1 mm posterior to the limbus for approximately 1 minute till the visible ice ball forms. It produces non-specific necrosis of all tissues, hence associated with more complications such as postoperative inflammation, hypotony, etc. Hence, it is not preferred mode of treatment.
2. *Cyclophotocoagulation:* It includes use of laser to cause photocoagulation of the ciliary epithelium. The common methods employed are:
   a. Transscleral photocoagulation by using Nd-YAG laser or diode laser done through transscleral route similar to cryotherapy.
   b. Endoscopic laser photocoagulation by using diode laser.

Because of more complications, cryotherapy is not popular. Cyclophotocoagulation is associated with less severe complications, as transscleral photocoagulation causes selective destruction of the pigmented ciliary epithelium, as laser energy is more specifically absorbed by pigmented epithelium of the ciliary body. Endoscopic photocoagulation is performed with visualization of the ciliary processes by an endoscope passed through limbal incision or pars plana incision.

GIST BOX 9.7

- Glaucoma leads to irreversible visual loss because of progressive damage of the optic nerve. Reduction of intraocular pressure (IOP) is the only effective known treatment available to prevent the progression of the disease. The aim of treatment is to reduce the IOP and monitor the changes in optic disk and visual fields at regular intervals to prevent the progression of the disease.
- The treatment options available are medical treatment by using antiglaucoma drugs, laser treatment and glaucoma surgeries. Generally, antiglaucoma drugs are the first line of management.

FREQUENTLY ASKED QUESTIONS (FAQs)

*Short Answers

1. Mention the functions of aqueous humor.
2. Production of aqueous humor.
3. Drainage of aqueous humor.
4. Mention the structures of the angle of the anterior chamber.
5. Grading of the angle of the anterior chamber.
6. Mention the methods of measurement of intraocular pressure (IOP).
7. Mention the anatomical basis of glaucomatous visual field defects.
8. Buphthalmos.
9. Treatment of congenital glaucoma.
10. Mention the risk factors for primary open-angle glaucoma.
11. Mention the drugs used for neuroprotection in glaucoma.
12. Ocular hypertension.
13. Mention the risk factors for primary angle-closure glaucoma.
14. Treatment of absolute glaucoma.
15. Classify primary angle-closure glaucoma.
16. Mention the clinical stages of primary angle-closure glaucoma.
17. Mention the causes for secondary glaucoma.
18. Ghost-cell glaucoma.
19. Schwartz's syndrome.
20. Mention the causes for neovascularization of iris and neovascular glaucoma.
21. Mention the indication for laser peripheral iridotomy/surgical peripheral iridectomy.
22. Mention non-penetrating glaucoma surgeries.
23. Mention the role of antimetabolites in trabeculectomy.

**Short Essays

1. Define IOP. Describe the factors influencing IOP.
2. Tonometry.
3. Describe the pathogenesis of optic nerve damage in glaucoma.
4. Define and classify glaucoma.
5. Primary congenital glaucoma.
6. Describe the clinical features and treatment of congenital glaucoma.
7. Optic disk changes in primary open-angle glaucoma.
8. Visual field changes in primary open-angle glaucoma.
9. Antiglaucoma drugs.
10. Normal-tension glaucoma.
11. Pathogenesis of primary angle-closure glaucoma.
12. Absolute glaucoma.
13. Colored halos.
14. Treatment of acute congestive glaucoma.
15. Define secondary glaucoma. Mention the causes for secondary glaucoma.
16. Pigmentary glaucoma.
17. Pseudoexfoliation glaucoma.
18. Steroid-induced glaucoma.
19. Inflammatory glaucoma.
20. Traumatic glaucoma.
21. Angle-recession glaucoma.
22. Neovascular glaucoma.
23. Malignant glaucoma.
24. Trabeculectomy.

***Long Essays

1. Define Glaucoma. Classify glaucoma. Describe clinical features and management of congenital glaucoma.
2. Describe etiology, clinical features and management of primary open-angle glaucoma.
3. Describe etiology, clinical features and management of primary angle-closure glaucoma.
4. Describe etiology, clinical features and management of acute angle-closure glaucoma.
5. Mention the differential diagnosis of acute red eye. Describe the management of acute congestive glaucoma.

BIBLIOGRAPHY

1. Agarwal R, Gupta SK, Agarwal P, et al. Current concepts in the pathophysiology of glaucoma. Indian J Ophthalmol. 2009;57(4):257-66.
2. Aref AA, Sayyad FE, Mwanza JC, et al. Diagnostic specifities of retinal nerve fiber layer, optic nerve head, and macular ganglion cell-inner plexiform layer measurements in myopic eyes. J Glaucoma. 2014;23(8):487-93.
3. Bodh SA, Kumar V, Raina UK, et al. Inflammatory glaucoma. Oman J Ophthalmol. 2011;4(1):3-9.
4. Bruce SM, Rand AR, Karim FD, et al. Shields' Textbook of Glaucoma, 5th edition. Lippincott Williams & Wilkins.
5. Chua B, Goldberg I. Neuroprotective agents in glaucoma therapy: recent developments and future directions. Expert Rev Ophthalmol. 2010;5(5):627-36.
6. Cook C, Foster P. Epidemiology of glaucoma: what's new? Can J Ophthalmol. 2012;47(3):223-6.
7. Dada T, Nair S, Dhawan M. Steroid-induced glaucoma. Journal of Current Glaucoma Practice. 2009;3(2):33-8.
8. Fasih U, Fehmi MS, Shaikh N, et al. Secondary glaucoma: causes and management. Pak J Ophthalmol. 2008;24(2).
9. Foster PJ, Buhrmann RR, Quigley HA, et al. The definition and classification of glaucoma in prevalence surveys. Br J Ophthalmol. 2002;86:238-42.
10. Goel M, Picciani RG, Lee RK, et al. Aqueous humor dynamics: a review. Open Ophthalmol J. 2010;4:52-9.
11. Hayreh SS. Neovascular glaucoma. Prog Retin Eye Res. 2007;26(5):470-85.
12. Johnson DH, Johnson M. How does nonpenetrating glaucoma surgery work? Aqueous outflow resistance and glaucoma surgery. J Glaucoma. 2001;10(1):55-67.
13. Kanski JJ. Clinical Ophthalmology, 5th edition. Butterworth Heinemann.
14. Koerber N. Canaloplasty: a new approach to nonpenetrating glaucoma surgery. Techniques in Ophthalmology. 2007;5(3):102-6.
15. Le A, Mukesh BN, McCarty CA, et al. Risk factors associated with the incidence of open-angle glaucoma: the visual impairment project. Invest Ophthalmol Vis Sci. 2003;44(9):3783-9.
16. Mandal AK, Chakrabarti D. Update on congenital glaucoma. Indian J Ophthalmol. 2011;59(Suppl 1):S148-57.
17. Marsh BC, Cantor LB. Assessing the configuration of the anterior chamber angle. Glaucoma Today. 2005;22-5.
18. Marsh BC, Cantor LB. The Spaeth Gonioscopic Grading System. Glaucoma Today. 2005;22.
19. Morrison JC, Pollack IP. Glaucoma Science and Practice. Thieme.
20. Moster M, Ichhpujani P. Episcleral venous pressure and glaucoma. Journal of Current Glaucoma Practice. 2009;3(1):5-8.
21. Pan Y, Varma R. Natural history of glaucoma. Indian J Ophthalmol. 2011;59:19-23.
22. Primus S, Harris A, Siesky BA, et al. Diabetes a risk factor for glaucoma. Br J Ophthalmol. 2011;95:1621-2.
23. Rathi A, Sharma R, Jha B, et al. Role of lens extraction in primary angle closure disease. Journal of Current Glaucoma Practice. 2011;5(1):20-5.

24. Shahid H, Salmon JF. Malignant glaucoma: a review of the modern literature. J Ophthalmol. 2012;2012:852659.
25. Singh P, Kuldeep K, Tyagi M, et al. Glaucoma drainage devices. J Clin Ophthalmol Res. 2013;1(2).
26. Thomas R, Braganza A, Chandrasekhar G, et al. The role of artificial drainage devices in glaucoma surgery. Indian J Ophthalmol. 1998;46:41-6.
27. Vasudevan SK, Gupta V, Crowston JG. Neuroprotection in glaucoma. Indian J Ophthalmol. 2011;59:102-13.
28. Yanoff M, Duker JS. Ophthalmology, 3rd edition. Mosby.
29. Zimmerman TJ, Kooner KS. Clinical Pathways in Glaucoma. Thieme.

SECTION 10

Vitreous

CHAPTER

10.1 Anatomy and Congenital Anomalies of Vitreous

ANATOMY OF VITREOUS

Vitreous is an inert, transparent, gel-like structure situated between the lens and the retina. Vitreous accounts for 75–80% of the entire volume of the eye with a volume of 4.5 mL. It is composed of collagen fibrils interspersed with hyaluronic acid (Fig. 10.1.1).

Attachments of Vitreous

Vitreous is attached to surrounding structures:

1. The strongest attachment of vitreous is to vitreous base. Vitreous base lies in ora serrata extending about 2 mm into pars plana anteriorly and 2 mm posteriorly into peripheral retina.
2. Optic disk.
3. Posterior capsule of lens.
4. Macula.
5. Retinal blood vessels.

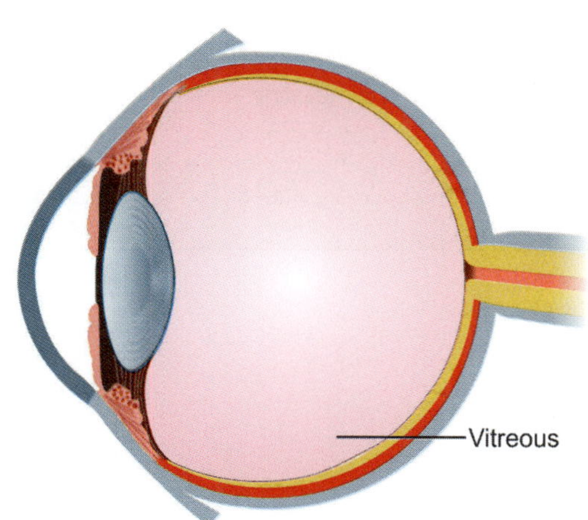

FIG. 10.1.1: Vitreous

Composition of Vitreous

Vitreous constitutes of 99% water and the remaining 1% by collagen (type 2 collagen is the main constituent), hyaluronic acid, sugars and amino acids.

FUNCTIONS OF VITREOUS*

- Being transparent, it forms part of refractive media of the eye
- It accounts for 75–80% of the volume of the entire eyeball, thus providing structural support to the eyeball.

EMBRYOLOGY OF VITREOUS

1. *Primary vitreous:* Arises from mesoderm and it usually involutes by 2nd month of gestation. Primary vitreous is vascular in nature. Persistence of primary vitreous gives rise to persistent hyperplastic primary vitreous (PHPV), which is described below.

2. *Secondary vitreous:* Develops from neuroectoderm and it represents adult vitreous. Unlike primary vitreous, secondary vitreous is avascular.
3. *Tertiary vitreous:* It also develops from neuroectoderm mainly in the ciliary region differentiating as zonules of lens.

PERSISTENT HYPERPLASTIC PRIMARY VITREOUS*

Definition

Persistent hyperplastic primary vitreous is a rare congenital anomaly characterized by persistence of primary vitreous and hyaloid vasculature.

Pathogenesis

The condition is due to failure of involution of primary vitreous and hyaloid vasculature, which normally occurs by 2nd month of gestation. During development of the eye, primary vitreous fills the vitreous cavity, and the hyaloid vessels run between the optic disk and the lens nourishing the lens and the anterior segment structures. Persisting primary vitreous and hyaloid vasculature opacifies, which result in diminution of vision.

Clinical Features

Depending on the amount and site of PHPV, clinical manifestations vary. Mittendorf's dot and Bergmeister's papilla represent mild variety. Leukocoria with retrolenticular membrane represent the severe variety. Mittendorf's dot is a small opacity present on the posterior capsule of lens representing the remnant of anterior end of hyaloid artery.

Bergmeister's papilla is a small flake of glial tissue present on the optic disk representing the remnant of posterior end of hyaloid artery.

Differential Diagnosis

Severe variety of PHPV presenting with leukocoria should be differentiated from other causes of leukocoria such as retinoblastoma, retinopathy of prematurity, etc.

Treatment

Treatment is required in moderate-to-severe cases causing visual impairment. Visual prognosis is poor in severe cases because of associated complication such as retinal detachment.

GIST BOX 10.1

- Vitreous is an inert, transparent, gel-like structure situated between the lens and the retina. Vitreous accounts for 75–80% of the entire volume of the eye with a volume of 4.5 mL.
- Persistent hyperplastic primary vitreous (PHPV) is a rare congenital anomaly characterized by persistence of primary vitreous and hyaloid vasculature. It is due to failure of involution of primary vitreous and hyaloid vasculature, which normally occurs by 2nd month of gestation.

CHAPTER

10.2 Diseases of Vitreous

POSTERIOR VITREOUS DETACHMENT**

Definition

Separation of vitreous from retina is called posterior vitreous detachment (PVD).

Etiopathogenesis

1. With the increasing age because of liquefaction, vitreous separates from retina at the sites of weak attachments (optic disk, macula and retinal blood vessels) excluding the strongest attachment, which is at the vitreous base.
2. About 75% of people above 75 years of age will have PVD. People with pathological myopia are at higher risk for development of PVD.

Clinical Features

Posterior vitreous detachment presents with sudden onset of flashes of light and floaters (Fig. 10.2.1).

Weiss ring represents ring-shaped opacity formed due to detachment of the vitreous from the optic disk.

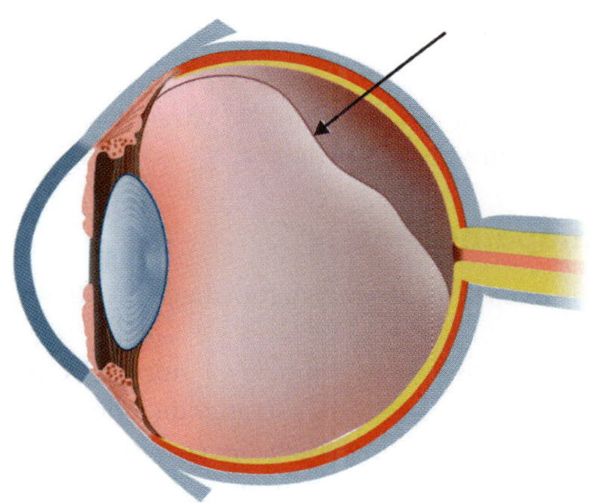

FIG. 10.2.1: Posterior vitreous detachment

Complications

No complications occur in most eyes and symptoms will subside over a period of time. It may lead to retinal tear in about 10% of eyes at sites of abnormally strong vitreoretinal adhesions and rarely may cause vitreous hemorrhage because of avulsion of retinal blood vessel.

Treatment

Treatment is required in cases associated with retinal tear. Retinal tear is treated by prophylactic laser photocoagulation or cryotherapy to prevent development of retinal detachment.

Synchysis of Vitreous

Liquefaction of the vitreous gel is called synchysis. It is due to age-related degeneration of the vitreous gel. Pathological causes for synchysis of vitreous are pathological myopia, post-trauma or inflammation.

Syneresis of Vitreous

Collapse of the vitreous because of liquefaction or synchysis is called syneresis of vitreous.

VITREOUS HEMORRHAGE**

Definition

Presence of blood within the vitreous cavity is called vitreous hemorrhage.

Etiopathogenesis*

The causes of vitreous hemorrhage are divided into:

1. Bleeding from rupture of normal retinal blood vessels. This category includes:
   a. Trauma including direct trauma to the eye or indirect trauma as in Terson's syndrome (intraocular hemorrhage associated with intracranial hemorrhage).
   b. Postsurgery as a complication of surgeries of the posterior segment, e.g. retinal detachment surgery.
   c. Rupture of retinal blood vessel as in posterior vitreous detachment.
   d. Hemorrhage seen in bleeding disorders, rupture of retinal artery macroaneurysm.
2. Bleeding from new fragile blood vessels seen in retinal vascular diseases associated with ischemia. This category includes:
   a. Proliferative diabetic retinopathy.
   b. Ischemic central retinal vein occlusion.
   c. Eales' disease.
   d. Retinopathy of prematurity.
   e. Proliferative sickle cell retinopathy.

Clinical Features

Symptoms

Patient usually presents with sudden onset of floaters or sudden diminution of vision in massive vitreous hemorrhage.

Signs

Examination of posterior segment of the eye by indirect ophthalmoscopy shows collection of blood in the vitreous.

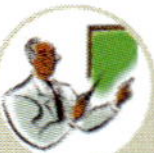

Clinical Types of Vitreous Hemorrhage

Intravitreal Hemorrhage (Figs 10.2.2A and B)

- Presence of blood within the vitreous body. It clots readily and it takes long time to clear.

Subvitreal Hemorrhage (Figs 10.2.3A and B)

- Presence of blood between the posterior hyaloid face and internal limiting membrane of retina.
- It is also known as preretinal hemorrhage or subhyaloid hemorrhage. The blood remains unclotted and shifts with change of posture.
- It usually assumes boat shape with concave inferior border and straight superior border. It is commonly seen in diabetics.

Complications

Complete absorption of blood in the vitreous may occur slowly over a period of 8 weeks. Long-standing non-clearing vitreous hemorrhage may lead to complications as follows:

- Ghost cell glaucoma
- Hemosiderosis bulbi
- Retinal damage because of retinitis proliferans or proliferative vitreoretinopathy.

Investigations

B-scan ultrasonography for confirmation of diagnosis and to look for associated retinal pathologies in case of retinal detachment.

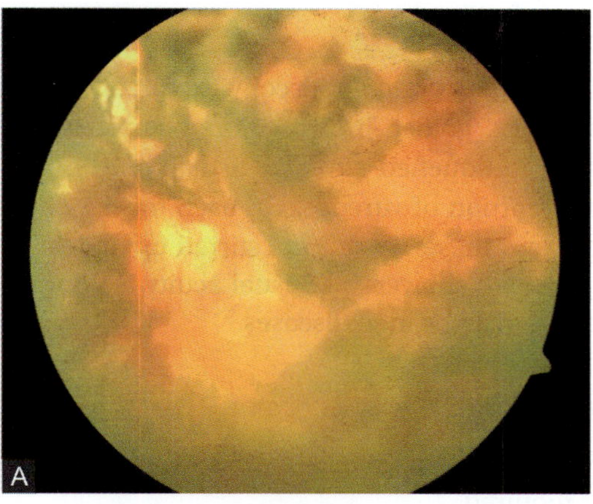

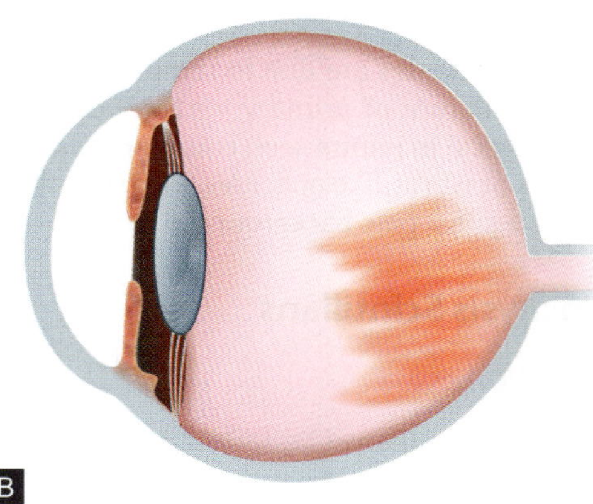

FIGS 10.2.2A and B: Intravitreal hemorrhage. **A.** Photograph; **B.** Diagrammatic representation.

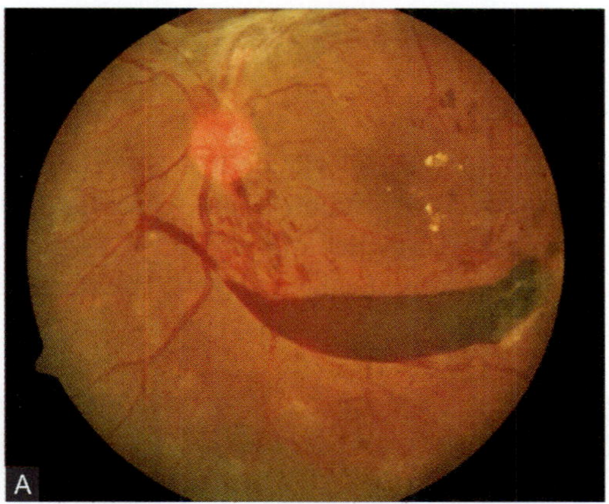

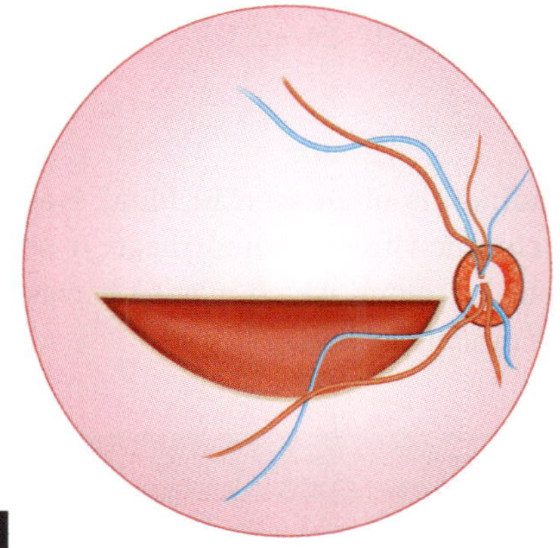

FIGS 10.2.3A and B: Subvitreal hemorrhage. **A.** Photograph; **B.** Diagrammatic representation.

Laboratory tests to rule out common underlying diseases such as diabetes mellitus, Eales' disease, etc.

Treatment*

1. Conservative medical line of management in the form of bedrest with head end elevation and oral vitamin C supplementation for faster absorption of blood. Once the vitreous hemorrhage starts resolving, examination of the retina is done to know the underlying cause. Laser photocoagulation is required in cases associated with new blood vessels.
2. Surgical treatment in the form of vitrectomy is indicated in:
   a. Nonclearing of vitreous hemorrhage even after 3 months.
   b. Vitreous hemorrhage associated with retinal detachment.

VITREOUS OPACITIES

Vitreous is a transparent structure, opacities in vitreous can be seen because of trauma, inflammation, degeneration and congenital anomalies.

Muscae Volitantes

Muscae volitantes are due to remnants of hyaloid vasculature of primary vitreous. They are physiological in nature seen commonly as minute dots or worm-like opacities, best seen when viewed against pale background.

Synchysis Scintillans*

Definition

Synchysis scintillans (Table 10.2.1) is a degenerative condition characterized by deposition of flat, angular crystals composed of cholesterol in liquefied vitreous. It is also known as cholesterosis bulbi (Figs 10.2.4A to C).

Etiology

The condition is often seen in blind eyes following chronic vitreous hemorrhage. It occurs in liquefied vitreous, which may be because of trauma or inflammation.

Clinical Features

On indirect ophthalmoscopy examination, flat, angular, golden-brown-colored crystals are seen in liquefied vitreous, usually in the inferior portion of vitreous. On each movement of the eye, these crystals are stirred up appearing as golden shower fall. Visual acuity is poor because of associated diseases.

Treatment

Since it is often seen in blind eyes, no treatment is required.

Asteroid Hyalosis*

Definition

Asteroid hyalosis (refer Table 10.2.1) is a degenerative condition of the vitreous, characterized by deposition of calcium pyrophosphate globules in the form of spherical white opacities in the vitreous (Figs 10.2.5A to C).

TABLE 10.2.1: Differences between asteroid hyalosis and synchysis scintillans

Clinical features	*Asteroid hyalosis*	*Synchysis scintillans*
Definition	Deposition of calcium pyrophosphate globules in the form of spherical white opacities in the vitreous	Deposition of flat, angular crystals composed of cholesterol in liquefied vitreous
Etiology	Unilateral condition seen in elderly people	Bilateral condition seen in young individuals
Associated diseases/disorder	Diabetes mellitus may be associated condition	Secondary to ocular inflammation or trauma
Golden shower fall	Not seen	Seen on movements of the eye
Status of vitreous	Normal	Liquefied
Treatment	In asymptomatic cases, treatment is not required and vitrectomy is indicated in cases causing diminution of vision	Not required, as it usually occurs in damaged and blind eyes

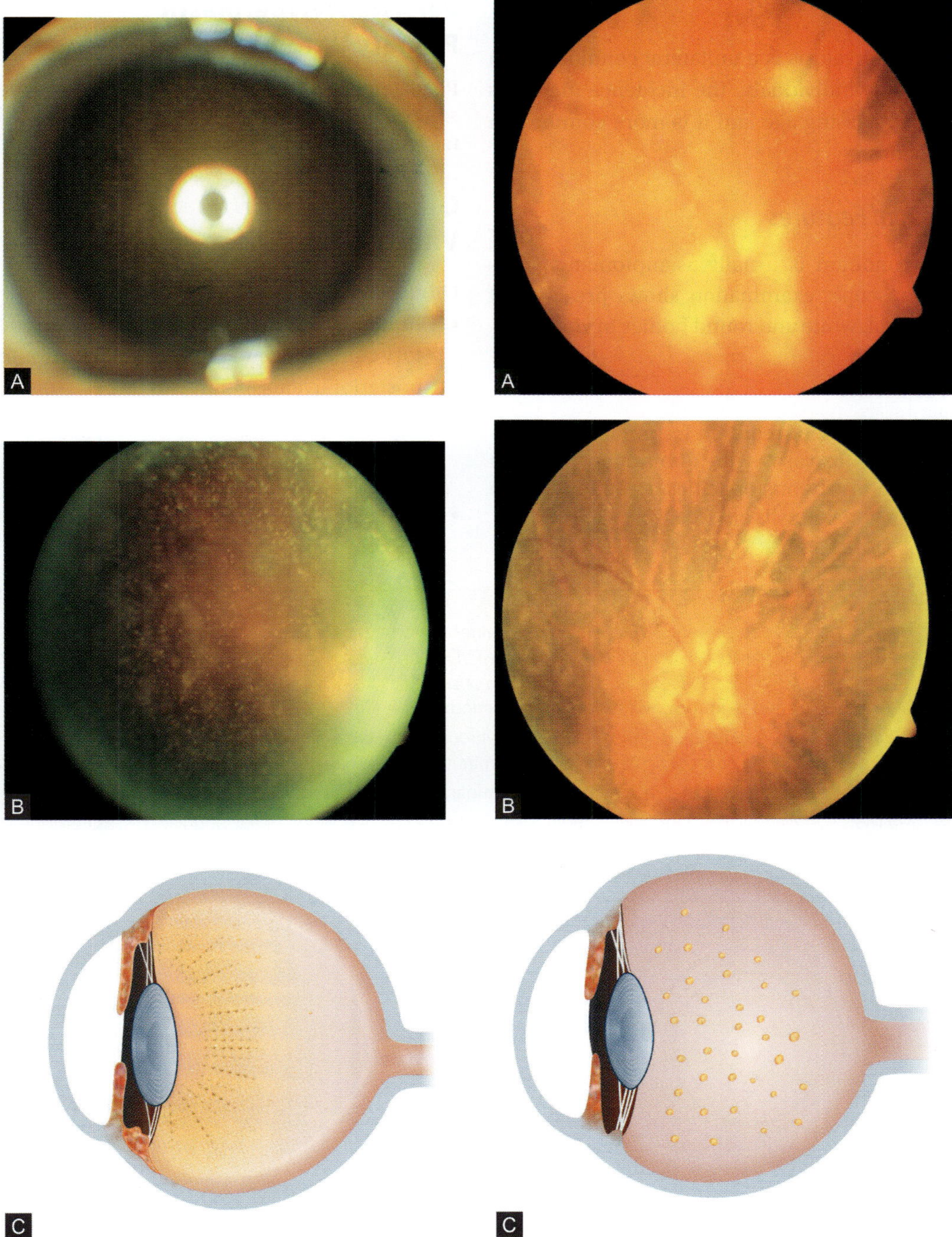

FIGS 10.2.4A to C: Synchysis scintillans. **A and B.** Photograph; **C.** Diagrammatic representation. (*Note:* Angular crystals in vitreous).

FIGS 10.2.5A to C: Asteroid hyalosis. **A and B.** Photograph; **C.** Diagrammatic representation.

Etiology

Asteroid hyalosis is a unilateral condition seen in elderly individuals. The incidence increases with increasing age and it is more common in diabetics.

Clinical Features

The condition is usually asymptomatic. Ophthalmoscopic examination shows presence of spherical, white and round bodies in vitreous.

Treatment

Treatment is not required for mild asymptomatic cases. In cases with diminution of vision because of vitreous opacities, treatment in the form of vitrectomy is advised.

Persistent Hyperplastic Primary Vitreous

Persistent hyperplastic primary vitreous is described in Chapter 10.1 'Anatomy and Congenital Anomalies of Vitreous.'

Other Causes for Vitreous Opacities

Other causes include:

- Inflammatory opacities seen in inflammatory conditions such as intermediate uveitis, posterior uveitis, panuveitis, etc.
- Tumor cells from the intraocular tumors such as retinoblastoma and malignant melanoma
- Amyloidosis.

GIST BOX 10.2

- Posterior vitreous detachment (PVD): Separation of vitreous from retina is called posterior vitreous detachment. About 75% of people above 75 years of age will have PVD. People with pathological myopia are at higher risk for development of PVD. The PVD presents with sudden onset of flashes of light and floaters. No complications occur in most eyes and symptoms will subside over a period of time. It may lead to retinal tear in about 10% of eyes.
- Vitreous hemorrhage: Presence of blood within the vitreous cavity is called vitreous hemorrhage. Patient usually presents with sudden onset of floaters or sudden diminution of vision in massive vitreous hemorrhage.
- Muscae volitantes are opacities in vitreous due to remnants of hyaloid vasculature of primary vitreous.
- Synchysis scintillans is a degenerative condition characterized by deposition of flat, angular crystals composed of cholesterol in liquefied vitreous. Asteroid hyalosis is a degenerative condition of the vitreous characterized by deposition of calcium pyrophosphate globules in the form of spherical white opacities in the vitreous.

FREQUENTLY ASKED QUESTIONS (FAQs)

*Short Answers

1. Functions of vitreous.
2. Persistent hyperplastic primary vitreous.
3. Causes of vitreous hemorrhage.
4. Treatment of vitreous hemorrhage.
5. Asteroid hyalosis.
6. Synchysis scintillans.

**Short Essays

1. Posterior vitreous detachment.
2. Vitreous hemorrhages.

BIBLIOGRAPHY

1. Jack J Kanski. Clinical Ophthalmology: A Systematic Approach, 5th edition. Philadelphia: Butterworth Heinemann; 2003.
2. Jerry, Sebag. Vitreous anatomy and pathology. In: Myron Yanoff, Jay S Duker (Eds). Ophthalmology, 3rd edition. China: Mosby Elsevier Inc; 2006.
3. Khurana AK, Khurana I. Anatomy and Physiology of Eye, 2nd edition. New Delhi: CBS Publishers & Distributors Pvt Ltd; 2010.
4. Saxena S, Jalali S, Verma L, et al. Management of vitreous hemorrhage. Indian J Ophthalmol. 2003;51(2):189-96.

SECTION 11

Retina

CHAPTER

11.1 Anatomy of Retina

INTRODUCTION

Retina is the innermost layer of the eyeball. It is light sensitive layer of and it converts light impulses into neural impulses, which travel along the optic nerve to reach the visual cortex.

The word retina is derived from a Latin word 'rete' meaning 'net'.

GROSS ANATOMY

The retina is a thin, delicate, transparent membrane extending from ora serrata to the optic disk. It appears purplish red in color, because of the presence of rhodopsin pigment and underlying vascular choroid. The thickness of retina is not uniform and it is thickest near the optic disk in macula measuring about 0.4 mm, and thin as it reaches the periphery with a thickness of about 0.08 mm.

The retina is divided into central retina and peripheral retina with both being separated by retinal equator. The central retina is also called posterior pole, as it is the part of the retina, which lies posterior to the equator. The equator of retina corresponds to the equator of eyeball and lie in line with exit of the four vortex veins (Fig. 11.1.1). The posterior pole of the retina includes optic disk and macula lutea.

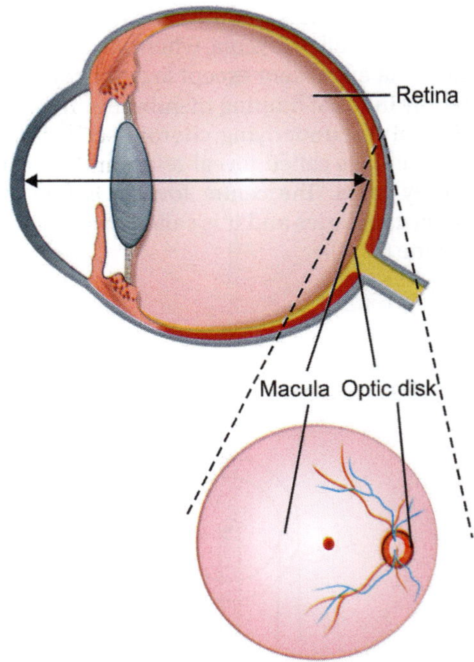

FIG. 11.1.1: Anatomy of retina

Optic Disk

Optic disk is also called optic nerve head. It is circular or slightly vertically oval in shape measuring about 1.5 mm in diameter. It represents the beginning of the optic nerve. At the optic disk, the nerve fiber layer of the retina continues as optic nerve and the remaining layers of the retina including the layer of rods and cones are absent at the optic disk.

Macula Lutea*

The word macula lutea is derived from Latin word macula meaning 'spot' and lutea meaning 'yellow'. It is so-called because of the presence of lutein and zeaxanthin, the yellow xanthophyll carotenoids. It is situated temporal to the optic disk in the posterior pole of the retina and is responsible for central vision. It measures about 5.5–6 mm in diameter. Macula lutea is subdivided into fovea, parafovea and perifovea (Fig. 11.1.2).

Fovea

Fovea is the central depressed part of the macula measuring about 1.5 mm in diameter. The word fovea means 'pit' in Latin. The center of the fovea is called foveola, where all the layers of the retina are absent except layer of cones covered by internal limiting membrane. The bright reflex of the underlying choroid seen through the foveola is called foveal reflex and indicates healthy fovea. The center foveola is free from retinal capillaries and it is called foveal avascular zone (FAZ).

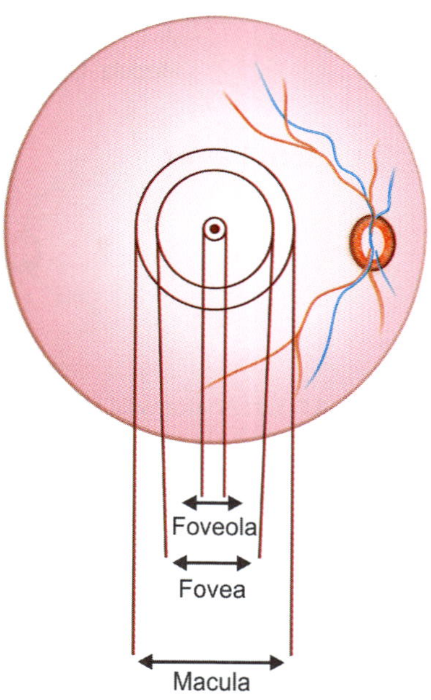

FIG. 11.1.2: Anatomy of macula

Parafovea and Perifovea

The parafovea and perifovea surround the fovea and they contain multiple layers of ganglion cells.

The foveal reflex appears as cherry-red spot in diseases such as central retinal artery occlusion, lipid storage diseases, etc. which leads to whitening of the surrounding macula as the foveal reflex stands out against the surrounding white retina.

Periphery of Retina

The periphery of retina extends from equator of the retina to ora serrata. It is divided into near periphery, measuring about 1.5 mm wide; midperiphery, measuring about 3 mm wide and far periphery, measuring about 10 mm temporally and 15 mm nasally. Ora serrata is the junction between retina and ciliary body.

MICROSCOPIC ANATOMY*

The retina consists of 10 layers (Fig. 11.1.3).

Retinal Pigment Epithelium

Retinal pigment epithelium (RPE) is the outermost layer of the retina and it is firmly attached to the Bruch's membrane of choroid. It consists of a single layer of melanin pigment containing flattened hexagonal cells. It forms the outer blood retinal barrier and takes part in visual cycle.

Layer of Rods and Cones

Layer of rods and cones are the photoreceptors or end organs of vision. The highest density of rods is in the periphery and they are absent in the fovea, whereas cones are found in high density in fovea. There are about 120 million rods and they are responsible for peripheral vision and scotopic vision. There are about 6 million cones and they are responsible for central vision, color vision and photopic vision.

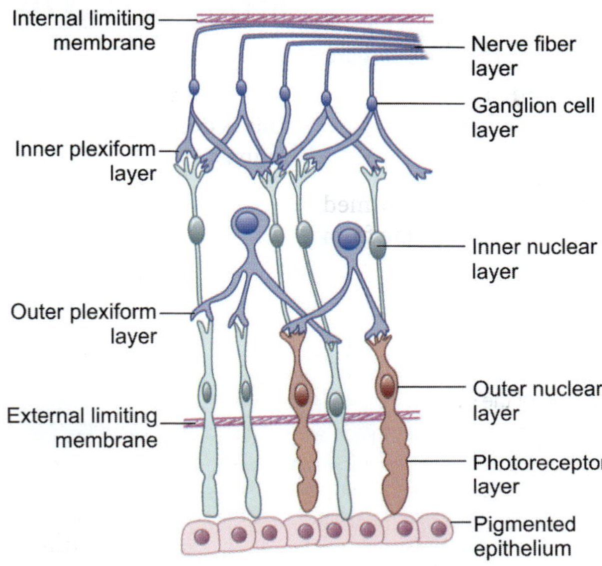

FIG. 11.1.3: Microscopic anatomy of retina

External Limiting Membrane

External limiting membrane is formed by the Müller's fibers and the processes of rods and cones pass through it.

Outer Nuclear Layer

The outer layer consists of nuclei of rods and cones.

Outer Plexiform Layer

The outer plexiform layer consists of synapses of axons of rods and cones with dendrites of bipolar cells, horizontal cells and amacrine cells. The outer plexiform layer is thickest in the fovea where the cones are arranged obliquely and it is called Henle's layer.

Inner Nuclear Layer

Inner nuclear layer consists of bipolar cells, amacrine cells and horizontal cells. Bipolar cells are the first-order neurons.

Inner Plexiform Layer

The inner plexiform layer consists of synapses of axons of bipolar cells with dendrites of ganglion cells along with amacrine cells and Müller's cells.

Ganglion Cell Layer

The ganglion cell layer consists of ganglion cells, the second order neurons. This layer shows single layer of ganglion cells in the rest of the retina, except in the parafovea and perifovea where it shows multiple layers of the ganglion cells.

Nerve Fiber Layer

The nerve fiber layer consists of axons of ganglion cells, which forms the optic nerve.

Internal Limiting Membrane

Internal limiting membrane layer is formed from Müller's fibers and it separates retina from vitreous.

BLOOD SUPPLY OF RETINA

The blood is supplied to retina from two sources, retinal circulation and choroidal circulation. This is described under vascular diseases of the retina.

GIST BOX 11.1

- Retina is the innermost layer of the eyeball.
- The retina is a thin, delicate, transparent membrane extending from ora serrata to the optic disk.
- The retina is divided into central retina and peripheral retina with both being separated by retinal equator. The central retina is also called posterior pole, and it includes optic disk and macula.
- The retina consists of 10 layers—retinal pigment epithelium, layer of rods and cones, external limiting membrane, outer nuclear layer, outer plexiform layer, inner nuclear layer, inner plexiform layer, ganglion cell layer, nerve fiber layer and internal limiting membrane.
- The blood supply of retina is derived from two sources, retinal circulation and choroidal circulation.

CHAPTER

11.2 Congenital Anomalies of Retina

EMBRYOLOGY OF RETINA

Retina develops from neuroectoderm. Retinal pigment epithelium and rest of the retina called sensory retina develop from outer wall and inner wall of the optic cup, respectively.

> Retinal detachment occurs because of separation of the neurosensory retina from the pigmented epithelium of retina as these are embryologically derived from different layers of the optic cup.

CONGENITAL ANOMALIES

The congenital anomalies are classified into four categories as follows.

Congenital Anomalies of Optic Disk and Nerve Fibers

The congenital anomalies of optic disk and nerve fibers are described under Section 12 Optic Nerve.

Congenital Anomalies of Macula/Fovea

1. Aplasia or hypoplasia of macula: It is usually seen associated with other ocular anomalies such as aniridia and ocular albinism. It is because of failure of in differentiation of retina, which normally occurs by 8 months of intrauterine life. Clinically, it presents as gross diminution of vision, amblyopia in uniocular cases, nystagmus, etc. This condition is diagnosed by absence of foveal reflex.
2. Congenital cyst of macula.

Congenital Anomalies of Retinal Vessels

Congenital tortuosity of retinal vessels: It is a rare condition and presents with tortuosity of the retinal vessels. The patients with tortuosity of retinal vessels are at risk of spontaneous retinal hemorrhages.

Congenital retinal telangiectasia: It is also called Coats' disease. It is described in Chapter 11.5 'Vascular Diseases of Retina'.

Congenital Anomalies of Retina

1. *Coloboma of retina:* It is seen in association with the coloboma of the uveal tract as a result of failure in fusion of the choroidal fissure.
2. *Congenital folds of retina:* It is a rare congenital condition characterized by the presence of fold of retina projecting into vitreous.

3. *Congenital hypertrophy of retinal pigment epithelium:* It is a common condition presenting as a flat-pigmented lesion due to increased pigmentation of the retinal pigment epithelium.
4. *Leber's congenital amaurosis:* It is a rare condition of the eye, which is present at birth and inherited as an autosomal recessive trait. The basic pathology is maldevelopment of the photoreceptors.
5. It presents with diminution of vision with diminished pupillary reflexes and normal appearance of fundus initially, hence the disease is called congenital amaurosis (amaurosis means loss of vision without any detectable lesion). Pigmentary retinopathy is seen later in the disease.
6. The characteristic finding is repeated rubbing or pressing of the eyes called oculodigital sign. The diagnosis is made by electroretinogram (ERG), which is nondetectable or nonrecordable.
7. The other congenital diseases of the retina such as congenital retinoschisis, congenital night blindness, Coats' disease, retinal dystrophies, etc. are described in Chapter 11.5' 'Vascular Diseases of Retina' and Chapter 11.6 'Retinal Dystrophies and Degenerations'.

GIST BOX 11.2

- Aplasia or hypoplasia of macula is usually seen associated with other ocular anomalies such as aniridia and ocular albinism.
- Coloboma of retina is seen in association with the coloboma of the uveal tract as a result of failure in fusion of the choroidal fissure.
- Leber's congenital amaurosis is a rare condition of the eye, which is present at birth and inherited as an autosomal recessive trait. The basic pathology is maldevelopment of photoreceptors.

CHAPTER

11.3 Retinal Detachment

DEFINITION

Retinal detachment (RD) is the separation of sensory retina from the retinal pigment epithelium (RPE) by subretinal fluid.

> Retinal pigment epithelium is firmly attached to the underlying choroid and loosely attached to rest of the retina (sensory retina) as these two layers are embryologically derived from different layers. Hence, retinal detachment can be better called retinal separation.

TYPES

- Rhegmatogenous RD or primary RD
- Non-rhegmatogenous RD or secondary RD:
  - Tractional RD
  - Exudative RD.

RHEGMATOGENOUS RETINAL DETACHMENT**

The word rhegma means break. RD associated with break in the retina is called rhegmatogenous detachment.

Definition

Retinal detachment due to break in the sensory layer of retina allowing fluid from the vitreous cavity (synchitic or liquefied vitreous gel) to seep in between sensory retina and RPE, and separate them is called rhegmatogenous RD (Figs 11.3.1A and B, Figs 11.3.2A and B).

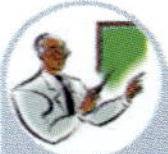

> **Retinal Break**
>
> A full thickness defect in the sensory retina is called retinal break. It can be retinal tear or retinal hole:
> - A retinal break caused by dynamic vitreoretinal traction is called retinal tear.
> - A retinal break caused by chronic atrophy of the sensory retina is called retinal hole.

Etiology

The incidence of rhegmatogenous RD is 1 in 10,000 and it is bilateral in 10% of cases. Myopia, trauma, peripheral retinal degenerations, aphakia are the common predisposing factors. Myopia and lattice degeneration are seen in about 40% of eyes with RD.

Pathogenesis

Development of rhegmatogenous RD is related to:

1. Changes in the fibrillar structure of the vitreous as a result of age-related changes or diseases such as myopia resulting in posterior vitreous detachment (PVD).
2. Persistent vitreoretinal traction and peripheral degenerations predisposing to retinal tear formation.

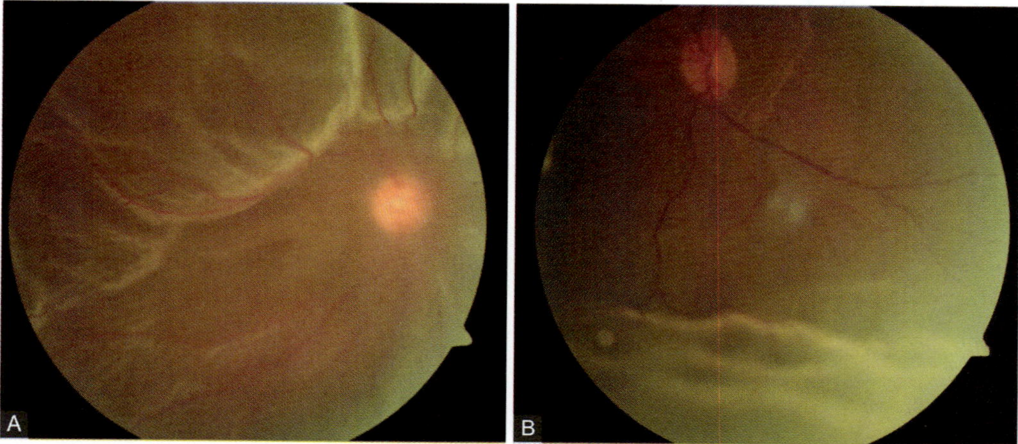

FIGS 11.3.1A and B: Rhegmatogenous retinal detachment (*Note:* Convex configuration and corrugated appearance of the detached retina).

3. Liquefied vitreous seeps through retinal break separating sensory retina from RPE resulting in rhegmatogenous RD.

Posterior Vitreous Detachment*

Separation of vitreous from retina is called posterior vitreous detachment. With the increasing age, because of liquefaction vitreous separates from retina. About 75% of people above 75 years of age will have posterior vitreous detachment. People with pathological myopia are at higher risk for development of posterior vitreous detachment.

Posterior vitreous detachment presents with sudden onset of flashes of light and floaters. Weiss ring represents ring-shaped opacity formed due to detachment of the vitreous from the optic disk and is detected on indirect ophthalmoscopic examination.

No complications occur in most eyes and symptoms will subside over a period of time. It may lead to retinal tear in about 10% of eyes at sites of abnormally strong vitreoretinal adhesions and rarely may cause vitreous hemorrhage, because of avulsion of retinal blood vessel.

Peripheral Retinal Degenerations

Lattice degeneration, snail track degeneration, degenerative retinoschisis, white without pressure are some of the peripheral retinal degenerations, which predispose to the formation of retinal breaks. About 60% of retinal breaks develop in areas of peripheral retinal degeneration.

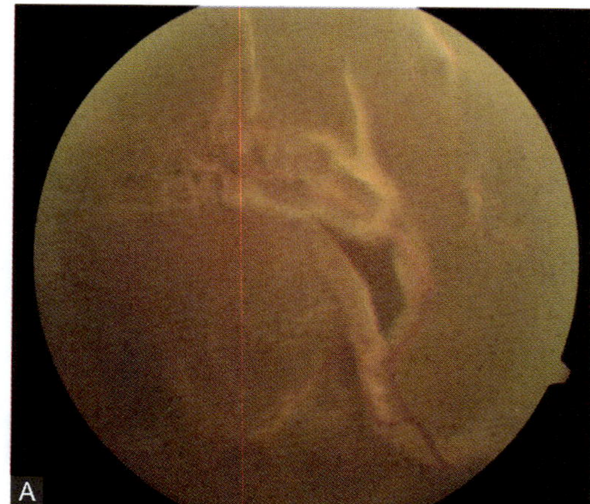

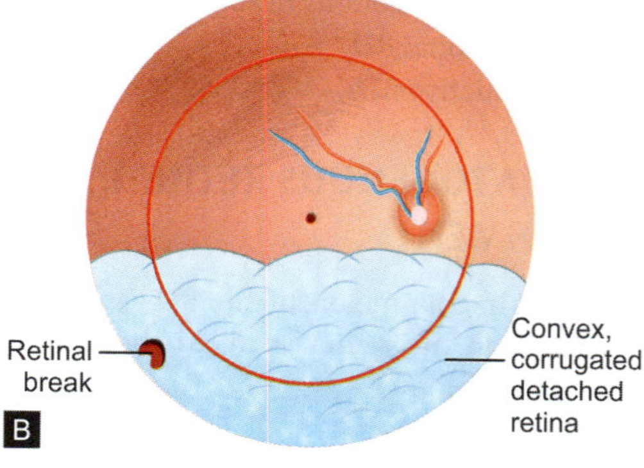

FIGS 11.3.2A and B: Retinal tear with rhegmatogenous retinal detachment. **A.** Photograph; **B.** Diagrammatic representation.

Clinical Features

Symptoms

- The prodromal symptoms are seen in more than half of patients with rhegmatogenous RD and are in the form of:
  - Floaters because of vitreous degeneration
  - Photopsia because of vitreoretinal traction.
- The rest of the patients may remain asymptomatic for a long time unless it is:
  - Complicated by involvement of the macula resulting in sudden painless diminution of vision
  - Spread of RD posterior to the equator resulting in visual field defect perceived by patient as a curtain in the visual field.

Signs

On examination it is found:

- Diminution of vision is seen in cases involving the macula
- Relative afferent pupillary defect is seen in eyes with extensive RD
- Intraocular pressure may be decreased.

  Fresh retinal detachment:
- Slit examination shows pigmentation/ tobacco dusting in the anterior vitreous called Shafer's sign
- Ophthalmoscopic examination shows:
  - Gray reflex instead of red reflex
  - Detached retina with convex configuration, corrugated appearance, undulating freely with eye movements.

  Long-standing retinal detachment:
- Ophthalmoscopic examination shows:
  - Detached retina shows thinning, intraretinal cysts, subretinal demarcation lines and fibrosis.

Complications

Complications of long-standing RD show proliferative vitreoretinopathy, chronic uveitis, chronic hypotony, phthisis bulbi, etc.

Investigations

Ultrasonography by B-scan examination is a useful investigation for diagnosis of RD particularly in eyes with hazy media where ophthalmoscopic examination cannot be made.

Treatment

The treatment of rhegmatogenous RD is by:

- Searching the retinal break
- Sealing the retinal break
- Subretinal fluid drainage
- Maintenance of chorioretinal apposition.

Searching the Retinal Break

Indirect ophthalmoscopy with scleral indentation is the most commonly used method for searching the retinal break.

Lincoff rule helps in determining the retinal break. It states that the position of the retinal break can be determined from the shape of detachment as subretinal fluid spreads in a predictable manner from the retinal break:

- In superior nasal or temporal RDs, the retinal break will lie within 1 hour 30 minutes of the highest border of the detachment
- In inferior RD, the higher border indicates the side of retinal break
- In total or superior RDs, (which cross the midline) the break will lie within a triangle whose apex is at 12 O'clock at the ora with sides extending posteriorly on both the sides toward 10.30 and 1.30 meridians.

Sealing the Retinal Break

The retinal breaks once localized are sealed by cryotherapy or laser photocoagulation or diathermy.

Subretinal Fluid Drainage

Subretinal fluid drainage is done by sclerotomy or by inserting a needle through the sclera and choroid into the subretinal space.

Maintenance of Chorioretinal Apposition

The maintenance of the chorioretinal apposition is done by external tamponade or internal tamponade. External tamponade is provided by scleral buckling and internal tamponade is provided by pneumatic retinopexy or pars plana vitrectomy with internal tamponade:

1. *Scleral buckling:* It is a surgical procedure, which involves suturing an explant material to the sclera to create inward indentation of sclera. Scleral buckling once was the gold standard in the treatment of RD, but with the recent advancements in vitrectomy, scleral buckling is slowly becoming less popular. It is still indicated in RD caused by large tears and dialysis of retina.
2. *Pneumatic retinopexy:* It is a surgical procedure, which involves injection of expanding gases such as sulfur hexafluoride (SF_6) or perfluoropropane (C_3F_8) is injected into the vitreous cavity as a tamponade. It is indicated in RD with retinal break in the superior clock hours.
3. *Pars plana vitrectomy with internal tamponade by expanding gases or by silicone oil*: It is now increasingly used in all types of rhegmatogenous and tractional RD.

Prophylactic Treatment

Prophylactic treatment is done by treating retinal breaks and high-risk peripheral retinal degenerations. The treatment is compulsory in high-risk patients such as myopics, aphakics, RD in the other eye. The treatment is by laser photocoagulation or by cryotherapy.

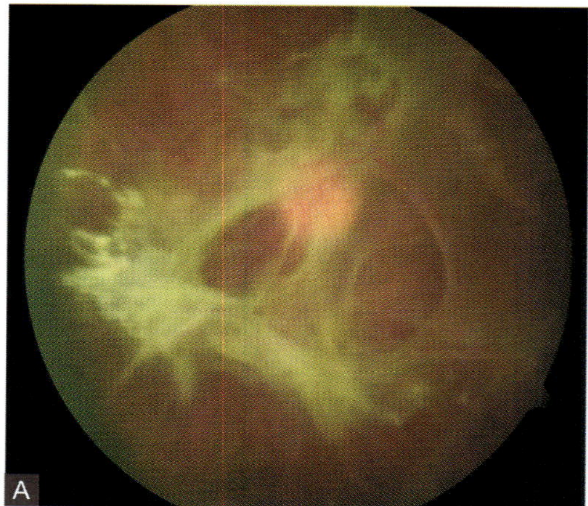

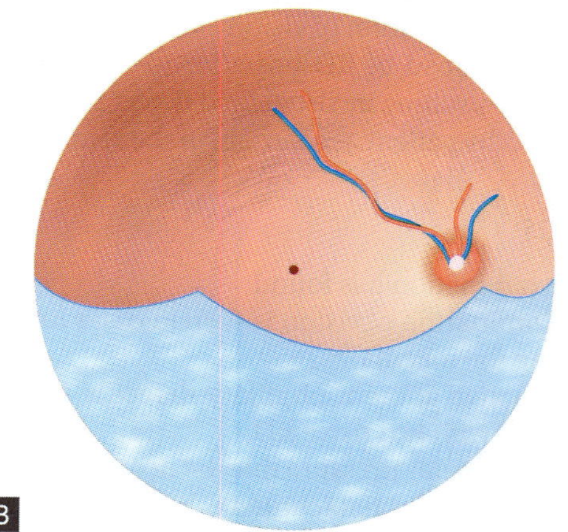

FIGS 11.3.3A and B: Tractional retinal detachment. **A.** Photograph; **B.** Diagrammatic representation. (*Note:* Concave configuration of detached retina).

TRACTIONAL RETINAL DETACHMENT**

Definition

Retinal detachment caused by tractional membranes (vitreoretinal membranes) from inflammatory or vascular causes on the surface of the retina pulling the sensory retina away from RPE is called tractional RD (Figs 11.3.3A and B).

Etiology

The common causes for tractional RD are proliferative diabetic retinopathy, Eales' disease, familial exudative vitreoretinopathy, sickle cell retinopathy, retinopathy of prematurity, penetrating and perforating injuries involving retina, etc.

Pathogenesis

Tractional RD is because of pulling of the sensory retina away from the RPE by fibrovascular membranes.

Clinical Features

1. Tractional RD is slowly progressive hence causes gradual progressive loss of visual field or vision.
2. The signs and symptoms of the underlying diseases are seen.
3. The prodromal symptoms of floaters and photopsia are absent.
4. The configuration of RD is concave with reduced mobility and absence of retinal breaks.

Treatment

The treatment of the condition is by pars plana vitrectomy to relieve the vitreoretinal tractional membranes.

EXUDATIVE RETINAL DETACHMENT**

Definition

Retinal detachment caused by exudation from choriocapillaries, which seeps into the subretinal space through damaged RPE thus separating it from sensory retina is called exudative RD (Fig. 11.3.4).

Etiology

Exudative retinal detachment is seen in ocular and systemic conditions, which lead to exudation from the choriocapillaries. The ocular conditions are:

1. Congenital conditions such as nanophthalmos, uveal effusion syndrome, Coats' disease, etc.
2. Inflammatory conditions such as posterior uveitis, posterior scleritis, sympathetic ophthalmitis, etc.
3. Tumors of the eye such as choroidal hemangioma, choroidal melanoma, etc.

The systemic conditions are pregnancy-induced hypertension, renal hypertension, etc.

Clinical Features

1. The exudative retinal detachment presents with diminution of vision or metamorphopsia, because of involvement of macula.
2. The detached retina is convex in configuration with smooth appearance with shifting of subretinal fluid and absence of retinal breaks.

Treatment

The treatment of the exudative RD is by management of the underlying cause.

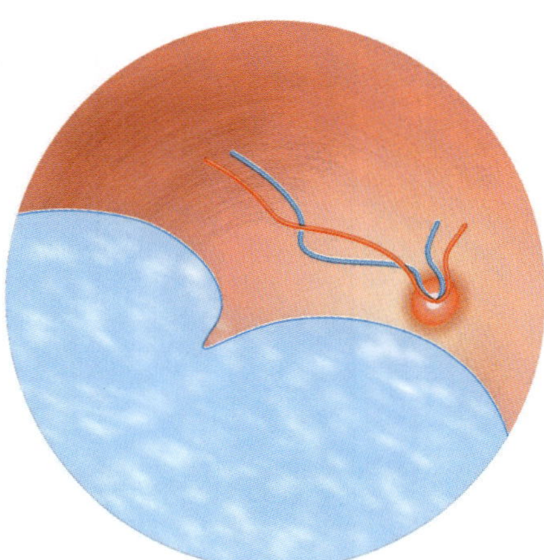

FIG. 11.3.4: Exudative retinal detachment (*Note:* Convex configuration of detached retina, which is noncorrugated and bullous).

GIST BOX 11.3

- Retinal detachment is the separation of sensory retina from the retinal pigment epithelium by subretinal fluid.
- Retinal detachment associated with break in the retina is called rhegmatogenous detachment.
- Retinal detachment caused by tractional membranes (vitreoretinal membranes) from inflammatory or vascular causes on the surface of the retina pulling the sensory retina away from RPE is called tractional retinal detachment.
- Retinal detachment caused by exudation from choriocapillaries, which seeps into the subretinal space through damaged retinal pigment epithelium thus separating it from sensory retina is called exudative retinal detachment.

CHAPTER

11.4 Inflammatory Diseases of Retina

RETINITIS

Definition

Retinitis is defined as inflammation of retina. The inflammation of retina is usually associated with inflammation of the surrounding choroid; hence it is called chorioretinitis. However, isolated inflammation of the retina can be seen.

Classification

Retinitis is classified into:

1. *Acute purulent retinitis:* It is usually seen in septicemia and it is caused by metastatic infection caused by pyogenic organisms. It can lead to metastatic endophthalmitis.
2. *Subacute retinitis:* It is usually seen in patients with bacterial endocarditis, because of septic emboli from the cardiac source. It is sometimes called septic retinitis of Roth, characterized by white-centered retinal hemorrhages. However, Roth's spots are non-specific signs, which are also seen in blood dyscariasis such as anemia.
3. *Chronic specific retinitis:* It is usually caused by bacterial infections such as tuberculosis, syphilis, etc. and in viral causes like varicella-zoster virus, herpes virus, cytomegalovirus (CMV), etc. parasitic causes such as toxoplasma, Toxocara, onchocerca, etc. and they are described under posterior uveitis and panuveitis.

RETINAL VASCULITIS

Definition

Inflammation of the blood vessels of the retina is called retinal vasculitis.

Etiology

Retinal vasculitis can be primary or secondary depending on the mode of involvement:

1. In primary retinal vasculitis, retinal vessels are the primary sites of inflammation, the causes are:
   a. Ocular causes such as frosted branch angiitis, pars planitis, idiopathic retinal vasculitis, etc.
   b. Systemic causes such as giant cell arteritis, Wegener's granulomatosis, polyarteritis nodosa, etc.
2. In secondary vasculitis, retinal vessels are involved secondary to inflammation of the surrounding structures, the causes are:
   a. Ocular causes: Ocular tuberculosis, ocular toxoplasmosis, etc.
   b. Systemic causes: Sarcoidosis, Behcet's disease, systemic lupus erythematosus, tuberculosis, syphilis, etc.

Clinical Features

1. It remains asymptomatic in the initial stages.
2. Floaters are seen because of associated vitritis.

3. Diminution of vision is seen because of complications such as cystoid macular edema, macular ischemia, etc.
4. Fundus examination shows sheathing of the vessels with associated vitritis.

Complications

Complications include ocular neovascularization, proliferative retinopathy, recurrent vitreous hemorrhage, neovascular glaucoma, retinal artery or vein occlusion.

Investigations

Fundus fluorescein angiography (FFA) is the investigation of choice for confirmation of diagnosis and it shows characteristic leakage of the affected vessel along with staining.

Common blood tests such as complete blood count (CBC), differential count, erythrocyte sedimentation rate (ESR), C-reactive protein and specific tests such as fluorescent treponemal antibody test, serological tests for toxoplasma, chest X-ray, Mantoux test for tuberculosis and tests to rule out autoimmune disorders such as antinuclear antibody test, antiphospholipid antibody, etc. are carried out depending on the clinical suspicion.

Treatment

1. Corticosteroids are the mainstay of treatment of retinal vasculitis along with the treatment of underlying disease.
2. Immunosuppressive agents are indicated in patients not responding to steroids or as steroid-sparing drugs.

EALES' DISEASE**

Definition

Eales' disease is defined as an idiopathic inflammatory obliterative vasculopathy involving the peripheral retina.

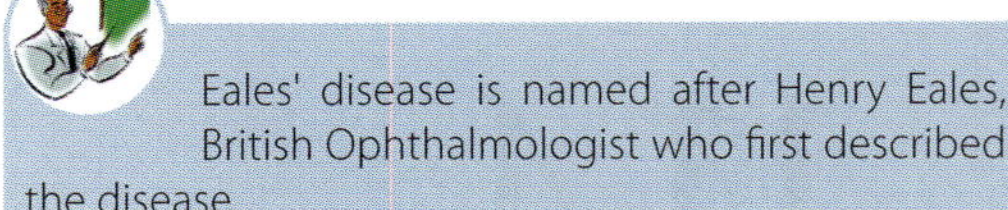

Etiopathogenesis

Eales' disease commonly affects young adults with males being affected more commonly than females. It is more commonly seen in India and other countries of Asia.

The pathogenesis is still not properly understood. The most commonly proposed etiological factor is hypersensitivity reaction to tuberculoprotein. Individuals with particular human leukocyte antigen (HLA) such as HLA-B5 are more predisposed to develop Eales' disease as a result of hypersensitivity reaction to antigen of Mycobacterium.

The disease usually runs in three stages, characterized by:

1. Stage of inflammation of retinal veins.
2. Stage of occlusion of retinal veins.
3. Stage of retinal neovascularization.

Clinical Features

The disease is usually bilateral in nature and the symptoms are floaters and decreased visual acuity. The decreased vision is because of either associated macular edema or vitreous hemorrhage.

Fundus examination shows periphlebitis of retinal veins in the form of tortuous veins with vascular sheathing and perivascular exudates in the initial stages.

The later stage of the disease shows occlusion of retinal veins manifesting as areas of retinal nonperfusion.

Neovascularization of the retina in the form of neovascularization of disk (NVD) or neovascularization elsewhere (NVE) is seen in advanced stages of the disease.

Complications

Recurrent episodes of vitreous hemorrhage and macular edema are the frequent complications seen and they are responsible for decreased visual acuity. Tractional retinal detachment may be seen in untreated cases.

Investigations

Fundus fluorescein angiography is useful to demonstrate the areas of retinal nonperfusion, NVD and NVE.

Treatment

1. Corticosteroids administered in the form of systemic or periocular route are the main stay of treatment in the inflammatory stage.
2. Photocoagulation of the non-perfused retina is carried out in the stage of occlusion.
3. Vitrectomy is indicated in non-resolving vitreous hemorrhage or in cases complicated with tractional retinal detachment.

GIST BOX 11.4

- Retinitis is defined as inflammation of retina. The inflammation of retina is usually associated with inflammation of the surrounding choroid; hence, it is called chorioretinitis.
- Inflammation of the blood vessels of the retina is called retinal vasculitis.
- Eales' disease is defined as an idiopathic inflammatory obliterative vasculopathy involving the peripheral retinal detachment.

CHAPTER

11.5 Vascular Diseases of Retina

RETINAL CIRCULATION*

1. The blood supply of retina is derived from two sources, retinal circulation and choroidal circulation. Retinal circulation is from central retinal artery, a branch of ophthalmic artery and choroidal circulation is from posterior ciliary arteries, again branches of ophthalmic artery.
2. Central retinal artery divides into four branches with each branch supplying a quadrant and named superotemporal, superonasal, inferotemporal and inferonasal branches. Each branch is an end artery with no anastomosis and gives rise to retinal capillaries.
3. Retinal capillaries supply the inner six layers of the retina. The outer four layers of the retina get its blood supply from choriocapillaries derived from choroidal circulation. However, about 20–25% of people show cilioretinal artery arising from posterior ciliary circulation and supply the macula.
4. The venous drainage is from central retinal veins, which drain into cavernous sinus.

The eye is the only site in our body where blood vessels can be seen directly with the help of instruments such as ophthalmoscope, thus allow studying the changes in the vessels induced by various diseases. Thus, changes in the retinal blood vessels as in diseases such as hypertension, diabetes, etc. allow to grade the changes occurring in the blood vessels in other parts of the body also.

OCCLUSIVE DISEASES AFFECTING THE ARTERIAL CIRCULATION

Occlusive diseases are classified depending on the site of obstruction into:

- Central retinal artery occlusion (CRAO)
- Branch retinal artery occlusion (BRAO)
- Ophthalmic artery occlusion
- Cilioretinal artery occlusion
- Ocular ischemic syndrome (OIS).

CENTRAL RETINAL ARTERY OCCLUSION**

Definition

Occlusion of central retinal artery resulting in hypoxic damage of the retina is called central retinal artery occlusion (CRAO) (Fig. 11.5.1).

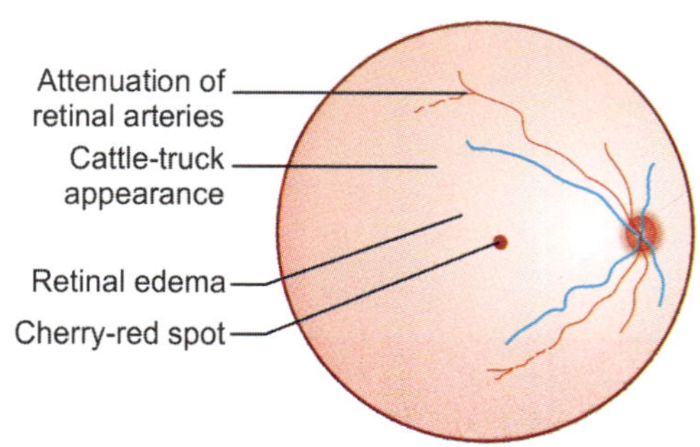

FIG. 11.5.1: Central retinal artery occlusion

Central retinal artery occlusion is an ocular emergency and requires immediate treatment, if not almost always leads to gross diminution of vision.

Central retinal artery occlusion can be compared to myocardial infarction or cerebral stroke. The risk factors are same for all the conditions. Infact all patients with central retinal artery occlusion should be evaluated for risk of myocardial infarction or cerebral stroke.

Etiology

Central retinal artery occlusion is caused by thrombosis, embolism or vasculitis of the central retinal artery:

1. The most common cause is thrombosis or thromboembolus, obstructing the central retinal artery as a result of atherosclerosis. It accounts for 75–80% of cases of CRAO. The most common site of obstruction is proximal to the lamina cribrosa.
2. The second common cause is embolism accounting for about 20% of cases and the source of emboli can be carotid arteries or from the cardiac etiology.
3. The less common causes are:
    a. Vasculitis involving the central retinal artery.
    b. Giant cell arteritis.
    c. Periarteritis associated with systemic lupus erythematosus (SLE), polyarteritis nodosa, Wegener's granulomatosis, etc.
    d. Thrombophilic disorders such as hyperhomocysteinemia, antiphospholipid antibody syndrome, etc.
    e. Susac syndrome named after John Susac, who first described the disease, characterized by triad of retinal artery occlusion, encephalopathy and hearing loss.
    f. Systemic coagulopathies.

It is more commonly seen in males with highest incidence in sixth decade. Diabetes, hypertension, hypercholesterolemia, ischemic heart disease, cerebrovascular diseases are the common risk factors associated with CRAO.

Pathogenesis

Occlusion of central retinal artery leads to hypoxic damage of inner layers of the retina resulting in edema, ischemic necrosis and opacification of the retinal layers.

Clinical Features

Symptoms

1. Sudden painless gross diminution of vision is the presenting complaint.
2. The visual acuity may be produced up to hand movements or perception of light.
3. The prodromal symptom of amaurosis fugax is seen in 5–10% of cases.
4. Patients with additional cilioretinal artery supplying the macula may have good central vision.
5. Complete loss of vision with perception of light being negative is seen in ophthalmic artery occlusion.

Signs

On examination:

1. Relative afferent pupillary pathway defect is usually present on the affected side and it is the earliest sign to appear.
2. Fundus examination shows:*
    a. Retinal arteries are markedly narrowed with thread-like appearance with retinal veins being normal.
    b. The retina appears white in color, because of edema resulting in opacification. It develops after 15 minutes to a few hours after obstruction and resolves over 4–6 weeks with restoration of circulation. The retinal whitening is denser at the posterior pole as the nerve fiber layer is thicker in the posterior pole.
    c. Cherry-red spot at the macula is because of normal choroidal appearance as choroidal circulation remains intact in CRAO. This shines through the fovea and stands out against the surrounding

edematous white retina giving rise to appearance of cherry-red spot.

d. Box-carring or segmentation of blood in the retinal vessels rise to cattle-truck appearance is seen in severe obstruction.
e. Patients with additional cilioretinal artery supplying the macula show macular sparing with normal appearance of the macula.

Clinical Course

1. Irreversible injury to the retinal cells occurs in cases where the ischemia, because of obstruction of blood supply persists for more than 100 minutes. The retinal edema resolves by 4–6 weeks with restoration of circulation by establishment of collateral vessels. The arteries will remain narrow and relative afferent pupillary pathway defect persists and eventually optic disk becomes pale because of optic atrophy.
2. The amount of visual loss depends on the severity and duration of ischemia induced by arterial obstruction.
3. Complications such as ocular neovascularization including rubeosis iridis. Neovascularization of optic disk are not uncommon and are seen in small percentage of people.

Investigations

1. Fundus fluorescein angiography (FFA) shows compromised retinal blood flow with normal choroidal flow.
2. Electroretinography (ERG) shows reduced b-wave and normal a-wave indicating that ischemia is limited only to inner layers of the retina.
3. All patients with CRAO need evaluation to find out the risk factors and modification of them as they are at increased risk of cerebrovascular and cardiovascular diseases.
4. The common laboratory investigations done are carotid artery studies, lipid profile, cardiac evaluation by electrocardiogram and echocardiogram, prothrombin time, erythrocyte sedimentation rate (ESR), etc.

Treatment

The visual prognosis is poor for CRAO as the retina goes for ischemic necrosis as early as within few hours of occlusion of the artery. The treatment has to be started as early as possible and unfortunately no definitive treatment exists. The treatment options are:

1. Immediate reduction of intraocular pressure to improve the retinal artery perfusion by:
   a. Intravenous mannitol, acetazolamide and other antiglaucoma drugs.
   b. Anterior chamber paracentesis.
   c. Ocular massage.
2. Vasodilatation to improve the blood supply by:
   a. Sublingual isosorbide dinitrate.
   b. Hyperbaric oxygen.
   c. Breathing of carbogen, a mixture of 95% carbon dioxide and 5% oxygen.
   d. Rebreathing into a polythene bag to increase the carbon dioxide level in blood to cause vasodilatation.
3. Reduction of retinal edema by:
   a. Intravenous methylprednisolone is very effective in artery occlusions associated with giant cell arteritis.
4. Thrombolytic therapy to cause thrombolysis is still not used commonly as conclusive evidence is not available. Thrombolysis is done by:
   a. Intravenous heparin, streptokinase, tissue plasminogen activator.
   b. Neodymium: yttrium aluminum garnet (Nd:YAG) laser embolectomy.

Differential Diagnosis of Cherry-Red Spot at Macula*

Cherry-red spot is seen in diseases, which cause opacification of the layers of the retina involving the posterior pole as in:

- Central retinal artery occlusion as described in this chapter.
- Lipid storage disorders, because of accumulation of abnormal material in the layers of retina.

Contd...

Contd...

> Since the inner nerve fiber layers are absent at the fovea, the underlying choroidal reflex stands out against the surrounding white retina giving rise to the appearance of cherry-red spot. The various lipid storage diseases are:
> - Tay-Sachs disease
> - Niemann-Pick disease
> - Sandhoff disease
> - Mucolipidosis
> - Hurler's syndrome
> - Farber's disease
> - Gangliosidosis.
>
> Pseudo cherry-red spot is seen in conditions such as macular hemorrhage and macular hole with retinal detachment.

BRANCH RETINAL ARTERY OCCLUSION

Definition

Occlusion of a branch of central retinal artery resulting in hypoxic damage corresponding part of retina, which is supplied by that particular branch is called BRAO (Fig. 11.5.2).

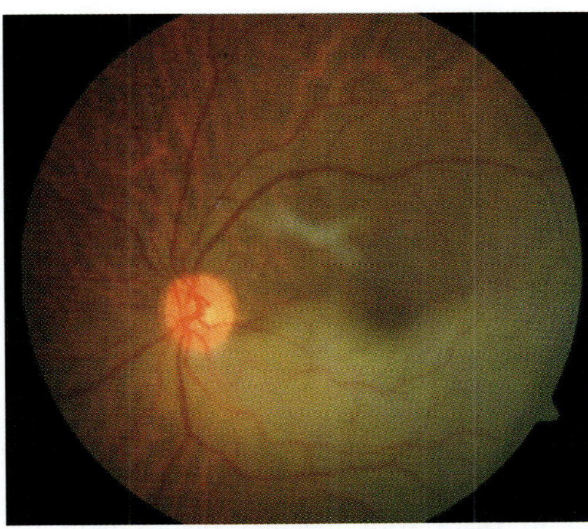

FIG. 11.5.2: Inferotemporal branch retinal artery occlusion (*Note:* Narrowing of the retinal arteries and retinal whitening in the inferotemporal quadrant).

Etiopathogenesis

Branch retinal artery occlusion is similar to CRAO and it is also seen more commonly in males with highest incidence in sixth decade. It is less commonly seen than CRAO and emboli are responsible for 75% of cases of BRAO.

Atherosclerosis, which accounts for majority of CRAO does not have role in the pathogenesis of CRAO as atherosclerosis does not involve the branch retinal arteries as they lack internal elastic lamina. The emboli can be:

1. Cholesterol emboli called Hollenhorst plaque arising from atheromatous plaques of the carotid arteries and appear as golden-yellow refractile crystal.
2. Calcific emboli usually arise from calcified heart valves and appear as white non-refractile opaque body.
3. Fibrin-platelet emboli are usually multiple gray-white colored plugs like and arise following myocardial infarction or atrial fibrillation.

The obstruction usually occurs at the site of bifurcation of arteries and more commonly affecting the temporal retina than nasal retina probably, because of increased branching on the temporal side.

Clinical Features

1. It presents with sudden painless partial loss of vision in a particular sector or quadrant with visual field defect in that corresponding sector or quadrant.
2. The amount of loss of visual acuity remains variable depending on the involvement of macula.
3. A relative afferent pupillary pathway defect is often present.

Examination of Retina

Examination of retina shows:

1. Markedly narrowed retinal arteries in the affected segment with retinal veins being normal.

2. The retina appears white in color, because of edema resulting in opacification in the corresponding quadrant or sector.
3. Box-carring or segmentation of blood in the retinal vessels giving rise to cattle-truck appearance may be seen.
4. Emboli may be seen in one or more branches of the central retinal artery.

Treatment

1. It is mainly aimed at identifying the risk factors by systemic evaluation and correcting them.
2. In cases with macular involvement the treatment is similar to that of CRAO.

OPHTHALMIC ARTERY OCCLUSION

Definition

Occlusion of the ophthalmic artery resulting in obstruction of both retinal and choroidal circulations resulting in complete loss of vision is called ophthalmic artery occlusion.

Etiopathogenesis

The etiology is similar to CRAO. Since both retinal choroidal circulations are affected this leads to gross diminution of vision, often perception of light negative. It does not lead to cherry-red spot as choroidal circulation is also affected.

Clinical Features

1. It presents with sudden painless complete loss of vision with perception of light being negative.
2. Pupil of the affected side shows total afferent pupillary pathway defect.
3. Fundus examination shows severe retinal edema and cherry-red spot is usually absent.
4. Electroretinogram shows reduced a- and b-wave indicating involvement of all the layers of retina.
5. Fundus fluorescein angiography shows compromised retinal and choroidal blood flow.

Treatment

No satisfactory treatment is available and eye becomes totally blind because of secondary optic atrophy.

CILIORETINAL ARTERY OCCLUSION*

Cilioretinal artery is seen in up to 25% of people; it arises from posterior ciliary arteries and supplies macula (Fig. 11.5.3).

Occlusion of cilioretinal arteries results in edema of the retina temporal to the optic disk in the papillomacular bundle, which corresponds to the area supplied by the artery and variable amount of visual loss depending on the area of retina supplied by it.

The etiology and risk factors are similar to CRAO. Isolated cilioretinal artery occlusion is seen in about 40% of eyes, associated with central retinal vein occlusion in 40% of eyes and associated with anterior ischemic optic neuropathy in 20% of eyes. The visual prognosis is good in isolated cilioretinal artery occlusion.

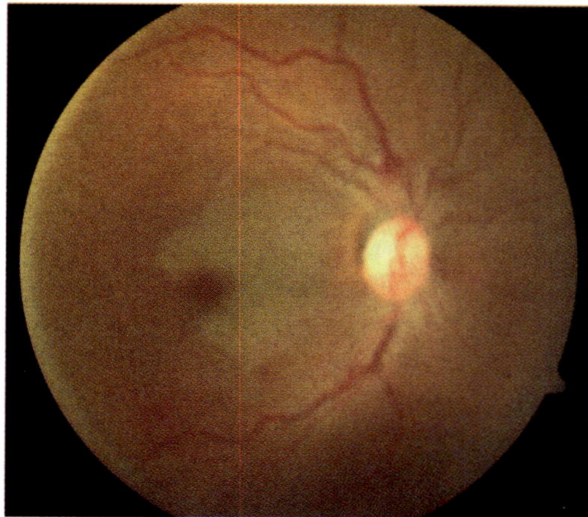

FIG. 11.5.3: Cilioretinal artery occlusion (*Note:* Whitening of the retina because of retinal edema temporal to the optic disk in the papillomacular bundle).

OCULAR ISCHEMIC SYNDROME**

Definition

Ocular ischemic syndrome is a clinical condition characterized by chronic ocular hypoperfusion occurring secondary to ipsilateral obstruction of the carotid artery resulting in ocular ischemia.

Etiopathogenesis

1. Ocular ischemic syndrome is seen in elderly people with mean age of presentation being more than 65 years with a male female ratio of 2:1.
2. The most common underlying etiology is atherosclerosis of the carotid artery thereby reducing the size of the lumen of the artery. The obstructions reducing the lumen by more than 90% are associated with ocular ischemic syndrome.
3. The other less common etiologies are giant cell arteritis, trauma, fibrovascular dysplasia, Takayasu's arteritis, aortic arch syndrome, etc.
4. The pathogenesis of the condition is because of chronic ischemia caused by reduced ocular perfusion and hence involves structures of both anterior and posterior segments.

Clinical Features

Symptoms

1. Gradual progressive painful loss of vision over weeks or months is the common presenting complaint, however few patients can complain repeated episodes of amaurosis fugax and sudden diminution of vision.
2. Ocular pain commonly called ocular angina.
3. Prolonged recovery time after exposure to bright light called bright-light amaurosis fugax.

Signs

1. On examination, the anterior segment shows:
   a. Iris neovascularization or rubeosis iridis.
   b. Anterior chamber cells and flare.
2. The posterior segment shows:
   a. Retinal hemorrhages, dot and blot in type situated in the deeper layers of the retina.
   b. Narrowing of retinal arteries.
   c. Dilatation of the retinal veins without beading or tortuosity.
   d. Cotton-wool spots.
   e. Neovascularization of optic disk.

Investigations

1. Fundus fluorescein angiography shows delayed choroidal filling, prominent arterial staining and prolonged arteriovenous (AV) transit time.
2. Color Doppler imaging of the carotid artery shows obstruction and reduced flow on the affected side.

Differential Diagnosis

Ocular ischemic syndrome has to be differentiated from the following.

Diabetic Retinopathy

Diabetic retinopathy is usually a bilateral condition. In addition to the features of ocular ischemic syndrome, it shows hard exudates and venous beading, which are absent in ocular ischemic syndrome. The FFA shows normal choroidal filling and AV transit time, which are typically prolonged in ocular ischemic syndrome.

Non-ischemic Central Retinal Vein Occlusion

Non-ischemic central retinal vein occlusion is also a unilateral condition such as ocular ischemic syndrome; it shows tortuous veins with superficial flame-shaped hemorrhages. FFA shows normal choroidal filling with prolonged AV transit time and prominent venous staining.

Treatment

1. Panretinal photocoagulation (PRP) is indicated in cases associated with rubeosis iridis or neovascular glaucoma.
2. Systemic treatment in the form of carotid artery endarterectomy or angioplasty or stenting for the underlying carotid artery stenosis.

OCCLUSIVE DISEASES AFFECTING THE VENOUS CIRCULATION

Occlusive diseases affecting the venous circulation are:
- Central retinal vein occlusion (CRVO)
- Hemiretinal vein occlusion
- Branch retinal vein occlusion (BRVO)
- Tributary retinal vein occlusion.

CENTRAL RETINAL VEIN OCCLUSION**

Definition

Occlusion or obstruction of the central retinal vein at the lamina cribrosa and resulting in occlusion retinopathy is called central retinal vein occlusion.

Central retinal vein occlusion is the second common vascular disorder affecting retina, the most common being diabetic retinopathy.

Etiology

Central retinal vein occlusion occurs most commonly in the fifth or sixth decade of life with males being affected more commonly.

Diabetes mellitus, hypertension, hyperlipidemia, bleeding and clotting disorders, vasculitis, use of oral contraceptives and atherosclerotic cardiovascular diseases are the most commonly associated conditions. The obstruction is caused by formation of thrombus at the lamina cribrosa.

The central retinal vein and the artery share common adventitia hence arteriosclerosis or atherosclerosis of the artery can compress the central retinal vein as both pass through the narrow lamina cribrosa. The compression is known to cause endothelial cell proliferation in the vessel wall resulting in the formation of thrombus. The causes for thrombus formation in the vein are:
1. Stasis of blood because of hypotension or external compression as explained above.
2. Hypercoagulable states such as protein C or protein S deficiency, antithrombin deficiency, hyperhomocysteinemia, polycythemia, etc.
3. The inflammation of the vessel wall as in phlebitis is caused by diseases such as Behçet's syndrome, sarcoidosis, Wegener's granulomatosis.

Pathogenesis

The occlusion of the vein results in hypoxia because of stagnation of blood flow. The hypoxic damage leads to damage of capillary endothelial cells and extravasation of blood constituents.

Clinical Features*

Based on the clinical features, CRVO is classified into ischemic CRVO and non-ischemic CRVO (Figs 11.5.4A and B, Figs 11.5.5A and B, Table 11.5.1).

*Clinical Course**

1. The retinal hemorrhages are absorbed over a period of 3 months. The amount of visual loss depends on the complications, which follow CRVO.
2. Macular edema, ocular neovascularization, neovascular glaucoma and vitreous hemorrhage are the causes for visual impairment following CRVO.

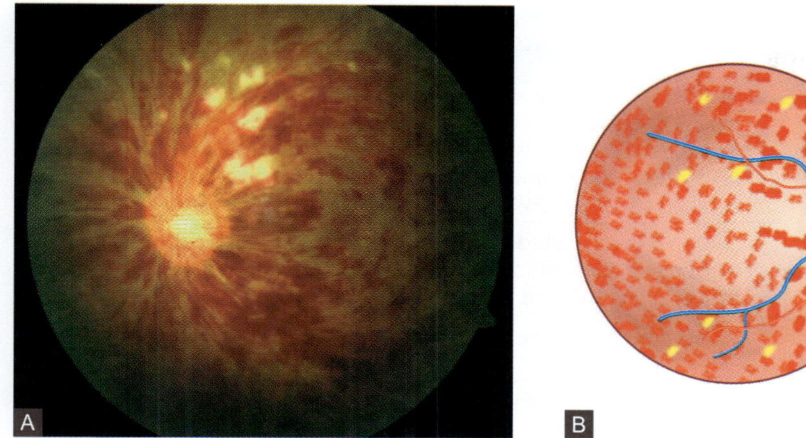

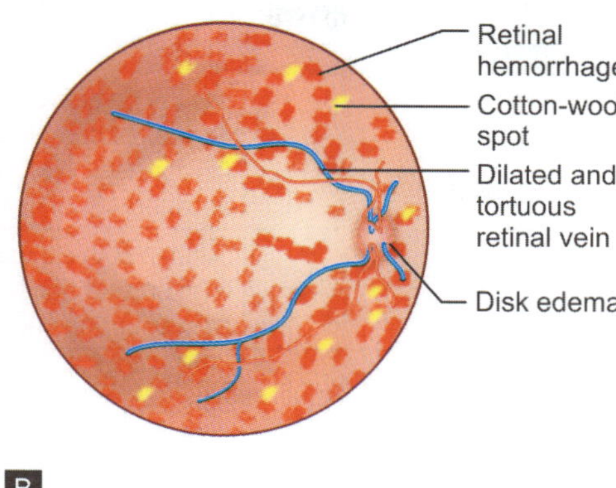

FIGS 11.5.4A and B: Ischemic central retinal vein occlusion. **A.** Photograph; **B.** Diagrammatic representation.

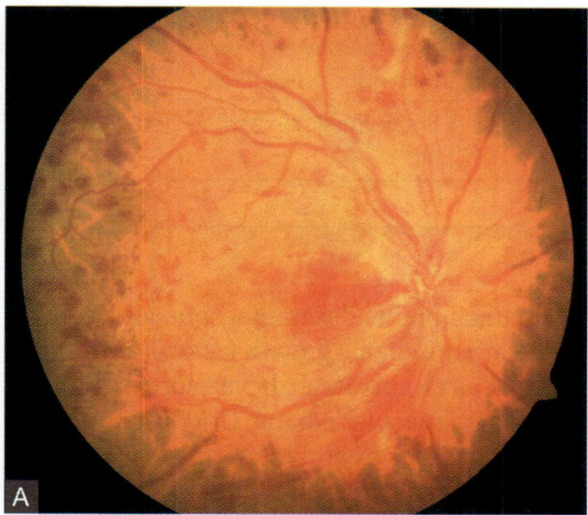

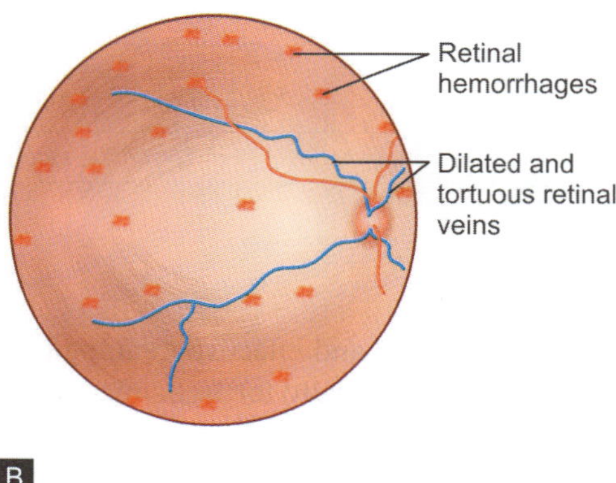

FIGS 11.5.5A and B: Non-ischemic central retinal vein occlusion. **A.** Photograph; **B.** Diagrammatic representation.

3. Macular edema is the most common cause for visual impairment following CRVO. It is usually because of focal leak or because of diffuse leakage from capillaries.
4. Neovascular glaucoma is seen in more than 50% of cases of ischemic CRVO and the mean time for development of glaucoma is after 3 months. It is called 100 days glaucoma. Neovascular glaucoma is seen in less than 5% of cases of non-ischemic CRVO.

Investigations

All patients with CRVO should undergo evaluation to look for the associated systemic diseases and high-risk factors such as diabetes, hypertension, lipid profile, cardiac evaluation, thrombophilia screening, etc.

Fundus fluorescein angiography is required to differentiate ischemic from non-ischemic CRVO, and to look for areas of capillary non-perfusion and neovascularization of retina, the risk factors for neovascular glaucoma, and thus to decide on requirement for PRP. FFA is done after about 3 months to have good visibility as the hemorrhages would have cleared by then.

Optical coherence topography (OCT) is done to identify, quantify and to treat macular edema, the most common cause for loss of vision in the initial stages.

TABLE 11.5.1: Differences between ischemic and non-ischemic CRVO*

Clinical features	*Ischemic CRVO*	*Non-ischemic CRVO*
Definition	It is the severe variety of CRVO also called complete CRVO or hemorrhagic retinopathy and accounts for 25% of CRVO	It is the mild variety of CRVO also called incomplete CRVO or venous stasis retinopathy and accounts for 75% of CRVO
Visual acuity	Sudden painless marked visual loss with presenting visual acuity of less than counting fingers at 3 meter	Sudden painless mild-to-moderate visual loss with presenting visual acuity of better than 6/60
Random amplified polymorphic deoxyribonucleic acid	Always present in severe form	Present in mild form or absent
Fundus	Venous engorgement and tortuosity Widespread retinal hemorrhages involving all the four quadrants and called blood and thunder fundus Cotton-wool spots Marked optic disk edema Macular edema and hemorrhages	Venous congestion and tortuous veins Dot and blot, flame-shaped hemorrhages few in number involving all the four quadrants and hemorrhages involve periphery of the retina more than the posterior pole Mild optic disk edema
FFA†	Shows extensive capillary non-perfusion areas	Shows minimal capillary non-perfusion areas

*CRVO, central retinal vein occlusion; †FFA, fundus fluorescein angiography.

Treatment

There is no proven and effective treatment option for CRVO especially for ischemic variety. Hence, the main treatment option considered are identifying the risk factors and treating them, and treatment of complications.

Non-ischemic Central Retinal Vein Occlusion

1. No treatment is required in patients with good vision without involvement of macula. However, regular follow-up is advised to look for signs of neovascular glaucoma or macular edema.
2. Macular edema was treated in the past by oral steroid drugs and oral acetazolamide with limited success. The recent pharmacological drugs and investigations such as OCT have led to rapid treatment of CRVO with better visual prognosis. The recent treatment includes use of intravitreal steroids such as triamcinolone, dexamethasone and antivascular endothelial growth factors (anti-VEGF) such as ranibizumab, bevacizumab for treatment of macular edema. Grid laser photocoagulation for treatment of macular edema is not as effective as it is for BRVO.
3. Ocular neovascularization as noticed on fundus examination or preferably by FFA is treated by PRP.

Ischemic Central Retinal Vein Occlusion

There is no satisfactory treatment for ischemic variety as the damage is severe and ischemia is severe, response to treatment is minimal resulting in irreversible visual loss. Intravitreal steroids and anti-VEGF are usually ineffective in treating macular edema. Hence, main treatment is aimed at preventing the development of neovascular glaucoma. It is done by prophylactic PRP after 2–3 months when the retinal hemorrhages are cleared to prevent neovascular glaucoma.

Surgical modalities of treatment: Choroidoretinal anastomosis and radial optic neurotomy are the proposed mode of surgical treatments for CRVO.

HEMIRETINAL VEIN OCCLUSION

Definition

Occlusion of one of the trunks of central retinal vein in people who have two-trunked central retinal vein as congenital anomaly (Fig. 11.5.6).

> About 20% of people show the presence of this hemicentral retinal vein proximal to the lamina cribrosa. Hence, hemiretinal vein occlusion is a relatively rare event.

Etiology

The etiology and pathogenesis are similar to CRVO. It also presents in two varieties, ischemic and nonischemic.

Clinical Features

The involved retina shows venous engorgement and tortuosity, retinal hemorrhages, cotton-wool spots associated with optic disk edema, macular edema and hemorrhages. The visual acuity depends on the macular involvement. Clinical course, investigations and treatment are similar to CRVO.

BRANCH RETINAL VEIN OCCLUSION**

Definition

Occlusion of a branch of central retinal vein resulting in involvement of the corresponding part of retina, which is supplied by that particular branch is called BRVO (Fig. 11.5.7).

Etiopathogenesis

Branch retinal vein occlusion is more common than CRVO. The etiology is similar to CRVO; it is more common in fifth or sixth decade of life with males being affected more commonly.

Diabetes mellitus, hypertension, hyperlipidemia, bleeding and clotting disorders, vasculitis, use of oral contraceptives and atherosclerotic cardiovascular diseases are the most commonly associated conditions.

Branch retinal vein occlusion is usually precipitated by compression of the retinal vein by an arteriosclerotic artery, which results in turbulent blood flow and endothelial damage resulting in thrombosis and occlusion of the vein.

The superotemporal branch, followed by inferotemporal branch of the retinal vein is more commonly involved probably because of

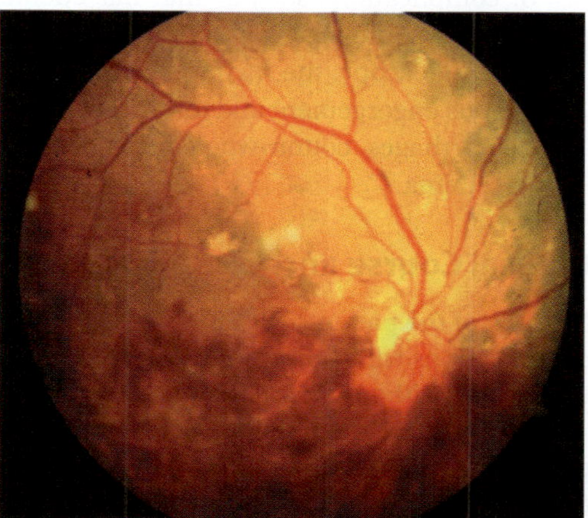

FIG. 11.5.6: Hemiretinal vein occlusion

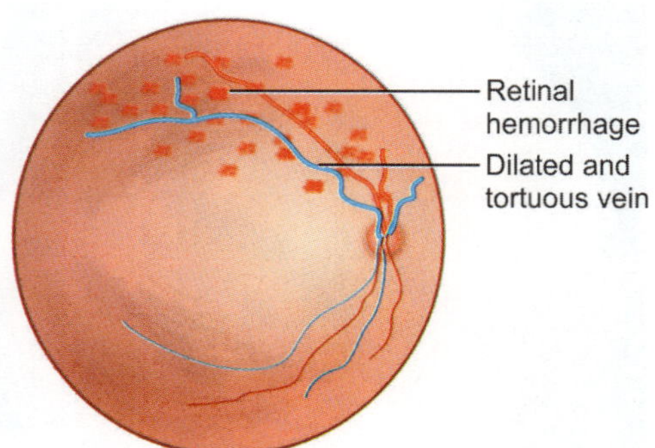

FIG. 11.5.7: Branch retinal vein occlusion (*Note:* Dilated and tortuous vein in the superotemporal quadrant associated with retinal hemorrhages in the affected quadrant).

presence of more AV crossings in the superotemporal quadrant of the retina. The superotemporal branch is involved in approximately 50% of cases (Figs 11.5.8A and B).

The site of occlusion can be seen involving a major branch or a peripheral branch called tributary retinal vein occlusion.

Clinical Features

1. Sudden painless loss of vision in the affected segment presenting as visual field defect is the presenting complaint.
2. Central vision is affected in cases of involvement of macular branch or because of complications such as macular edema, macular hemorrhage, etc.
3. On fundoscopy, the involved retina shows venous engorgement and tortuosity, retinal hemorrhages, cotton-wool spots with retinal edema.

Clinical Course and Complications

Majority of the patients with BRVO without any complications will show improvement in visual acuity even without treatment by 3–6 months.

Occlusion of the circulation leads to ischemia and inflammation leading to complications. The complications responsible for visual impairment and which require treatment are:

- Macular edema
- Macular ischemia
- Epiretinal membrane
- Neovascularization leading to neovascular glaucoma, vitreous hemorrhage.

Treatment

1. In patients with normal visual acuity and without involvement of the macula, observation and follow-up is sufficient.
2. In patients with visual impairment because of macular edema:
   a. Conventional management: Observation till 3 months for doing FFA to decide the mode of management depending on the presence or absence of macular ischemia. 3 months waiting is for clearing of retinal hemorrhages to have good visibility during FFA. Macular ischemia is a contraindication for laser treatment. Macular edema without ischemia is treated by macular grid laser photocoagulation.
   b. Recent advances in management: OCT is performed to know the presence of macular edema, and the recent treatment includes use of intravitreal steroids such as triamcinolone, dexamethasone and antivascular endothelial growth factors (ranibizumab and bevacizumab).

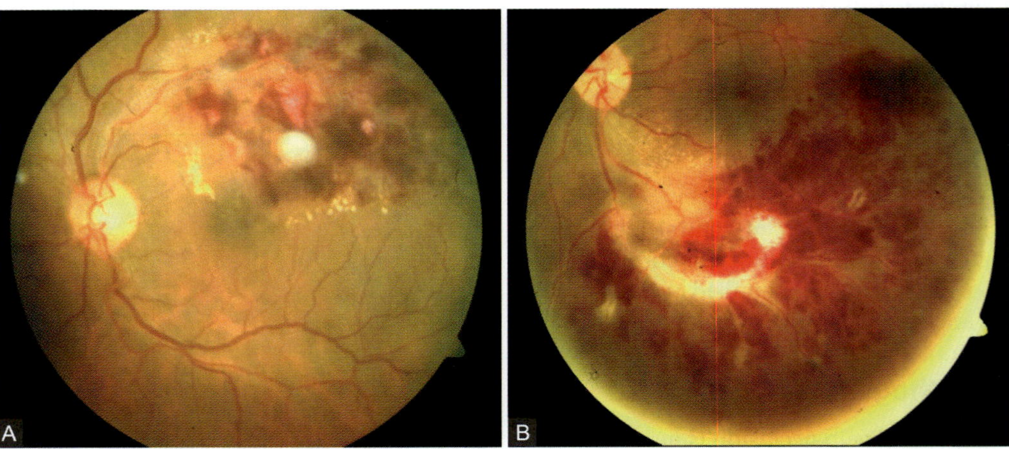

FIGS 11.5.8A and B: Branch retinal vein occlusion (BRVO). **A.** Superotemporal BRVO; **B.** Inferotemporal BRVO.

c. In patients with ocular neovascularization and neovascular glaucoma: This usually develops by 3–6 months. This is treated by PRP of the involved segment of retina only. Neovascular glaucoma is treated with antiglaucoma drugs.

TRIBUTARY RETINAL VEIN OCCLUSION

Definition

Occlusion of peripheral branch of the central retinal vein is called tributary retinal vein occlusion (Fig. 11.5.9).

Etiology

The etiology is same as branch retinal vein occlusion.

Clinical Features

The clinical features are same as BRVO, with the retinal hemorrhages and venous tortuosity limited to area of the retina drained by the affected branch. Occlusion of the macular branch results in severe visual impairment.

Management

The investigations and treatment are similar to BRVO.

COMBINED RETINAL ARTERY AND RETINAL VEIN OCCLUSION

Occlusion of the retinal artery and retinal vein are known to occur together. The common etiologies associated with combined artery and vein occlusion include systemic and ocular causes. Systemic causes are antiphospholipid syndrome, hypertension, diabetes, hyperhomocysteinemia, coagulopathies, autoimmune diseases (e.g. SLE) malignancies such as non-Hodgkin's lymphoma, leukemia, etc. Ocular causes are orbital trauma, orbital cellulitis, complications of retrobulbar injections, etc.

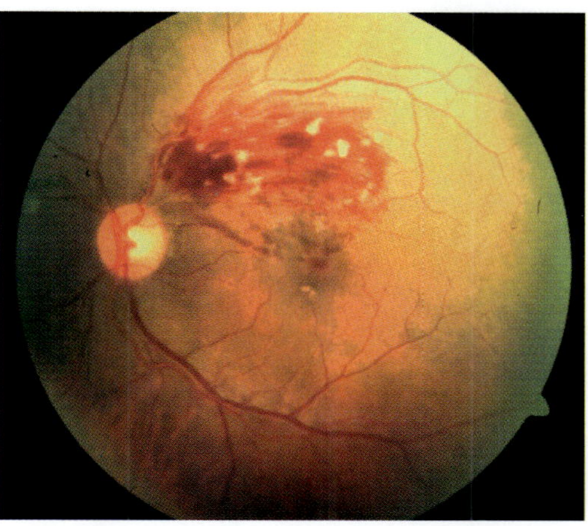

FIG. 11.5.9: Tributary retinal vein occlusion

Patients with combined retinal artery and vein occlusion present with sudden painless diminution of vision or loss of vision with fundoscopy showing features of both artery and vein occlusion in the form of retinal edema with retinal hemorrhages and dilated, tortuous veins (Fig. 11.5.10).

The common combinations of artery and vein occlusion seen are:

- Combined central retinal artery and CRVO
- Combined branch retinal artery and CRVO
- Combined cilioretinal artery and CRVO.

Though the artery and vein occlusion of the retina have got similar etiology, they vary in their clinical features and treatment. The probable causes found are given in Table 11.5.2.

DIABETIC RETINOPATHY***

Definition

Retinopathy seen in patients with diabetes mellitus is called diabetic retinopathy. It is a microangiopathy predominantly affecting the smaller blood vessels such as arterioles, venules and capillaries.

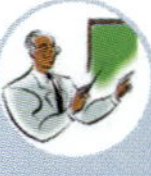

Diabetic retinopathy is one of the leading causes of blindness worldwide.

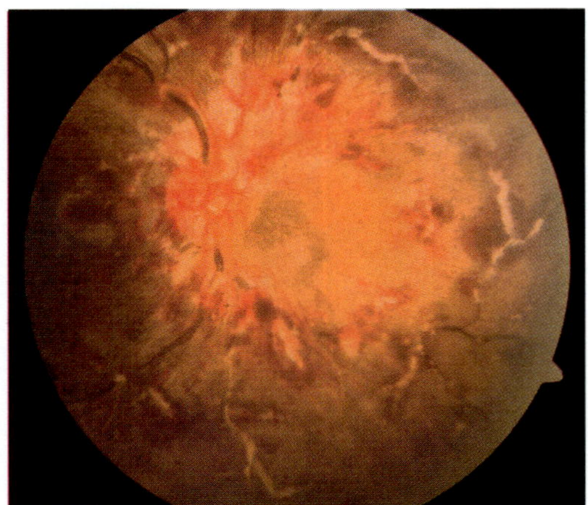

FIG. 11.5.10: Combined central retinal artery occlusion and central retinal vein occlusion

Etiopathogenesis

The important risk factors are given below.

Duration of Diabetes

Duration of diabetes is the most important risk factor associated with development of diabetic retinopathy. Increase in the duration of diabetes is associated with increased incidence of diabetic retinopathy. The incidence of diabetic retinopathy is about 90% after duration of 30 years of diabetes, whereas it is 50% after 10 years of diabetes.

Age

Diabetic retinopathy is rarely seen before puberty. Earlier the age of onset of diabetes, more common is the incidence of diabetic retinopathy as the duration of diabetes is more likely to be longer. Hence, more incidence of diabetic retinopathy is seen in patients with onset of diabetes before 40 years of age.

Control of Diabetes

Strict control of glycemic levels is associated with lesser incidence of diabetic retinopathy.

Hypertension

Hypertension especially uncontrolled when associated with diabetes is known to increase the progression of the diabetic retinopathy.

Nephropathy

Presence of diabetic nephropathy is associated with increased risk of diabetic retinopathy.

TABLE 11.5.2: Differences between artery and vein occlusion—clinical features and treatment

Artery occlusion	*Vein occlusion*
Artery occlusion leads to rapid ischemic damage to the inner layers of retina causing edema and white appearance The retina appears white because of lack of blood and arteries appear thin or attenuated	Vein occlusion leads to gradual onset ischemia leading to development of capillaries with weak walls, which rupture leading to retinal hemorrhages The retina appears full of blood because of impaired drainage with veins dilated and tortuous
As rapid ischemic damage leads to death of retinal cells, no satisfactory treatment is available after permanent damage has occurred	As ischemic damage occurs slowly, treatment options such as intravitreal steroids or anti-VEGF drugs have a role in treatment in vein occlusion at least in non-ischemic variety
Because of rapid ischemic damage, angiogenic factors may not be released hence it has low incidence of ocular neovascularization and neovascular glaucoma, and hence anti-VEGF* drugs have no role in treatment	Because of slow ischemic damage angiogenic factors are released, hence it has high incidence of ocular neovascularization and neovascular glaucoma, and hence anti-VEGF drugs have a definite role in treatment

*VEGF, vascular endothelial growth factor

Pregnancy

Pregnancy is known to increase the progression of diabetic retinopathy.

Hyperlipidemia

Hyperlipidemia is known to increase the progression of diabetic retinopathy.

Family History

A family history of diabetic retinopathy is associated with increased risk of developing diabetic retinopathy.

Pathogenesis

Diabetic retinopathy is a microangiopathy characteristically affecting the arterioles, venules and capillaries resulting in retinal ischemia. The resulting retinal ischemia results in the characteristic features of diabetic retinopathy.

Pathology

The pathological abnormalities seen in diabetic retinopathy are thickening of capillary basement membrane and pericyte dropout. Microaneurysms appear in areas of absence of pericytes. These microaneurysms are permeable leading to accumulation of lipids, fluids and hemorrhages in the retina.

Clinical Features

Symptoms

Diabetic retinopathy presents with visual impairment in patients with diabetes. The degree of visual impairment depends on the severity of diabetic retinopathy and presence of associated complications such as involvement of macula and vitreous hemorrhage.

Signs

Depending on the severity of signs, diabetic retinopathy is classified into different stages.

Classification

The most widely followed classification based on signs is by Early Treatment of Diabetic Retinopathy Study (ETDRS) group:**

- Non-proliferative diabetic retinopathy (NPDR)
- Proliferative diabetic retinopathy (PDR)
- Diabetic maculopathy
- Clinically significant macular edema
- Advanced diabetic eye disease.

Non-proliferative Diabetic Retinopathy

Symptoms and signs

Non-proliferative diabetic retinopathy shows (Figs 11.5.11A and B):

1. *Microaneurysms:* They are localized dilatation of the capillary wall seen because of absence of pericytes. They appear as red dots on fundoscopy.
2. *Retinal hemorrhages:* They are of two types:*
   a. Superficial retinal hemorrhages occurring as a result of bleeding from precapillary arterioles and are flame shaped as a result of spreading along the nerve fiber layer.
   b. Deep retinal hemorrhages occurring as a result of bleeding from capillaries are seen in the middle layers of the retina and are called dot and blot hemorrhages.

Dot and blot hemorrhages are typical of diabetic retinopathy.

3. *Hard exudates:* They are collection of lipids within the layers of retina. Increased hard exudates are seen in association with hyperlipidemia.
4. *Cotton-wool spots:* They are also known as soft exudates. They represent infarcts of nerve fiber layer of retina and are caused by swelling of the nerve fibers as a result of obstruction axoplasmic flow.
5. *Venous beading:* It is beading of the vein and it indicates hypoxia of the retina. Dilatation and

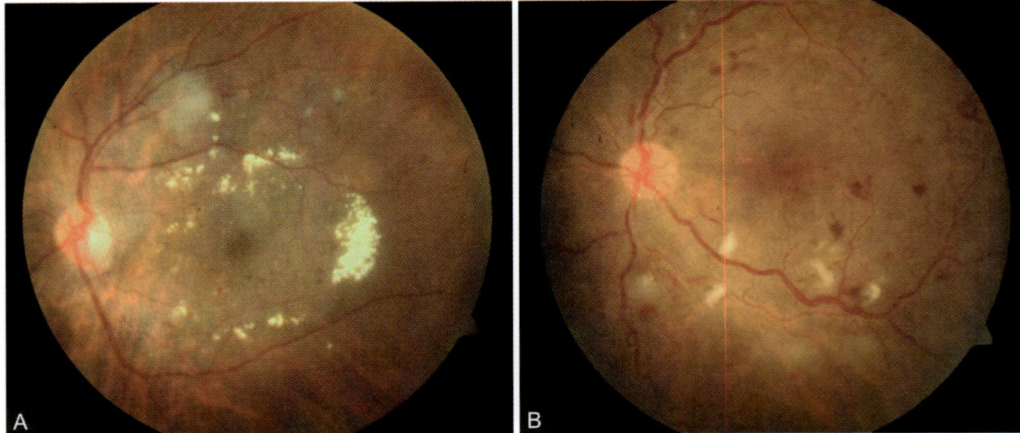

FIGS 11.5.11A and B: Non-proliferative diabetic retinopathy

tortuosity of the veins are the other changes seen in the veins.

6. *Intraretinal microvascular abnormalities:* They represent arteriovenular shunts that running from retinal arterioles to venules, bypassing the capillary bed. They are seen adjacent to areas of marked capillary hypoperfusion.

Classification

Non-proliferative diabetic retinopathy is classified into the following.

Very mild NPDR: Shows microaneurysms only.

Mild NPDR: Shows microaneurysms, retinal hemorrhages and hard exudates in one or two quadrants.

Moderate NPDR: Shows microaneurysms, retinal hemorrhages and hard exudates in three quadrants. Cotton-wool spots and venous beading may be present.

Severe NPDR: Shows one or more of 4-2-1 rule:

- Microaneurysms, retinal hemorrhages and hard exudates in all the four quadrants
- Venous beading in more than two quadrants
- Intraretinal microvascular abnormalities in more than one quadrant.

Very severe NPDR: Shows two or more of 4-2-1 rule:

- Microaneurysms, retinal hemorrhages and hard exudates in all the four quadrants
- Venous beading in more than two quadrants
- Intraretinal microvascular abnormalities in more than one quadrant.

*Proliferative Diabetic Retinopathy***

Proliferative diabetic retinopathy is characterized by the formation of new blood vessels involving the disk or elsewhere in the retina (Figs 11.5.12A and B).

Classification

Proliferative diabetic retinopathy is further classified into the following:

1. Early PDR, which is characterized by:
   a. New vessels on the retina either on the optic disk called new vessels on the disk (NVD) or elsewhere called new vessels elsewhere (NVE).
   b. With absence of the high-risk characteristics.
2. High-risk PDR, which is characterized by:
   a. New vessels on the disk of one fourth to one third or more of the disk area.
   b. New vessels on optic disk of less than one fourth of disk area or NVE with vitreous hemorrhage or preretinal hemorrhage.

Treatment

Proliferative diabetic retinopathy is treated by PRP. It is based on the principle that ischemia of

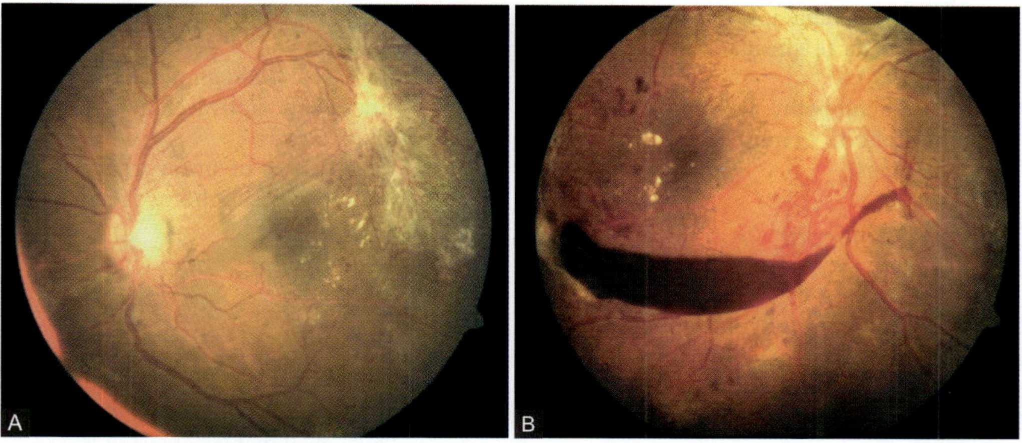

FIGS 11.5.12A and B: Proliferative diabetic retinopathy. **A.** Proliferative diabetic retinopathy with neovascularization; **B.** Proliferative diabetic retinopathy with preretinal hemorrhage.

the retinal layers is responsible for neovascularization and by destroying the peripheral retina away from macula the risk of neovascularization and progression of PDR is reduced. Thus, PRP preserves central vision at the cost of peripheral vision. Following PRP peripheral vision is impaired because of destruction of the retina by laser energy. The indications for PRP are:

1. PDR with high-risk characteristics.
2. Very severe NPDR/PDR without high-risk characteristics, but with risk factors such as extensive capillary nonperfusion or with risk factors, which accelerate the progression such as nephropathy, pregnancy, poor control of diabetes, requiring cataract surgery, requiring YAG laser capsulotomy, poor patient compliance, etc.

Panretinal photocoagulation is done by placing about 2,000 laser burns from posterior pole to the periphery of the fundus avoiding the macula and retinal vessels. The spot size is usually 500 µm and exposure time is 0.1 second. Usually, PRP is completed in 2–4 settings.

Follow-up is required after PRP, to look for appearance of new vessels or lack of regression of new vessels. These patients are treated by additional or add PRP.

Surgical management

Proliferative diabetic retinopathy is done in the form of vitrectomy and is indicated in patients with complications such as:

1. Non-resolving vitreous hemorrhage of more than 3 months duration.
2. Tractional retinal detachment.

*Diabetic Maculopathy***

Diabetic maculopathy is characterized by accumulation of fluids between outer plexiform and inner nuclear layers of the retina in the macula. It is the major cause of visual impairment in diabetic retinopathy. It is caused by either diffuse leakage or focal leakage from the microaneurysms.

It is classified into:

1. Diffuse maculopathy: It is characterized by diffuse retinal thickening or retinal edema caused by diffuse leakage from the affected capillaries.
2. Focal maculopathy: It is characterized by focal retinal thickening or retinal edema caused by focal leakage from the affected capillaries.
3. Ischemic maculopathy: It is characterized by minimal retinal thickening and maximal

visual impairment. It is caused by ischemia of the macula as a result of capillary hypoperfusion.
4. Mixed maculopathy: It is characterized by features of one or more of the above mentioned types.

Clinically Significant Macular Edema

Clinically significant macular edema (CSME) is defined by the presence of anyone of the following criteria:
1. Presence of retinal thickening within 500 µm from the center of the macula.
2. Presence of hard exudates within 500 µm of the center of the macula associated with surrounding retinal thickening.
3. Presence of retinal thickening one disk area or larger, a part of which is within one disk diameter from the center of the macula.

Treatment

Clinically significant macular edema in any stage of NPDR/PDR should be considered for treatment.

Depending on the type of leakage, focal or diffuse as obtained from FFA, the treatment is as follows:
1. Focal photocoagulation is considered for focal maculopathy with focal leakage. It is done by applying the laser burns directly to the leaking microaneurysms avoiding fovea and an area of 300 µm from the center of the macula. The spot size is usually 100 µm and exposure time is 0.1 second.
2. Grid photocoagulation is considered for diffuse maculopathy with diffuse leakage. It is done by applying laser burns to the area of retinal thickening avoiding fovea and an area of 500 µm from the center of the macula. The spot size is 100 µm and exposure time is 0.1 second.
3. Argon laser and frequency-doubled neodymium-doped yttrium aluminum garnet (Nd-YAG) laser are most commonly used for laser photocoagulation.
4. The other recent modes of treatment for CSME are:
   - Intravitreal triamcinolone
   - Intravitreal antivascular endothelial growth factors
   - Combination of intravitreal injections followed by laser photocoagulation.

Advanced Diabetic Eye Disease

Advanced diabetic eye disease is seen in people with inadequate treatment for PDR or because of failure in treatment for PDR. It is characterized by complete loss of vision because of one or more complications such as tractional retinal detachment, neovascular glaucoma or persistent vitreous hemorrhage or preretinal hemorrhage.

For hand-drawn fundus diagrams of diabetic retinopathy refer Author's textbook *Clinical Methods in Ophthalmology*, Chapter 11 'Examination of Retina'.

Investigations

The diagnosis of diabetes and status of its control is made by blood investigations such as fasting blood sugar (FBS), postprandial blood sugar and glycosylated hemoglobin (HbA1c). The ocular investigations frequently required are:
1. Fundus fluorescein angiography: It is helpful in demonstrating capillary nonperfusion and neovascularization. In maculopathy, it shows site of leakage and can differentiate focal leakage from diffuse leakage.
2. Ocular coherence tomography: It is helpful to measure retinal thickness and retinal edema, and important tool to assess the response to treatment.

Treatment
1. General management is by control of diabetes and maintaining the HbA1c below 7.
2. Treatment of the associated factors such as hypertension, hyperlipidemia, etc. which influence the course of diabetic retinopathy.

3. The treatment of diabetic retinopathy depends on the stage and severity. Regular follow-up is necessary in all the stages of retinopathy with treatment required in PDR and in diabetic maculopathy.
4. Follow-up schedule is given in Table 11.5.3.

TABLE 11.5.3: Follow-up schedule for advanced diabetic eye disease

Schedule	*Types of diabetic retinopathy*
Follow-up once in a year	No diabetic retinopathy Very mild NPDR* Mild NPDR
Follow-up once in 6 months	Moderate NPDR
Follow-up once in 4 months	Severe NPDR
Follow-up once in 3 months	Very severe NPDR
Follow-up once in 2 months	PDR without high-risk characteristics

*NPDR, non-proliferative diabetic retinopathy

HYPERTENSIVE RETINOPATHY***

Definition

Retinopathy occurring as a result of changes in the retinal vasculature, because of systemic hypertension is called hypertensive retinopathy (Fig. 11.5.13).

Etiopathogenesis

Hypertensive retinopathy is seen in:

1. Uncontrolled chronic systemic/essential hypertension.
2. Malignant hypertension in association with hypertensive choroidopathy and hypertensive optic neuropathy (malignant hypertension is a condition characterized by rapid elevation of blood pressure in the range of 200/140 mm Hg).
3. Hypertensive retinopathy is seen in about 10–15% of people with systemic hypertension.

The pathogenesis depends on the underlying cause, chronic hypertension or malignant hypertension.

In chronic hypertension, the chronically elevated blood pressure focal and generalized constriction of retinal arterioles because of autoregulation. This can lead to breakdown of the blood retinal barrier and vascular leakage.

In malignant hypertension, there is fibrinoid necrosis and focal occlusion of the choriocapillaries leading to choroidopathy. The ischemia of the optic nerve head leads to stasis of axoplasmic flow resulting in optic disk edema. The breakdown of blood retinal barrier leads to vascular leakage.

Clinical Features

Symptoms

1. Ocular symptoms are usually absent in patients with hypertensive retinopathy because of essential hypertension.
2. Ocular symptoms in the form of visual disturbances associated with headache

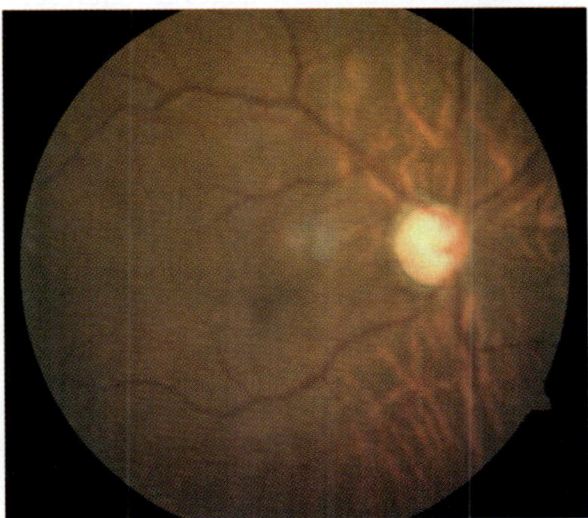

FIG. 11.5.13: Grade II hypertensive retinopathy

are commonly seen in cases of hypertensive retinopathy as a result of malignant hypertension.

Signs

The fundus findings depend on the type of hypertensive retinopathy.

Chronic hypertensive retinopathy: It is characterized by:

1. Focal or generalized narrowing or constriction of the retinal arterioles.
2. Arteriosclerosis or thickening of the vessel wall of the retinal arteries. It is because of endothelial hyperplasia and hyalinization in the lumen of the vessel wall.
3. Arteriovenous crossing changes in the form of change in the path of the vein at the site of crossing over arteries, dilatation of the vein distal to the crossing. These changes are seen as both artery and vein share common adventitial sheath at the site of crossing. AV crossing changes are highly specific for chronic hypertensive retinopathy (Fig. 11.5.14).
4. Cotton-wool spots because of retinal hypoxia and features of vascular leakage such as retinal edema, hard exudates and flame-shaped retinal hemorrhages are rarely seen. These changes are very common in case of malignant hypertensive retinopathy.

Malignant hypertensive retinopathy: It is characterized by:

1. Hypertensive retinopathy:
   - Focal narrowing of the retinal arterioles
   - Features of vascular leakage such as cotton-wool spots, retinal edema, hard exudates, flame-shaped hemorrhages, etc.
2. Hypertensive choroidopathy:
   - Focal occlusion of the choriocapillaries presenting as Elschnig spots; Elschnig spots appear as black lesions surrounded by yellow halos
   - Pigmentation extending along the choroidal arteries indicating fibrinoid necrosis called Siegrist streaks
   - Exudative retinal detachment.
3. Hypertensive optic neuropathy:
   - Disk edema because of ischemia resulting in stasis of axoplasmic flow.

Grading of Hypertensive Retinopathy**

Keith-Wagner-Barker Classification

Grade I: Mild generalized arteriolar attenuation.

Grade II: Moderate to marked generalized narrowing and focal attenuation of arterioles associated with AV nipping.

Grade III: Changes in the grade II plus copper wiring of arterioles, AV crossing changes, flame-shaped hemorrhages, cotton-wool spots and hard exudates (Figs 11.5.15A and B).

Grade IV: This consists of all changes of grade III plus silver wiring of arterioles and disk edema.

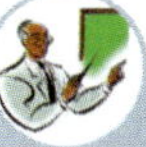

Arteriovenous Crossing Changes*

Gunn's sign: Tapering of vein on either side of arteriovenous crossing.

Salus' sign: Deflection of vein at arteriovenous crossing.

Bonnet's sign: Venous banking distal to the arteriovenous crossing.

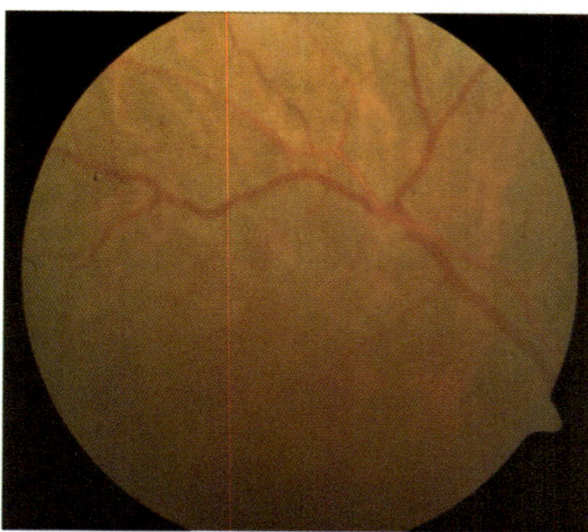

FIG. 11.5.14: Arteriovenous crossing changes

Scheie's Classification

Scheie's classification takes arteriosclerosis changes into consideration for grading hypertensive retinopathy along with the hypertensive changes (Table 11.5.4).

Treatment

Hypertensive retinopathy rarely affects vision; hence main treatment is by systemic treatment to control the hypertension.

In malignant hypertensive retinopathy, the blood pressure should be reduced slowly to prevent ischemia and damage to the vital organs. Slow reduction will allow time for autoregulation thereby prevents ischemic damage.

Hypertensive retinopathy is regarded as an indicator of systemic mortality and morbidity. This risk is defined by the Wong-Mitchell classification. It states that:

1. Mild retinopathy is characterized by generalized narrowing and focal attenuation of arterioles associated with AV nicking. The nicking is associated with modest risk of systemic morbidity in the form of cerebrovascular diseases (stroke) and cardiovascular diseases (coronary heart disease).
2. Moderate retinopathy characterized by AV crossing changes, flame-shaped hemorrhages, cotton-wool spots and hard exudates is associated with strong risk of morbidity in the form of cerebrovascular diseases like stroke and cardiovascular diseases like coronary heart disease.
3. Malignant retinopathy is characterized by all the changes of moderate retinopathy with disk edema has got strong association with systemic mortality.

For hand-drawn fundus diagrams of hypertensive retinopathy refer Author's textbook *Clinical Methods in Ophthalmology* Chapter 11 'Examination of Retina'.

PREGNANCY-INDUCED HYPERTENSION RETINOPATHY

Definition

Retinopathy occurring secondary to pregnancy-induced hypertension is called pregnancy-induced hypertension retinopathy (Fig. 11.5.16).

Etiopathogenesis

The incidence of ocular symptoms in pregnancy-induced hypertension is about 50%, whereas about 40% of people show retinal changes. The spasm

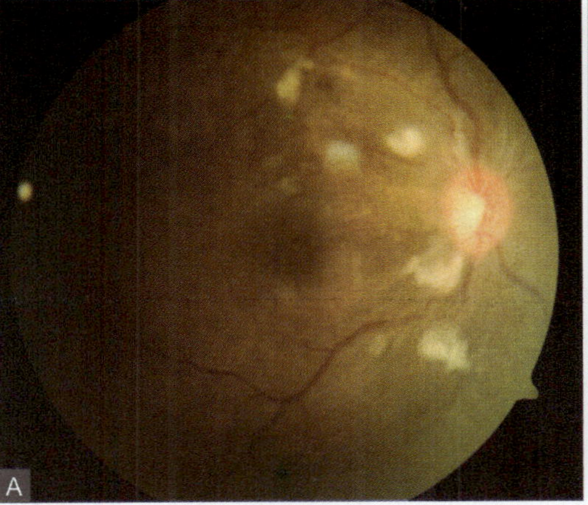

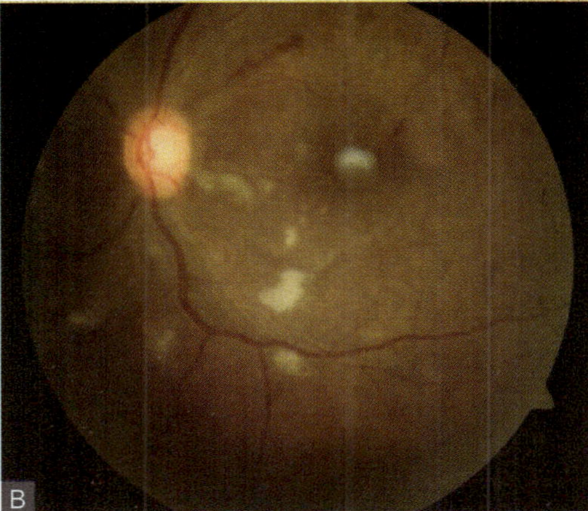

FIGS 11.5.15A and B: Grade III hypertensive retinopathy

TABLE 11.5.4: Scheie's classification

Classification	*Hypertensive features*	*Arteriosclerotic features*
Grade I	Generalized arteriolar narrowing	Broadening of light reflex with no or minimal AV* compression
Grade II	Marked generalized narrowing and focal attenuation of arterioles	Broadening of light reflex with moderate AV compression
Grade III	Generalized and focal narrowing of arterioles with retinal hemorrhages and hard exudates	Copper wire appearance of arterioles with marked AV compression
Grade IV	All the above features along with disk edema	Silver wire appearance of arterioles with marked and severe AV compression

*AV, arteriovenous

of the retinal arterioles associated with raised hypertension followed by retinal ischemia leading to vascular leakage is the proposed mechanisms for development of pregnancy-induced hypertension retinopathy.

Clinical Features

The retinal features are similar to those seen in hypertensive retinopathy and include:

- Spasm of retinal arterioles
- Retinal hemorrhages
- Cotton-wool spots
- Hard exudates
- Serous detachment of retina
- Macular edema.

About 50% of patients with pregnancy-induced hypertension will present with ocular symptoms in the form of blurring of vision, amaurosis, scotoma, etc.

The causes for sudden loss of vision in pregnancy are exudative retinal detachment with an incidence of up to 10% in eclampsia associated with pregnancy-induced hypertension.

Cortical blindness with an incidence of up to 15% in eclampsia associated with pregnancy-induced hypertension.

Treatment

The visual prognosis is good for retinopathy associated with pregnancy-induced hypertension as the changes reverse in the postpartum period following delivery. Hence the main treatment is directed toward control of hypertension.

However, onset of ischemic retinopathy characterized by cotton-wool spots, disk edema is associated with increased mortality; hence termination of pregnancy should be considered.

RETINOPATHY IN HEMATOLOGICAL DISEASES

Retinopathy is commonly seen in hematological diseases such as anemia, leukemia, lymphoma and hemoglobinopathies.

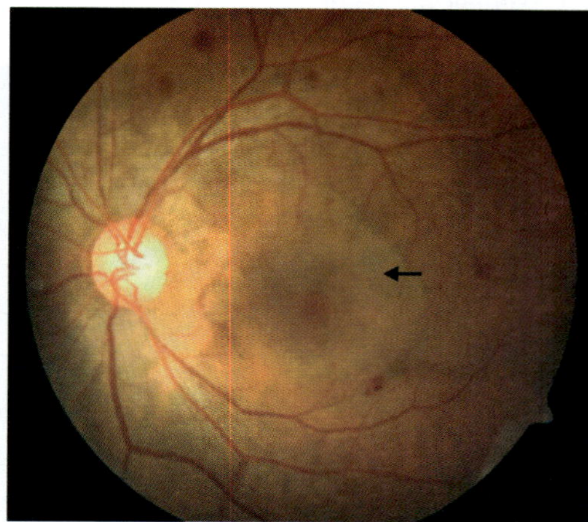

FIG. 11.5.16: Pregnancy-induced hypertension retinopathy with retinal hemorrhages and exudative detachment of retina involving the macula.

Anemic Retinopathy

Anemic retinopathy is seen in severe anemia and is caused by retinal hypoxia. The fundus picture shows venous tortuosity, cotton-wool spots, flame-shaped retinal hemorrhages, retinal edema and white-centered hemorrhages called Roth's spots (Figs 11.5.17A and B).

Optic neuropathy and optic atrophy are the other features seen.

Leukemic Retinopathy

Leukemic retinopathy is characterized by retinal hemorrhages, white-centered retinal hemorrhages, cotton-wool spots, venous tortuosity, optic nerve infiltration, sea-fan neovascularization affecting the peripheral retina, etc.

Choroidal deposits appearing as leopard skin is seen in chronic leukemias.

Sickle Cell Retinopathy

Sickle cell retinopathy includes proliferative retinopathies seen because of retinal hypoxia in sickling hemoglobinopathies. The fundus picture shows peripheral arterial occlusions and neovascularization of sea-fan configuration. Vitreous hemorrhage and retinal detachment are the common complications seen in advanced stages.

COATS' DISEASE**

Definition

Coats' disease is an abnormal telangiectatic condition characterized by intraretinal and subretinal exudation.

Etiopathogenesis

Coats' disease was first described by George Coats and it is named after him. It is usually seen as a unilateral condition predominantly in childhood affecting boys more than girls. The etiology is not known and it is supposed to be idiopathic in nature. It is characterized by abnormal vascular development resulting in intraretinal and subretinal exudation, which may lead to exudative retinal detachment.

Clinical Features

Coats' disease presents as leukocoria because of retinal detachment or squint in children. Fundus examination shows aneurysmal dilatations of the retinal vessels with extensive intraretinal and subretinal exudates. The disease runs through five stages:

- Stage I is characterized by abnormal blood vessels
- Stage II is characterized by abnormal blood vessels with exudation

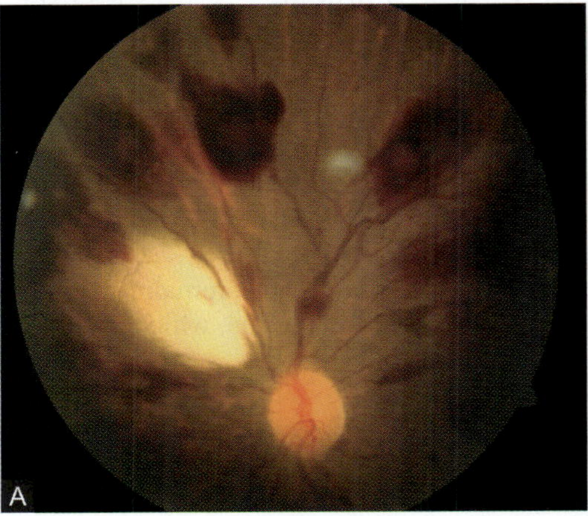

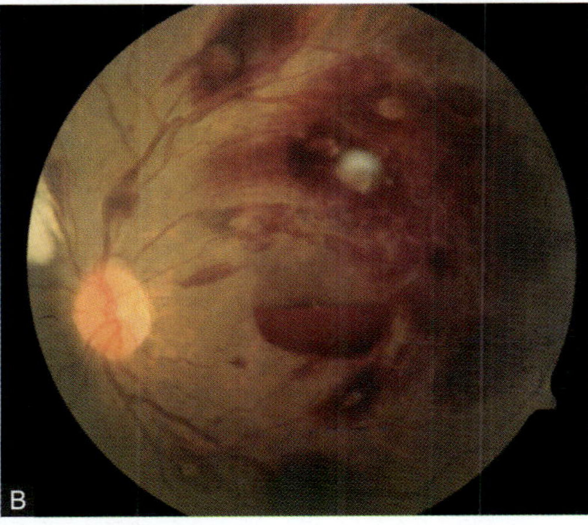

FIGS 11.5.17A and B: Anemic retinopathy

- Stage III is characterized by exudative retinal detachment
- Stage IV is characterized by total retinal detachment and glaucoma
- Stage V is characterized by painful blind eye.

The adult onset type of Coats' disease is less severe and it presents in limited form, and the cause for visual loss is because of cystoid macular edema.

Differential Diagnosis

Coats' disease has to be differentiated from other causes of leukocoria such as retinoblastoma, congenital cataract, toxocara endophthalmitis, etc.

The adult type has to be differentiated from diabetic retinopathy, branch retinal vein occlusion and other causes associated with exudation.

Investigations

Fundus fluorescein angiography aids in diagnosing the vascular abnormalities and severity of the diseases in the initial stages of the disease.

Treatment

- Laser photocoagulation/Cryotherapy of the abnormal telangiectatic vessels is indicated in the initial stages of the disease in stage I and II
- Retinal detachment surgery is indicated in stage III
- Treatment for glaucoma and retinal detachment surgery is indicated in stage IV
- Enucleation is indicated in stage V with painful blind eye.

RETINOPATHY OF PREMATURITY***

Definition

Retinopathy of prematurity (ROP) is defined as a proliferative retinopathy seen in prematurely born babies with low birth weight. It was called retrolental fibroplasia.

Etiopathogenesis

Retinopathy of prematurity is because of the fact that the retinal vessels are immature in premature babies. The blood supply of the inner retina starts at 16th week of gestational age. The blood supply starts as spindle cells arising from the hyaloid artery. These spindle cells start from the optic disk and migrate to reach the ora serrata, the periphery of the retina. They reach the nasal ora serrata by 36th week of gestation and temporal retina by 40th week of gestation at birth. This disparity is because of the fact that the temporal ora serrata is at a greater distance from the optic disk.

The pathogenesis is explained by the spindle cell theory. It says that exposure of immature spindle cells to the relatively hyperoxic outside environment from hypoxic intrauterine environment leads to spindle cell damage. This is because of the incapability of immature spindle cells to scavenge the oxygen free-radicals resulting in the pathological changes and proliferative retinopathy.

Risk Factors

- Low gestational age and low birth weight
- Supplemental oxygen administration.

Clinical Features

The clinical features and progression depend on the location of ROP. The retina is divided into three zones (Fig. 11.5.18):

1. Zone I includes circular area with optic disk as center and twice the disk fovea distance as the radius.
2. Zone II includes circular area outside the zone I with optic disk to nasal ora serrata as the radius.
3. Zone III includes the remaining crescent area of temporal retina, which lies outside the zone II.

Clinical Features Based on ROP Stages

International classification of ROP has classified ROP into five stages:*

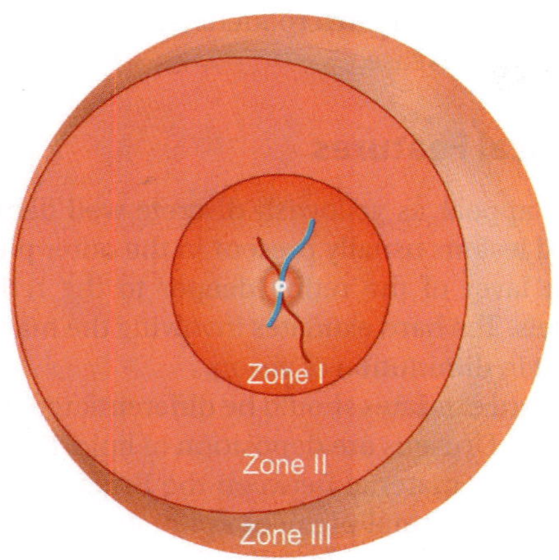

FIG. 11.5.18: Zones of retinopathy of prematurity

1. Stage I is characterized by the presence of demarcation line separating the avascular anterior retina from the vascularized posterior retina.
2. Stage II is characterized by progression of the demarcation line to form ridge with height, width and volume.
3. Stage III is characterized by presence of fibrovascular proliferation extending into the vitreous.
4. Stage IV is characterized by progressive fibrovascular proliferation leading to subtotal retinal detachment. It is further subdivided into stage IVA with subtotal retinal detachment not involving macula and stage IVB with subtotal retinal detachment involving the macula.
5. Stage V is characterized by the total retinal detachment.

Plus Disease

Plus disease refers to the presence of dilated and tortuous vessels in at least two quadrants of the posterior pole. It is associated with other ocular features such as poor dilatation of the pupil because of vascular engorgement of the iris and vitreous haze. Plus disease signifies that the disease is progressing.

Threshold Disease

Threshold disease refers to the presence of stage III and ROP in zone I or II involving five contiguous clock hours or eight non-contiguous clock hours of retina. The presence of threshold disease indicates compulsory treatment failing, where more than 50% of cases progress to retinal detachment.

Prethreshold Retinopathy of Prematurity

Prethreshold retinopathy is of two types, type 1 and type 2. Treatment is indicated in prethreshold type 1 and in prethreshold type 2 follow-up is required.

Prethreshold type 1 includes:

- Stage I and II ROP in zone I with plus disease
- Stage III ROP in zone I without plus disease
- Stage III ROP in zone II with plus disease.

Prethreshold type 2 includes:

- Stage I or II ROP in zone I without plus disease
- Stage III ROP in zone II without plus disease.

Natural History

About 80% of patients with ROP show spontaneous resolution, whereas 20% show cicatricial complications. The cicatricial complications include retinal pigmentary disturbances, straightening of the vessels with dragging of macula and optic disk, falciform retinal fold, partial retinal detachment and total retinal detachment.

Differential Diagnosis

Retinopathy of prematurity with retinal detachment has to be differentiated from other causes of leukocoria such as retinoblastoma, congenital cataract, toxocara endophthalmitis, etc.

Treatment

1. The principle of treatment is to remove the ischemic stimulus by ablating the hypoxic retina. Treatment is indicated in threshold ROP and prethreshold ROP type 1.

2. The treatment modalities used are laser photocoagulation and cryotherapy.
3. Surgical management in the form of vitrectomy is indicated in cases presenting with stage IV and V.
4. Antivascular endothelial growth factors such as bevacizumab is the recent advance in the treatment of ROP. They act by preventing angiogenesis.

*Screening**

The incidence of ROP is increased with availability of better neonatal care as more and more premature infants are surviving. However, the disease can be prevented by screening these premature infants who are at high risk of developing this disease. The screening is indicated in:

1. Premature infants who are born at or before 31 weeks, or with birth weight of less than 1,500 g.
2. The screening is performed after 4 weeks from birth or at a postconceptional age of 32 weeks, whichever is earlier. The next screening is performed at 35–37 weeks and the last screening at 39–42 weeks.

HARD EXUDATES*

Definition

Hard exudates are collection of lipids in the middle layers of the retina (Fig. 11.5.19).

Etiopathogenesis

Hard exudates are because of aggregation of lipids as a result of chronic leakage of plasma from the damaged vessels and they are almost always because of microvascular retinal disease. The common causes for hard exudates are:

- Diabetic retinopathy
- Hypertensive retinopathy
- Radiation retinopathy
- Retinal venous obstructions
- Retinal artery macroaneurysm
- Coats' disease.

Clinical Features

They appear as yellowish discrete well demarcated lesions usually present in the outer plexiform layer of the retina deeper to the retinal vessels. The hard exudates involving the macula result in diminution of vision.

Hard exudates should be differentiated from drusen. Drusens are deposition of lipid-rich extracellular material between the Bruch's membrane and retinal pigment epithelium, and are seen in elderly people and in age-related macular degeneration.

Clinical Course

The hard exudates disappear when the leakage from the vessel stops as they are phagocytosed by the macrophages.

Treatment

The treatment is by underlying causative microvascular disease. Hard exudates involving macula threatening vision is treated by laser photocoagulation of the leaking vessel.

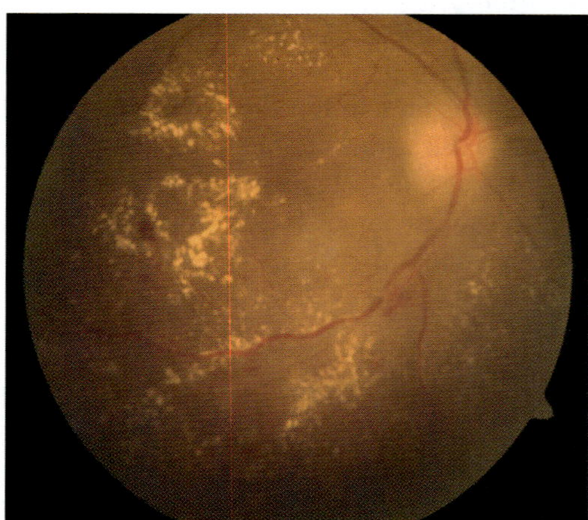

FIG. 11.5.19: Hard exudates

SOFT EXUDATES OR COTTON-WOOL SPOTS*

Definition

Soft exudates or cotton-wool spots are infarcts of nerve fiber layer of retina (Fig. 11.5.20).

Etiopathogenesis

Soft exudates are caused by swelling of the nerve fibers as a result of obstruction axoplasmic flow because of infarction of the nerve fiber layer of the retina. The common causes for cotton-wool spots are:

- Diabetic retinopathy
- Hypertensive retinopathy
- Collagen vascular diseases
- Carotid artery occlusive diseases
- Human immunodeficiency virus (HIV) retinopathy
- Anemia
- Papilledema
- Retinopathies associated with hematological diseases such as anemia and leukemia.

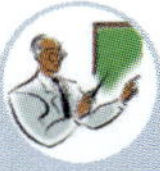

Roth Spot

- Roth spots (Fig. 11.5.21) are defined as white-centered retinal hemorrhages.
- They represent cotton-wool spots surrounded by retinal hemorrhages.
- Roth spots are seen in the following conditions:
  - Bacterial endocarditis
  - Anemic retinopathy
  - Leukemic retinopathy
  - Diabetic retinopathy
  - HIV retinopathy.

Clinical Features

The cotton-wool spots appear as superficial yellowish or white patches with ill-defined margins.

Treatment

Cotton-wool spots are treated by treatment of the underlying causative disease.

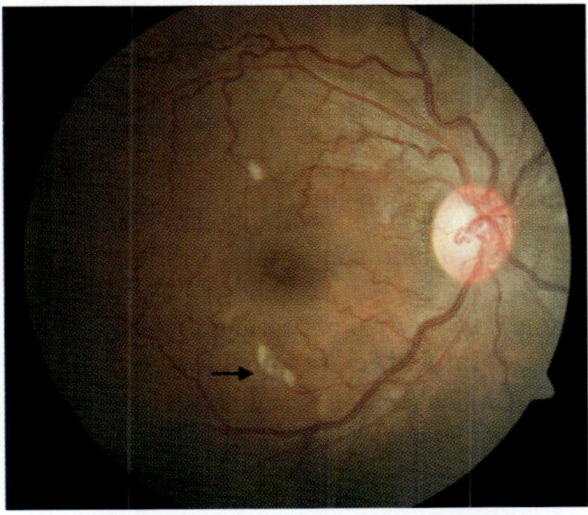

FIG. 11.5.20: Cotton-wool spots

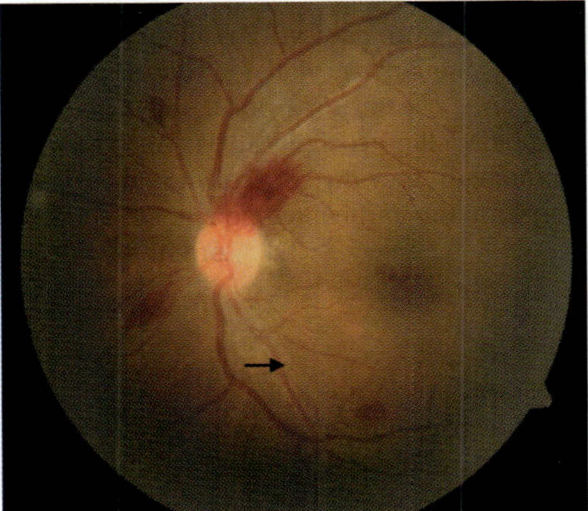

FIG. 11.5.21: Roth spots

GIST BOX 11.5

- Occlusion of the central retinal artery resulting in hypoxic damage of the retina is called central retinal artery occlusion.
- Central retinal artery occlusion is an ocular emergency and requires immediate treatment, if not, almost always leads to gross diminution of vision.
- Occlusion of a branch of central retinal artery resulting in hypoxic damage corresponding part of retina, which is supplied by that particular branch is called branch retinal artery occlusion.
- Occlusion of the ophthalmic artery resulting in obstruction of both retinal and choroidal circulations, resulting in complete loss of vision is called ophthalmic artery occlusion.
- Ocular ischemic syndrome is a clinical condition characterized by chronic ocular hypoperfusion occurring secondary to ipsilateral obstruction of the carotid artery, resulting in ocular ischemia.
- Occlusion/Obstruction of the central retinal vein at the lamina cribrosa resulting in occlusion retinopathy is called central retinal vein occlusion.
- Occlusion of one of the trunks of central retinal vein in people in whom the two-trunked central retinal vein persists as congenital anomaly is called hemiretinal vein occlusion.
- Occlusion of a branch of central retinal vein resulting in involvement of the corresponding part of retina, which is supplied by that particular branch is called branch retinal vein occlusion.
- Retinopathy seen in patients with diabetes mellitus is called diabetic retinopathy. It is a microangiopathy predominantly affecting the smaller blood vessels such as arterioles, venules and capillaries.
- Retinopathy occurring as a result of changes in the retinal vasculature because of systemic hypertension is called hypertensive retinopathy.
- Retinopathy occurring secondary to pregnancy-induced hypertension is called pregnancy-induced hypertension retinopathy.
- Coats' disease is an abnormal telangiectatic condition characterized by intraretinal and subretinal exudation.
- Retinopathy of prematurity is defined as a proliferative retinopathy seen in prematurely born babies with low birth weight.

CHAPTER

11.6 Retinal Dystrophies and Degenerations

RETINITIS PIGMENTOSA**

Definition

Retinitis pigmentosa is a genetically determined dystrophy of the retina affecting photoreceptors characterized by progressive degeneration of the photoreceptors with predominant involvement of the rods (Figs 11.6.1A to I).

> Retinitis pigmentosa is the most common hereditary retinal dystrophy with a prevalence of 1:3,500–1:5,000.

Epidemiology

Retinitis pigmentosa is worldwide in its distribution and it is one of the common retinal causes of blindness in India. Males are affected more than females probably because of presence of X-linked inheritance with females acting as carriers. The inheritance pattern can be sporadic, autosomal dominant, autosomal recessive or X-linked recessive. Autosomal recessive is the most common mode of inheritance. X-linked recessive is the least common type of inheritance pattern, but leads to most severe form of disease.

Pathogenesis

The retinitis pigmentosa affects rods more than cones resulting in rod-cone dystrophy. It characteristically leads to degeneration of rod photoreceptors resulting in progressive loss of peripheral visual field and night blindness. It typically affects both the eyes symmetrically.

Clinical Features

Symptoms

1. Night blindness, delayed dark adaptation and diminution of vision in dim illumination are the most common symptoms. The symptoms usually begin in second to third decade of life.
2. Progressive loss of visual field, the visual field loss usually starts in the midperiphery, and progresses both toward center and periphery, finally resulting in tunnel vision.
3. Decreased central vision is seen because of involvement of macula in the form of cystoid macular edema.

*Signs**

The characteristic signs are:

1. Retinal pigment epithelial changes in the form of bone corpuscle pigmentation, characteristically perivascular in nature, and beginning in the midperiphery and extend gradually anteriorly and posteriorly.
2. Narrowing or attenuation of retinal arterioles.
3. Pale waxy pallor of the optic disk with consecutive optic atrophy in advanced stages.

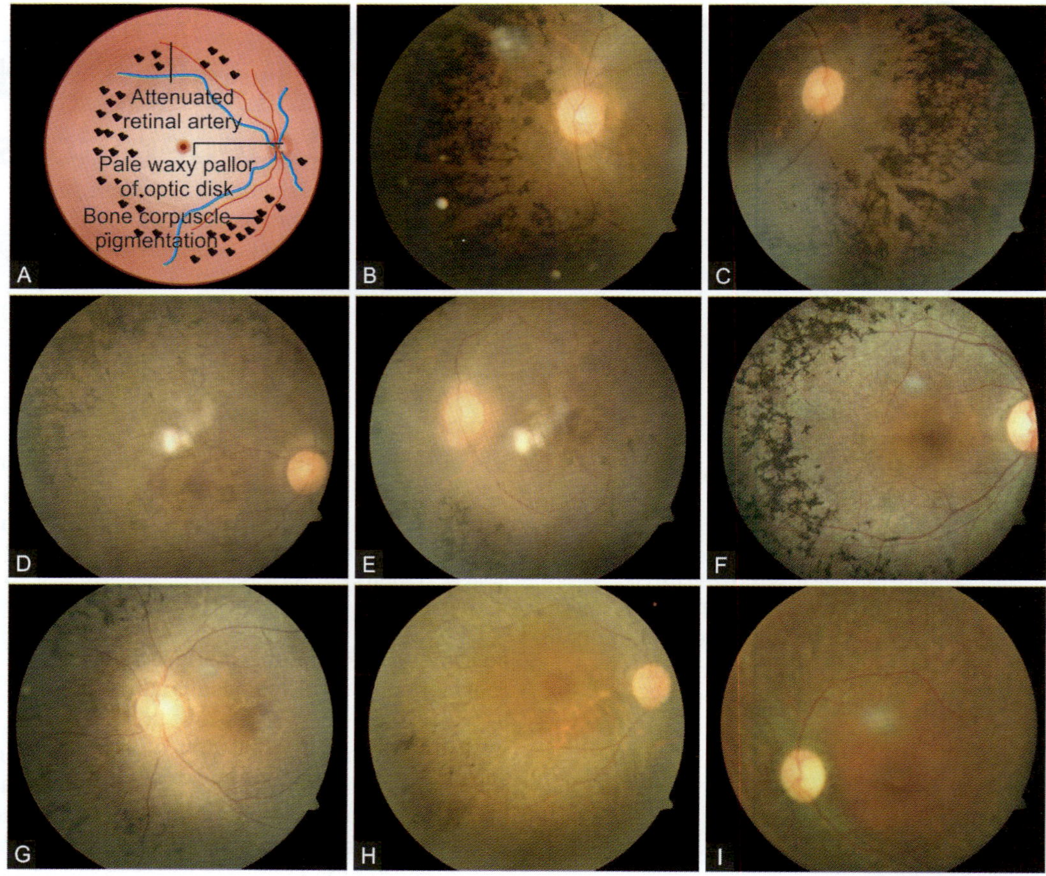

FIGS 11.6.1A to I: Retinitis pigmentosa

4. Associated changes in the macula such as cystoid macular edema, epiretinal membrane, macular hole, macular atrophy, etc.

Ocular Associations

Posterior subcapsular cataract, myopia, primary open-angle glaucoma, optic disk drusen and keratoconus are the usual ocular associations.

Systemic Associations*

1. *Usher's syndrome:* It is an autosomal recessive condition characterized by retinitis pigmentosa and deafness.
2. *Laurence-Moon-Bardet-Biedl syndrome:* It is a syndrome characterized by retinitis pigmentosa, mental retardation, obesity, hypogonadism and polydactyly.
3. *Kearns-Sayre syndrome:* It is characterized by chronic progressive external ophthalmoplegia, heart block and retinitis pigmentosa.
4. *Bassen-Kornzweig syndrome:* It is characterized by fat malabsorption, abetalipoproteinemia, ataxia and pigmentary retinopathy resembling retinitis pigmentosa.
5. *Refsum's syndrome:* It is characterized by cerebellar ataxia, polyneuropathy, deafness and pigmentary retinopathy resembling retinitis pigmentosa.

Atypical Forms of Retinitis Pigmentosa

1. *Sectorial retinitis pigmentosa:* It is characterized by involvement of one quadrant, most commonly one of the inferior quadrants. It usually shows slow progression, hence associated with good vision.
2. *Retinitis pigmentosa sine pigmento:* It is characterized by absence of pigment accumulation and presence of remaining features of retinitis pigmentosa.
3. *Retinitis punctata albescens:* It is characterized by the presence of yellowish white spots instead of bone corpuscle pigments and presence of rest all features of retinitis pigmentosa.
4. *Retinitis pigmentosa inversa:* It is also called central retinitis pigmentosa, as it involves the central part of the retina and macula earlier resulting in early loss of central vision.

Investigations

Investigations and examination are required for confirmation of diagnosis, to look for ocular and systemic associations, to document progression of the disease, and to decide on treatment and visual prognosis:

1. *Visual fields:* These show annular or ring-shaped scotoma, peripheral field constriction and tunnel vision in the advanced stages.
2. *Electroretinography:* It measures the functional status of the photoreceptors and in retinitis pigmentosa, it is subnormal or not detectable.

Treatment

There is no cure for retinitis pigmentosa as of now, and hence treatment depends on the steps to correct associated factors causing loss of vision and to stop the progression of the disease:

1. Measures to improve the vision by correcting associated eye conditions such as myopia, treatment of cataract, glaucoma, macular edema, epiretinal membrane, etc.
2. Measures to stop progression of the disease by supplementation of vitamin A, vitamin E, lutein and zeaxanthin, and treatment by vasodilators, electroacupuncture therapy, etc.
3. Measures to improve vision by use of low visual aids.
4. Gene therapy, retinal chip implant and retinal transplantation are still under research stage, and when available, can be a boon to patients with retinitis pigmentosa.
5. A retinal prosthesis by name Argus retinal prosthesis is available in some countries such as UK, USA, etc. has shown promising results in treatment of retinitis pigmentosa.

CONGENITAL STATIONARY NIGHT BLINDNESS

Congenital stationary night blindness (CSNB) includes a group of diseases characterized by presence of stationary night blindness from birth. It is of three types:

1. Congenital stationary night blindness with normal fundus.
2. Congenital stationary night blindness with abnormal fundus:
   a. Oguchi disease: It is characterized by golden-yellow color of the fundus in light-adapted state.
   b. Fundus albipunctatus: It is characterized by presence of white spots in the fundus.

HEREDITARY DYSTROPHIES OF FUNDUS AND MACULA

The hereditary dystrophies of fundus and macula are detailed in Table 11.6.1.

PERIPHERAL RETINAL DEGENERATIONS**

The degenerative conditions involving the periphery of the retina are commonly seen in clinical practice, though majority of them are clinically insignificant, they are important because a few are associated with increased risk of retinal detachment. The common peripheral degenerations are detailed as follows.

TABLE 11.6.1: Hereditary dystrophies of fundus and macula

Dystrophy	*Inheritance*	*Clinical features*	*Visual prognosis*
Stargardt disease (Figs 11.6.2A and B)* Fundus flavimaculatus (Fig. 11.6.3)	Autosomal recessive	• In first to second decade with gradual impairment of central vision • Initially macula shows non-specific mottling, beaten bronze appearance in later stages and geographical atrophy in advanced stages • It is a variant of Stargardt disease characterized by presence of white flecks in the posterior pole of the retina	Poor
Best macular dystrophy (Figs 11.6.4A and B)	Autosomal dominant	• Onset in early childhood • Macula shows yellow yolk-like lesion	Good
Familial dominant drusen	Autosomal dominant	• Onset in third to fourth decade • Macula shows presence of drusen	Good in cases of extrafoveal drusen and poor visual prognosis is seen in cases associated with secondary choroidal neovascularization
North Carolina macular dystrophy	Autosomal dominant	• Onset in first decade • Macula shows confluent macular deposits progressing to atrophic macular lesions in advanced stages	Poor
Sorsby pseudoinflammatory dystrophy	Autosomal dominant	• Onset in third to fifth decade • Fundus shows drusen-like deposits with hemorrhages in the periphery • Vision loss occurs because of exudative maculopathy	Poor
Dominant cystoid macular edema	Autosomal dominant	• Onset is in first to second decade • Macula shows cystoid macular edema	Poor
Butterfly-shaped macular dystrophy	Autosomal dominant	• Onset is in second to third decade • Macula shows yellowish pigment arranged in triradiate manner resembling butterfly	Good
Central areolar choroidal dystrophy	Autosomal dominant	• Onset in third to fourth decade • Macula shows granular deposits in the initial stages and geographical atrophy with prominent choroidal vessels in the advanced stages	Poor
Pigmented paravenous chorioretinal atrophy	Autosomal dominant	• Onset in third to fourth decade • Fundus shows paravenous pigmentation and chorioretinal atrophy along the retinal veins	Good
Familial benign fleck retina	Autosomal recessive	• Fundus shows presence of yellowish white flecks sparing the fovea	Good
Bietti corneoretinal crystalline dystrophy	Autosomal recessive	• Onset in third to fourth decade • Deposition of yellowish white crystals in periphery of cornea and retina	Poor
Progressive cone dystrophy	Autosomal dominant/ 'X' linked	• Onset in second to third decade with loss of central vision and color vision • Macula shows pigmentary changes initially and geographic atrophy in advanced stages • Few cases show typical Bull's eye maculopathy	Poor

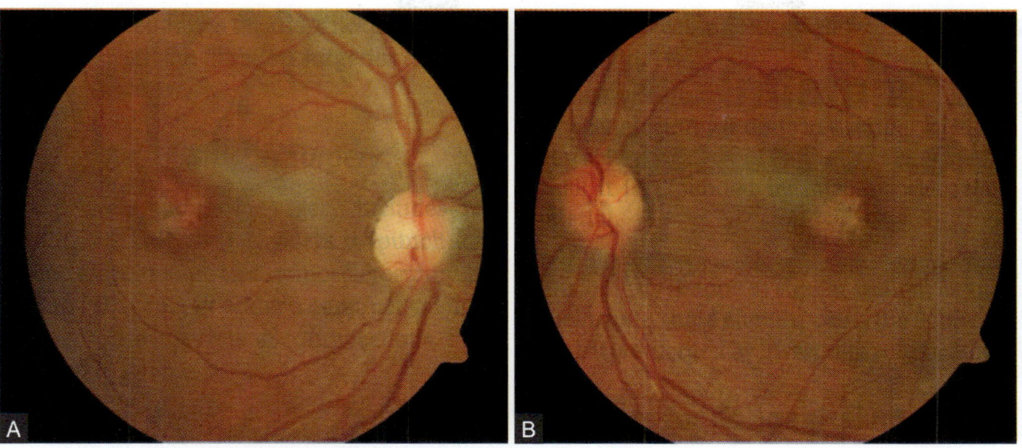

FIGS 11.6.2A and B: Stargardt dystrophy

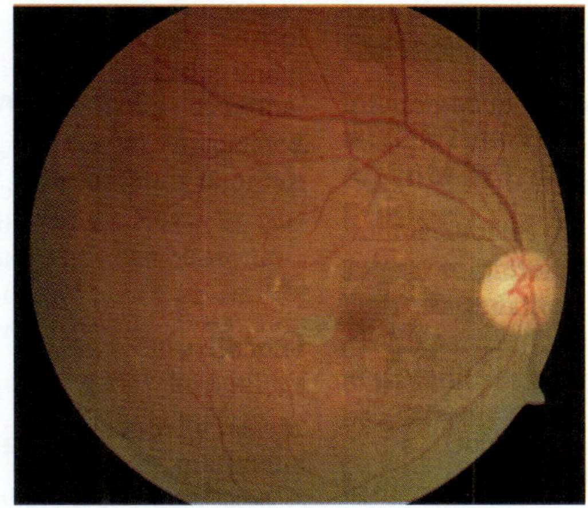

FIG. 11.6.3: Fundus flavimaculatus

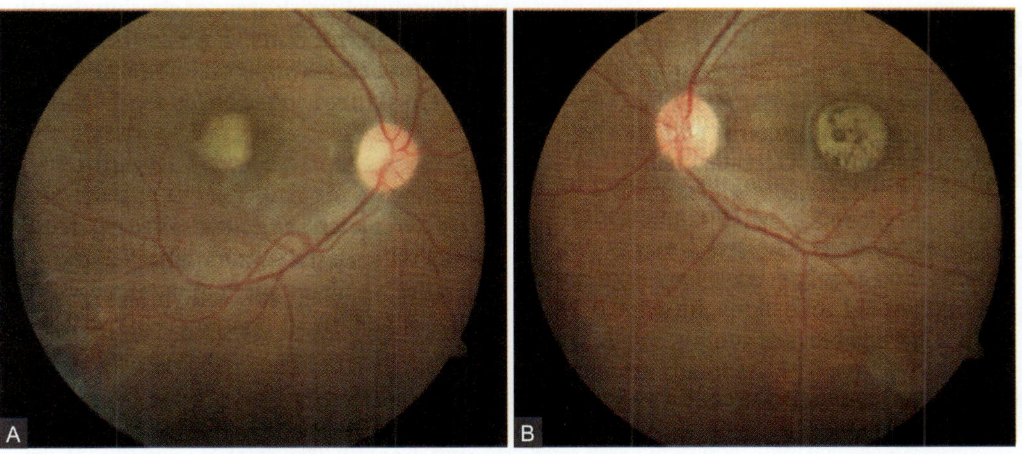

FIGS 11.6.4A and B: Best macular dystrophy

Lattice Degeneration*

Lattice degeneration is a common degenerative condition of the peripheral retina characterized by patches of thinning of retina.

> Lattice degeneration is the most common degeneration associated with rhegmatogenous retinal detachment with 40% of eyes with rhegmatogenous retinal detachment showing lattice degeneration.

Lattice degeneration is seen in about 10% of general population and in about 15% of people with myopia. Typical lattice degeneration presents as a spindle shaped, circumferentially oriented area of retinal thinning with a network of arborizing white lines within the thinned area. Sometimes, a lattice presents as radially oriented area of retinal thinning and is called atypical lattice, and it is seen in syndromes such as Stickler's syndrome.

Lattice degeneration can become complicated by development of atrophic retinal hole or retinal tear, which may give rise to rhegmatogenous retinal detachment. Treatment by prophylactic laser photocoagulation is indicated in lattice degeneration associated with retinal tear or retinal hole and in individuals with retinal detachment in other eye.

Snail Track Degeneration

Snail track degeneration is a peripheral retinal degeneration characterized by presence of sharply demarcated areas of snowflake appearance. They are usually associated with atrophic retinal holes.

White with Pressure and White without Pressure

White with pressure is a peripheral degeneration of the retina characterized by whitish appearance of the peripheral retina on examination by scleral depression.

White without pressure is a peripheral degeneration of the retina characterized by whitish appearance of the peripheral retina without any depression. It is usually seen in myopics. It can predispose to formation of retinal tear and retinal detachment.

Degenerative Retinoschisis

Degenerative retinoschisis is a peripheral retinal degeneration characterized by splitting of neurosensory retina either at the outer plexiform layer or at the inner nerve fiber layer. It is more common in hypermetropes. It may be occasionally associated with retinal breaks and retinal detachment.

Paving-stone Degeneration

Paving-stone degeneration is a peripheral retinal degeneration characterized by the presence of discrete yellowish areas of chorioretinal thinning and atrophy. It does not appear to predispose to retinal detachment, hence no treatment is required.

GIST BOX 11.6

- Retinitis pigmentosa is a genetically determined dystrophy of the retina affecting photoreceptors characterized by progressive degeneration of the photoreceptors with predominant involvement of the rods. Retinitis pigmentosa affects rods more than cones resulting in rod-cone dystrophy. It characteristically leads to degeneration of rod photoreceptors, resulting in progressive loss of peripheral visual field and night blindness.
- The degenerative conditions involving the periphery of the retina are commonly seen in clinical practice, though majority of them are clinically insignificant, they are important because few are associated with increased risk of retinal detachment.
- The common peripheral degenerations are lattice degeneration, snail track degeneration, white with pressure, white without pressure, paving-stone degeneration, etc.
- Lattice degeneration is the most common degeneration associated with rhegmatogenous retinal detachment with 40% of eyes with rhegmatogenous retinal detachment showing lattice degeneration.

CHAPTER

11.7 Acquired Diseases of Macula

AGE-RELATED MACULAR DEGENERATION***

Definition

Age-related macular degeneration (ARMD) is a degenerative condition usually affecting people older than 50 years, characterized by retinal pigment epithelium changes and drusen deposition in the macula.

Etiopathogenesis

Age-related macular degeneration is the leading cause of blindness in people aged over 50 years particularly in developed countries.

The condition is bilateral, but often asymmetrical and seen in elderly people with the incidence increasing with increasing age.

The risk factors associated with ARMD are:*

- Age
- Family history
- Smoking
- Hypertension
- Atherosclerosis
- Obesity
- Hypercholesterolemia
- Increased exposure to sunlight
- Light iris color
- Genetic factors like defects in *ABCR* gene, which encodes for retinal rod protein.

The pathogenesis of ARMD is because of oxidative stress and damage of the retinal photoreceptors. The photoreceptors, because of high rate of metabolism, are highly susceptible to oxidative stress. The age-related changes, which occur in the retinal pigment epithelium such as decrease in the melanin (that protects macula by absorbing free radicals) and increase in the concentration of lipofuscin (a product of phagocytosis of outer segments of the photoreceptors) along with age-related changes in the Bruch's membrane (e.g. thickening and calcification) predispose to the development of ARMD.

Normally, the nutrients and oxygen to the macula are supplied by diffusion from choroid across the Bruch's membrane, and the toxic products of metabolism are transported into choroid across this membrane.

Classification

The ARMD is classified into two types depending on the pathogenesis:

1. Dry ARMD or non-exudative ARMD.
2. Wet ARMD or exudative ARMD.

Dry Age-related Macular Degeneration

Dry ARMD is because of accumulation of waste products of metabolism arising from incomplete degradation of rods and cones in the retinal pigment epithelial (RPE) cells. This is also due to impairment of transportation of toxic products of metabolism across the Bruch's membrane in the form of drusen.

Drusen are defined as deposition of lipid-rich extracellular material between the Bruch's membrane and retinal pigment epithelium. They are found in elderly people and in ARMD. There are two types of drusen, hard drusen and soft drusen.

Hard drusen are well defined and appear as yellow nodules measuring less than half width of retinal vein.

Soft drusen are ill defined and appear as yellow plaques, and measure twice or thrice the size of hard drusen.

Wet Age-related Macular Degeneration

Wet ARMD is because of increase in vascular endothelial growth factor as a result of separation of retinal pigment epithelium from choroid resulting in formation of new choroidal blood vessels invading the macula resulting in the formation of choroidal neovascular membrane (CNVM). This results in further separation of Bruch's membrane from retinal pigment epithelium resulting in retinal thickening, bleeding from new vessels and ultimately resulting in death of photoreceptors and fibrosis with loss of visual acuity.

Clinical Features

Dry Age-related Macular Degeneration

Dry ARMD is the common type of ARMD and it accounts for about 85–90% of cases. It presents with insidious onset of impairment of vision, with difficulty to read in dim light being the initial symptom. Distorted vision or metamorphopsia, central or paracentral scotomas with reduction of central vision are seen in later stages (Fig. 11.7.1).

On examination by ophthalmoscopy, macula shows the following:

- Deposition of drusen, discrete drusen in initial stages and confluent drusen in later stages
- Pigmentary changes of the retinal pigment epithelium with atrophy are seen in later stages
- Geographical atrophy is seen in advanced stages.

Wet Age-related Macular Degeneration

Wet ARMD is less common type accounting for less than 10–15% of cases, but causes more impairment of vision. It presents with metamorphopsia and sudden reduction of central vision (Fig. 11.7.2).

On examination by ophthalmoscopy, macula shows neovascularization of the macula usually because of ingrowth of choroidal vessels called choroidal neovascularization. Neovascularization of the macula is the characteristic feature of wet ARMD.

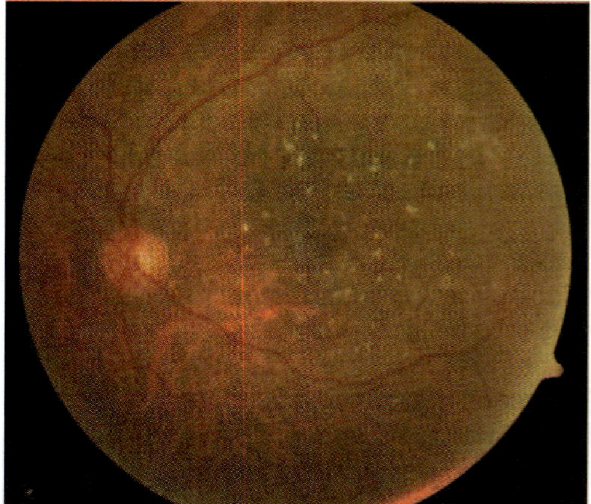

FIG. 11.7.1: Dry age-related macular degeneration

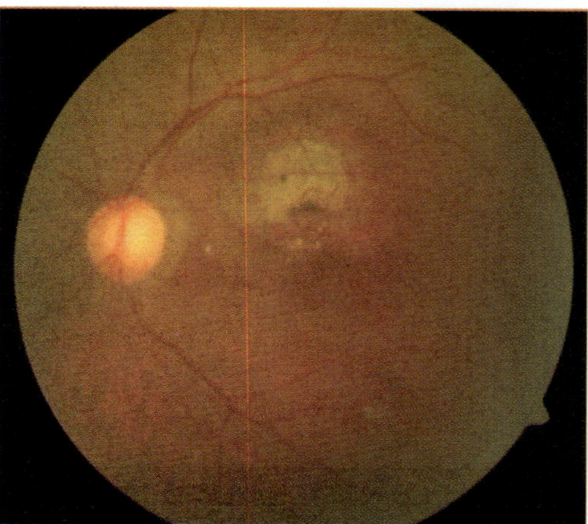

FIG. 11.7.2: Wet age-related macular degeneration with choroidal neovascular membrane

A wet ARMD shows features such as:

- Choroidal neovascular membrane appearing as grayish or yellowish membrane
- Retinal pigment epithelial detachment either serous, fibrovascular, drusenoid or hemorrhagic in nature
- Retinal pigment epithelial tear
- Retinal or subretinal lipid exudates or hemorrhages
- Subretinal fibrosis or scar formation is seen in advanced stages.

Age-related Eye Disease Study

Age-related eye disease study (AREDS) has categorized ARMD into four categories for the purpose of monitoring clinical progression and treatment:

1. *Category I:* No ARMD characterized by presence of few drusen in macula with each drusen measuring less than 63 microns.
2. *Category II:* Early ARMD characterized by presence of few drusen in macula with each drusen measuring 63–124 microns and retinal pigment epithelium abnormalities in the form of hyperpigmentation or hypopigmentation.
3. *Category III:* Intermediate ARMD characterized by extensive drusen in macula with at least one large drusen measuring more than 125 microns and non-foveal geographic atrophy.
4. *Category IV:* Advanced ARMD characterized by geographical atrophy involving fovea and CNVM.

Investigations

Fundus Fluorescein Angiography

Fundus fluorescein angiography (FFA) helps in confirming CNVM. It shows classical CNVM as a well-defined area, which in the early phase of FFA, fluoresces brightly and leaks the dye around CNVM in 1–2 minutes. It also classifies classical CNVM into:

1. Extrafoveal, where CNVM is situated more than 200 microns from the center of the fovea.
2. Juxtafoveal, where CNVM is situated in between 1 and 200 microns from the center of the fovea.
3. Subfoveal, where CNVM is situated exactly below the fovea.

Occult Choroidal Neovascular Membrane

Poorly defined membrane with ill-defined limits is called occult CNVM. It is further classified as fibrovascular pigment epithelial detachment and late leakage of undetermined source.

Indocyanine Green Angiography

Indocyanine green angiography (ICG) is more sensitive than FFA in determining the CNVM and it shows CNVM as a hyperfluorescent spot. It is indicated in cases of occult CNVM. It also differentiates CNVM from other pathologies of choroid such as idiopathic polypoidal choroidal vasculopathy, retinal angiomatous proliferation, etc.

Ocular Coherence Tomography

Ocular coherence tomography is helpful in assessing the response to treatment and in follow-up.

Treatment**

Dry Age-related Macular Degeneration

There is no effective treatment for dry ARMD, except for nutritional supplements to prevent complications and progression. AREDS has recommended vitamin C 500 mg, vitamin E 400 IU, beta carotene 15 mg, zinc oxide 80 mg and copper 2 mg/day. They are indicated in patients with category III disease and in those with advanced ARMD in one eye.

Wet Age-related Macular Degeneration

1. Laser photocoagulation is indicated in extrafoveal and juxtafoveal CNVM.
2. Verteporfin photodynamic treatment is indicated in subfoveal CNVM and in occult CNVM. Transpupillary thermotherapy and

radiation treatment are the alternative modes of treatment for subfoveal CNVM. Submacular surgery in the form of surgical removal of CNVM and macular translocation, as treatment modalities for subfoveal CNVM are still in experimental stages.

3. The recent mode of treatment in the form of antivascular endothelial growth factors such as pegaptanib, bevacizumab and ranibizumab administered as intravitreal injection. The advantage is that they can be used in all types of CNVM. This has become the widely used mode of treatment.
4. Low visual aids are indicated in patients with end-stage disease presenting as macular scarring (Fig. 11.7.3).

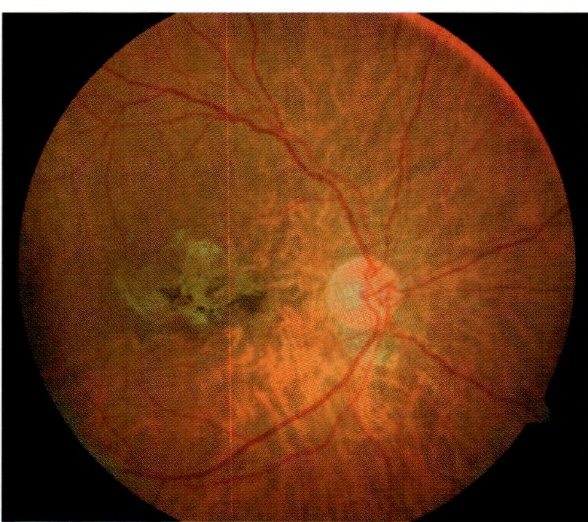

FIG. 11.7.3: End-stage age-related macular degeneration with macular scar

Age-related macular disease is seen because of ageing changes in the macula with potential risk factors as described earlier. The basic lesions are drusen, which are accumulation of lipid-rich extracellular matter between Bruch's membrane and retinal pigment epithelium. It presents in two forms, dry ARMD with only drusen and wet ARMD with formation of CNVM because of progression of the disease.

Since macula is affected, the central vision is affected in ARMD. In dry ARMD, the vision loss is slow and it takes years to progress. In wet ARMD, the vision loss is more dramatic and it progresses quickly.

The treatment for dry ARMD is mainly by observation and by nutritional supplements.

The treatment for wet ARMD is by treating the CNVM:

1. Laser photocoagulation is used to destroy the CNVM in cases, when it is away from fovea as in extrafoveal or juxtafoveal CNVM.
2. Verteporfin photodynamic treatment is used to selectively destroy the CNVM in cases of subfoveal CNVM.
3. The recent mode of treatment in the form of antivascular endothelial growth factors such as pegaptanib, bevacizumab and ranibizumab can be used in all types of CNVM. They act by binding with the vascular endothelial growth factor thereby retarding and reversing the CNVM.

MACULAR HOLE

Definition

Full thickness defect/loss of the neuroretinal tissue in the macula involving the fovea is called macular hole.

Etiopathogenesis

Idiopathic macular hole is the most common cause of macular hole. It is usually seen in elderly individuals in sixth or seventh decade of life.

The other causes for macular hole are:

- Blunt injury
- Diabetic retinopathy
- Hypertensive retinopathy
- Epiretinal membrane
- Cystoid macular edema
- Pathological myopia
- Vitreomacular traction syndrome
- Rhegmatogenous retinal detachment.

The pathogenesis of idiopathic macular hole is proposed to be abnormal vitreous traction on the fovea because of persistent vitreofoveal attachment following perifoveal vitreous separation. The pathogenesis for other macular holes depends on the underlying disease.

Gass Staging of Formation of Macular Hole

1. *Stage 1a:* Impending macular hole, characterized by loss of foveal depression.
2. *Stage 1b:* Occult macular hole, characterized by cyst-like space because of foveal detachment.
3. *Stage 2:* Small full thickness macular hole, characterized by macular hole measuring about 100–300 microns.
4. *Stage 3:* Full thickness macular hole, characterized by macular hole measuring more than 400 microns.
5. *Stage 4:* Full thickness macular hole with posterior vitreous detachment.

Clinical Features

Macular hole is usually a unilateral condition and presents with symptoms of distorted vision, metamorphopsia, central scotoma and loss of central vision. On examination by ophthalmoscopy, a full thickness defect involving the macula is seen.

Investigations

1. Simple test by focusing a horizontal or vertical beam of light onto the macula by using a Goldmann fundus contact lens and the patient is said to say about the status of the line. A patient with macular hole will say that the line is broken. This is called Watzke-Allen test.
2. Ocular coherence tomography is useful in demonstrating the stage and clinical diagnosis of macular hole.

Treatment

Conservative management in the form of observation and follow-up is indicated in stage 1 macular holes, as approximately half of them are known to undergo spontaneous resolution.

Surgical management in the form of vitrectomy and relieving of vitreomacular traction are indicated in macular holes of stage 2 or more.

CENTRAL SEROUS RETINOPATHY**

Definition

Central serous retinopathy (CSR) is an idiopathic disease characterized by serous detachment of the neurosensory retina in the macular region (Figs 11.7.4A and B). It is also called central serous chorioretinopathy.

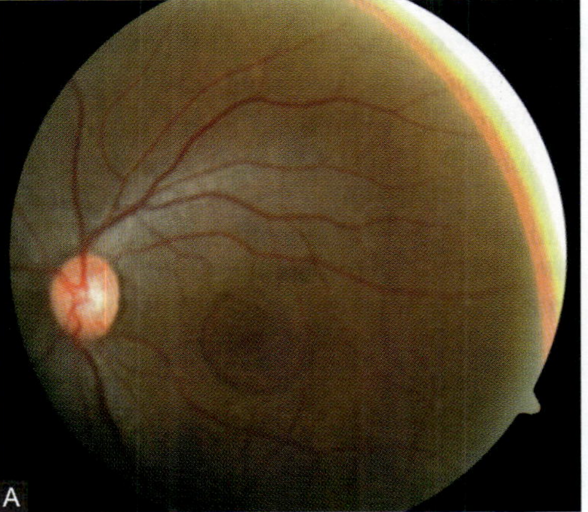

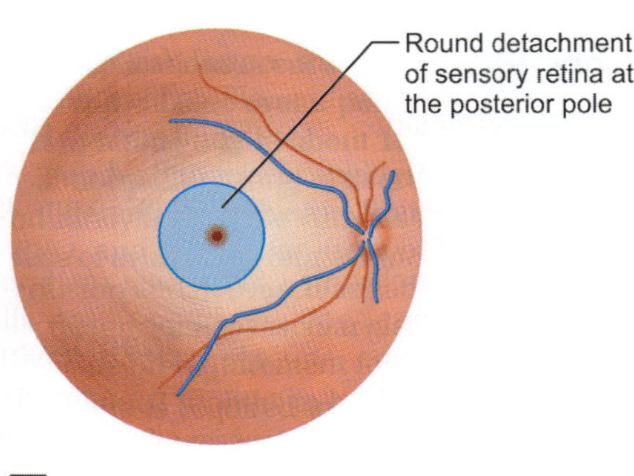

FIGS 11.7.4A and B: Central serous retinopathy. **A.** Photograph; **B.** Diagrammatic representation.

Etiopathogenesis

Central serous retinopathy is usually seen in middle-aged adults with males being more commonly affected than females.

Type A personality, emotional stress and systemic hypertension are frequently associated with risk factors. This may be explained from the fact that increased level of cortisol in these conditions affecting the autoregulation of choroidal circulation. The drugs associated with CSR are corticosteroids, sympathomimetics and sildenafil citrate.

The neurosensory detachment of the retina occurs because of exudation, which is because of hyperpermeability of retinal pigment epithelium in association with alteration in the choroidal circulation. The alteration in the choroidal circulation is caused by inflammation or choroidal ischemia.

Clinical Features

Symptoms

1. It usually presents with unilateral involvement in the form of distorted vision or metamorphopsia. Dyschromatopsia and altered contrast sensitivity are usually associated features.
2. Visual acuity is usually mildly impaired and it will be in the range of better than 6/18, refraction shows hypermetropia because of elevation of neurosensory retina.

Signs

1. On examination, in case of typical or classical CSR, a circumscribed solitary well-defined neurosensory detachment involving the macula is seen.
2. Atypical or chronic CSR is seen in about 5–10% of cases and present as diffuse ill-defined edema, and are associated with cystic intraretinal changes and poor visual prognosis compared to classical type of CSR. The chronic form is usually in elderly individuals and in patients receiving steroids.
3. Subretinal lipid deposits appearing as yellow spots or subretinal fibrin deposits appearing as grayish white membrane can be seen in typical and atypical CSR.

Clinical Course and Complications

1. Majority of typical CSR show spontaneous resolution and improvement of visual acuity by 3–6 months.
2. Majority of atypical CSR cases and few cases of typical CSR may show chronic course lasting for more than 1 year and may show RPE degeneration and permanent visual impairment.

Investigations

1. Fundus fluorescein angiography: It shows most commonly ink-blot type pattern with a hyperfluorescent dot, which expands slowly into large dot in the later stages. Few cases may show smoke stack pattern with a hyperfluorescent dot, which progresses to form a vertical column.
2. Indocyanine green angiography: It shows areas of hyperfluorescence because of leakage from the dilated choroidal vessels.
3. Ocular coherence tomography: It shows neurosensory elevation.

Differential Diagnosis

Central serous retinopathy has to be differentiated from secondary CSR as seen in:

- Age-related macular degeneration
- Posterior scleritis
- Optic disk pit
- Idiopathic uveal effusion syndrome
- Systemic diseases such as malignant hypertension, Vogt-Koyanagi-Harada syndrome and sarcoidosis
- Chorioretinitis seen in tuberculosis, syphilis and histoplasmosis.

Cases with secondary CSR show diffuse edema involving whole of the macula, and are associated with progressive visual loss with signs and symptoms of the underlying disease.

Treatment

There is no effective medical treatment available for treatment of CSR. Steroids are contraindicated and should not be used. Since majority of patients show spontaneous resolution, regular follow-up is indicated. Treatment is required in:

- Unresolving CSR by 3 months
- Recurrent CSR.

Treatment options are:

- Laser photocoagulation in patients with extrafoveal leak on FFA
- Photodynamic therapy (PDT) is done in patients with foveal leakage or diffuse leakage.

CYSTOID MACULAR EDEMA**

Definition

Accumulation of fluid in the outer plexiform layer and inner nuclear layer of the retina in macula resulting in the formation of cystic spaces in the macula is called cystoid macular edema (Figs 11.7.5A and B).

Etiopathogenesis

Cystoid macular edema is because of breakdown of blood retinal barrier in a variety of conditions including:

- Inflammatory conditions such as posterior uveitis, intermediate uveitis, retinal vasculitis, Eales' disease, etc.
- Vascular conditions such as diabetic retinopathy, vascular occlusions of retinal veins, etc.
- Following surgeries such as cataract surgery, keratoplasty, glaucoma surgery, etc.
- Inherited conditions such as retinitis pigmentosa, etc.
- Drugs such as epinephrine, topical prostaglandins, etc.

Breakdown of blood retinal barrier because of various causes leads to accumulation of fluid in the outer plexiform layer and inner nuclear layer of the retina in macula resulting in the formation of cystic spaces in the macula.

> The thinness of fovea centralis (provides little protection against inflammatory exudates that pass through vitreous) and the thickness of Henle's layer (because of its thickness, can absorb large quantities of fluid) are responsible for accumulation of inflammatory exudates at macular region.

Clinical Features

1. Diminution of central vision and distorted vision or metamorphopsia is the presenting symptoms.
2. Fundoscopic examination shows loss of foveal reflex and multiple cystoid areas in the macula. Cystoid macular edema is best examined by slit lamp biomicroscopic examination of retina by using fundus contact lenses because of stereoscopic vision.

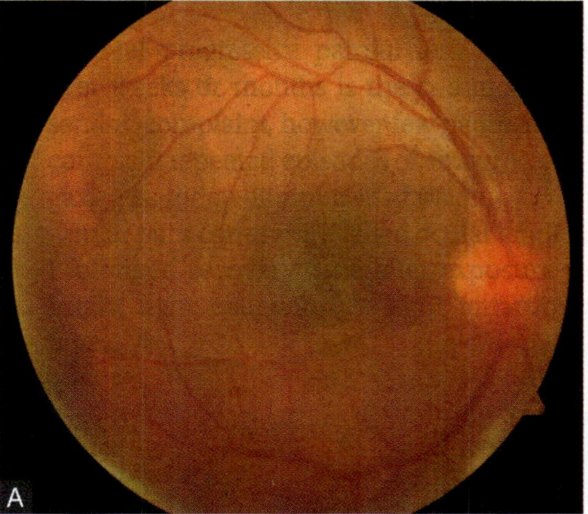

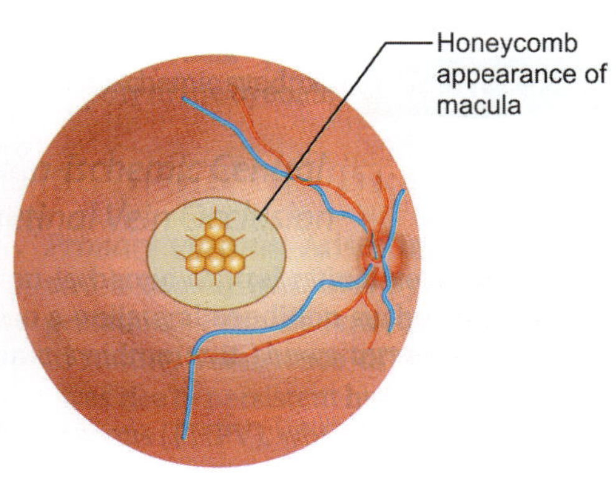

FIGS 11.7.5A and B: Cystoid macular edema. **A.** Photograph; **B.** Diagrammatic representation.

3. Long-standing cases may show complications such as lamellar macular hole.

Investigations

1. Fundus fluorescein angiography shows leakage of the dye and characteristic flower petaloid pattern as a result of accumulation of dye in the cystoid spaces.
2. Ocular coherence tomography shows cystoid spaces in the macula.

Treatment*

1. Topical antiprostaglandins such as ketorolac, indomethacin are used as initial treatment or as prophylactic treatment before cataract surgery to prevent development of cystoid macular edema.
2. Topical steroids, periocular steroids and systemic steroids are helpful in established cases.
3. Systemic carbonic anhydrase inhibitors such as acetazolamide are helpful in few cases.
4. Treatment of the underlying cause wherever possible should be done along with the above modes of treatment.

PHOTORETINITIS*

Definition

Photoretinitis is commonly called solar retinopathy. It includes a group of conditions characterized by damage to the macula as a result of exposure to solar radiation or other sources of ultraviolet light.

Etiopathogenesis

Photoretinitis is usually seen as:

1. Occupational injury in people engaged in occupations involving use of ultraviolet light such as welders.
2. Follows viewing solar eclipse or prolonged sun watching.

It is because of photochemical injury caused by the ultraviolet light.

Clinical Features

The symptoms occur within short period following exposure to solar radiation or exposure to a source of ultraviolet light. The common presenting symptoms are impairment of central vision with central scotoma, distorted vision or metamorphopsia, dyschromatopsia, etc.

On examination by ophthalmoscopy, a small yellow spot can be seen in the macula with associated macular edema. Later, the spot is replaced by a burnt hole with pigmentary abnormalities.

Treatment

There is no effective treatment for the condition. However, majority of the patients show spontaneous improvement in vision by 6 months to 1 year. The prophylaxis is by using protective glasses to prevent occupational exposure to ultraviolet light and for viewing solar eclipse.

GIST BOX 11.7

- The age-related macular degeneration (ARMD) is a degenerative condition usually affecting people older than 50 years, characterized by retinal pigment epithelium changes and drusen deposition in the macula. ARMD is the leading cause of blindness in people aged more than 50 years, particularly in developed countries.
- Dry ARMD is the common type of ARMD and it accounts for about 85–90% of cases.
- Wet ARMD is less common type accounting for less than 10–15% of cases, but causes more impairment of vision.
- Full-thickness defect/loss of the neuroretinal tissue in the macula involving the fovea is called macular hole.
- Central serous retinopathy is an idiopathic disease characterized by serous detachment of the neurosensory retina in the macular region.
- Accumulation of fluid in the outer plexiform layer and inner nuclear layer of the retina in macula resulting in the formation of cystic spaces in the macula is called cystoid macular edema.
- Photoretinitis or solar retinopathy includes a group of conditions characterized by damage to the macula as a result of exposure to solar radiation or other sources of ultraviolet light.

FREQUENTLY ASKED QUESTIONS (FAQs)

*Short Answers

1. Macula lutea.
2. Mention the layers of retina/microscopic anatomy of retina.
3. Posterior vitreous detachment.
4. Blood supply of retina.
5. Cherry-red spot at macula.
6. Fundus picture of central retinal artery occlusion.
7. Fundus picture of cilioretinal artery occlusion.
8. Fundus picture of ischemic retinal vein occlusion.
9. Mention the differences between ischemic CRVO and non-ischemic CRVO.
10. Mention the complications of CRVO.
11. Mention the arteriovenous crossing changes in hypertensive retinopathy.
12. Fundus picture of hypertensive retinopathy.
13. Screening of ROP.
14. Mention the stages of ROP.
15. Fundus picture of retinitis pigmentosa.
16. Mention the ocular and systemic associations of retinitis pigmentosa.
17. Stargardt disease.
18. Lattice degeneration.
19. Mention the risk factors for ARMD.
20. Treatment of CME.
21. Photoretinitis.
22. Hard exudates.
23. Retinal hemorrhages.
24. Soft exudates/Cotton-wool spots.

**Short Essays

1. Rhegmatogenous retinal detachment.
2. Exudative retinal detachment.
3. Tractional retinal detachment.
4. Eales' disease.
5. Central retinal artery occlusion.
6. Ocular ischemic syndrome.
7. Central retinal vein occlusion.
8. Branch retinal vein occlusion.
9. ETDRS classification of diabetic retinopathy.
10. Diabetic maculopathy.
11. Proliferative diabetic retinopathy.
12. Hypertensive retinopathy.
13. Classification/Grading of hypertensive retinopathy.
14. Coats' disease.
15. Retinitis pigmentosa.
16. Treatment of ARMD.
17. Central serous retinopathy.
18. Cystoid macular edema.

***Long Essays

1. Define and classify retinal detachment. Describe etiology, clinical features and management of rhegmatogenous retinal detachment.
2. Describe etiopathogenesis, classification and management of diabetic retinopathy.
3. Describe etiopathogenesis, classification and management of hypertensive retinopathy.
4. Describe etiopathogenesis, classification, clinical features and management of retinopathy of prematurity.
5. Describe etiopathogenesis, classification, clinical features and management of ARMD.

BIBLIOGRAPHY

1. Abu El-Asrar AM, Herbort CP, Tabbara KF. Differential diagnosis of retinal vasculitis. Middle East Afr J Ophthalmol. 2009;16(4):202-18.
2. Barbara Terelak-Borys, Katarzyna Skonieczna, Iwona Grabska-Liberek. Ocular ischemic syndrome—A systematic review. Med Sci Monit. 2012;18(8):RA138–RA144.
3. Biswas J, Ravi RK, Naryanasamy, et al. Eales' disease—current concepts in diagnosis and management. J Ophthalmic Inflamm Infect. 2013;3(1):11.
4. Clare Porte. Pathogenesis and management of age-related macular degeneration. Scottish Universities Medical Journal. 2012;1(2):141-53.
5. Cugati S, Varma DD, Chen CS, et al. Treatment options of central retinal artery occlusion. Curr Treat Options Neurol. 2013;15(1):63-77.
6. Das T. Guidelines for the management of rhegmatogenous retinal detachment. Indian J Ophthalmol. 1993;41(1):37-40.
7. Dutta LC. Modern Ophthalmology, vol 3, 3rd edition. New Delhi: Jaypee Brothers Medical Publishers (P) Ltd;2005.
8. Gass JD. Idiopathic senile macular hole. Its early stages and pathogenesis. Arch Ophthalmol. 1988;106(5):629-39.
9. Grosso A, Veglio F, Porta M, et al. Hypertensive retinopathy revisited: some answers, more questions. Br J Ophthalmol. 2005;89(12):1646-54.
10. Jack J Kanski. Clinical Ophthalmology: A Systematic Approach, 5th edition. China: Butterworth Heinemann; 2003.
11. Jefferies AL. Canadian Paediatric Society, Fetus and Newborn Committee. Retinopathy of prematurity: Recommendations for screening. Paediatr Child Health. 2010;15(10):667-74.
12. Myron Yanoff, Jay S Duker. Ophthalmology, 3rd edition. China: Mosby Elsevier; 2008.
13. Rameez Hussain, Giridhar A, Mahesh G. Pregnancy and Retinal Diseases. Kerala Journal of Ophthalmology. 2011.
14. Saxena S, Lincoff H. Finding the retinal break in rhegmatogenous retinal detachment. Indian J Ophthalmol. 2001;49(3):199-202.
15. Schmidt D. Comorbidities in combined retinal artery and vein occlusions. Eur J Med Res. 2013;18:27.
16. Suvarna JC, Hajela SA. Cherry-red spot. J Postgrad Med. 2008;54(1):54-7.

SECTION 12

Optic Nerve

CHAPTER

12.1 Anatomy of Optic Nerve

Optic nerve is the II cranial nerve. It is the continuation of the nerve fiber layer of the retina consisting of about 1.2 million axons derived from the retinal ganglion cells.

Though optic nerve is included in the list of cranial nerves, optic nerve is not a true nerve, but it is a continuation of brain and it is considered as sensory tract because:

- Embryologically optic nerve develops from diencephalon
- Optic nerve is covered by myelin sheath unlike peripheral nerves, which are covered by neurilemma
- Optic nerve is covered by dura mater, arachnoid and pia mater—the three meningeal layers
- Optic nerve does not regenerate once damaged, unlike other cranial nerves.

ANATOMY OF OPTIC NERVE

Optic nerve starts from the optic disk as acontinuation of nerve fiber layer of retina and extends up to optic chiasm. At the optic chiasm the nasal fibers decussate or crossover to the opposite side and the temporal fibers remain on the same side. Optic nerve measures about 50 mm and is divided into four parts (Fig. 12.1.1):

1. Intraocular part (1 mm).
2. Intraorbital part (25 mm).
3. Intracanalicular part (9 mm).
4. Intracranial part (15 mm).

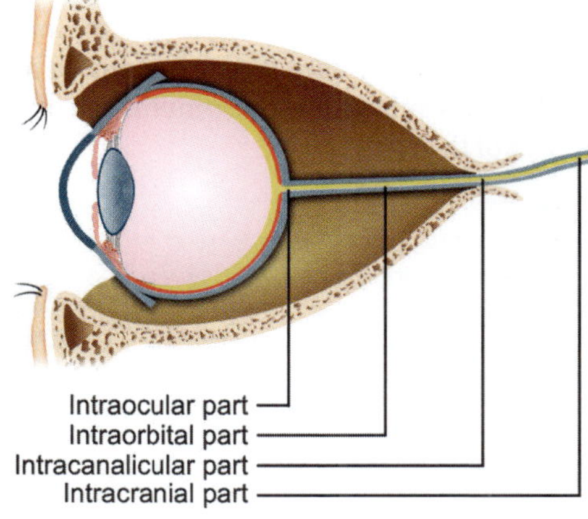

FIG. 12.1.1: Parts of optic nerve

Intraocular Part

Intraocular part is called optic disk or optic nerve head. It is circular or slightly vertically oval in shape measuring about 1.5 mm in diameter. It represents the beginning of the optic nerve. At the optic disk the nerve fiber layer of the retina continues as optic nerve and the remaining layers of the retina including the layer of rods and cones are absent at the optic disk. Intraocular part of optic nerve consists of superficial nerve fiber layer, prelaminar region, laminar region and retrolaminar region. Laminar region corresponds to the portion of the optic nerve passing through the lamina cribrosa. The myelination of the nerve fibers of optic nerve begins in the retrolaminar region.

Though optic nerve is responsible for vision, optic disk appears as blind spot in the visual field as rods and cones; the end organs of vision are absent in the optic disk.

Normally blind spot in the visual field is not experienced by us because during binocular vision the visual fields of both eyes overlap and during uniocular vision visual cortex is able to mask the blind spot by filling the missing portion of the image falling on the blind spot.

Intraorbital Part

Intraorbital part extends from posterior aspect of the globe to optic foramen present at the apex of the orbit. The intraorbital part of the optic nerve is covered by dura mater, arachnoid and pia mater. It is surrounded by annulus of Zinn at the apex of the orbit.

Intraorbital part of the optic nerve is redundant by 8 mm, thus it allows the movements of the eyeball and allows proptosis of eye up to 8 mm without any damage to optic nerve.

Intracanalicular Part

Intracanalicular part is the portion of the optic nerve in the optic canal. It lies lateral to sphenoid and ethmoidal sinuses; they are separated from optic nerve by a thin bone. This close proximity to the sinuses is responsible for sinusitis being a common cause of the retrobulbar neuritis.

Intracanalicular portion of the optic nerve is enclosed tightly in the optic canal as a result of which it is easily susceptible to injury because of compression in the optic canal.

Intracranial Part

Intracranial part extends from posterior end of the optic canal to optic chiasm. The intracranial portion of the optic nerve lies above the cavernous sinus.

Blood Supply

The prelaminar region of the intraocular part is supplied by short posterior ciliary arteries and the laminar, and retrolaminar part of the optic nerve is supplied by circle of Zinn. The intraorbital part of the optic nerve is supplied by pial vessels, intracanalicular part is supplied by ophthalmic artery and intracranial part is supplied by pial vessels.

GIST BOX 12.1

- Optic nerve is the II cranial nerve. It is the continuation of the nerve fiber layer of the retina consisting of about 1.2 million axons derived from the retinal ganglion cells.
- Though optic nerve is included in the list of cranial nerves, optic nerve is not a true nerve, but it is a continuation of brain and it is considered as sensory tract.
- Optic nerve starts from optic disk as continuation of nerve fiber layer of retina and extends up to optic chiasm. At the optic chiasm, the nasal fibers decussate or crossover to the opposite side and the temporal fibers remain on the same side. Optic nerve measures about 50 mm and is divided into four parts, i.e. intraocular part (1 mm), intraorbital part (25 mm), intracanalicular part (9 mm) and intracranial part (15 mm).

CHAPTER

12.2 Congenital Anomalies of Optic Nerve

EMBRYOLOGY OF OPTIC NERVE

Optic nerve develops from optic stalk, a part of optic vesicle. The optic nerve fibers are derived from the nerve fibers of retina. The neuroectodermal cells and mesenchyme surrounding the optic stalk gives rise to glial cells and sheaths of the optic nerve respectively. Myelination of the optic nerve fibers is seen up to retrolaminar part of the optic nerve.

CONGENITAL ANOMALIES OF OPTIC NERVE

Congenital anomalies of the optic nerve are as follows:

- Optic nerve aplasia
- Optic nerve hypoplasia
- Myelinated nerve fibers
- Excavated optic disk anomalies including optic disk coloboma, optic disk pit, morning glory disk anomaly and megalopapilla
- Congenital tilted disk syndrome
- Aicardi syndrome.

Optic Nerve Aplasia

Optic nerve aplasia is a rare congenital condition characterized by complete absence of optic nerve head or optic disk. It is associated with absence of retinal ganglion cells, retinal nerve fiber layer and retinal vessels. It may be unilateral or bilateral. It may be associated with other congenital defects of the eye such as coloboma, microphthalmos and persistent hyperplastic primary vitreous.

Optic Nerve Hypoplasia

Optical disk hypoplasia is a congenital condition characterized by the decreased number of optic nerve axons with normal mesodermal and glial tissues.

On examination, the optic disk appears small and pale in color on ophthalmoscopy with characteristic double-ring sign. Double-ring sign is the characteristic appearance of peripapillary halo with ring of pigmentation on either side.

Optic disk hypoplasia is the most common congenital anomaly of the optic disk.

De Morsier syndrome: Optic disk hypoplasia may be associated with De Morsier syndrome or septo-optic dysplasia characterized by midline brain malformations because of absence of septum pellucidum and agenesis of corpus callosum presenting as hypopituitarism.

Growth hormone deficiency, thyroid-stimulating hormone deficiency (presents as neonatal jaundice) and corticotrophin hormone deficiency (presents as neonatal hypoglycemia) are the most common endocrinological abnormalities. It should be suspected in infants presenting with signs of hypothalamic dysfunction or hypopituitarism such as neonatal jaundice and recurrent attacks of hypoglycemia with poor vision development.

Children diagnosed with optic nerve hypoplasia should be investigated to rule out the central nervous system (CNS) anomalies by magnetic resonance imaging (MRI) and endocrinological studies.

The visual prognosis depends on the extent of hypoplasia of optic nerve axons. The management of the patient is by evaluation for associated CNS anomalies and treatment by multidisciplinary approach to treat the endocrinological abnormalities.

Myelinated Nerve Fibers*

Myelinated never fibers is a condition characterized by presence of myelinated nerve fibers on the optic disk. Normally the myelination of nerve fibers begins in the retrolaminar part of the optic nerve.

The exact pathogenesis of myelinated fibers is not known. It may be explained by the presence of defective lamina cribrosa allowing the oligodendrocytes to enter the retina or by the presence of oligodendrocyte-like cells in the retina and produce myelin (Figs 12.2.1A to C).

The ocular associations associated with unilateral myelinated nerve fibers are high myopia and amblyopia. The myelinated nerve fibers are associated with systemic disease such as Gorlin syndrome.

Myelinated nerve fibers by themselves will not cause diminution of vision. Myelinated nerve fibers produce enlargement of blind spot when present on the optic disk and scotoma when isolated myelinated nerve fibers are present in retina.

Optic Disk Coloboma*

Optic disk coloboma is a congenital anomaly characterized by presence of excavation in the optic disk because of defective closure of the embryonic fissure. It may occur as an isolated condition or along with coloboma of the uveal tract (Fig. 12.2.2).

The associated systemic conditions include CHARGE syndrome characterized by **C**oloboma of the eye, **H**eart defects, **A**tresia of the nasal choanae, growth **R**etardation, **G**enital anomalies and **E**ar anomalies; other condition such as Goldenhar syndrome, Aicardi syndrome, etc.

Optic Disk Pit

Optic disk pit is a congenital anomaly characterized by the presence of localized excavation in the optic disk. Optic disk pits are usually unilateral and present as grayish round or oval depression in the optic disk.

Optic disk pits are usually asymptomatic unless complicated by serous retinal detachment involving the macula. About 50% of optic disk pits are known to be associated with this complication.

Treatment is by laser photocoagulation applied at temporal disk margin to prevent the entry of subretinal fluid from optic disk. Non-responsive cases require vitrectomy and gas tamponade.

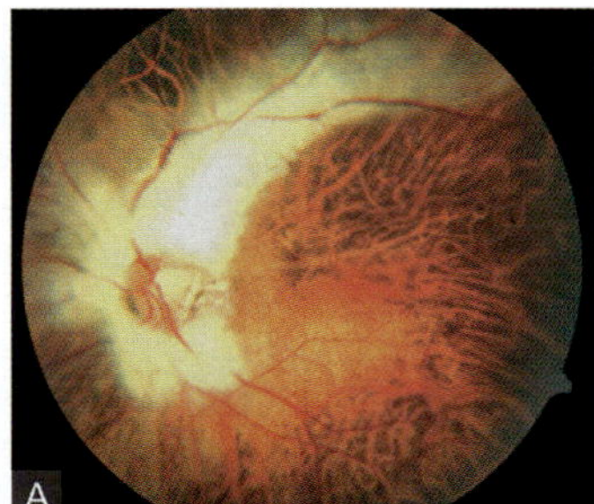

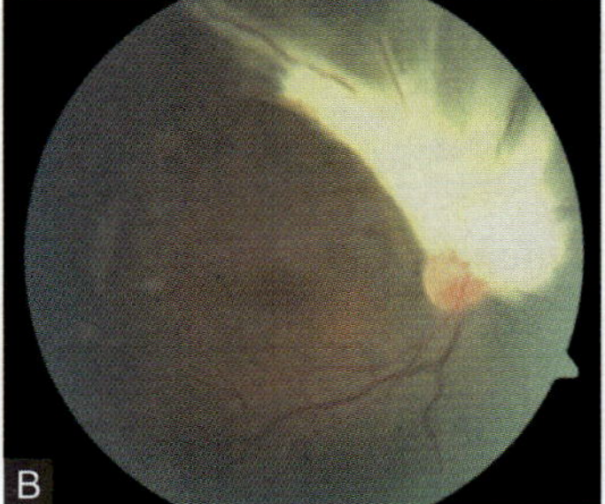

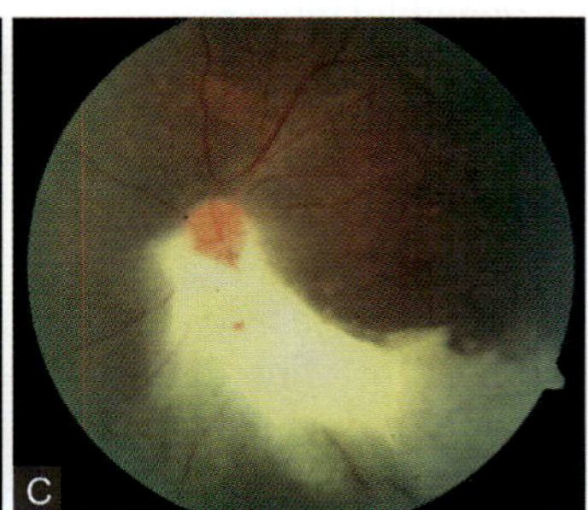

FIGS 12.2.1A to C: Myelinated nerve fibers

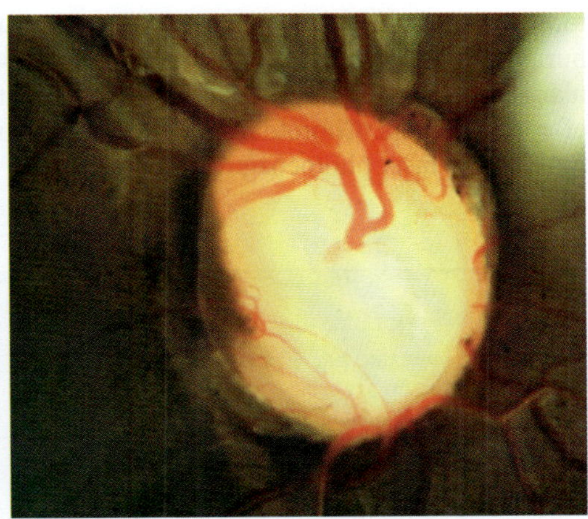

FIG. 12.2.2: Optic disk coloboma

Morning Glory Disk Anomaly

Morning glory disk anomaly is a congenital condition characterized by excavation of the retina involving the optic disk. It is characterized by the presence of hyperplastic glial tissue in the center of the optic disk and abnormal retinal vasculature in the form of abnormally straight vessels arising from the disk margin.

It is differentiated from optic disk coloboma from the fact that, in optic disk coloboma excavation lies within the optic disk and in morning glory disk anomaly optic disk lies within the excavation (Fig. 12.2.3).

Congenital Tilted Disk Syndrome

Congenital tilted disk syndrome is a condition characterized by inferonasal tilting of the optic disk probably because of malclosure of the embryonic optic fissure.

It produces characteristic visual field defect of superotemporal hemianopsia, resembling the visual field defect produced by chiasmal lesions.

Aicardi Syndrome

Aicardi is a rare congenital disease characterized by agenesis of corpus callosum, infantile spasms and ophthalmoscopy showing multiple depigmented chorioretinal lacunae around the optic disk. It is because of mutation of X chromosome and seen only in females.

Optic Disk Drusen

Optic disk drusen is a congenital condition characterized by abnormal deposition of proteins and calcium salts in the optic nerve head and presenting as pseudoelevation of the disk with indistinct lumpy margins (Fig. 12.2.4).

Optic disk drusens are not visible in childhood, they become visible by second to third decade. Most of the patients are asymptomatic and the condition is diagnosed during routine

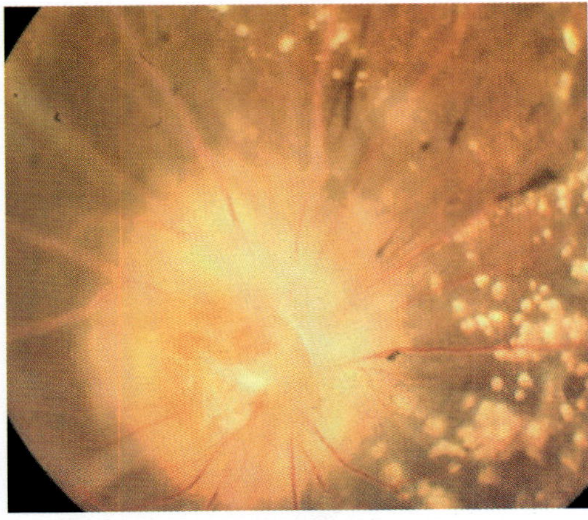

FIG. 12.2.3: Morning glory disk anomaly

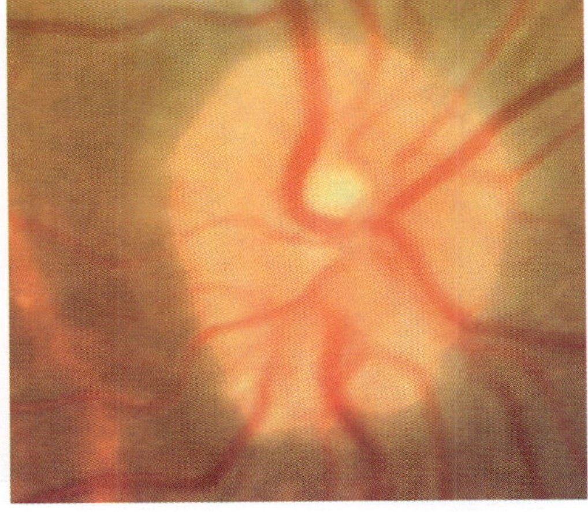

FIG. 12.2.4: Optic disk drusen

funduscopic examination. Optic disk drusen are rarely associated complications, i.e. choroidal neovascularization.

Optic disk drusen show autofluorescence on fluorescein angiography. B-scan or computed tomography (CT) scan is helpful in diagnosis of buried drusen. Treatment is by follow-up by regular fundus examination to look for development of complications. Choroidal neovascularization is treated by laser photocoagulation.

GIST BOX 12.2

- Optic disk hypoplasia is the most common congenital anomaly of the optic disk.
- Myelinated nerve fibers is a condition characterized by presence of myelinated nerve fibers on the optic disk.
- Optic disk coloboma is a congenital anomaly characterized by presence of excavation in the optic disk because of defective closure of the embryonic fissure. It may occur as an isolated condition or along with coloboma of the uveal tract.
- Optic disk drusen is a congenital condition characterized by abnormal deposition of proteins and calcium salts in the optic nerve head and presenting as pseudoelevation of the disk with indistinct lumpy margins.

CHAPTER

12.3 Optic Neuritis and Optic Neuropathies

OPTIC NEURITIS***

Definition

Optic neuritis is defined as inflammation of the optic nerve.

Etiology

Idiopathic causes are demyelinating diseases such as multiple sclerosis, neuromyelitis optica, Schilder's disease and encephalitis periaxialis concentrica. Infectious causes such as syphilis, tuberculosis, cat scratch fever, Lyme disease, cryptococcal meningitis in patients with acquired immunodeficiency syndrome (AIDS), sinus-related infections, etc. Parainfectious causes following viral infections such as mumps, measles or following immunization against measles, rubella, etc. Systemic autoimmune diseases such as sarcoidosis, systemic lupus erythematosus, etc.

Pathogenesis

Optic neuritis is probably because of delayed type IV hypersensitivity induced by activated T cells following inflammatory process causing destruction of myelin, neuronal cell death and degeneration of the axons.

Clinical Features

Optic neuritis is commonly seen in young females in the age group of 20–50 years with female-to-male ratio of 3:1. The incidence of optic neuritis is 1–5 in 100,000 per year.

> Acute demyelinating optic neuritis is the most common cause of unilateral painful diminution or loss of vision in young adults. Optic neuritis may present as the initial presentation of multiple sclerosis.

Symptoms

Acute onset of sudden progressive diminution of vision or loss of vision progressing over 1 week associated with periocular pain on ocular movements and altered color vision are the three classical symptoms of optic neuritis.

Signs

On examination:

1. Visual acuity shows moderate-to-severe reduction or even perception of light negative.
2. Relative afferent pupillary defect (RAPD).
3. Dyschromatopsia.

4. Visual field changes such as central scotoma, centrocecal scotoma, arcuate defects, etc.
5. Decreased contrast sensitivity.
6. Photopsia or flashes of light more commonly with ocular movements.
7. Uhthoff's phenomenon characterized by worsening of the visual symptoms by increased body temperature induced by exposure to heat or by physical exercise; this is explained by the fact that increased temperature altering the metabolic environment of the axon, thereby decreasing the neuronal conduction of visual impulses.
8. Pulfrich phenomenon is characterized by altered depth perception because of delay in transmission of visual impulses from the affected nerve to the visual cortex.
9. Ophthalmoscopic appearance depends on the subtype of optic neuritis, which is described under classification.

Classification

Based on the anatomical site of inflammation and ophthalmoscopic appearance, optic neuritis is classified as follows.

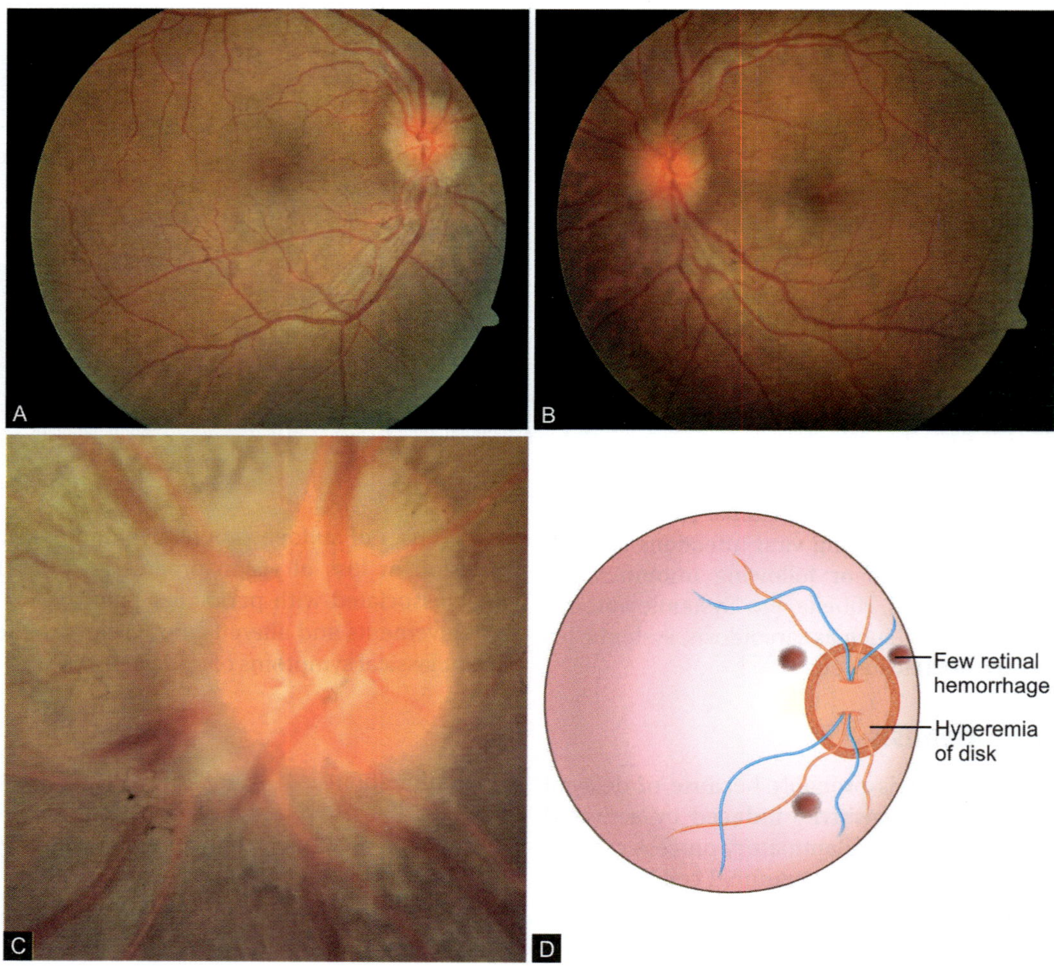

FIGS 12.3.1A to D: Papillitis. **A to C:** Photograph; **D.** Diagrammatic representation.

Papillitis

Papillitis refers to the inflammation of the optic disk and is characterized by hyperemia and edema of the optic disk on ophthalmoscopy (Figs 12.3.1A to D).

*Retrobulbar Neuritis***

Retrobulbar neuritis refers to inflammation of the posterior part of the optic nerve in the retrobulbar region behind the globe and is characterized by normal appearance of the optic disk on ophthalmoscopy.

*Neuroretinitis***

Neuroretinitis refers to the inflammation of the optic disk along with retinal nerve fiber layer in the adjacent macula and is characterized by hyperemia and edema of the optic disk along with exudates in the macular area on ophthalmoscopy (Figs 12.3.2A to C).

Depending on the clinical features, optic neuritis is classified as typical optic neuritis and atypical optic neuritis (Table 12.3.1).

Differential Diagnosis

Optic neuritis has to be differentiated from:

1. Ischemic optic neuropathies such as anterior ischemic optic neuropathy (AION), posterior ischemic optic neuropathy, diabetic papillopathy, etc. Compressive optic neuropathies caused by primary tumors, metastatic tumors and aneurysms. Hereditary optic neuropathies such as Leber's hereditary optic neuropathy.
2. Toxic and nutritional optic neuropathies such as tobacco-alcohol amblyopia, methyl alcohol amblyopia, quinine amblyopia and ethambutol amblyopia.

Investigations

The diagnosis of optic neuritis is mainly by clinical diagnosis; however investigations are required to rule out other causes of optic neuropathy.

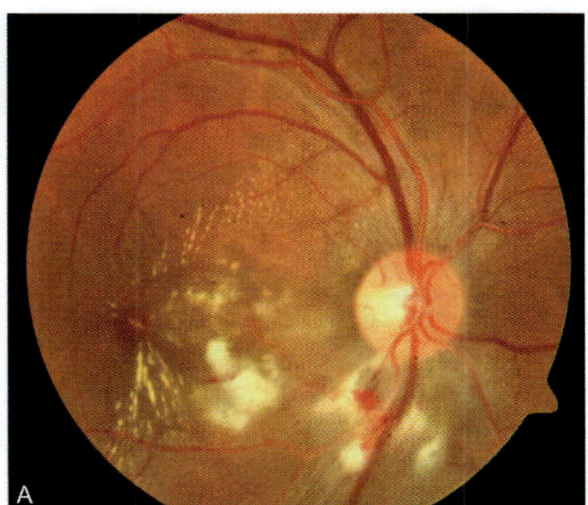

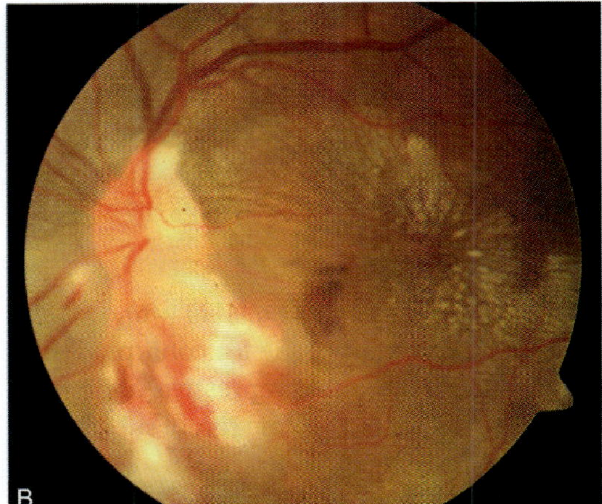

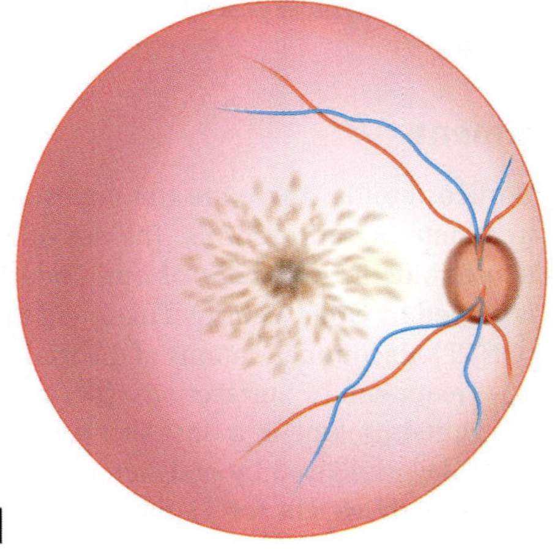

FIGS 12.3.2A to C: Neuroretinitis. **A and B:** Photograph; **C.** Diagrammatic representation.

TABLE 12.3.1: Clinical features of typical and atypical optic neuritis

Typical optic neuritis	*Atypical optic neuritis*
It usually occurs as an isolated disease of idiopathic nature or in association with multiple sclerosis	It usually occurs in association with systemic disease either infective or inflammatory or autoimmune in nature other than multiple sclerosis
It presents in the age group of 20–50 years	It presents in the age group of less than 12 years or more than 50 years
Unilateral	Bilateral disease or sequentially occurring in both the eyes
Acute onset of sudden progressive unilateral diminution of vision progressing over several hours to 1 week	The vision loss will be severe in the form of negative perception of light and its progression extends more than 2 weeks
Periocular pain on ocular movements is characteristically present during the acute phase, which extends for 1 week	Periocular pain on ocular movements is characteristically absent and if present, it extends for more than 2 weeks
Spontaneous improvement in vision within 5 weeks of onset of disease even without treatment	No improvement in vision within 5 weeks of onset of disease
No deterioration in vision after stopping treatment by steroids	Deterioration in vision after stopping treatment by steroids
Ocular examination shows mild-to-moderate disk edema with hyperemia of the optic disk and mild posterior uveitis and mild periphlebitis	Ocular examination shows severe anterior uveitis or posterior uveitis, severe periphlebitis, severe disk edema associated with disk hemorrhages and macular star

Magnetic resonance imaging (MRI) with gadolinium enhancement: It is done for confirmation of diagnosis, to rule out compressive optic neuropathies and to find out the risk of subsequent development of multiple sclerosis.

Lumbar puncture and cerebrospinal fluid analysis: It is required in atypical cases to rule out infectious causes.

Treatment

1. Corticosteroids: These are the mainstay of treatment of optic neuritis. The use of corticosteroids in treatment of optic neuritis is guided by Optic Neuritis Treatment Trial (ONTT). Recommendations of the trial are:
   a. Treatment by intravenous (IV) methylprednisolone in a dose of 1 g/day for 3 days, followed by oral steroids 1 mg/kg body weight for 11 days. This regimen speeds up the recovery of vision improvement without affecting the final visual prognosis. It also reduces the risk of development of multiple sclerosis within 2 years in patients in whom MRI shows one or more white matter lesions. Hence, this regimen is indicated in those patients with MRI abnormalities and in patients with normal MRI findings in case of involvement of only normal eye or bilateral involvement for faster visual recovery.
   b. Oral steroids alone should not be used as it is associated with increased recurrence rate.
2. Immunomodulatory therapy: It is indicated to prevent axonal damage in the patients with high risk of developing multiple sclerosis as indicated by presence of two or more white matter lesions, with each white matter lesion being 3 mm or larger in diameter situated in periventricular areas of the white matter.

3. It is done by drugs such as interferon β-1a (Avonex and Rebif), interferon β-1b (Betaferon).
4. The Controlled High-Risk Avonex Multiple Sclerosis Prevention Study (CHAMPS) and Controlled High-Risk Avonex Multiple Sclerosis Prevention Study in Ongoing Neurological Surveillance (CHAMPIONS) advice treatment with interferon β-1a (Avonex) 30 μg intramuscularly once a week.
5. Early Treatment of Multiple Sclerosis Study, i.e. ETOMS, advises treatment with interferon β-1a (Rebif) 22 μg subcutaneously once a week. Betaferon in Newly Emerging Multiple Sclerosis for Initial Treatment, i.e. BENEFIT, advises treatment by interferon β-1b (Betaferon) 250 μg subcutaneously every alternative day.

Clinical Course and Visual Outcome

Optic neuritis is known to recur either in same eye or contralateral eye. The recurrence rate is about 28% for 5 years and 35% for 10 years as indicated from ONTT trial. The recurrences are common in patients who are treated with only oral steroids and in patients who develop multiple sclerosis.

Patients with acute optic neuritis with abnormal MRI are at increased risk of developing multiple sclerosis. The risk is expected to be at 75% for females and 30% for males in 15 years.

Pallor of the optic disk is seen after 6 weeks of onset of the disease and it correlates with the severity of inflammation.

Spontaneous improvement in vision is seen in more than 90% of typical optic neuritis within 5 weeks of onset of disease even without treatment. It begins after 2–3 weeks and extends to 6 months to 1 year. Though the improvement in vision occurs in more than 90% of cases, it is only visual acuity, which improves, whereas defects involving the other components of vision such as contrast sensitivity, color vision, visual fields, depth perception persist. RAPD may disappear with complete visual recovery or it may persist in case of severe axonal loss causing optic atrophy.

ISCHEMIC OPTIC NEUROPATHY**

Definition

Optic neuropathy resulting from ischemia of the optic nerve is called ischemic optic neuropathy.

Classification

Depending on the part of the optic nerve involved, ischemic optic neuropathy is classified into anterior ischemic optic neuropathy and posterior ischemic optic neuropathy (PION).

Anterior Ischemic Optic Neuropathy

Anterior ischemic optic neuropathy is because of involvement of the anterior part of the optic nerve (intraocular part), optic disk or optic nerve head and is characterized by disk edema. It is further classified into arteritic AION and non-arteritic AION (Table 12.3.2).

Arteritic anterior ischemic optic neuropathy: It is an acute optic neuropathy resulting from ischemia of the short posterior ciliary arteries, which supply the optic nerve head. It is associated with giant cell arteritis. It is a medical emergency and requires immediate treatment with high-dose steroids to prevent loss of vision.

Non-arteritic anterior ischemic optic neuropathy: It is a subacute optic neuropathy resulting from ischemia of the small vessels distal to the short posterior ciliary arteries, which supply the optic nerve head. It is more common than AION. It is caused by ischemia distal to the short posterior ciliary arteries. Unlike arteritic anterior ischemic optic neuropathy, it runs a subacute course and the improvement in vision occurs in half of the cases.

Posterior Ischemic Optic Neuropathy

Posterior ischemic optic neuropathy is because of involvement of the posterior part of the optic nerve (intraorbital or intracanalicular, or intracranial parts) and is characterized by absence of disk edema.

TABLE 12.3.2: Differences between arteritic anterior ischemic optic neuropathy (AION) and non-arteritic AION

Arteritic AION	*Non-arteritic AION*
• It is caused by ischemia of the short posterior ciliary artery	• It is caused by ischemia distal to the short posterior ciliary arteries
• It is seen in elderly individuals with the mean age of 70 years, more common in females when compared to males	• It is more common than arteritic AION and is seen about a decade earlier than arteritic AION, with mean age of 60 years; the incidence is same in both males and females
• It is secondary to vasculitis of the short posterior ciliary arteries and it is usually associated with giant cell arteritis and symptoms such as headache, jaw claudication, amaurosis fugax, etc. • Other causes for vasculitis associated with arteritic AION are rheumatoid arthritis, relapsing polychondritis, herpes zoster, systemic lupus erythematosus, etc.	• It is secondary to non-inflammatory small vessel disease affecting the smaller vessels distal to the short posterior ciliary arteries • It is not associated with giant cell arteritis and usually symptoms are absent
• It presents with moderate-to-severe loss of vision with presenting visual acuity worse than 6/60	• It presents with mild-to-moderate loss of vision with presenting visual acuity better than 6/60
• Examination of the eye shows relative afferent pupillary defect (RAPD) and optic disk shows edema with pallor more than hyperemia • Visual field shows characteristic altitudinal defect involving the inferior visual field more commonly	• Examination of the eye shows presence or absence of RAPD and optic disk shows edema with hyperemia more than pallor • Visual field shows altitudinal defect similar to arteritic AION
• Examination of the fellow eye is normal with normal optic disk	• Examination of the fellow eye shows small cup-to-disk ratio called disk at risk, thereby causing overcrowding of the nerve fibers predisposing to compression of the capillaries and small blood vessels
• Erythrocyte sedimentation rate (ESR) is grossly elevated more than 70 mm/h	• Erythrocyte sedimentation rate is usually normal
• Fundus fluorescein angiography shows delayed filling of optic disk and choroid	• Fundus fluorescein angiography shows delayed filling of optic disk
• Fundus fluorescein angiography shows delayed filling of optic disk and choroid	• No effective known treatments are found; the proposed treatment modalities are: – Antiplatelet drugs, e.g. aspirin, anticoagulants and thrombolytics – Vasodilators, e.g. nicotinic acid – Corticosteroids
• The risk of involvement of the fellow eye is about 90%	• The risk of involvement of the fellow eye is about 30%

LEBER'S HEREDITARY OPTIC NEUROPATHY

Leber's hereditary optic neuropathy is a mitochondrial genetic disease characterized by hereditary optic neuropathy affecting young adult males.

The clinical features include sudden onset of painless diminution of vision associated with impairment of color vision with normal pupillary reflexes. Optic disk shows telangiectasia of the blood vessels around the optic disk and tortuosity of the retinal vessels. Optic disk in the later stages becomes pale because of optic atrophy. The clinical features become bilateral either simultaneously or sequentially.

The treatment is mainly by providing low-visual aids. Medical treatment by drugs, i.e. idebenone belonging to quinone group is under trial to arrest the progression of the disease by preventing the degeneration of the retinal ganglion cells.

TOXIC AND NUTRITIONAL OPTIC NEUROPATHIES**

Definition

The toxic and nutritional optic neuropathies include a group of diseases characterized by damage to the papillomacular fibers of the optic nerve resulting in visual impairment secondary exposure to certain toxins or because of deficiency of essential nutrients. Toxic optic neuropathies are also called toxic amblyopia.

Etiology

Common Causes for Toxic Optic Neuropathy

- Methyl alcohol
- Ethyl alcohol
- Quinine
- Chloroquine
- Isoniazid
- Ethambutol
- Digitalis
- Amiodarone
- Tobacco.

Common Causes for Nutritional Optic Neuropathy

Deficiency of vitamin B complex group including:

- Vitamin B_{12} (cyanocobalamin)
- Vitamin B_6 (pyridoxine)
- Vitamin B_1 (thiamine)
- Vitamin B_3 (niacin).

Pathogenesis

The basic pathology is damage to the papillomacular bundle because of impairment in the mitochondrial oxidative phosphorylation secondary to toxins and deficiency of essential nutrients.

> Papillomacular bundle is preferentially affected because the impairment of mitochondrial oxidative phosphorylation damages the nerve fibers with rapid rate of firing; narrow caliber, absence of myelin sheath and papillomacular nerve fibers show all these characteristics.

Clinical Features

The symptoms are:

1. Painless, symmetrical diminution of vision in both the eyes.
2. Dyschromatopsia out of proportion to diminution of vision.

On examination:

1. Visual acuity is decreased depending on the severity of damage; it can be perception of light negative in cases of methyl alcohol toxicity.
2. Pupillary reflexes are normal until late in the disease, till optic atrophy sets in the advanced stages of the disease.
3. Optic disk shows temporal pallor and optic atrophy in advanced stages.
4. Visual field examination shows typical centrocecal scotoma.

Investigations

Toxic and nutritional optic neuropathies are diagnosed by medical history and supportive investigations, e.g. serum vitamin B_{12} assay and electrophysiological tests, i.e. visual evoked potential. MRI is done to rule out intracranial space occupying lesions.

Treatment

Treatment is done by stopping the causative agent, improving the nutrition and multivitamin supplementation.

Tobacco-alcohol Amblyopia

1. Tobacco-alcohol amblyopia is seen in individuals who are chronic users of tobacco or alcohol. Since, tobacco and alcohol addiction is commonly associated both optic neuropathies are commonly seen together. Hence, it is described as tobacco-alcohol amblyopia.
2. The underlying mechanism is attributed to excessive cyanide levels in blood resulting from smoking, decreased cyanide detoxification due to deficiency of sulfur-rich proteins commonly seen in alcoholics and deficiency of vitamin B_{12} seen in smokers and alcoholics, which results in excessive cyanide levels in the blood. Excessive cyanide levels in blood results in damage to papillomacular bundle and characteristic visual impairment.
3. Treatment is by complete cessation of use of tobacco and alcohol, improvement of nutrition and supplementation of multivitamins and vitamin B_{12}. Vitamin B_{12} or cyanocobalamin acts by conversion of cyanide to cyanocobalamin.

Ethyl Alcohol Amblyopia

1. Ethyl alcohol amblyopia is seen the in individuals who are chronic alcoholics, but nonsmokers.
2. Its mechanism, clinical features and treatment are similar to the tobacco-alcohol amblyopia.

Quinine Amblyopia

1. Quinine is an antimalarial drug and it is known to cause optic neuropathy in susceptible individuals even with small doses.
2. It is known to cause sudden and complete loss of vision with fixed and dilated pupils in the initial stage. The vision is known to recover on discontinuing the drug, but in some cases loss of vision can be permanent.
3. The initial ophthalmoscopic picture shows absence of foveal reflex. In the advanced stages, maculopathy develops resembling the bull's eye lesion similar to chloroquine maculopathy.

Chloroquine Amblyopia

1. Chloroquine is a commonly used drug for treatment of malaria, rheumatoid arthritis and it is known to cause maculopathy and optic neuropathy on long-term usage.
2. The risk of toxicity depends on cumulative dose and the risk of toxicity increases with cumulative dose of more than 300 g.
3. The fundus picture shows absence of foveal reflex in the initial stages and later stages are characterized by atrophy of the retinal pigment epithelium in the macula resulting in the characteristic appearance of bull's eye lesion. The periphery of the retina shows attenuation of the retinal arterioles and accumulation of pigments similar to retinitis pigmentosa.
4. Corneal changes such as keratopathy are also seen in long-term usage of the drug.

Isoniazid and Ethambutol Amblyopia

Isoniazid and ethambutol are commonly used antitubercular drugs and they are known to cause ocular complications such as optic neuritis, bitemporal hemianopia and optic neuropathy.

Methyl Alcohol Amblyopia

1. Methyl alcohol amblyopia follows accidental or suicidal ingestion of methyl alcohol. It is common in people from low-socioeconomic status who consume adulterated beverages.

2. Formic acid resulting from the metabolism of methyl alcohol is responsible for the toxic symptoms.
3. Nausea, vomiting, abdominal pain are seen in acute phase following consumption of methyl alcohol. The patient may rapidly go into coma and die; if the patient survives in the acute phase, he/she will be left with permanent blindness.
4. Optic disk shows optic disk edema, hyperemia in the initial phase and optic atrophy later with permanent loss of vision.
5. Treatment is by:
   a. Gastric lavage to remove unabsorbed methyl alcohol.
   b. Sodium bicarbonate to correct metabolic acidosis.
   c. Antidote such as ethyl alcohol or fomepizole to prevent the metabolism of methyl alcohol.
6. Chronic methyl alcohol poisoning is seen in industrial workers where methyl alcohol is used by absorption across skin or by inhalation. Chronic methyl alcohol poisoning presents as slowly progressive loss of vision.

TRAUMATIC OPTIC NEUROPATHY**

Definition

Optic neuropathy following direct or indirect trauma to the optic nerve is called traumatic optic neuropathy.

Etiopathogenesis

Traumatic optic neuropathy occurs following primary or secondary mechanism:

1. Primary mechanism is by direct trauma to the optic nerve causing transaction of optic nerve or interruption of vascular supply as a result of shearing forces of trauma.
2. Secondary mechanism is by indirect trauma to the optic nerve by edema or hemorrhage following trauma.

> The intracanalicular portion of the optic nerve is easily susceptible to both direct and indirect trauma because of tight adherence of the optic nerve to periosteum of optic canal.

Clinical Features

Patients with traumatic optic neuropathy present with diminution of vision or loss of vision depending on the severity of injury. On examination, RAPD is present in all cases.

Signs of injury to the optic nerve such as hemorrhage on the optic disk are seen in injury to the anterior part of the optic nerve. In cases of injury to the posterior part of the optic nerve, optic disk appears normal and only finding will be RAPD. Optic atrophy is not present on initial presentation, but develops later.

Investigations

Computed tomography (CT) is done in all cases of traumatic optic neuropathies to find out the mode of injury, primary or secondary.

Treatment

Traumatic optic neuropathy following secondary mechanism is treatable, whereas traumatic optic neuropathy following primary mechanism leads to permanent loss of vision.

High-dose steroids and surgical optic nerve decompression are the modes of treatment to prevent indirect trauma to optic nerve by edema or hemorrhage following injury. High-dose steroids called mega dose should be administered within 8 hours of injury. The treatment is by IV methylprednisolone 30 mg/kg is administered over 30 minutes, followed by 15 mg/kg after 2 hours and 15 mg/kg four times a day for 24–48 hours. Precaution should be executed in patients with associated head injury, while using mega dose of steroids.

If the patient responds to mega dose of steroids in the form of improvement of vision, steroids are tapered over period of 2–3 weeks. If the patient does not show response to steroids optic nerve decompression is considered.

Orbital decompression in the form of cantholysis is sufficient for cases associated with orbital hemorrhage. The cases associated with optic nerve sheath hemorrhage may require optic nerve decompression.

GIST BOX 12.3

- Inflammation of the optic nerve is called optic neuritis.
- Acute demyelinating optic neuritis is the most common cause of unilateral painful diminution or loss of vision in young adults; optic neuritis may present as the initial presentation of multiple sclerosis.
- Papillitis, it refers to the inflammation of the optic disk and is characterized by hyperemia and edema of the optic disk on ophthalmoscopy.
- Retrobulbar neuritis, it refers to inflammation of the posterior part of the optic nerve in the retrobulbar region behind the globe and is characterized by normal appearance of the optic disk on ophthalmoscopy.
- Neuroretinitis, it refers to the inflammation of the optic disk along with retinal nerve fiber layer in the adjacent macula and is characterized by hyperemia and edema of the optic disk along with exudates in the macular area on ophthalmoscopy.
- Optic neuropathy resulting from ischemia of the optic nerve is called ischemic optic neuropathy.
- Leber's hereditary optic neuropathy is a mitochondrial genetic disease characterized by hereditary optic neuropathy affecting young adult males.
- Toxic and nutritional optic neuropathies include a group of diseases characterized by damage to the papillomacular fibers of the optic nerve resulting in visual impairment secondary to exposure to certain toxins or because of deficiency of essential nutrients.

CHAPTER

12.4 Papilledema

DEFINITION***

Papilledema is defined as passive edema of the optic disk secondary to raised intracranial pressure (ICP).

Papilledema must be differentiated from disk edema. Disk edema includes all the cases of swelling of disk, both active and passive, and may be unilateral or bilateral. Papilledema includes passive edema of the optic disk, secondary to raised ICP and it is almost always bilateral.

ETIOLOGY

The causes for papilledema include those, which cause rise of ICP and the list of causes include:

1. Intracranial tumors, which tend to increase the ICP because of obstruction to the flow of cerebrospinal fluid (CSF) through the aqueduct of Sylvius. Hence, papilledema is seen more frequently in infratentorial tumors.
2. Intracranial infections such as meningitis, encephalitis because of obstruction of the CSF pathway.
3. Intracranial hemorrhages including intracerebral hemorrhage, subarachnoid hemorrhage and subdural hemorrhage.
4. Intracranial space occupying lesions other than tumors such as aneurysms, cerebral abscess, tuberculoma, cysticercosis cyst, etc.
5. Cerebral edema following any head injury or infarction.
6. Benign intracranial hypertension or pseudotumor cerebri.
7. Cerebral venous sinus thrombosis.
8. Congenital causes such as craniosynostosis, mucopolysaccharidosis, aqueductal stenosis, etc.

Papilledema is not common in infants, as the cranial sutures are not fused and fontanels are open at this age, hence the cranial cavity can expand before causing rise in ICP.

PATHOGENESIS

Papilledema is caused by stasis of axoplasmic flow. Axoplasmic flow is the flow of organelles produced in the neurons and it is essential for normal functioning of the neurons (Fig. 12.4.1).

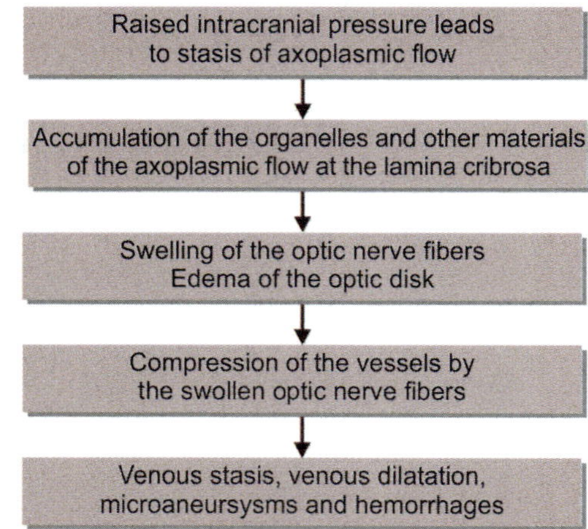

FIG. 12.4.1: Pathogenesis of papilledema

Papilledema is almost always bilateral and unilateral papilledema is seen in.

Foster Kennedy syndrome: Optic atrophy in one eye and papilledema in other eye seen in frontal lobe tumors is called Foster Kennedy syndrome. It is because of simultaneous compression of the ipsilateral optic nerve directly by the tumor resulting in ipsilateral optic atrophy and rise in ICP resulting in contralateral papilledema. The associated features seen in Foster Kennedy syndrome are ipsilateral anosmia because of compression of the ipsilateral olfactory nerve and frontal lobe signs such as memory loss and emotional liability.

Pre-existing optic atrophy involving one optic nerve: Since the optic nerve fibers are atrophied in optic atrophy, edema because of blockage of axoplasmic flow can never develop.

Pseudo-Foster Kennedy syndrome: Unilateral optic disk swelling and contralateral optic atrophy in the absence of an intracranial mass causing compression of the optic nerve is called pseudo-Foster Kennedy syndrome. This syndrome is caused by bilateral sequential optic neuritis or bilateral ischemic optic neuropathy.

SYMPTOMS

The symptoms are secondary to raised ICP and include.

Headache: It is typically worse in the morning and exacerbated by Valsalva maneuver.

Nausea and vomiting: They are secondary to raised ICP and vomiting is typically projectile in nature.

Visual Symptoms

1. Visual acuity is fairly good until late in the disease and loss of vision is seen in advanced stage of the disease because of optic atrophy.
2. Transient loss of vision or amaurosis fugax is the most commonly seen visual symptom and is characterized by transient blurring obscuration of vision lasting for 5 seconds or less, seen because of transient ischemia of the optic nerve because of compression of the optic nerve.

SIGNS

On examination:

1. Anterior segment examination is normal; relative afferent pupillary defect (RAPD) is seen late in disease because of optic atrophy.
2. Posterior segment examination shows variable degrees of disk edema depending on the stage of papilledema.
3. Visual field changes include enlargement of blind spot in early stages of papilledema and constriction of visual field in the advanced stage.
4. Decreased perception of colors and loss of color vision are seen in advanced stage.
5. Diplopia may be seen because of VI cranial nerve palsy secondary to the raised ICP.

STAGES OF PAPILLEDEMA**

Papilledema is graded into four stages.

Incipient Papilledema

Incipient papilledema (Fig. 12.4.2) is characterized by the obscuration and elevation of disk margins, (nasal margin is the earliest to be affected and temporal margin is affected last) disk hyperemia and absence of spontaneous venous pulsation.

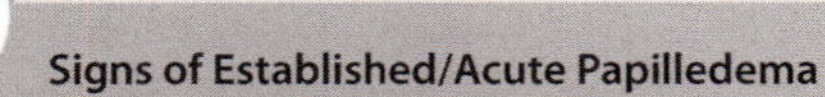

Signs of Established/Acute Papilledema

Acute papilledema or fully established papilledema is characterized by 10 signs, including 5 each of vascular and mechanical signs.

Vascular signs of papilledema are:

1. Hyperemia of optic disk.
2. Hemorrhages.
3. Hard exudates.
4. Cotton wool spots.
5. Congestion of the retinal vessels.

Mechanical signs of papilledema are:

1. Elevation of the optic disk > 3 diopters.
2. Edema of the nerve fiber layer.
3. Obscuration of the disk margins.
4. Obliteration of the physiological cup.
5. Folds of retina and/or choroid. Retinal folds seen on the temporal side of the optic disk, early in papilledema are called Paton's lines.

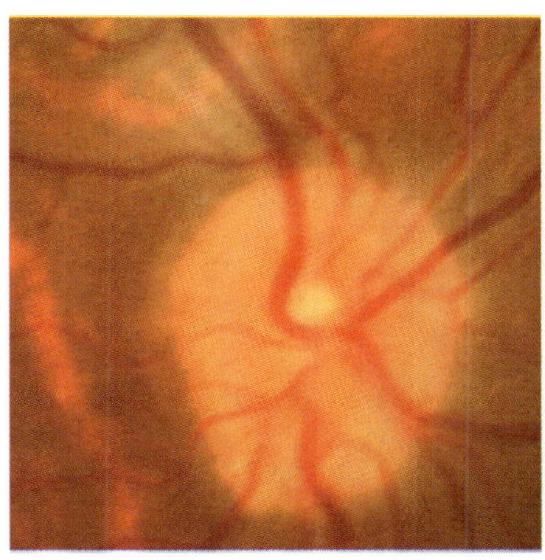

FIG. 12.4.2: Incipient papilledema

Established Papilledema

Established papilledema (Figs 12.4.3A and B) is characterized by marked hyperemia of the optic disk, complete obliteration of the normal physiological cup of the optic disk, marked elevation of the optic disk with dome-shaped configuration, obscuration of retinal vessels on the surface of the optic disk, dilated and tortuous retinal veins with peripapillary hemorrhages, cotton wool spots and hard exudates.

Chronic Papilledema

Chronic papilledema (Fig. 12.4.4) is characterized by round and elevated appearance of the

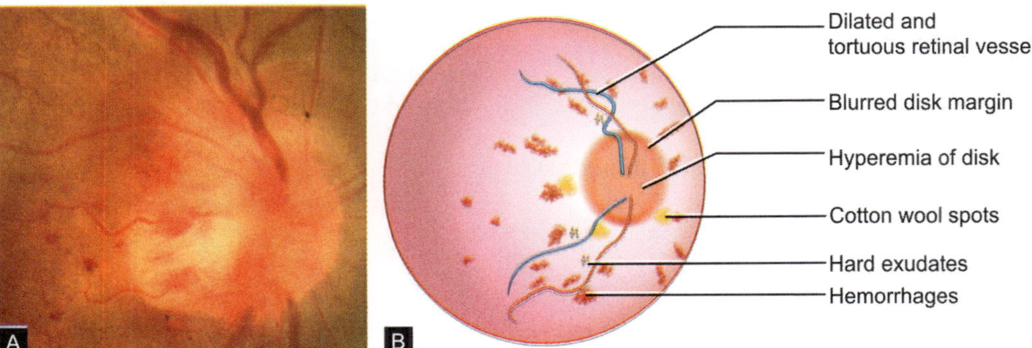

FIGS 12.4.3A and B: Established papilledema. **A**. Photograph; **B**. Diagrammatic respresentation.

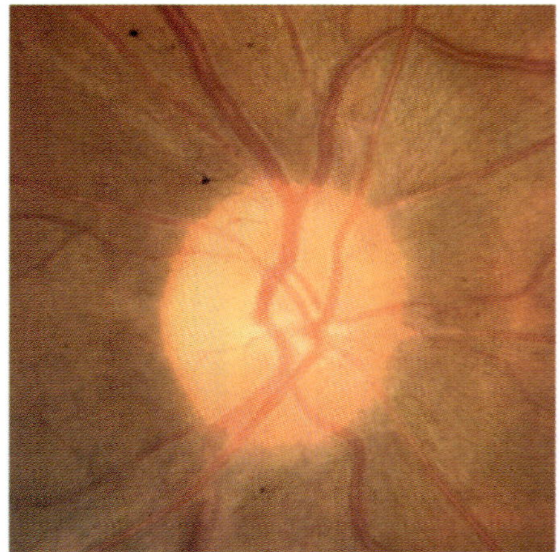

FIG. 12.4.4: Chronic papilledema

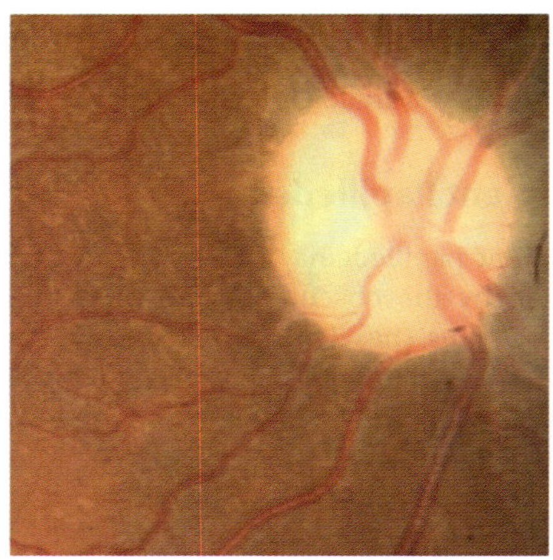

FIG. 12.4.5: Atrophic papilledema

optic disk resembling champagne cork. The hemorrhages and hard exudates are resolved; hyperemia of the disk is decreased. Visual acuity is decreased with visual fields showing enlargement of blind spot and constriction of visual field.

Atrophic Papilledema

Atrophic papilledema (Fig. 12.4.5) is characterized by features of secondary optic atrophy. Visual acuity is markedly decreased with development of RAPD and visual fields are markedly constricted.

Optic disk appears dirty white in color with poorly delineated disk margins because of excessive gliosis. The retinal vessels show attenuation and perivascular sheathing.

DIFFERENTIAL DIAGNOSIS*

Papilledema has to be differentiated from disk edema and pseudopapilledema.

Disk edema: It includes all the cases of swelling of disk both active and passive, and may be unilateral or bilateral. The causes for disk edema are:
- Intraocular diseases such as posterior uveitis, posterior scleritis, central retinal vein occlusion, ocular hypotony, etc. Diseases of the optic nerve such as optic neuritis, neuroretinitis, anterior ischemic optic neuropathy, tumors of the optic nerve, etc. Orbital diseases such as thyroid ophthalmopathy, tumors of the orbit.
- Systemic conditions such as malignant hypertension, pregnancy-induced hypertension, grade IV hypertensive retinopathy.
- All the causes of papilledema.

Pseudopapilledema:* It is also called pseudoedema of disk or pseudopapillitis. It includes a group of conditions, which present with false elevation of the optic disk appearing similar to papilledema or disk edema. The causes of pseudopapilledema are:
- Congenital conditions such as optic nerve head drusen, tilted disk, hypoplasia of optic nerve, medullated nerve fibers, etc.
- Hypermetropia.

INVESTIGATIONS

All patients with papilledema should be examined for any underlying cause of raised ICP. Neuroimaging is done preferably by a magnetic resonance imaging (MRI). The patient requires neurological and neurosurgical references.

TREATMENT

The principle of treatment is to treat the underlying cause for papilledema and to prevent loss of vision because of optic atrophy.

Treatments of the underlying cause such as intracranial tumor, intracranial space occupying lesion, intracranial infection, etc. are as follows:

1. Medical treatment is by carbonic anhydrase inhibitors such as acetazolamide and repeated lumbar punctures.
2. Surgical treatment is indicated in cases not responding to medical treatment and presenting with worsening of the visual symptoms. Surgical treatment is in the form of lumboperitoneal shunt or ventriculoperitoneal shunt to bypass CSF drainage and optic nerve sheath decompression.

Benign or idiopathic intracranial hypertension: It is an idiopathic condition characterized by raised ICP because of raised CSF pressure with normal neuroimaging studies and normal composition of CSF. As the condition presents with symptoms similar to intracranial tumor it is called pseudotumor cerebri.

It is commonly seen in obese females in second and third decade. Patients usually presents with symptoms of headache and transient loss of vision. Bilateral papilledema is the characteristic clinical sign seen on fundoscopy.

Neuroimaging by computed tomography (CT) scan or MRI will be negative for space occupying mass lesions and may show slit-like lateral ventricles.

Though pseudotumor cerebri is idiopathic in nature, associated conditions, which can cause elevated ICP have to be ruled out. The conditions include:

- Endocrine diseases such as hypoparathyroidism, Addison's disease and Cushing's syndrome.
- Drugs such as nitrofurantoin, nalidixic acid, vitamin A, steroid withdrawal, phenytoin and tetracycline.
- Iron-deficiency anemia, obstructive sleep apnea, autoimmune diseases such as multiple sclerosis, sarcoidosis.

Treatment is on similar lines as for papilledema. Weight reduction in obese patients is known to be beneficial.

GIST BOX 12.4

- Papilledema is defined as passive edema of the optic disk secondary to raised intracranial pressure (ICP).
- Papilledema is graded into four stages, i.e. incipient papilledema, established papilledema, chronic papilledema and atrophic papilledema.
- Papilledema has to be differentiated from disk edema and pseudopapilledema.
- All patients with papilledema should be examined for underlying cause for raised ICP. Neuroimaging is done preferably by a magnetic resonance imaging (MRI). The patient requires neurological and neurosurgical references. The principle of treatment is to treat the underlying cause for papilledema and to prevent loss of vision because of optic atrophy.

CHAPTER

12.5 Optic Atrophy

DEFINITION**

Optic atrophy is defined as degeneration of the axons of the optic nerve and loss of function of the optic nerve as a result of lesions of the anterior visual pathway extending from retinal ganglion cell layer to lateral geniculate body resulting in loss of retinal ganglion cells.

It is not a proper disease, but the end result of various pathologic processes involving the anterior visual pathway, which result in loss of retinal ganglion cells.

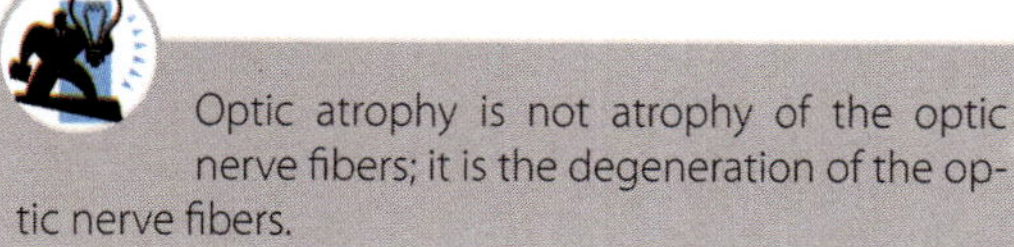

Optic atrophy is not atrophy of the optic nerve fibers; it is the degeneration of the optic nerve fibers.

Histologically, optic atrophy is characterized by decrease in the diameter of optic nerve, loss of axons and varying degree of gliosis. Ophthalmoscopically optic atrophy shows characteristic pallor of the optic disk because of decrease in the number of capillaries and gliosis.

CLASSIFICATION**

Depending on the ophthalmoscopic appearance of the optic disk, optic atrophy is classified as:

1. Primary optic atrophy.
2. Secondary optic atrophy.

Primary Optic Atrophy*

Primary optic atrophy occurs without antecedent swelling of optic disk (Figs 12.5.1A and B).

Characteristics

Primary optic atrophy is characterized by:

- Pale optic disk with sharply delineated margins of the optic disk
- Reduction in the number of small blood vessels on the optic disk. This is called Kestenbaum sign
- Normal physiological cup
- Normal retinal vessels and the surrounding retina.

Causes

Primary optic atrophy is caused by lesions involving retrolaminar part of the optic nerve to lateral geniculate body. The causes include:

- Retrobulbar neuritis
- Hereditary optic neuropathy
- Toxic and nutritional optic neuropathies
- Traumatic optic neuropathy
- Demyelinating diseases (e.g. multiple sclerosis)
- Compressive optic neuropathies, which are caused by intracranial tumors and space-occupying lesions.

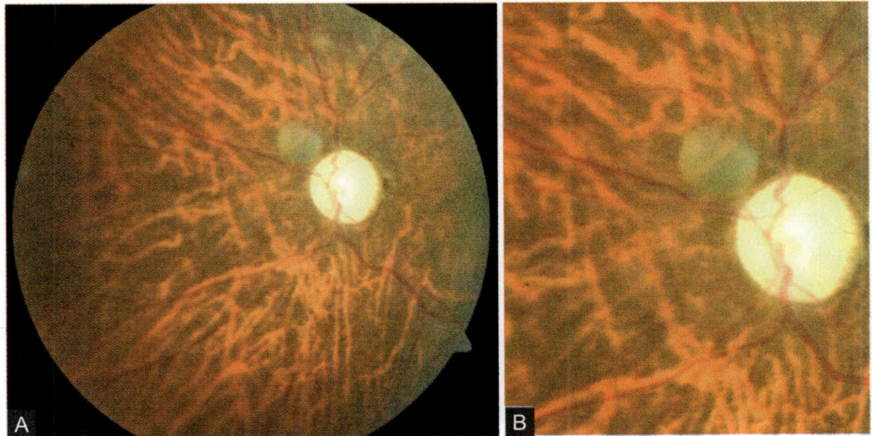

FIGS 12.5.1A and B: Primary optic atrophy

Secondary Optic Atrophy*

Secondary optic atrophy occurs with antecedent swelling of optic disk as a result of long-standing disk edema. Since it is commonly seen following papilledema or papillitis, it is called postpapilledema optic atrophy or postneuritic optic atrophy (Figs 12.5.2A and B).

Characteristics

Secondary optic atrophy is characterized by:
- Dirty white appearance of the optic disk with poorly delineated margins of the optic disk because of excessive gliosis
- Obliteration of the physiological cup
- Attenuation of retinal vessels and perivascular sheathing.

Causes

Secondary optic atrophy is caused by lesions, which cause long-standing disk edema:
- Papilledema
- Papillitis
- Neuroretinitis
- Anterior ischemic optic neuropathy.

Consecutive Optic Atrophy*

Consecutive optic atrophy occurs as a consequence of destruction of the ganglion cells of the retina by diseases of the retina and choroid (Fig. 12.5.3).

Characteristics

Consecutive optic atrophy is characterized by:
- Yellow waxy pallor of the optic disk
- Surrounding retina showing the evidence of diseases of retina or choroid.

Causes

Consecutive optic atrophy is caused by:
- Degenerative diseases of retina such as retinitis pigmentosa, pathological myopia
- Inflammatory diseases of retina and choroid such as chorioretinitis
- Vascular diseases of the retina such as central retinal artery occlusion, central retinal vein occlusion.

Glaucomatous Optic Atrophy

Glaucomatous optic atrophy is described in Chapter 9.4 'Primary Open-angle Glaucoma'.

Pathological Classification

Depending on the gliosis and the pathological process following the destruction of the retinal ganglion cells optic atrophy is classified into following.

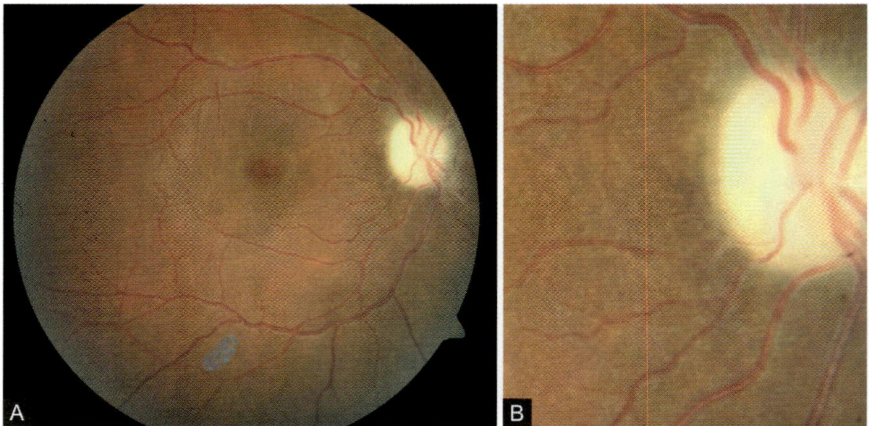

FIGS 12.5.2A and B: Secondary optic atrophy

Ascending optic atrophy: It is seen in diseases involving the retina, choroid and optic disk, and the destruction of axons of optic nerve ascends from optic disk to lateral geniculate body. It is characterized by gliosis in excess of the destruction of the axons of the optic nerve. It is responsible for secondary optic atrophy and consecutive optic atrophy.

Descending optic atrophy: It is seen in diseases involving the optic tract, optic chiasm and retrolaminar portion of the optic nerve, and the destruction of the ganglions of the optic nerve descend toward optic disk from optic tract, optic chiasm or retrolaminar portion of the optic nerve.

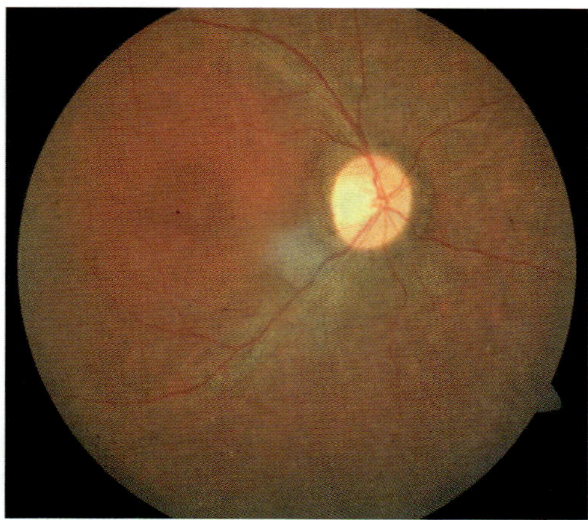

FIG. 12.5.3: Consecutive optic atrophy

Since this type of descending degeneration of the axons of the optic nerve is slow, the astrocytes replacing them arrange in a uniform pattern called columnar gliosis and the gliosis is uniform, and in proportion to destruction of the axons. It is responsible for primary optic atrophy.

Cavernous optic atrophy: It is seen in diseases causing chronic vascular insufficiency of the optic nerve, i.e. chronic glaucoma. It is characterized by negligible amount of gliosis and macular degeneration of the glial tissue resulting in the formation of lacunae.

CLINICAL FEATURE

The clinical features depend on the cause of optic atrophy. The clinical features of optic atrophy are diminution of vision of variable degree, relative afferent pupillary pathway defect, pallor of the optic disk and characteristic visual field defects.

DIFFERENTIAL DIAGNOSIS

Pallor of the optic disk seen in optic atrophy, should be differentiated from other causes of pale optic disk such as:

- Axial myopia
- Congenital anomalies of the optic disk such as optic nerve hypoplasia, myelinated nerve fibers, optic disk coloboma, optic disk pit and congenital tilted disk syndrome.

INVESTIGATION

Investigations depend on the medical history and findings of clinical examination. Investigations carried out are:

- Imaging procedures such as computed tomography (CT) or magnetic resonance imaging (MRI) to rule out intracranial space occupying lesions
- Hematological assessment such as total count, differential count, blood sugar, Venereal Disease Research Laboratory (VDRL) test to rule out syphilis, vitamin B_{12} assay, etc.

TREATMENT

There is no effective proven treatment for optic atrophy as optic nerve will not regenerate once damaged. The principle of treatment is to prevent the development of optic atrophy by treatment of underlying causative disease.

For hand written fundus diagrams of various types of optic atrophy are described in detail in Chapter 11 'Examination of Retina' in Author's textbook *'Clinical Methods in Ophthalmology'.*

GIST BOX 12.5

- Optic atrophy is defined as degeneration of the axons of the optic nerve and loss of function of the optic nerve as a result of lesions of the anterior visual pathway extending from retinal ganglion cell layer to lateral geniculate body resulting in loss of retinal ganglion cells.
- It is not a disease proper, but it is the end result of various pathologic processes involving the anterior visual pathway, which result in loss of retinal ganglion cells.
- Primary optic atrophy occurs without antecedent swelling of optic disk.
- Secondary optic atrophy occurs with antecedent swelling of optic disk as a result of long-standing disk edema. Since it is commonly seen following papilledema or papillitis, it is called postpapilledema optic atrophy or post-neuritic optic atrophy.
- Consecutive optic atrophy occurs as a consequence of destruction of the ganglion cells of the retina by diseases of the retina and choroid.

CHAPTER

12.6 Optic Nerve Tumors

Optic nerve tumors are broadly classified into primary and secondary tumors.

PRIMARY OPTIC NERVE TUMOR

Tumors arising in the optic nerve or in the meningeal sheaths covering the optic nerve are called primary tumors of the optic nerve. Optic nerve glioma and optic nerve sheath meningioma are the most common primary tumors of the optic nerve.

Optic Nerve Glioma

Optic nerve glioma is the most common primary tumor of the optic nerve. It is a benign tumor of the optic nerve commonly arising from the astrocytes. It usually affects children in the first decade, more commonly affecting girls.

Optic nerve glioma may occur in association with neurofibromatosis type 1. About 30% of patients with neurofibromatosis type 1 show optic nerve gliomas.

It presents as gradually progressive loss of vision followed by proptosis. Optic disk examination shows disk edema in the initial phase and optic atrophy later in the disease.

Diagnosis is by clinical presentation and by computed tomography (CT) scan findings, which shows fusiform enlargement of the optic nerve.

Treatment depends on the growth of the tumor. Tumors showing slow growth without causing any visual symptoms do not require treatment and they are followed up by frequent examinations. Tumors increasing in size or those causing visual symptoms are treated by surgical resection. Tumors with intracranial extension, where surgical resection is not possible, are treated by radiotherapy and chemotherapy.

Malignant Glioma

Malignant glioma of the optic nerve is relatively rare, but aggressive and fatal tumor. It arises from malignant astrocytes. It usually affects middle-aged adults unlike that of benign glioma, which affects children.

It usually affects the intracranial portion of the optic nerve and spreads rapidly to involve the surrounding structures.

It presents with rapidly progressive loss of vision over a period of 8–10 weeks unlike that of benign glioma, which causes gradually progressive loss of vision. Neurological abnormalities such as ophthalmoplegia, convergence and gaze abnormalities are more commonly seen with malignant glioma. Malignant glioma is associated with a mortality of almost 100%.

Optic Nerve Sheath Meningioma

Optic nerve sheath meningioma is the second most common tumor of the optic nerve. It is a benign tumor arising from meningothelial cells of the arachnoid villi. It is most commonly seen in middle-aged females.

The clinical features of optic nerve sheath meningioma are characterized by triad of gradually progressive loss of vision, optociliary shunt vessels and optic atrophy.

Treatment is similar to optic nerve glioma. Treatment depends on the growth of the tumor. Tumors showing slow growth without causing any visual symptoms do not require any treatment and they are followed up by frequent examinations. Tumors increasing in size or those causing visual symptoms are treated by surgical resection. Tumors where surgical resection is not possible are treated by radiotherapy.

SECONDARY OPTIC NERVE TUMOR

Secondary optic nerve tumors are because of extension of the tumors from surrounding structures. Most common secondary tumors of the optic nerve are because of extension of intraocular tumors such as retinoblastoma, malignant melanoma, extension of the intracranial tumors and metastasis of hematopoietic malignancies, e.g. leukemia, lymphoma, etc.

GIST BOX 12.6

- Optic nerve glioma is the most common primary tumor of the optic nerve. It is a benign tumor of the optic nerve commonly arising from the astrocytes. It usually affects children in the first decade, more commonly affecting girls.
- Malignant glioma of the optic nerve is relatively rare, but aggressive and fatal tumor. It arises from malignant astrocytes. It usually affects middle-aged adults unlike that of benign glioma, which affects children.
- Optic nerve sheath meningioma is the second most common tumor of the optic nerve. It is a benign tumor arising from meningothelial cells of the arachnoid villi.
- Most common secondary tumors of the optic nerve are because of extension of intraocular tumors such as retinoblastoma, malignant melanoma, extension of the intracranial tumors and metastasis of hematopoietic malignancies such as leukemia and lymphoma.

FREQUENTLY ASKED QUESTIONS (FAQs)

*Short Answers

1. Myelinated nerve fibers.
2. Optic disk coloboma.
3. Differential diagnosis of papilledema.
4. Pseudopapilledema.
5. Primary optic atrophy.
6. Secondary optic atrophy.
7. Consecutive optic atrophy.

**Short Essays

1. Retrobulbar neuritis.
2. Neuroretinitis.
3. Ischemic optic neuropathy.
4. Toxic amblyopia/neuropathy.
5. Traumatic optic neuropathy.
6. Stages of papilledema.
7. Optic atrophy.
8. Classify optic atrophy.

***Long Essays

1. Define optic neuritis. Describe etiology, clinical features and management of optic neuritis.
2. Define papilledema. Describe etiology, clinical features and management of papilledema.

BIBLIOGRAPHY

1. Agarwal AK, Yadav P, Sharma RK, et al. Papilloedema (Choked Disc). Indian Academy of Clinical Medicine. 2000;1(3).
2. Agarwal S, Agarwal A, Apple DJ, Agarwal A, Alió JL, Pandey SK, Buratto L (Eds). Textbook of Ophthalmology, vol. 1. New Delhi: Jaypee Brothers Medical Publishers (P) Ltd; 2002.
3. Arnold AC. Ischemic optic neuropathy. In: Miller NR, Newman NJ, Biousse V, Kerrison JB (Eds). Walsh & Hoyt's Clinical Neuro-ophthalmology, 2nd edition. Philadelphia: Lippincott Williams & Wilkins; 2007.
4. Atkins EJ, Bruce BB, Newman NJ, et al. Treatment of nonarteritic anterior ischemic optic neuropathy. Surv Ophthalmol. 2010;55(1):47-63.
5. Bansal S, Dabbs T, Long V. Pseudo-Foster Kennedy Syndrome due to unilateral optic nerve hypoplasia: a case report. J Med Case Rep. 2008;2:86.
6. Borchert M, Garcia-Filion P. The syndrome of optic nerve hypoplasia. Curr Neurol Neurosci Rep. 2008;8(5):395-403.
7. Brodsky MC. Congenital anomalies of the optic disc. In: Miller NR, Newman NJ, Biousse V, Kerrison JB (Eds). Walsh & Hoyt's Clinical Neuro-ophthalmology, 2nd edition. Philadelphia: Lippincott Williams & Wilkins; 2007.
8. Brodsky MC. Congenital optic disc anomalies. In: Yanoff M, Duker JS (Eds). Ophthalmology, 3rd edition. China: Mosby; 2008.
9. Chaddah MR, Khanna KK, Chawla GD. Optic atrophy (review of 100 cases). Indian J Ophthalmol. 1971;19(4):172-6.

10. Guercio JR, Balcer LJ. Inflammatory optic neuropathies and neuroretinitis. In: Yanoff M, Duker JS (Eds). Ophthalmology, 3rd edition. China: Mosby; 2008.
11. Hoorbakht H, Bagherkashi F. Optic neuritis, its differential diagnosis and management. Open Ophthalmol J. 2012;6:65-72.
12. Man PY, Turnbull DM, Chinnery PF. Leber hereditary optic neuropathy. J Med Genet. 2002;39(3):162-9.
13. Shams PN, Plant GT. Optic neuritis: a review. Int MS J. 2009;16(3):82-9.
14. Sarma CM. Quinine amblyopia. Indian J Ophthalmol. 1972;20(4):187-8.
15. Sharma P, Sharma R. Toxic optic neuropathy. Indian J Ophthalmol. 2011;59(2):137-41.
16. Spoor TC. Traumatic optic neuropathies. In: Yanoff M, Duker JS (Eds). Ophthalmology, 3rd edition. China: Mosby; 2008.
17. Tarabishy AB, Alexandrou TJ, Traboulsi EI. Syndrome of myelinated retinal nerve fibers, myopia and amblyopia: a review. Surv Ophthalmol. 2007;52(6):588-96.
18. Voss E, Raab P, Trebst C, et al. Clinical approach to optic neuritis: pitfalls, red flags and differential diagnosis. Ther Adv Neurol Disord. 2011;4(2):123-34.
19. Vuori ML, Mäntyjärvi M. Tilted disc syndrome may mimic false visual field deterioration. Acta Ophthalmol. 2008:86(6):622-5.

SECTION 13

Lacrimal System

CHAPTER

13.1 Anatomy of Lacrimal System

Lacrimal system consists of secretory part including main lacrimal gland and accessory lacrimal gland, which secrete tears; and drainage part including punctum, canaliculi, lacrimal sac and nasolacrimal duct (NLD) that drain the tears (Fig. 13.1.1).

SECRETORY PART

Lacrimal Gland

Lacrimal gland is a serous acinous gland situated in the anterolateral part of the orbit. It consists of superior orbital part situated in the fossa for lacrimal gland on the orbital plate of frontal bone and inferior palpebral part situated in the upper eyelid. Lacrimal ducts of about 10–12 in number collect the secretions of the lacrimal gland and open onto the surface of the conjunctiva at the lateral part of the superior fornix.

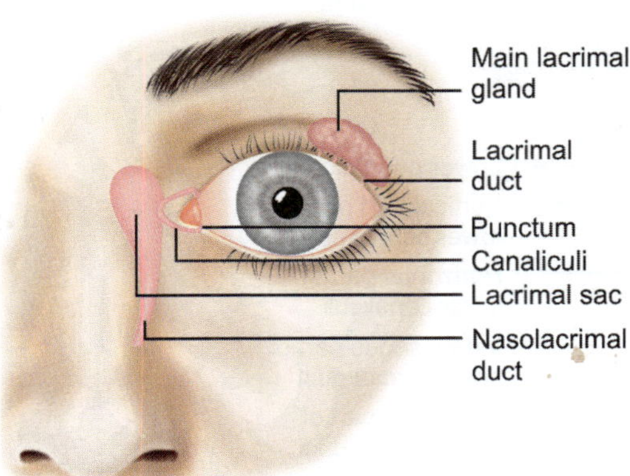

FIG. 13.1.1: Anatomy of lacrimal system

Accessory Lacrimal Glands of Krause and Wolfring

Accessory lacrimal glands of Krause are located deep in the stroma of the conjunctiva. There are about 40–42 glands of Krause in the superior fornix and 6–8 in the inferior fornix. Accessory lacrimal glands of Wolfring are situated along the upper border of tarsal plate. There are about 5 glands of Wolfring in upper eyelid and 3 in lower eyelid.

Both main lacrimal gland and accessory lacrimal glands secrete lacrimal secretions, which form the aqueous layer of the tear film. Main lacrimal glands are responsible for reflex secretions and accessory lacrimal glands are responsible for basal secretions.

Accessory lacrimal gland secretions are sufficient enough to meet the requirements of tear film even in the absence of main lacrimal gland.

Lacrimal gland gets its blood supply from lacrimal artery, a branch of ophthalmic artery. Nerve supply of lacrimal gland is from lacrimal nerve, a branch of trigeminal nerve. The secretomotor supply to lacrimal glands is from branches of facial nerve.

DRAINAGE PART*

The drainage part of the lacrimal system includes lacrimal punctum, lacrimal canaliculi, lacrimal sac and NLD (Fig. 13.1.2).

Lacrimal Punctum

Lacrimal punctum are two in number, situated one each in upper and lower eyelids. Lacrimal punctum are situated on the lid margin about 6 mm and 6.5 mm lateral to medial canthus in the upper and lower eyelids respectively.

Lacrimal Canaliculi

Lacrimal canaliculi extend from the punctum to lacrimal sac. Lacrimal canaliculi measure about 10 mm with vertical course of 1–2 mm and horizontal course of 6–8 mm. Superior and inferior canaliculi join together to form common canaliculi and open into the lateral wall of the lacrimal sac.

Lacrimal Sac

Lacrimal sac is situated in the lacrimal fossa or groove formed by lacrimal bone and frontal process of maxilla. It measures about 15 mm in length and 5 mm in breadth. The inner surface of the lacrimal sac is lined by stratified columnar epithelium containing mucus-secreting goblet cells. The lacrimal sac continues as NLD.

Nasolacrimal Duct

Nasolacrimal duct extends from lacrimal sac and opens into the inferior meatus of the nose. It measures about 15–20 mm in length and 3 mm in width. The NLD consists of intraosseous part lying in the bony nasolacrimal canal formed by maxilla and lacrimal bone, and intrameatal part lying in the inferior meatus. The intraosseous part measures about 13–14 mm and intrameatal part is about 5–6 mm.

Valves of the Lacrimal Drainage System

Valve of Rosenmüller is present at the site of entrance of common canaliculi into lacrimal sac. Valve of Hasner is present at the lower end of the NLD. The valves prevent the reflux entry of nasal secretions into the eyes.

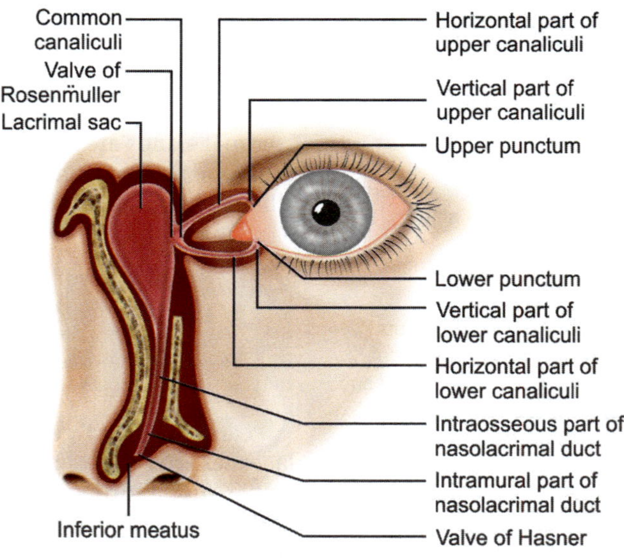

FIG. 13.1.2: Lacrimal drainage system

TEAR FILM**

Tear film is the liquid layer covering the cornea and conjunctiva. It is also called precorneal film or preocular film (Fig. 13.1.3).

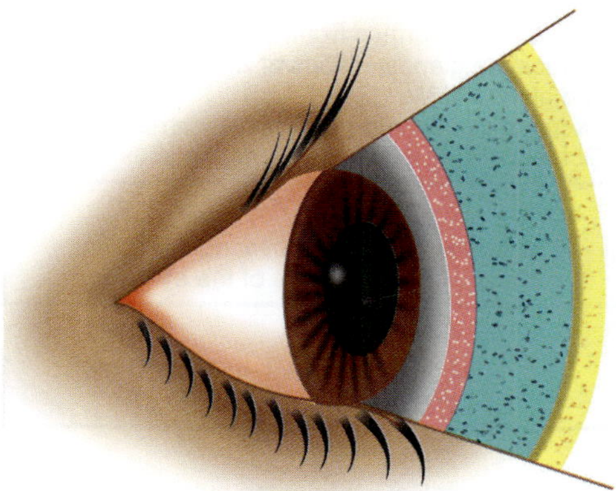

FIG. 13.1.3: Tear film

Functions of Tear Film*

- To provide a smooth optical refractive surface.
- To keep the ocular surface of cornea and conjunctiva moist.
- To provide protection against infection of the ocular surface by microbes because of presence of antimicrobial substances, e.g. lysozyme, lactoferrin and immunoglobulins.
- To wash away the metabolic waste products from the ocular surface.
- To provide glucose, oxygen and other essential nutrients to corneal epithelium.
- To lubricate the lid-cornea interface for smooth eyelid movements.

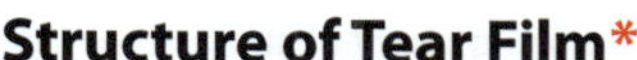

Structure of Tear Film*

Tear film consists of three layers (Fig. 13.1.4):

1. Outermost lipid layer.
2. Middle aqueous layer.
3. Inner mucus layer.

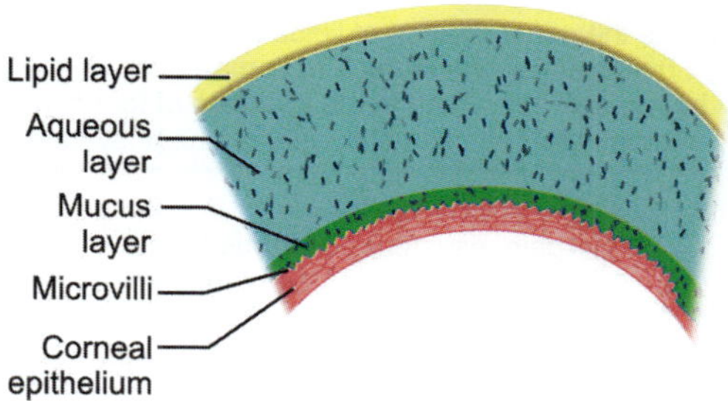

FIG. 13.1.4: Structure of tear film

Lipid Layer

Lipid layer is produced from meibomian glands, glands of Zeis and glands of Moll. It measures about 0.1 µm in thickness. The primary function of lipid layer is to prevent evaporation of tears.

Aqueous Layer

Aqueous layer is produced from lacrimal glands and accessory lacrimal glands. It measures about 7 µm in thickness, accounting for bulk of the tear film. It is responsible for all the functions of the tear film as mentioned above.

Mucus Layer

Mucus layer is produced from goblet cells, glands of Henle and glands of Manz. It measures about 0.05 µm in thickness. It is responsible for stability of the tear film by converting the hydrophobic surface of cornea to hydrophilic surface.

Physical Properties

- Thickness of tear film: 7–7.5 µm
- Volume of tear film: 8 mL
- Refractive index: 1.3
- Rate of tear secretion: 1.2 µL/min
- pH of tear film: 7–7.5.

Composition of Tear Film

- The lipid layer consists of fatty acids, cholesterol and lipids
- The aqueous layer consists of water accounting for about 98% and remaining 2% by solids, e.g. glucose, amino acids and electrolytes such as sodium, potassium, magnesium, calcium, etc.

The tear film is formed from secretions of the:
• Meibomian glands, glands of Zeis and glands of Moll
• Lacrimal glands and accessory lacrimal glands
• Goblet cells, glands of Henle and glands of Manz

↓

The tear film spreads covering the ocular surface with movements of the eyelids

↓

The tear film thins out first because of evaporation

↓

The lipid molecules from the outermost lipid layer migrate to the innermost mucus layer

↓

As the concentration of lipids increase in the mucus layer, the surface of cornea becomes hydrophobic resulting in the breaking of tear film, which is drained by the lacrimal drainage system

↓

Again, new tear film forms from the secretions of the glands

FIG. 13.1.5: Formation of tear film

- The mucus layer consists of mucins along with proteins, glucose and electrolytes.

Dynamics of Tear Film

Normal healthy ocular surface requires normal tear film, which depends on formation, retention and elimination of tear film. The formation of tear film is shown in Figure 13.1.5.

The rate of tear secretion is normally 1.2 μL/min. This rate is increased in cases of hyperlacrimation. The turnover rate of tear film is about 5 minutes. The tears reach the medial canthus and get collected as lacus lacrimalis. The tears collected in the lacus lacrimalis are drained by lacrimal drainage system by lacrimal pump mechanism. The lacrimal pump mechanism was proposed by Jones, which explains the drainage of tears by blinking movements of the eyelids.

Lacrimal Pump Mechanism (Fig. 13.1.6)

Closure of the eyelids during blinking results in contraction of preseptal and pretarsal fibers of orbicularis oculi, causing shortening of the canaliculi and distension of the lacrimal sac

↓

Entry of tears into lacrimal sac

↓

Opening of the eyelids during blinking results in relaxation of the preseptal and pretarsal fibers of orbicularis oculi causing collapse of the lacrimal sac

↓

Drainage of tears into nasolacrimal duct

FIG. 13.1.6: Lacrimal pump mechanism

GIST BOX 13.1

- Lacrimal system consists of secretory part including main lacrimal gland and accessory lacrimal gland, which secrete tears; and drainage part including punctum, canaliculi, lacrimal sac and nasolacrimal duct that drain tears.
- Tear film is the liquid layer covering the cornea and conjunctiva. It is also called precorneal film or preocular film. Tear film consists of three layers, i.e. outermost lipid layer, middle aqueous layer and inner mucus layer.

CHAPTER

13.2 Congenital Diseases of Lacrimal System

EMBRYOLOGY OF LACRIMAL SYSTEM

Lacrimal gland develops from surface ectoderm differentiating from solid epithelial cords of conjunctiva arising from the superolateral side.

The development of lacrimal drainage system begins as ectodermal invagination resulting in the formation of solid cord of ectoderm, which gets canalized by 7–8 months except for the valve of Hasner.

CONGENITAL ANOMALIES OF LACRIMAL SYSTEM

Anomalies of Lacrimal Gland

Congenital absence of the lacrimal gland is called alacrima. Lacrimal gland fistula, displacement of lacrimal gland leading to ectopic lacrimal gland and aberrant lacrimal gland are some of the congenital anomalies of lacrimal gland.

Patients with absence of lacrimal gland present with absence of reflex tear secretion; hence there will be absence of tears while crying. Usually, this will not develop dry eye because of presence of normal basal secretions by accessory lacrimal glands.

Anomalies of Lacrimal Punctum

Congenital atresia or absence of punctum and supernumerary or double punctum are some of the common congenital anomalies of the lacrimal punctum.

Anomalies of Lacrimal Canaliculi

Congenital stenosis or failure of canalization of the canaliculi is the most common anomaly of lacrimal canaliculi.

Anomalies of Lacrimal Sac

Congenital dacryocystocele, congenital fistula of lacrimal sac and congenital diverticulum are some of the common congenital anomalies of lacrimal sac.

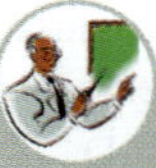

Dacryocystocele

Dacryocystocele is also called amniocele or mucocele. It is also called amniocele, as the amniotic fluid, which enters the lacrimal sac before birth gets accumulated in the lacrimal sac because of non-patent lacrimal drainage system.

Dacryocystocele is the cystic swelling because of distension of the lacrimal sac as a result of obstruction of the lacrimal sac proximally at the common canaliculi and distally at the nasolacrimal duct. It presents as a bluish swelling in medial-to-medial canthus present at birth. Dacryocystocele may be a secondary infection, leading to acute dacryocystitis.

Contd...

Contd...

Dacryocystocele has to be differentiated from other swellings that are seen in medial-to-medial canthus such as capillary hemangioma, dermoid cyst and encephalocele.

Congenital dacryocystocele may be associated with extension to nasal cavity and when the association is bilateral, it can cause neonatal respiratory distress, as neonates are nasal breathers.

Treatment is by conservative methods, i.e. lacrimal sac massage and observation for first 6 months. Surgical management in the form of probing is indicated in cases not responding to medical line of management. Endoscopic marsupialization of the nasal cyst is required in cases with nasal extension.

Anomalies of Nasolacrimal Duct

Incomplete canalization of the nasolacrimal duct (NLD) is the common congenital anomaly of the lacrimal system.

*Congenital Nasolacrimal Duct Obstruction (Dacryostenosis)**

Congenital NLD obstruction is also called dacryostenosis. It is the most common congenital anomaly of the common lacrimal system and is the most common cause of epiphora or watering in children.

It is because of failure of canalization of the NLD, which normally occurs by 8 months of gestation. Obstruction can be membranous occlusion or bony occlusion. The common cause is membranous occlusion by the imperforate valve of Hasner at the lower end of the NLD.

Up to 50–70% of newborns are born with imperforate valve of Hasner at the lower end of the nasolacrimal duct. Up to 70% of these patients undergo spontaneous resolution by 3 months of age and up to 90% by 1 year of age.

The affected children present with watering with or without mucoid discharge. The discharge may be mucopurulent or purulent in cases of secondary bacterial infection.

Though congenital nasolacrimal duct obstruction at birth is very common, symptoms of watering are seen only in about 5% of cases.

Treatment

Treatment is by conservative methods, i.e. lacrimal sac massage and observation for first 6 months. Surgical management in the form of probing is indicated in cases not responding to medical line of management. The treatment is described in detail under the treatment of congenital dacryocystitis.

*Congenital Dacryocystitis****

Definition

Inflammation of lacrimal sac as a result of congenital nasolacrimal obstruction seen in children is called congenital dacryocystitis.

The word congenital dacryocystitis is a misnomer, as the condition though called congenital, is not present at birth; but develops after birth and is not inflammation of the lacrimal sac, but is the infection of the retained secretions within the lacrimal sac.

Etiopathogenesis

Congenital dacryocystitis results because of infection of the lacrimal sac secretions. Stasis of secretions occur in the lacrimal sac as a result of congenital NLD obstruction. The common cause for this is the membranous occlusion by the imperforate valve of Hasner at the lower end of the NLD.

Staphylococcus aureus (S. aureus), Haemophilus influenzae (H. influenzae), Pneumococci and β-hemolytic streptococci are the common causative organisms for congenital dacryocystitis. Though congenital nasolacrimal obstructions are seen in 50–70% of neonates at birth, congenital dacryocystitis is seen only in 5% of them.

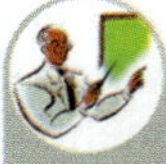

Congenital dacryocystitis usually presents as chronic dacryocystitis.

Acute variety of congenital dacryocystitis is very rare, accounting for < 1%. It is a serious condition because of the risk of spread of infection to the orbit resulting in orbital cellulitis, as the orbital septum is poorly developed in infants.

Clinical features

Chronic dacryocystitis is the most common type of presentation. Persistent epiphora (watering), mucoid or mucopurulent discharge from the eye and positive regurgitation test in the form of regurgitation of mucoid or mucopurulent discharge on applying pressure over the lacrimal sac area are the common features.

The initial symptom of congenital dacryocystitis is persistent epiphora. It starts from 2nd week, as the tears production from eyes starts only in 2nd week. Epiphora is followed by mucoid or mucopurulent discharge. Swelling of medial-to-medial canthus in the lacrimal sac area is seen in few infants.

Complications

- Acute dacryocystitis
- Lacrimal abscess
- Orbital cellulitis.

Differential diagnosis**

Congenital dacryocystitis has to be differentiated from:

- Ophthalmia neonatorum
- Congenital glaucoma.

Congenital dacryocystitis can be differentiated from ophthalmia neonatorum by negative regurgitation test and presence of clinical features of conjunctival inflammation, e.g. conjunctival congestion, chemosis of conjunctiva, etc. in ophthalmia neonatorum.

Congenital glaucoma can be differentiated from congenital dacryocystitis by the presence of other signs such as corneal edema, buphthalmos and raised intraocular pressure.

Investigations

Diagnosis of congenital dacryocystitis is done mainly by the presence of characteristic clinical features. Diagnosis can be confirmed by simple clinical tests, e.g. fluorescein dye disappearance test.

Treatment**

Conservative line of management

Conservative line of management is the treatment of choice for congenital dacryocystitis, as up to 90–95% of cases resolve spontaneously by 1 year of age. Conservative line of management is done by:

- Lacrimal sac massage
- Antibiotic eyedrops
- Lacrimal syringing.

Lacrimal sac massaging and antibiotic eyedrops instillation: Are done within the first 2 months of age. Lacrimal sac massaging acts by increasing the hydrostatic pressure within the lacrimal sac and opens up membranous lacrimal obstruction, which is the most common type of nasolacrimal obstruction. Lacrimal sac massaging is done three to four times per day. Topical antibiotic eyedrops are indicated in cases with mucopurulent discharge. The preferred antibiotic eyedrops are tobramycin, moxifloxacin, etc.

Lacrimal syringing: Can be done once the child crosses 2 months of age. Lacrimal syringing acts in a similar way to lacrimal sac massage by increasing the pressure within the lacrimal sac. Lacrimal syringing can be repeated once in a week.

Surgical management

Surgical management is indicated after the child reaches 6 months of age. Some ophthalmologists prefer to wait till child reaches 1 year of age continuing the conservative line of treatment. The surgical options are:

- Probing
- Silicone tube intubation
- Balloon catheter dilatation
- Dacryocystorhinostomy (DCR).

Probing**

Probing is the surgical treatment of choice for treatment of congenital dacryocystitis. It has got success rate of up to 95%. Younger the age of the patient, better are the results.

Probing is done between 6 months and 1 year of age. Early probing is indicated in children presenting with more symptoms and in those who require some other intraocular surgeries, e.g. cataract surgery. Probing after 18 months of age is associated with high failure rate.

Procedure

Probing is done by passing a Bowman's lacrimal probe through the punctum into nasolacrimal duct. It is done under short general anesthesia. Probing is done through upper punctum to prevent any irreversible damage, which may be caused by surgical trauma to lower punctum, as lower punctum drains about 90% of the tears.

A Bowman's lacrimal probe is passed through the upper punctum into the lacrimal sac along the direction of the lacrimal canaliculi. The probe is advanced till the probe touches the lacrimal bone, which is felt as hard stop. Then the probe is passed downward and laterally breaking any obstruction along the nasolacrimal duct. Lacrimal syringing is performed to confirm the patency of the nasolacrimal duct. It can be repeated after 2–3 months in cases of failure. Failure rate of probing is about 5–10%.

Silicone tube intubation and balloon catheter dilatation: These are done in children who present after 18 months of age when failure rates of probing is high or in cases of failed probing even on second time. Silicone tube stents are retained for at least 6 months.

Dacryocystorhinostomy: It is similar to that in adults is done in cases presenting after 4 years of age or in cases where probing, silicone tube intubation and balloon catheter dilatation are failed. DCR is usually performed after 4 years of age to allow normal anatomical development of the facial structures. DCR is usually difficult below 4 years of age because of the poor anatomical delineation of structures.

Management of Complications

Acute dacryocystitis is very rare, but potentially it is a dangerous complication because of the risk of spreading to orbit resulting in orbital cellulitis and cavernous sinus thrombosis, as the orbital septum is poorly developed in infants. Acute dacryocystitis has to be treated aggressively with intravenous (IV) antibiotics.

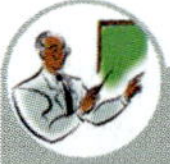

Summary of Management of Congenital Nasolacrimal Obstruction

Age of child	*Procedure*
< 2 month	Lacrimal sac massage and antibiotic eyedrops
2–6 month	Lacrimal sac massage, antibiotic eyedrops and lacrimal syringing
6–18 month	Probing
18 month to 4 year	Silicone tube intubation and balloon catheter dilatation
> 4 year	Dacryocystorhinostomy

Note: Children presenting with obstruction in the upper part of the lacrimal drainage pathway, e.g. punctual atresia or stenosis of canaliculi are treated by conjunctivo-canaliculocystorhinostomy or by insertion of prosthesis, e.g. Lester Jones tube.

GIST BOX 13.2

- Congenital nasolacrimal duct obstruction is also called dacryostenosis. It is the most common congenital anomaly of the common lacrimal system and is the most common cause of epiphora or watering in children. Treatment is by conservative methods, i.e. lacrimal sac massage and observation for first 6 months. Surgical management in the form of probing is indicated in cases not responding to medical line of management.
- Inflammation of lacrimal sac as a result of congenital nasolacrimal obstruction seen in children is called congenital dacryocystitis.

CHAPTER

13.3 Inflammatory Diseases of Lacrimal System

The common inflammatory diseases of the lacrimal system are:

- *Dacryocystitis*: Inflammation of the lacrimal sac
- *Canaliculitis*: Inflammation of the canaliculi
- *Dacryoadenitis*: Inflammation of the lacrimal gland.

DACRYOCYSTITIS

Definition

Inflammation of the lacrimal sac is called dacryocystitis.

Classification

Based on the age of onset, dacryocystitis is classified into congenital dacryocystitis and adult dacryocystitis. Depending on the clinical features, adult dacryocystitis is classified into acute dacryocystitis and chronic dacryocystitis. Congenital dacryocystitis is described in detail under the Chapter 13.2 'Congenital Diseases of Lacrimal System'.

Adult Dacryocystitis

Definition

Inflammation of lacrimal sac in adults is called adult dacryocystitis.

> Lacrimal sac infections are very common, as the epithelium lining of the lacrimal sac is in continuity with conjunctiva on one side and nasal mucosa on the other side. Both conjunctiva and nasal mucosa are colonized by bacteria, which can reach the lacrimal sac because of continuity.

Classification

Based on the clinical presentation, adult dacryocystitis is classified into chronic dacryocystitis and acute dacryocystitis. Chronic dacryocystitis is the common mode of presentation of adult dacryocystitis.

*Chronic dacryocystitis****

Definition

Chronic inflammation of the lacrimal sac is called chronic dacryocystitis. The clinical features are as follows:

1. Chronic dacryocystitis of adults is commonly seen in middle-age group in the fourth decade.
2. It is more common in females probably because of narrow nasolacrimal duct (NLD).
3. It is more common on left side with less commonly affecting the right side, probably because the tears are drained with more ease on right side compared to left side, as the NLD and lacrimal fossa form a greater angle on the right side.

4. It is more common in white races and rare in black races because of presence of shorter, straighter and wider NLD in blacks.
5. It is more common in individuals with narrow facial configuration compared to those with broad face because of presence of narrow bony nasolacrimal canal in individuals with narrow face.
6. It is more common in people with nasal tumors, nasal polyps, deviated nasal septum, hypertrophied inferior nasal turbinate, etc. because of obstruction to nasolacrimal outflow.
7. The source of infection is from either conjunctival sac or from nasal cavity and the infection spreads to lacrimal sac because of continuity of the epithelium lining.
8. Bacteria are the most common causative agents; common bacteria causing dacryocystitis are *Staphylococcus epidermidis* (*S. epidermidis*), *Staphylococcus aureus* (*S. aureus*), *Pseudomonas*, *Pneumococcus*, *Propionibacterium* and *Escherichia coli* (*E.* coli). Granulomatous inflammations, e.g. tuberculosis, syphilis and fungi such as *Aspergillus*, *Candida* are rare cause of dacryocystitis.

Etiopathogenesis

The process of chronic dacryocystitis is shown in Figure 13.3.1.

Chronic Dacryocystitis is More Common in:

- White race
- Middle age
- Females
- Left side
- Narrow facial configuration
- Associated nasal diseases, e.g. nasal tumors.

Clinical features

The disease usually progresses in three stages:

1. *Stage of catarrhal dacryocystitis*: It presents with epiphora and mucoid or mucopurulent discharge characterized by conspicuous absence of pain, redness and edema in the lacrimal sac region (Fig. 13.3.2).

Stagnation and stasis of tears in lacrimal sac because of slowing or obstruction to lacrimal outflow

↓

Infection of the stagnant secretions leading to inflammation of the lacrimal sac

↓

Inflammatory edema and fibrosis further reduce the lacrimal outflow, leading to increased stagnation and stasis, which further leads to increased inflammation and the vicious cycle sets in

FIG. 13.3.1: Etiopathogenesis of chronic dacryocystitis

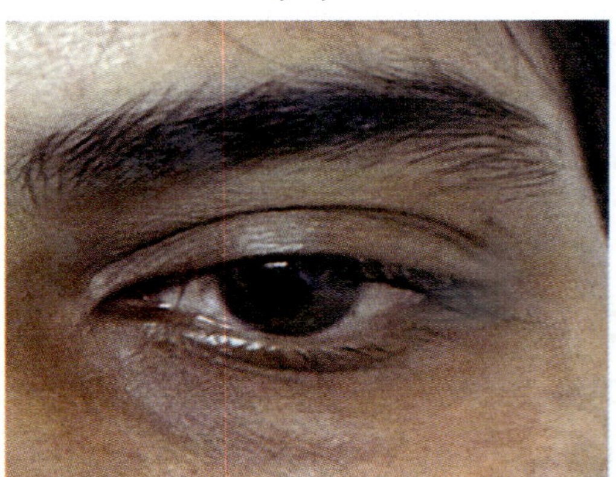

FIG. 13.3.2: Stage of chronic catarrhal dacryocystitis

2. *Stage of mucocele*: It is characterized by the formation of mucocele presenting as nontender cystic swelling with positive regurgitation test in the lacrimal sac region. It presents as epiphora and discharge from the eyes associated with swelling in the lacrimal sac region (Figs 13.3.3A and B).

   Stage of mucocele may become complicated because of secondary pyogenic infection resulting in the formation of

Encysted Mucocele

Encysted mucocele results from blockage of lacrimal sac at both the ends (above at the common canaliculi and below at the nasolacrimal duct). It presents as swelling in the lacrimal sac region with negative regurgitation test.

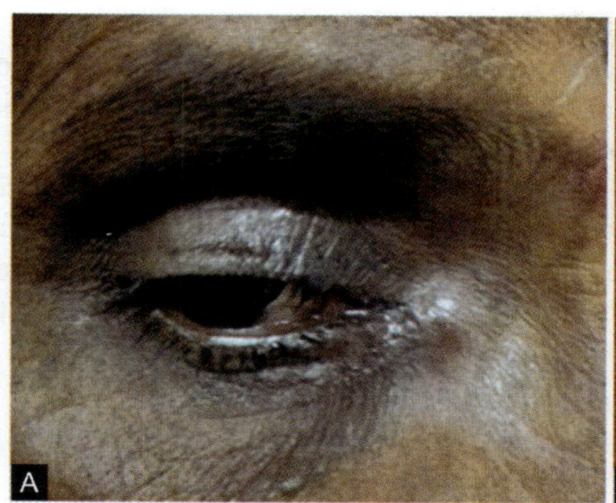

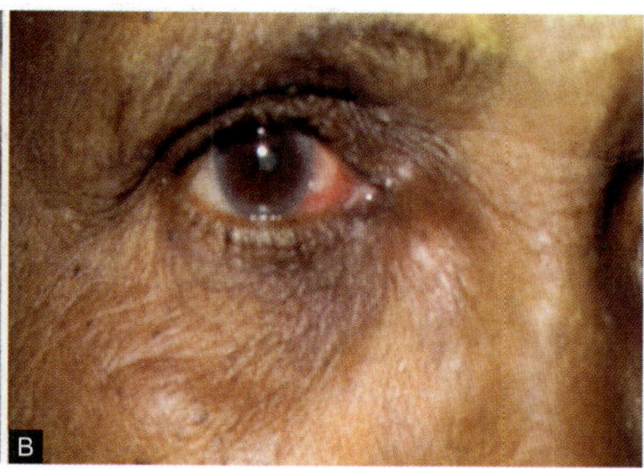

FIGS 13.3.3A and B: Stage of mucocele

pyocele similar to lacrimal abscess seen in the acute dacryocystitis.

3. *Stage of fibrosis*: It is the result of long-standing chronic inflammation or repeated acute exacerbations resulting in fibrosis of Sac. This stage presents as persistent epiphora with disappearance of the swelling.

Progression of chronic dacryocystitis

The progression of chronic dacryocystitis is shown in Figure 13.3.4.

Complications

- Acute dacryocystitis
- Intractable conjunctivitis
- Increased risk of hypopyon corneal ulcer following corneal abrasion
- Increased incidence of the postoperative endophthalmitis.

Investigations

Diagnosis of chronic dacryocystitis is usually made clinically; investigations are required to confirm the diagnosis and to find out the site of blockage in the lacrimal drainage pathway. The common investigations done are:

- Lacrimal syringing test
- Dacryocystography and dacryoscintigraphy
- Ear, nose and throat (ENT) examination to rule out nasal causes
- Investigations required before dacryocystectomy (DCT) or dacryocystorhinostomy (DCR) such as blood pressure measurement, blood sugar examination, bleeding time, clotting time, human immunodeficiency virus (HIV) and hepatitis B virus surface antigen (HBsAg).

Treatment

Surgery is the main treatment of chronic dacryocystitis. Medical management in the form of antibiotic eyedrops is advised to prevent acute exacerbation till surgery is done.

Dacryocystorhinostomy is the treatment of choice. DCT is done in cases where DCR cannot be done or DCR is contraindicated. Type of surgery depends on the site of obstruction in the lacrimal outflow tract (Table 13.3.1).

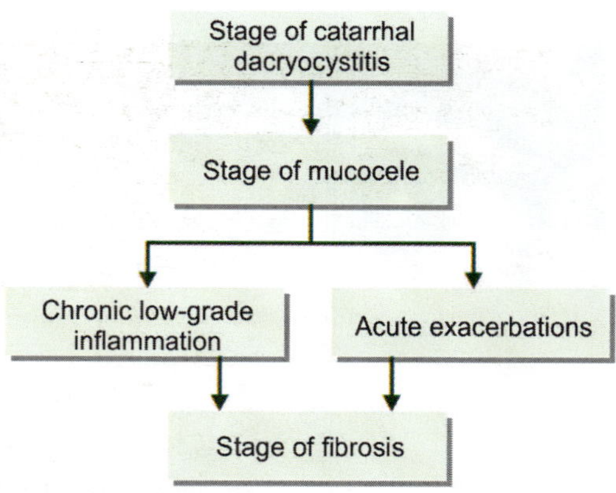

FIG. 13.3.4: Progression of chronic dacryocystitis

TABLE 13.3.1: Type of surgery on the basis of site of obstruction

Site of obstruction	*Surgery*
Lacrimal sac or nasolacrimal duct	Dacryocystorhinostomy
Common canaliculi	Canaliculodacryocystorhinostomy
Canaliculi or punctum	Conjunctivocanaliculocystorhinostomy

*Acute Dacryocystitis****

Definition

Acute suppurative inflammation of the lacrimal sac is called acute dacryocystitis.

Etiopathogenesis

The predisposing factors are same as for chronic dacryocystitis. Acute dacryocystitis can occur as a complication of chronic dacryocystitis or as primary acute infection because of infection from virulent pathogens. The common causative organisms are *Streptococcus pyogenes* (*S. pyogenes*), pneumococci and *S. aureus.* The source of infection is from paranasal sinuses and other surrounding structures. Ethmoiditis is a common source of infection.

Clinical features

Acute onset of pain, redness and swelling in the lacrimal sac region associated with epiphora are the initial presenting features of acute dacryocystitis.

The disease progresses to the stage of lacrimal abscess formation characterized by accumulation of pus in the lacrimal sac. The lacrimal abscess may burst open spontaneously resulting in the formation of lacrimal fistula.

Progression of acute dacryocystitis

1. Stage of acute inflammation (Figs 13.3.5A and B).
2. Stage of lacrimal abscess (Fig. 13.3.6).
3. Stage of lacrimal fistula.

Complications

- Acute conjunctivitis
- Preseptal cellulitis
- Orbital cellulitis
- Cavernous sinus thrombosis.

Differential diagnosis

Acute dacryocystitis has to be differentiated from pseudodacryocystitis. Inflammatory conditions of the structures surrounding lacrimal sac, i.e. acute ethmoiditis resembling the clinical picture of dacryocystitis are called pseudodacryocystitis. The differentiation can be made from absence of epiphora in pseudodacryocystitis. In doubtful cases, computed tomography

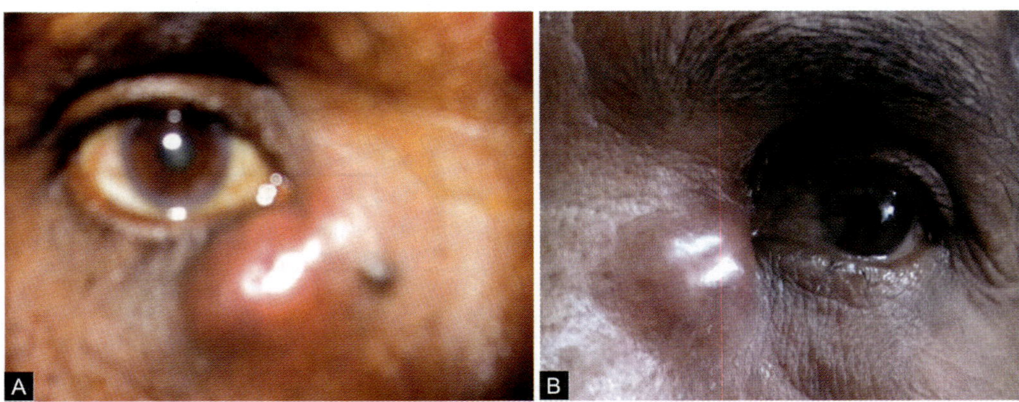

FIGS 13.3.5A and B: Acute dacryocystitis—stage of inflammation

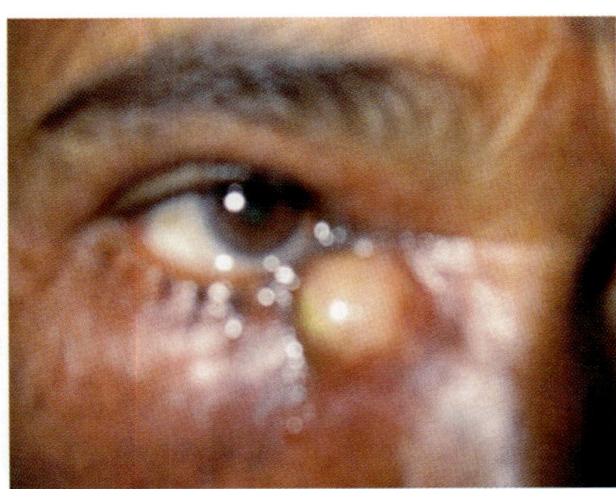

FIG. 13.3.6: Acute dacryocystitis—stage of lacrimal abscess

scan can be used to differentiate acute dacryocystitis from pseudodacryocystitis.

Investigations

The diagnosis is mainly clinical and the local investigation, for example, lacrimal syringing should be avoided, as it is very painful because of associated inflammation.

Treatment

Treatment is mainly by conservative methods and surgical treatment in the form of DCT or DCR should be avoided till the acute inflammation subsides.

Treatment is by topical antibiotic eyedrops, oral antibiotics and anti-inflammatory drugs. Intravenous antibiotics are indicated in patients with severe inflammation or with complications, e.g. orbital cellulitis. Lacrimal abscess, if seen in cases not responding to treatment is treated by incision and drainage.

Dacryocystorhinostomy**

Definition

Dacryocystorhinostomy is a surgical procedure done to re-establish the lacrimal drainage by connecting lacrimal sac to middle meatus of nose by making an ostium between lacrimal sac and nose (made by removing the lacrimal bone).

Indications*

Dacryocystorhinostomy is the surgery of choice except for the indications mentioned in DCT.

Types of Dacryocystorhinostomy

Lacrimal sac can be approached by three routes:

1. *Through canaliculi*: Canalicular DCR (laser DCR).
2. *Through skin over lacrimal sac area*: External DCR or conventional DCR.
3. *Through nose*: Nasal DCR (endonasal DCR).

External DCR has got more success rate compared to laser DCR and endonasal DCR. The success rate of external DCR is 90–95%.

Anesthesia for Dacryocystorhinostomy

Usually, it is done under local anesthesia. Local anesthesia is given by:

- Infiltration of the anesthetic agent along the skin incision over the lacrimal sac area
- Infratrochlear nerve block by inserting needle below trochlea
- Infraorbital nerve block by inserting the needle at the junction of inferior orbital margin with anterior lacrimal crest
- Anesthesia of nasal mucosa by packing nose with a gauze piece moistened with 4% lignocaine.

Steps of Surgery

1. Nasal package: Nose is packed with sterile gauze soaked in 4% lignocaine and adrenaline.
2. A straight vertical or curved incision is made within 3 mm or more than 8 mm medial to the inner canthus to avoid damage to angular vessels.

Incision for DCR or DCT should be made either within 3 mm or more than 9 mm medial-to-medial canthus, as normally angular vessels run between 3 and 9 mm medial-to-medial canthus.

3. Skin and fibers of orbicularis oculi are dissected to expose medial palpebral ligament. Below the medial palpebral ligament, lies the lacrimal sac. It is separated from medial wall and floor to expose the lacrimal fossa. The anterior lacrimal crest and the bone from the lacrimal fossa are removed.
4. Bowman's probe is introduced into the lacrimal sac and the sac is incised in an H-shaped manner to create two flaps.
5. A vertical incision is made in the nasal mucosa to create anterior and posterior flaps.
6. The posterior flaps and anterior flaps are sutured respectively.
7. The medial canthal tendon is resutured to periosteum and the skin incision is closed with interrupted sutures.

*Complications of Dacryocystorhinostomy**

- Hemorrhage from injury to angular vein or nasal mucosa is the most common intraoperative complication
- Blockage of ostium resulting in failure of the surgery is the most common late postoperative complication.

Cases with Failed DCR are Managed by:

- Repeat DCR
- Dacryocystorhinostomy with artificial implants, e.g. Pawar implant to prevent the closure of the ostium
- Lester Jones tube insertion.

Dacryocystectomy**

Definition

Dacryocystectomy is a surgical procedure where the lacrimal sac is removed completely.

*Indications**

- Elderly debilitated patient with shrunken and fibrosed sac
- Tumors or chronic granulomatous inflammations, e.g. tuberculosis, where sac has to be removed
- Nasal contraindications, e.g. atrophic rhinitis.

Anesthesia

Anesthesia is similar to DCR except anesthesia of nasal mucosa, which is not required.

Surgical Procedure

The surgical steps are similar to DCR till the exposure of the lacrimal sac. Once the lacrimal sac is exposed, it is cut and removed totally. Wound closure is similar to that of DCR.

Complications

- Intraoperative bleeding because of injury to angular vessels
- Recurrent dacryocystitis because of incomplete removal of lacrimal sac
- Persistent watering.

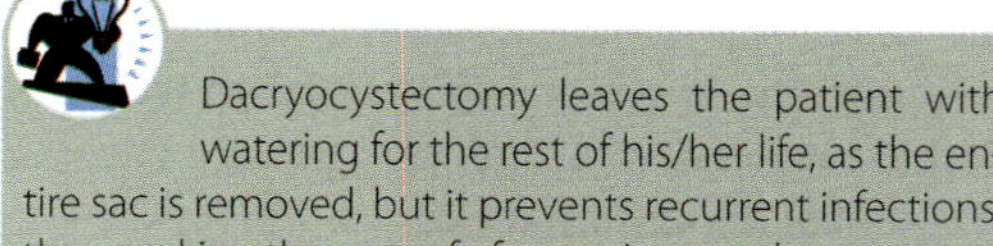

Dacryocystectomy leaves the patient with watering for the rest of his/her life, as the entire sac is removed, but it prevents recurrent infections; thus, making the eye safe for any intraocular surgeries.

CANALICULITIS*

Definition

Inflammation of the lacrimal canaliculi is called canaliculitis. It is a relatively rare condition and usually it presents as chronic inflammation.

Etiology

The most common causative agent is *Actinomyces israelii,* gram-positive anaerobic bacteria. The other causes include *Fusarium, Candida,* herpes simplex and *Propionibacterium.*

Clinical Features

Epiphora associated with mucoid or mucopurulent discharge is the presenting symptom. It can present as chronic mucopurulent or follicular conjunctivitis, which is not responding to treatment. On examination, the canaliculi show edema and erythema. Presence of pouting punctum with expression of discharge on applying pressure is, the characteristic feature of canaliculitis.

Complications

- Chronic intractable conjunctivitis
- Lacrimal stone or concretion formation.

Treatment

Treatment is by conservative management in the form of hot compress and topical antibiotic eyedrops and antibiotics according to the culture and sensitivity report.

Surgical treatment in the form of canaliculotomy is required particularly in cases associated with concretions. Canaliculotomy is done by incising the canaliculi from conjunctival side.

Dacryolith

Concretion in the nasolacrimal system is called dacryolith. It is also called lacrimal calculus or ophthalmolith.

Dacryoliths are seen in cases with chronic inflammation and obstruction of the lacrimal sac. They are caused by precipitation of calcium and phosphorus salts. Dacryolith presents as intermittent epiphora, canaliculitis and chronic dacryocystitis.

Treatment is done by surgical removal of the concretions.

DACRYOADENITIS*

Definition

Inflammation of the lacrimal gland is called dacryoadenitis.

Types

Dacryoadenitis is of two types:

1. Acute dacryoadenitis.
2. Chronic dacryoadenitis.

Acute Dacryoadenitis

Acute dacryoadenitis is inflammation of the lacrimal gland.

Etiopathogenesis

Acute dacryoadenitis is caused by obstruction of the lacrimal ductules and viral infections such as mumps, measles, influenza, mononucleosis, herpes and cytomegalovirus. Viral infections are responsible for dacryoadenitis in children. In adults, bacteria such as *Staphylococcus aureus, Neisseria gonorrhoeae* (*N. gonorrhoeae*) *Haemophilus influenzae* (*H. influenzae*) *and Chlamydia trachomatis* (*C. trachomatis*) are the usual causative agents.

The mode of spread of infection to the lacrimal gland is by hematogenous route, transneuronal, transconjunctival or by direct traumatic injury.

Clinical features

1. It presents as acute and painful swelling involving the upper and outer part of the orbit.
2. On examination, typical S-shaped swelling of the lid is seen because of swelling of the lateral one third of the upper eyelid. Conjunctiva may show congestion and chemosis in the upper and lateral palpebral conjunctiva.
3. Severe cases may present as eccentric proptosis with downward displacement of the globe.

Treatment

1. Acute dacryoadenitis because of viral infections is treated by symptomatic treatment in the form of hot compress and systemic anti-inflammatory drugs.
2. Acute dacryoadenitis because of bacterial infections are treated by systemic antibiotics, anti-inflammatory drugs and hot compress.

Chronic Dacryoadenitis

Chronic dacryoadenitis is chronic inflammation of the lacrimal gland.

Etiopathogenesis

Chronic dacryoadenitis is caused by chronic granulomatous inflammations such as tuberculosis, syphilis and autoimmune diseases such as sarcoidosis, Wegener's granulomatosis, Graves' disease, Sjögren's syndrome, etc.

Clinical features

- It presents as painless swelling of the lateral part of the upper eyelid
- Eccentric proptosis with downward displacement of the globe is seen in the severe cases.

Treatment

Management is by treatment of the underlying diseases such as tuberculosis and syphilis. Chronic dacryoadenitis caused by autoimmune diseases is treated by systemic steroids.

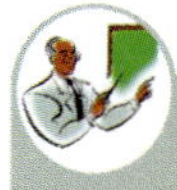

Mikulicz's Disease and Mikulicz's Syndrome*

Mikulicz's disease is a benign idiopathic disease characterized by bilateral enlargement of the lacrimal, parotid and salivary glands because of infiltration by lymphocytes.

Mikulicz's syndrome is bilateral enlargement of the lacrimal, parotid and salivary glands associated with systemic diseases such as tuberculosis, syphilis, sarcoidosis, leukemia, lymphosarcoma and Sjögren's syndrome.

GIST BOX 13.3

- Inflammation of the lacrimal sac is called dacryocystitis. Bacteria are the most common causative agents; common bacteria causing dacryocystitis are *Staphylococcus epidermidis, Staphylococcus aureus, Pseudomonas, Pneumococcus, Propionibacterium and E. coli.* Granulomatous inflammations, e.g. tuberculosis, syphilis and fungi such as *Aspergillus, Candida* are rare cause of dacryocystitis.
- Inflammation of the canaliculi is called canaliculitis. The most common causative agent is *Actinomyces israelii*, gram-positive anaerobic bacteria.
- Inflammation of the lacrimal gland is called dacryoadenitis. Acute dacryoadenitis is caused by viral infections, e.g. mumps, measles, influenza, mononucleosis, herpes and cytomegalovirus. Chronic dacryoadenitis is caused by chronic granulomatous inflammations, e.g. tuberculosis, syphilis, etc. and autoimmune diseases like sarcoidosis, Wegener's granulomatosis, Graves' disease, Sjögren's syndrome, etc.
- Dacryocystorhinostomy is a surgical procedure done to re-establish the lacrimal drainage by connecting lacrimal sac to middle meatus of nose by making an ostium between lacrimal sac and nose (made by removing the lacrimal bone).
- Dacryocystectomy is a surgical procedure, where the lacrimal sac is removed completely.

CHAPTER

13.4 Watery Eye

Watering from the eyes is a common symptom of the lacrimal system. It results from increased secretion of tears or due to decreased drainage of tears. The causes for watery eyes are included under two broad categories:

1. Hyperlacrimation.
2. Epiphora.

> Normally, the tear secretion rate (normal tear secretion rate is 1.2 μL/min) is equal to the rate of tear drainage and evaporation of tears. When the balance is disturbed either because of increased tear secretion or decreased drainage, tears overflow from the conjunctival sac resulting in watering eye.

Patients with watery eyes present with various symptoms, e.g. visual disturbances, ocular symptoms and watering from the eyes. The ocular symptoms may be due to any underlying disease responsible for watering the eyes.

HYPERLACRIMATION

Definition

Excessive secretion of lacrimal tears from lacrimal glands resulting in watering from the eyes with lacrimal drainage being normal is called hyperlacrimation.

Causes for Hyperlacrimation

1. Reflex hyperlacrimation, which occurs due to stimulation of the sensory nerve endings of trigeminal nerve is the common cause of hyperlacrimation. It occurs in a variety of the eye conditions such as trichiasis, entropion of eyelids and inflammatory diseases such as conjunctivitis, keratitis, episcleritis, scleritis, iridocyclitis, etc. Reflex lacrimation is because of reflex between the sensory trigeminal nerve and motor facial nerve.
2. Primary oversecretion of tears from the lacrimal glands is seen in inflammatory conditions, tumors of the lacrimal glands and cholinergic drugs because of stimulation of parasympathetic fibers.
3. Central hyperlacrimation is seen in supranuclear causes such as emotional stress and infranuclear causes such as aberrant regeneration of facial nerve.

EPIPHORA**

The word epiphora is derived from Greek word meaning downpour.

Definition

Epiphora refers to overflow of tears resulting in watering from the eyes because of obstruction in the lacrimal drainage system with secretion of tears being normal.

Causes for Epiphora*

The causes for epiphora may lie in punctum, canaliculi, lacrimal sac, nasolacrimal duct (NLD) or lacrimal pump.

Causes in Punctum

- Punctal obstruction because of congenital atresia or acquired stenosis following trauma, chronic use of drugs such as pilocarpine
- Punctal ectropion.

Causes in Canaliculi

Congenital stenosis or acquired stenosis following trauma and inflammation.

Causes in Lacrimal Sac

Congenital anomalies of lacrimal sac such as dacryocystocele and acquired causes such as dacryocystitis, lacrimal sac tumors, dacryolith, etc.

Causes in Nasolacrimal Duct

Congenital NLD obstruction and acquired causes such as inflammations, involutional stenosis and tumors.

Causes in Lacrimal Pump

Lacrimal pump weakness because of laxity of eyelids or weakness of orbicularis oculi.

Causes in Eyelids

Abnormalities in the eyelids such as ectropion and lagophthalmos.

EVALUATION AND INVESTIGATIONS

After thorough history regarding onset, duration, nature and associated symptoms, a patient with watering eye is evaluated below (Fig. 13.4.1).

Examination of the anterior segment of the eye to rule out:

- Causes for reflex hyperlacrimation
- Abnormalities of the eyelids as in ectropion, punctal ectropion or eversion and lagophthalmos

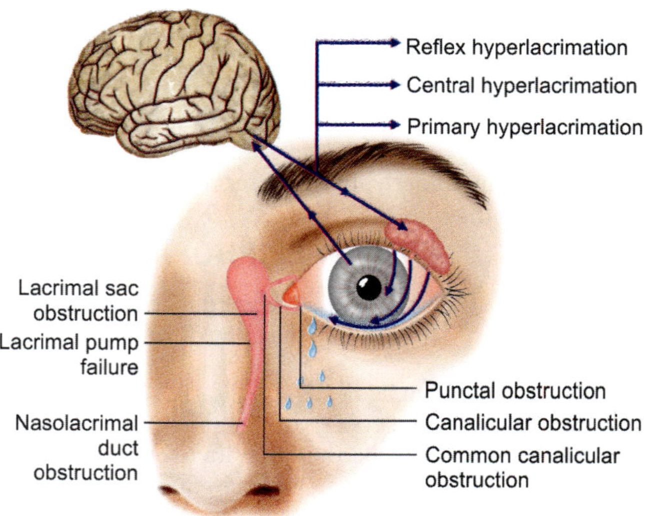

FIG. 13.4.1: Watery eye

- Lacrimal pump weakness because of laxity of the eyelids, weakness of orbicularis oculi
- Punctal abnormalities such as atresia of punctum, punctal ectropion
- Presence of swelling in the lacrimal sac indicating NLD obstruction.

Dye Disappearance Test

Fluorescein dye is instilled into conjunctival sac and tear meniscus is observed for disappearance of dye. Normally, no dye is seen in conjunctival sac after 5 minutes. Prolonged retention of the dye for more than 5 minutes indicates epiphora.

Regurgitation Test

Regurgitation test is done by applying pressure over the lacrimal sac area with either thumb or index finger. In cases with NLD obstruction such as chronic dacryocystitis, the contents of the sac regurgitate through the punctum.

Lacrimal Syringing Test*

Lacrimal syringing test is done to localize the site of obstruction in the lacrimal drainage system.

Procedure

Lacrimal syringing test is done under topical anesthesia by injecting normal saline into the lacrimal sac from lower or upper punctum with a lacrimal cannula fixed to syringe filled with saline. It is interpreted as follows:

- Saline is passing freely into the throat as seen by swallowing reflex and appreciation of salt taste by patient indicates normal patent lacrimal passage
- Fast regurgitation of clear fluid from same punctum indicates obstruction in same canaliculi (Fig. 13.4.2)
- Fast regurgitation of clear fluid from opposite punctum indicates obstruction at common canaliculi (Fig. 13.4.3)
- Slow regurgitation of mucoid or mucopurulent fluid from same and opposite punctum indicates obstruction in lacrimal sac or NLD (Fig. 13.4.4)

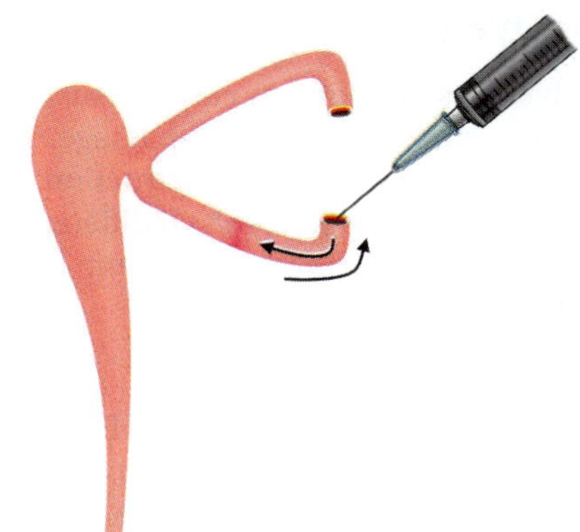

FIG. 13.4.2: Obstruction in the same canaliculi

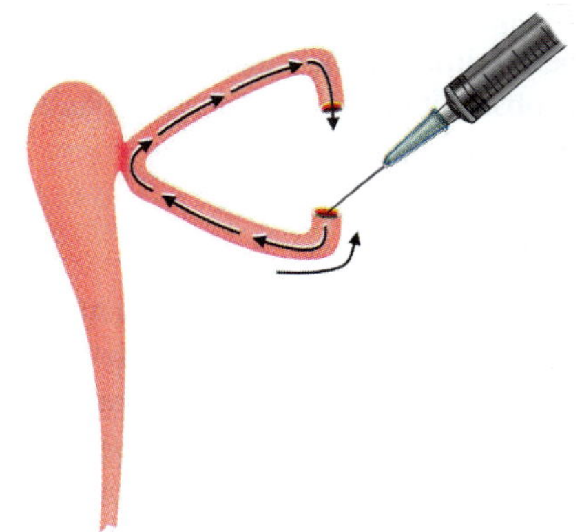

FIG. 13.4.3: Obstruction in the common canaliculi

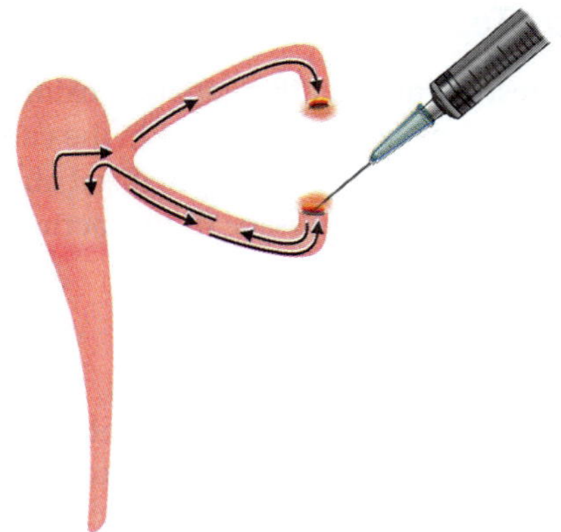

FIG. 13.4.4: Obstruction in the lacrimal sac

- Partial regurgitation of saline from punctum and partial saline going into throat indicates partial obstruction in the lacrimal passage.

Jones Dye Tests

Jones dye tests are done in cases of suspected partial obstruction of lacrimal passage. Jones test I differentiates partial obstruction from hyperlacrimation and Jones test II differentiates partial obstruction from lacrimal pump failure.

Jones Test I

Jones test I is done by instilling 2% fluorescein dye into conjunctival sac and placing a cotton bud in the inferior meatus. After 5 minutes, the cotton bud is inspected for staining with dye. Cotton bud stained with dye indicates that lacrimal passage is patent and the cause of watering is hyperlacrimation. A negative test indicates partial obstruction of the lacrimal passage or lacrimal pump failure.

Jones Test II

Jones test II is done in cases of negative Jones test I. Lacrimal syringing is done by following negative Jones test I. Cotton bud stained with dye after lacrimal syringing indicates partial obstruction of lacrimal passage. A negative Jones test II indicates lacrimal pump failure.

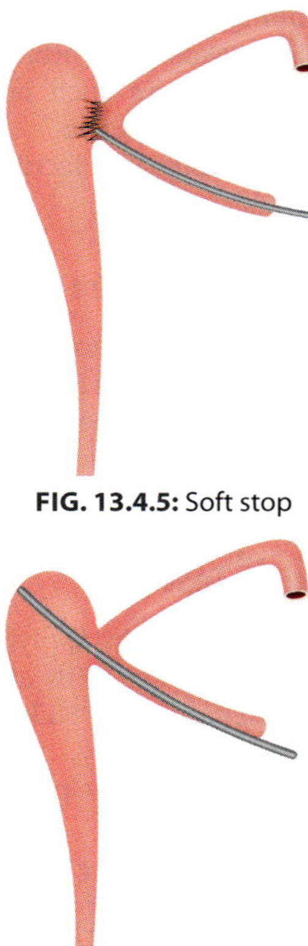

FIG. 13.4.5: Soft stop

FIG. 13.4.6: Hard stop

Probe Test

Probe test is done to differentiate proximal obstruction of the lacrimal passage in the canaliculi and common canaliculi from distal obstruction of the lacrimal passage in the lacrimal sac and NLD.

Procedure

A probe is passed into the lacrimal sac. Normally, probe can be advanced till it touches the medial wall of lacrimal sac and lacrimal bone, which is felt as hard stop. If the probe stops proximal to common canaliculi because of obstruction in canaliculi, soft stop is felt as the probe is pressed against the soft tissue of common canaliculus, lateral wall of lacrimal sac and medial wall of lacrimal sac before touching the lacrimal bone. Soft stop indicates obstruction in the canaliculi or common canaliculi (Figs 13.4.5 and 13.4.6).

Dacryocystography

Dacryocystography is performed by injecting radiopaque dye such as lipiodol into lacrimal passage and taking X-ray to visualize the passage of the dye. Dacryocystography localizes the site of obstruction in the lacrimal passage.

Dacryoscintigraphy

Dacryoscintigraphy is performed by instilling radioactive tracer such as technetium into conjunctival sac. The passage of the radioactive tracer is seen by gamma camera. Dacryoscintigraphy localizes the site of obstruction in the lacrimal passage.

TREATMENT OF WATERING EYE*

Hyperlacrimation is treated by treatment of the underlying cause:

1. Treatment of epiphora depends on the site of obstruction.
2. Obstruction in the punctum is treated by:
   - Punctoplasty and silicone tube intubation
   - Lester Jones tube insertion
   - Conjunctivocanaliculocystorhinostomy.
3. Obstruction in the canaliculi and common canaliculi is treated by:
   - Canaliculoplasty and silicone tube intubation
   - Canaliculodacryocystorhinostomy
   - Lester Jones tube insertion.
4. Obstruction in the lacrimal sac and NLD is treated by dacryocystorhinostomy.

GIST BOX 13.4

- Watering from the eyes is a common symptom of the lacrimal system. It results from increased secretion of tears or because of decreased drainage of tears.
- Excessive secretion of lacrimal tears from lacrimal glands resulting in watering from the eyes with lacrimal drainage being normal is called hyperlacrimation.
- Epiphora refers to overflow of tears resulting in watering from the eyes because of obstruction in the lacrimal drainage system with secretion of tears being normal.

CHAPTER

13.5 Dry Eye

International Dry Eye WorkShop has defined dry eye as a multifactorial disease involving tears and ocular surface accompanied by increased osmolarity of the tear film and inflammation of the ocular surface resulting in symptoms of ocular discomfort, disturbances in vision and tear film instability with potential damage to the ocular surface.

RISK FACTORS

- Increasing age, probably because of age-related decrease in the lacrimal secretions
- Postmenopausal women because of hormonal changes
- Autoimmune diseases because of infiltration of the lacrimal glands by the inflammatory cells resulting in lacrimal dysfunction
- Long-term contact lenses wear because of corneal hypoesthesia or decreased corneal sensation caused by it leading to reflex hyposecretion of tears
- Systemic anticholinergic drugs including antihistamines, antimuscarinic drugs, antiparkinsonian drugs, antidepressants, etc. that decrease tear production because of anticholinergic action
- Prolonged use of eyedrops (e.g. antiglaucoma drugs) containing preservatives such as benzalkonium chloride

History of Dry Eye

- Sjögren SC, a Swedish ophthalmologist, coined the term keratoconjunctivitis sicca describing the triad of dry eye, dry mouth and joint pain.
- Andrew de Roeth coined the term dry eye in the year 1950.
- National Eye Institute's definition of dry eye was framed in the year 1995, which defined dry eye as a disorder of tear film due to tear deficiency or excessive evaporation of tears resulting in damage to the ocular surface.
- International Dry Eye WorkShop revised the definition of National Eye Institute in the year 2007.

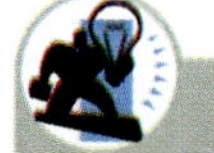

Dry eye disease or dry eye syndrome is one of the most commonly seen ocular diseases. About 25% of patients visit ophthalmologist for symptoms of dry eye.

Initially, dry eye was thought to be a disease involving the reduction of aqueous layer of tear film; the International Dry Eye WorkShop revised the definition to involve the role of inflammation of ocular surface and tear hyperosmolarity.

- Postcorneal surgeries such as keratoplasty, laser-assisted in situ keratomileusis (LASIK) because of damage to sensory nerve endings of V cranial nerve, which are afferent for lacrimal secretions
- Prolonged exposure to dry environment, wind, etc.
- Extensive viewing of computer screen, television, etc.
- Working environment with low humidity because of air conditioners (ACs).

CLASSIFICATION OF DRY EYE**

Dry eye is broadly classified into:
- Aqueous tear deficient dry eye
- Evaporative dry eye.

Aqueous Tear Deficient Dry Eye

Aqueous tear deficient dry eye is because of deficiency of aqueous layer of the tear film as a result of deficient lacrimal secretions. It is subdivided into:
- Sjögren's syndrome dry eye
- Non-Sjögren's syndrome dry eye.

Sjögren's Syndrome Dry Eye

Sjögren's syndrome is an autoimmune disease characterized by infiltration of lymphocytes in lacrimal glands and salivary glands resulting in aqueous deficient dry eye or keratoconjunctivitis sicca and dry mouth. Sjögren's syndrome may be primary or secondary.

Primary Sjögren's syndrome: It is characterized by dry eye and dry mouth and absence of systemic autoimmune diseases.

Secondary Sjögren's syndrome: It is characterized by dry eye and dry mouth associated with systemic autoimmune diseases, most commonly rheumatoid arthritis.

Non-Sjögren's Syndrome Dry Eye

Non-Sjögren's syndrome dry eye can result from the following conditions:
- Lacrimal gland dysfunction as a result of congenital causes such as congenital alacrima and acquired causes such as infections, inflammations, autoimmune diseases, tumors, trauma and surgical removal of the lacrimal gland
- Obstruction of the ducts of the lacrimal gland as in cicatricial conjunctivitis and trachoma
- Reflex hyposecretion because of defect in the afferent or efferent pathway as in surgeries of cornea such as refractive corneal surgeries, keratoplasty, Riley-Day syndrome
- Systemic anticholinergic drugs.

Evaporative Dry Eye

Evaporative dry eye is because of excessive evaporation of tears with normal lacrimal secretory function. The causes for evaporative dry eye are:
- Improper closure of the eyelids or improper lid-globe apposition as in proptosis, lagophthalmos, ectropion and symblepharon
- Meibomian gland dysfunction as seen in posterior blepharitis or meibomitis leading to deficiency of lipids in the tear film
- Mucin deficiency due to loss of goblet cells as in chemical burns, vitamin A deficiency, Stevens-Johnson syndrome and ocular cicatricial pemphigoid
- Ocular surface damage as in prolonged contact lens wear, epitheliopathies because of toxic causes such as prolonged use of eyedrops with preservatives and various types of keratoconjunctivitis.

PATHOGENESIS OF DRY EYE

Tear film instability again leads to increase in osmolarity of tear film, which in turn leads to activation of inflammation and it starts the vicious cycle (Fig. 13.5.1).

CLINICAL FEATURES

Symptoms

The symptoms of dry eye include dryness or grittiness of eyes, foreign body sensation, burning, redness and tiredness of eyes.

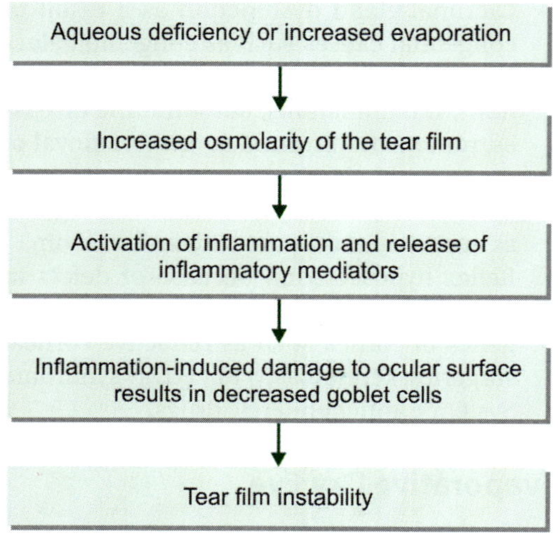

FIG. 13.5.1: Pathogenesis of dry eye

The symptoms of dry eye are worsened on exposure to dry environment, extensive viewing of computers or television, working environment with low humidity because of ACs.

Dry eye may present as watering eye paradoxically because of reflex hyperlacrimation in cases of evaporative dry eye caused by ocular surface damage.

Signs

On examination, the dry eyes show lusterless ocular surface with decreased corneal sheen, reduced tear meniscus and the increased tear debris.

Corneal changes such as epithelial erosions, filamentary keratitis and punctate keratopathy are seen in advanced stages of dry eye.

INVESTIGATIONS

Schirmer's Test*

Schirmer's test is done to determine the quantity of tear film secretions. Various types of Schirmer's tests are described below.

Schirmer's Test I

Schirmer's test I measures the total tear secretions. It is performed by a Schirmer's test strip, a Whatman filter paper measuring 5 × 35 mm, which is folded at 5 mm and kept in lower conjunctival fornix at the junction of lateral one thirds and medial two thirds. The test strip is kept in the lower fornix for 5 minutes and the amount of wetting of the filter paper is noted. Normally, the wetting of the filter paper is seen up to 15 mm, wetting between 10 mm and 15 mm is taken as borderline or mild dry eye, wetting between 5 and 10 mm as moderate dry eye and wetting less than 5 mm as severe dry eye.

Schirmer's Test II

Schirmer's test II is done to measure reflex secretions. It is performed in similar way as first test except that nasal mucosa is rubbed by a cotton bud to irritate it to measure reflex secretions.

Schirmer's Basal Secretion Test

Schirmer's basal secretion test is performed similar to test I except that conjunctival fornix is anesthetized before performing the test to measure the basal secretions.

Tear Film Breakup Time

Tears are stained with fluorescein dye and the time interval between a complete blink to the first appearance of dry spot in the tear film is taken as tear film breakup time (TBUT). Normal value is 15–30 seconds. Less than 10 seconds indicates abnormal tear film.

Conjunctival Impression Cytology

Conjunctival impression cytology is done to determine the abnormalities in the conjunctiva such as goblet cell loss and squamous metaplasia. It is done by collecting superficial conjunctival cells by applying and peeling a cellulose acetate paper on the bulbar conjunctiva. The cells are fixed and stained on a slide and studied under microscope. Normal count of goblet cells is more than 500 cells/mm^2; goblet cell count of less than 100 cells/mm^2 is taken as abnormal.

Ocular Mucus Ferning Test

Ocular mucus ferning test is done by studying the ferning pattern of the conjunctival mucus. It is done by pressing a coverslip over the bulbar conjunctiva and allowing it to dry. It is then observed under a microscope to see the ferning pattern. Incomplete ferning or absence of ferning indicates abnormal tear film.

Rose Bengal Staining

Rose Bengal is a vital stain and it stains the devitalized cells. It is done by instilling 1% rose Bengal dye. Ocular surface is divided into three zones, e.g. cornea, nasal bulbar conjunctiva and temporal bulbar conjunctiva. Depending on the density of staining, scoring is given as '0' for no staining, '1' for mild staining, '2' for moderate staining and '3' for severe staining. A total score of more than '3' is taken as indicative for dry eye. A score of '9' indicates severe dry eye.

Tear lysozyme Assay

Normal level of tear lysozyme is 2–4 mg/mL. Dry eye is associated with the decreased tear lysozyme level.

Tear Osmolarity

Normal tear osmolarity is 300–310 mOsm/L. An increase in the tear osmolarity is considered as the hallmark of dry eye according to the recent pathogenesis of dry eye.

TREATMENT*

Tear Substitutes

Tear substitutes in the form of artificial tears are indicated in treatment of all varieties of dry eye and they are the mainstay of treatment of aqueous deficient dry eye.

Artificial tears are composed of compounds such as chondroitin sulfate, sodium hyaluronate, polyvinyl alcohol and cellulose derivatives (e.g. hydroxymethyl cellulose, carboxymethyl cellulose). They are available as drops, gels, ointments and ocular inserts. Artificial tears containing preservatives should be avoided, as they are known to cause ocular surface damage and exaggerate dry eye symptoms on long-term use.

Preservation of Tears

The preservation of existing tears can be done by reducing the evaporation of the tears by reduction of room temperature, using room humidifiers, moisture chamber glasses and punctal occlusion. Temporary punctal occlusion can be done by using punctal plugs. Permanent punctal occlusion can be done by using thermal cautery or diode laser, or argon laser.

Stimulation of Tear Secretion

Cholinergic drugs can be used to stimulate lacrimal glands, but because of systemic side effects of cholinergic drugs, they are not commonly used. Cevimeline, a muscarinic acetylcholine receptor agonist, is found to be effective in treatment of dry eye.

Anti-inflammatory Agents

Treatment by anti-inflammatory agents is considered as the right treatment, as it is aimed at the basic pathology unlike others, which are aimed at symptoms of dry eye.

Topical Cyclosporine

Cyclosporine is an immunosuppressant drug; it acts by preventing T-cell activation and production of inflammatory cytokines. It is available as eyedrops in 0.05% and 0.1% concentrations.

Topical Steroids

Topical steroids are used because of potent anti-inflammatory action. They are preferably used in low doses to prevent steroid-related adverse effects, e.g. glaucoma.

Systemic Tetracycline

Systemic tetracycline is not used for antibacterial action, but because of anti-inflammatory action of tetracycline. It acts by inhibiting the action of matrix metalloproteinase and inflammatory cytokines.

Treatment of Underlying Diseases of the Eyelids and Ocular Surface

Treatment of underlying diseases of the eyelids and ocular surface is done by treatment of the diseases such as proptosis, lagophthalmos, ectropion, symblepharon, blepharitis, etc. and modification of the risk factors by discontinuing the use of contact lenses and eyedrops with preservatives.

GIST BOX 13.5

- International Dry Eye WorkShop has defined dry eye as a multifactorial disease involving tears and ocular surface accompanied by increased osmolarity of the tear film and inflammation of the ocular surface resulting in symptoms of ocular discomfort, disturbances in vision and tear film instability with potential damage to the ocular surface.
- Dry eye is broadly classified into aqueous tear deficient dry eye and evaporative dry eye.
- Aqueous tear deficient dry eye is because of deficiency of aqueous layer of the tear film as a result of deficient lacrimal secretions. It is subdivided into Sjögren's syndrome dry eye and non-Sjögren's syndrome dry eye.
- Sjögren's syndrome is an autoimmune diseases characterized by infiltration of lymphocytes in lacrimal glands and salivary glands resulting in aqueous deficient dry eye or keratoconjunctivitis sicca and dry mouth.
- The symptoms of dry eye include dryness or grittiness of eyes, foreign body sensation, burning, redness and tiredness of eyes.
- Tear substitutes in the form of artificial tears are indicated in treatment of all varieties of dry eye and they are the mainstay of treatment of aqueous deficient dry eye.

CHAPTER

13.6 Tumors of Lacrimal System

TUMORS OF LACRIMAL GLAND

Lacrimal gland tumors account for 10% of all orbital tumors. About 50–80% of all lacrimal gland tumors are non-epithelial tumors including pseudotumor and lymphoid tumors. Epithelial tumors account for rest of the lacrimal gland tumors.

Pleomorphic adenoma is the most common benign epithelial tumor of lacrimal gland. Adenoid cystic carcinoma is the most common malignant epithelial tumor of lacrimal glands.

Benign Tumors of Lacrimal Gland

Dacryops

Dacryops is also called lacrimal ductal cyst. It is because of obstruction of the lacrimal ducts resulting in cystic dilatation of the lacrimal gland because of retention of lacrimal gland secretions.

Dacryops presents as cystic swelling in the superotemporal conjunctival fornix with positive transillumination. Treatment is by drainage of the affected lacrimal duct.

Pleomorphic Adenoma

Pleomorphic adenoma is the most common benign epithelial tumor of the lacrimal gland. It is also known as benign mixed tumor. The tumor presents as painless swelling in the superotemporal part of the orbit with inferonasal displacement of the globe. It is commonly seen in fourth decade. Pleomorphic adenoma is well encapsulated and it is present in pseudocapsule. Incisional biopsy should be avoided, as this may lead to spread of tumor.

Treatment is by complete surgical excision along with the pseudocapsule. Incomplete removal leads to recurrence of the tumor.

Malignant Tumors of Lacrimal Gland

Adenoid cystic carcinoma is the most common malignant epithelial tumor of lacrimal glands. Malignant mixed tumor is the malignant variety of benign mixed tumor. Acinic cell carcinoma, malignant rhabdoid tumor and sebaceous carcinoma are the other rare malignant tumors of lacrimal gland.

TUMORS OF LACRIMAL DRAINAGE SYSTEM

Lacrimal sac tumors are the most common tumors of lacrimal drainage system.

Lacrimal Sac Tumors**

Lacrimal sac tumors are relatively rare, but more than 70% of them are malignant and are frequently associated with morbidity and mortality. The common benign tumors of lacrimal sac are squamous papilloma, transitional papilloma, oncocytoma, hemangiopericytoma, lipoma and neurofibroma. Squamous cell carcinoma, transitional cell carcinoma, adenocarcinoma and mucoepidermoid carcinoma are the common malignant tumors of lacrimal sac.

Squamous cell carcinoma is the most common malignant tumor of the lacrimal sac and transitional cell carcinoma is the most invasive malignant tumor of the lacrimal sac.

Clinical Features*

- Lacrimal sac tumors are seen usually in elderly patients with peak incidence in sixth and seventh decade
- Lacrimal sac tumors present as epiphora, recurrent dacryocystitis and a blockage or mass in the lacrimal sac area.

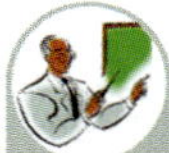

Masquerade Syndrome

Lacrimal sac tumors usually masquerade as chronic dacryocystitis; hence, high index of suspicion is required for early diagnosis of lacrimal sac tumors.

Malignancy should be suspected in patients presenting with:

- Firm and non-compressible mass above the medial palpebral ligament
- Presence of epistaxis or blood-stained tears
- Cervical lymphadenopathy
- Presence of ulceration over the lacrimal sac mass.

Investigations

Computed tomography (CT) scan and magnetic resonance imaging (MRI) show characteristic features such as lacrimal sac mass with erosion, and destruction of the lacrimal fossa and the surrounding structures.

Treatment

Treatment is by wide surgical excision followed by radiotherapy and chemotherapy.

GIST BOX 13.6

- Lacrimal gland tumors account for about 10% of all orbital tumors. Pleomorphic adenoma is the most common benign epithelial tumor of lacrimal gland. Adenoid cystic carcinoma is the most common malignant epithelial tumor of lacrimal glands.
- Lacrimal sac tumors are relatively rare, but more than 70% of them are malignant and are frequently associated with morbidity and mortality.
- Lacrimal sac tumors usually masquerade as chronic dacryocystitis; hence, high index of suspicion is required for early diagnosis of lacrimal sac tumors. Malignancy should be suspected in patients presenting with:
  - Firm and non-compressible mass above the medial palpebral ligament
  - Presence of epistaxis or blood-stained tears
  - Cervical lymphadenopathy
  - Presence of ulceration over the lacrimal sac mass.

FREQUENTLY ASKED QUESTIONS (FAQs)

*Short Answers

1. Lacrimal drainage system.
2. Mention the layers of tear film.
3. Mention the functions of tear film.
4. Structure of tear film.
5. Congenital nasolacrimal duct obstruction.
6. Mention the indications and contraindications for dacryocystorhinostomy (DCR).
7. Mikulicz's syndrome.
8. Canaliculitis.
9. Dacryoadenitis.
10. Mention the complications of DCR.
11. Mention the causes for epiphora.
12. Lacrimal syringing test.
13. Treatment of watering eye.
14. Treatment of dry eye.
15. Schirmer's test.
16. Clinical features and treatment of lacrimal sac tumors.

**Short Essays

1. Tear film.
2. Describe the differential diagnosis and treatment congenital dacryocystitis.
3. Lacrimal probing.
4. Clinical features and treatment of chronic dacryocystitis.
5. Clinical features and treatment of acute dacryocystitis.
6. Dacryocystorhinostomy.
7. Dacryocystectomy.
8. Epiphora.
9. Classify dry eye.
10. Lacrimal sac tumors.

***Long Essays

1. Describe the etiology, clinical features and management of congenital dacryocystitis.
2. Describe the etiology, clinical features and management of chronic adult dacryocystitis.
3. Describe the etiology, clinical features and management of acute adult dacryocystitis.
4. Define dry eye. Describe etiology, pathogenesis and management of dry eye.

BIBLIOGRAPHY

1. Aydin U, Hastar E, Yildirim D. Dacryolith: two case reports. Dentomaxillofac Radiol. 2007;36(4):237-9.
2. Amato J, Hartstein ME. Evaluation of the tearing patient. The Lacrimal System. 2006;66-73.
3. Amrith S, Goh PS, Wang SC. Tear flow dynamics in the human nasolacrimal ducts—a pilot study using dynamic magnetic resonance imaging. Graefes Arch Clin Exp Ophthalmol. 2005;243(2):127-31.
4. Bhavsar AS, Bhavsar SG, Jain. A review on recent advances in dry eye: Pathogenesis and management. Oman J Ophthalmol. 2011;4(2):50-6.
5. Crigler LW. The treatment of congenital dacryocystitis. Journal of American Medical Association. 1923;81(1):23-4.
6. Carneiro RC, Macedo EM, Oliveira PP. [Canaliculitis: case report and management]. Arq Bras oftalmol. 2008;71(1):107-9.

7. Derr C, Shah A. Bilateral dacryoadenitis. J Emerg Trauma Shock. 2012;5(1):92-4.
8. Fussell JN, Wilson T, Pride H. Case report: Congenital dacryocystocele and dacryocystitis. Pediatr Dermatol. 2011;28(1):70-2.
9. Gayton JL. Etiology, prevalence and treatment of dry eye disease. Clin Ophthalmol. 2009;3:405-12.
10. Lemp MA. Report of the National Eye Institute/ Industry Workshop on Clinical Trials in Dry Eyes. CLAO J. 1995;21(4):221-32.
11. Maheshwari R. Management of congenital nasolacrimal duct obstruction. Journal of the Bombay Ophthalmologists' Association. 2005;14(1):44-7.
12. Murthy R. Dacryocystitis. Kerala Journal of Ophthalmology. 2011;23(1):64-70.
13. Parmar DN, Rose GE. Management of lacrimal sac tumours. Eye (Lond). 2003;17(5):599-606.
14. Price KM, Richard MJ. The tearing patient: diagnosis and management. In: Scott IU, Fekrat S (Eds). Ophthalmic Pearls: External Disease.
15. Patel S, Blades KJ. The Dry Eye: A practical approach. Butterworth-Heinemann; 2003.
16. Stefanyszyn MA, Hidayat AA, Pe'er JJ, et al. Lacrimal sac tumors. Ophthal Plast Reconstr Surg. 1994;10(3):169-84.
17. Shields CL, Langer PD, Kim HJ. Lacrimal Sac Tumors: Diagnosis and Treatment. Smith and Nesi's Ophthalmic Plastic and Reconstructive Surgery, New York: Springer; 2012. pp. 609-14.
18. Shields CL, Shields JA, Eagle RC, et al. Clinicopathologic review of 142 cases of lacrimal gland lesions. Ophthalmology. 1989;96(4):431-5.
19. Singh R, Joseph A, Umapathy T, et al. Impression cytology of the ocular surface. Br J Ophthalmol. 2005;89(12):1655-9.
20. Tsubota K, Fujita H, Tsuzaka K, et al. Mikulicz's disease and Sjögren's syndrome. Invest Ophthalmol Vis Sci. 2000;41(7):1666-73.
21. Tovilla-Canales JL, Ball S, Olvera O, et al. Diagnosis and treatment of lacrimal gland neoplasias: a better understanding of the nature of these tumors and advanced diagnostic technologies are improving management. Review of Ophthalmology. 2013.
22. The definition and classification of dry eye disease: report of the Definition and Classification Subcommittee of the International Dry Eye WorkShop. Ocul Surf. 2007;5(2):75-92.
23. Tu EY, Rheinstrom S. Dry eye. In: Yanoff M, Duker JS (Eds). Ophthalmology, 3rd edition. Saint Louis, MO: Mosby Elsevier; 2008.

SECTION 14

Orbit

CHAPTER

14.1 Anatomy of Orbit

FUNCTION OF ORBIT

The orbit is a bony cavity and the main function of the orbit is to protect the eyeball.

GROSS ANATOMY

- Orbit is a pear-shaped four-walled pyramidal bony cavity situated one on either side of the nose (Fig. 14.1.1)
- Orbit is formed by seven bones—frontal, maxilla, sphenoid, palatine, ethmoid, lacrimal and zygomatic (Fig. 14.1.2).

Walls of Orbit*

Orbit has four walls, superior wall or roof, medial wall, lateral wall and inferior wall or floor (Table 14.1.1).

Relations of Orbit

- Superior: Anterior cranial fossa
- Inferior: Maxillary sinus
- Medial: Ethmoidal sinus and sphenoid sinus
- Lateral: Temporal fossa and middle cranial fossa.

Contents of Orbit*

Eyeball, extraocular muscles, orbital fat, lacrimal gland, lacrimal sac, ophthalmic artery and vein, ciliary ganglion, III, IV, VI and first two divisions of V cranial nerves, orbital fascia.

Dimensions of Orbit

- Volume: 30 cc
- Vertical height: 35 mm
- Horizontal width: 40 mm
- Depth: 45 mm.

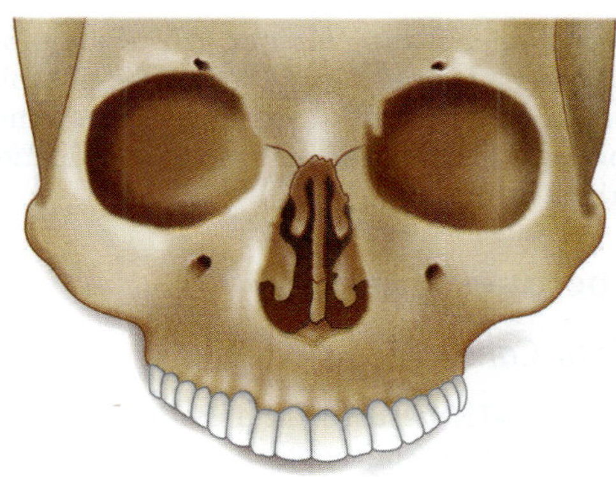

FIG. 14.1.1: Bony orbit

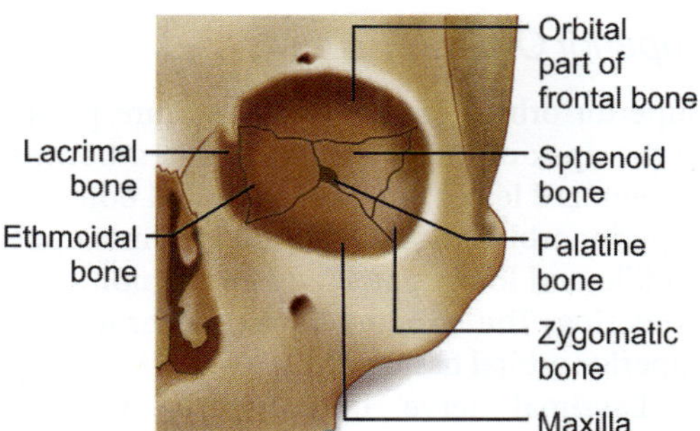

FIG. 14.1.2: Seven bones forming the orbit

TABLE 14.1.1: Walls of orbit

Walls	*Components*	*Features*
Superior wall	Made of frontal and sphenoid bones	• Fossa for lacrimal gland in the anterolateral part • Trochlear fossa for superior oblique muscle • Optic canal lies in the posterior part of the roof and it transmits optic nerve and ophthalmic artery
Inferior wall	Made of maxillary bone medially, zygomatic bone laterally and palatine bone posteriorly	• Infraorbital groove is present in the inferior wall for infraorbital nerve and vessels • It is most commonly involved in blowout fractures of orbit
Medial wall	Made of frontal process of maxilla, lacrimal bone, body of sphenoid bone and orbital plate of ethmoid bone	• It is the thinnest wall of the orbit, hence it is commonly destroyed by inflammatory lesions and tumors of the ethmoid sinuses • It has anterior and posterior ethmoidal foramina transmitting ethmoidal vessels
Lateral wall	Made of zygomatic bone and greater wing of sphenoid	• It covers only posterior half of the eyeball, as the anterior half of the eyeball is not covered from lateral wall; lateral orbitotomy is commonly done surgical approach for retrobulbar tumors

Orbital Apex

Orbital apex is the posterior end of the orbit formed by convergence of four walls of orbit. Orbital apex has two important apertures transmitting vital structures, optic canal and superior orbital fissure.

Apertures of Orbit*

Optic Canal

Optic canal is present in the posterior part of the roof, and it transmits optic nerve and ophthalmic artery. It connects orbit to the middle cranial fossa and it measures about 10 mm.

Superior Orbital Fissure

Superior orbital fissure is an aperture present in the apex of the orbit. It is situated between greater and lesser wings of sphenoid bone. The superior orbital fissure is subdivided into upper, middle and lower parts by the common tendinous ring. The structures passing through the superior orbital fissure are:

- Lacrimal nerve, frontal nerve, trochlear nerve superior ophthalmic vein through the upper part
- Oculomotor nerve, nasociliary nerve, abducens nerve through the middle part
- Inferior ophthalmic vein through the lower part.

Inferior Orbital Fissure

Inferior orbital fissure is present between the lateral wall of orbit and floor of orbit. The structures passing through the inferior orbital fissure are zygomatic nerve, infraorbital vessels, infraorbital nerve, pterygoid venous plexus and branches from sphenopalatine ganglion.

Orbital Fascia

The orbital fascia is divided into:

1. Fascia covering the globe called Tenon's capsule or fascia bulbi: It extends from the posterior aspect of the globe to fuse anteriorly at the limbus with conjunctiva. The space between the Tenon's capsule and the globe is called Tenon's space.
2. Fascia covering the extraocular muscles.
3. The membranous extensions of the extraocular muscles extending to the surrounding bone and eyelids called check ligaments.

4. Suspensory ligament of Lockwood: It is the extension of fascia of inferior rectus and inferior oblique. It is also called capsulopalpebral fascia and it is the retractor of lower eyelid analogous to levator aponeurosis complex of the upper eyelid.

Surgical Spaces of Orbit*

The important surgical spaces of orbit (Fig. 14.1.3) are the following.

Subperiosteal space: It is the space between the bones of the orbital wall and the periosteum.

Peripheral space or peribulbar space: It is the space between the periosteum and the four rectus extraocular muscles and intermuscular septa. The peribulbar space contains lacrimal gland, lacrimal sac, orbital fat, oblique muscles, lacrimal nerve, frontal nerve, trochlear nerve, superior and inferior ophthalmic veins.

Peribulbar injections are given in this space for peribulbar anesthesia. Space occupying lesions present in this space cause eccentric proptosis with the eyeball deviated in the direction opposite to the site of tumor or lesion.

Central space or retrobulbar space: It is the space behind the back of the globe and four rectus extraocular muscles and intermuscular septa. The retrobulbar space contains optic nerve, ophthalmic artery, ciliary ganglion, oculomotor nerve, abducens nerve, nasociliary nerve and orbital fat.

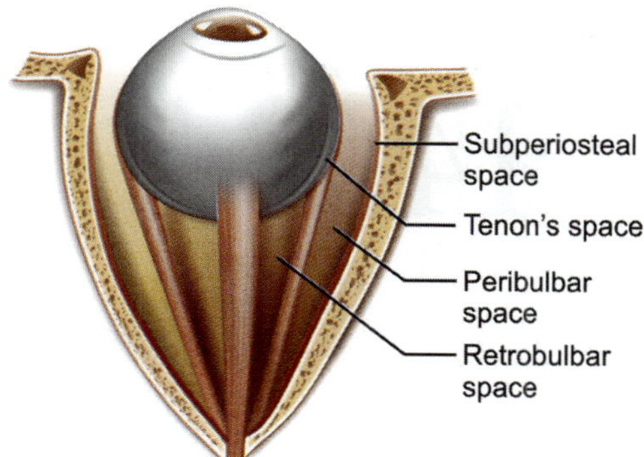

FIG. 14.1.3: Surgical spaces of orbit

Retrobulbar injections are given in this space for retrobulbar anesthesia. Space occupying lesions present in this space cause axial proptosis.

Tenon's space: It is the space between the sclera and Tenon's capsule. Sub-Tenon's injections are given in this space.

Blood Supply of Orbit

The arterial supply of orbit is by ophthalmic artery and venous drainage is by superior and inferior ophthalmic veins. There is no lymphatic supply for orbit.

GIST BOX 14.1

- Orbit is a pear-shaped four-walled pyramidal bony cavity situated one on either side of the nose.
- Orbit is formed by seven bones: Frontal, maxilla, sphenoid, palatine, ethmoid, lacrimal and zygomatic.
- Orbit has four walls: Superior wall or roof, medial wall, lateral wall and inferior wall or floor.
- Medial wall is the thinnest wall of the orbit; hence, it is commonly destroyed by inflammatory lesions and tumors of the ethmoid sinuses.
- Inferior wall is most commonly involved in blowout fractures of orbit.
- Orbital apex is the posterior end of the orbit formed by convergence of four walls of orbit. Orbital apex has two important apertures transmitting vital structures, optic canal and superior orbital fissure.
- The important surgical spaces of the orbit subperiosteal space, peribulbar space, retrobulbar space and Tenon's space.

CHAPTER

14.2 Congenital Anomalies of Orbit

EMBRYOLOGY

The orbit develops from the mesenchyme encircling the optic vesicle. Visceral mesoderm of the maxillary process gives rise to lower and lateral wall of the orbit, whereas the paraxial mesoderm gives rise to upper and medial wall of the orbit.

CONGENITAL ANOMALIES OF ORBIT

The congenital anomalies of orbit are usually associated with anomalies of the surrounding bones of the skull and face. The common congenital anomalies of the orbit are described below.

Craniosynostosis*

1. Premature closure or fusion of the bony sutures of the skull resulting in abnormal shape of the head is called craniosynostosis.
2. Sagittal, coronal, metopic and lambdoid are the sutures present in the skull (Fig. 14.2.1). The growth of the skull will be restricted perpendicular to the orientation of the suture. This is called Virchow's law.
3. Craniosynostosis can occur as an isolated condition or can be a part of a syndrome.
4. Because of premature closure of the bony sutures of the skull, the orbits become shallow, leading to proptosis, papilledema and optic atrophy. Associated extraocular muscle anomalies lead to variable amount of strabismus.

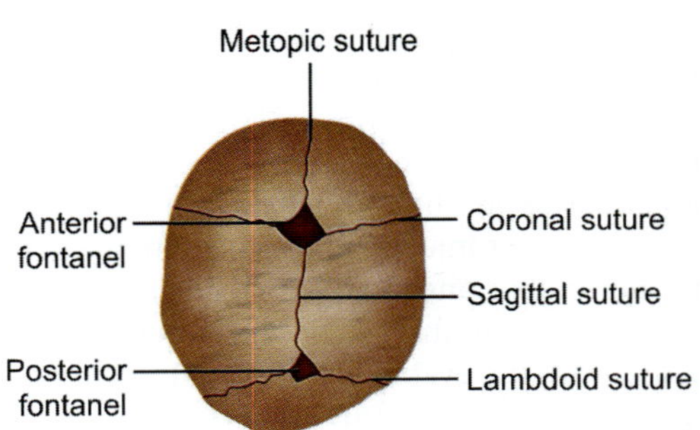

FIG. 14.2.1: Cranial sutures

5. Premature closure of the sutures can lead to secondary raised intracranial pressure and neurodevelopmental delay because of arrest in brain growth.
6. Treatment is by corrective craniectomies and external skull molding. Cerebral decompression is required in cases associated with increased intracranial pressure.
7. The shape of the skull is altered as a result of premature closure of the sutures and the shape depends on the involved suture and depending on this various types of the anomalies are described in Table 14.2.1.

Sagittal suture is most commonly involved in craniosynostosis; thus scaphocephaly is the most common type of craniosynostosis.

Crouzon's Syndrome

1. Crouzon's syndrome is craniofacial dysostosis and it shows brachycephaly and maxillary hypoplasia. It is named after

TABLE 14.2.1: Anomalies associated with craniosynostosis

Anomaly	*Suture involved*	*Shape of the skull*
Scaphocephaly (Figs 14.2.2A and B)	Sagittal suture	Boat-shaped skull
Trigonocephaly (Fig. 14.2.3)	Metopic suture	Egg-shaped or triangular skull
Oxycephaly (Fig. 14.2.4)	Coronal suture and lambdoid suture	Tower-shaped skull or high head
Brachycephaly	Bilateral coronal sutures	Short head
Anterior plagiocephaly	One coronal suture	Flat head
Posterior plagiocephaly	One lambdoid suture	Flat head or skull
Pansynostosis or Kleeblattschädel syndrome	All sutures	Cloverleaf skull

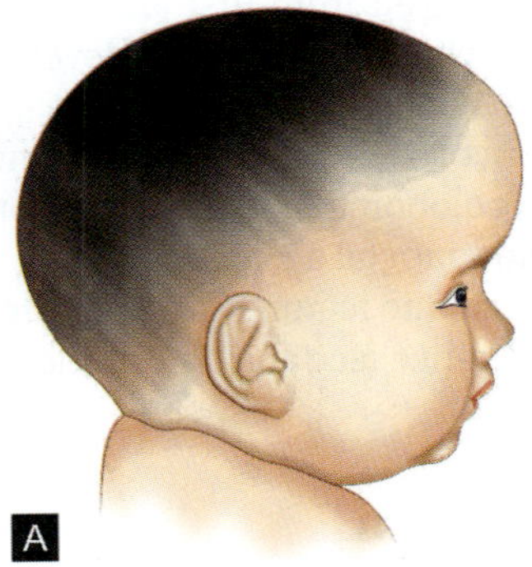

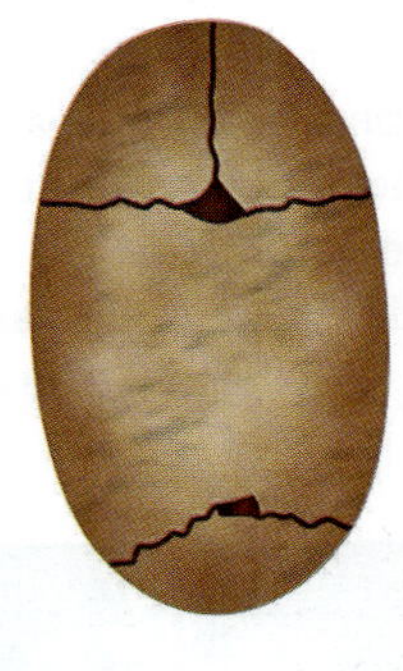

FIGS 14.2.2A and B: Scaphocephaly. **A.** An infant's image with scaphocephaly; **B.** Skull with scaphocephaly.

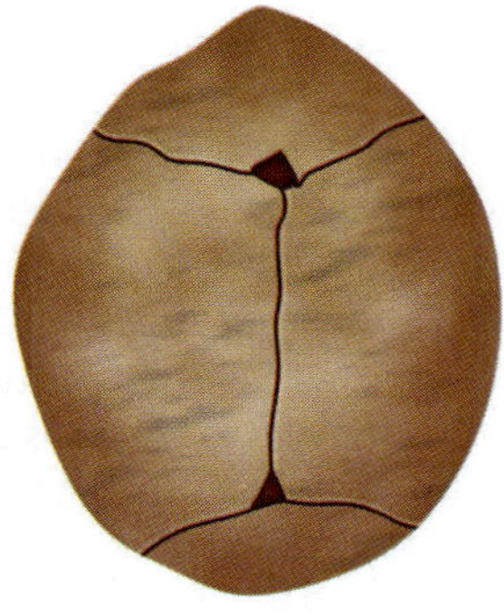

FIG. 14.2.3: Trigonocephaly

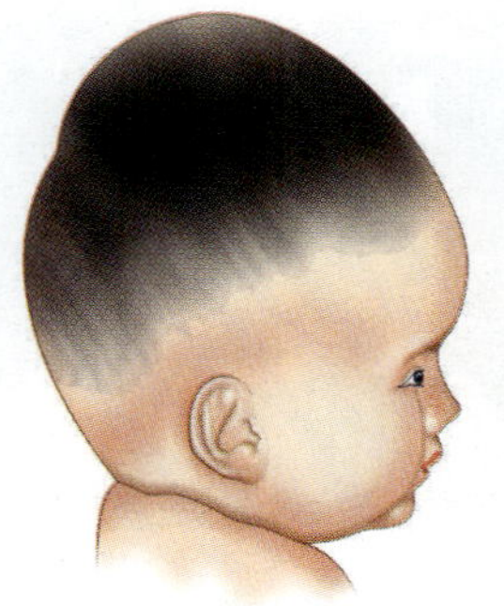

FIG. 14.2.4: Oxycephaly

Octave Crouzon, who first described the disease.
2. It shows autosomal dominant inheritance with defect of the fibroblast growth factor receptor 2 *(FGFR2)* gene located on chromosome 10.
3. The ocular features are proptosis, papilledema, strabismus, hypertelorism and optic atrophy.
4. The systemic features are frog-like face, parrot beak nose and variable degrees of mental retardation.
5. Treatment is by corrective craniectomies and external skull molding to prevent ocular complications such as papilledema and optic atrophy.

Apert's Syndrome (Fig. 14.2.5)

1. Apert's syndrome is also craniofacial dysostosis and it is involved oxycephaly associated with syndactyly of fingers and toes.
2. It is called acrocephalosyndactyly indicating oxycephaly and syndactyly, and it is named after Eugène Apert, who first described the syndrome.
3. The genetic defect is similar to Crouzon's syndrome with defect of the *FGFR2* gene.
4. The ocular features are similar to Crouzon's syndrome such as proptosis, papilledema, hypertelorism and optic atrophy. The other ocular features are antimongoloid slant, oculomotor palsies and congenital ptosis.
5. The systemic features are oxycephaly or brachycephaly, maxillary hypoplasia, and syndactyly of fingers and toes.
6. Treatment is by craniectomies or craniofacial surgery and external skull molding to prevent ocular complications such as papilledema and optic atrophy.

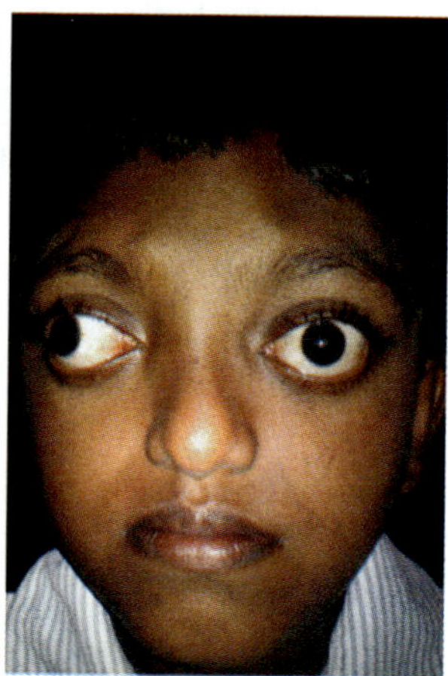

FIG. 14.2.5: Apert's syndrome

Mandibulofacial Dysostosis

1. Mandibulofacial dysostosis is also called Treacher Collins syndrome or Franceschetti syndrome.
2. It shows autosomal dominant inheritance with genetic defect on the chromosome 5. It is because of maldevelopment of structures derived from first and second branchial arches leading to maldevelopment of maxilla, mandible and zygoma.
3. The ocular features are antimongoloid slant, coloboma of lower eyelid, ptosis and inferior punctal agenesis.
4. The systemic features are high-arched palate, bird-like face and deformities of the external ear.

Hypertelorism*

1. Hypertelorism is defined as a condition in which the distance between the orbits is increased. Normal distance between the orbits is about 15 mm at birth and 25 mm in adults.
2. Hypertelorism should be differentiated from telecanthus in which the distance between two medial canthi is more because of abnormally long medial canthal tendons. In hypertelorism, interpupillary distance is increased, whereas in telecanthus the interpupillary distance is normal.
3. Hypertelorism is seen in association with craniosynostosis and meningoencephaloceles.

4. Treatment is by surgery to remove the excessive tissues present in between the two orbits.

Hemifacial Microsomia

1. Hemifacial microsomia presents with facial asymmetry as a result of unilateral abnormalities of mandible and ear.
2. Goldenhar syndrome: It is a variant of hemifacial microsomia presenting with unilateral abnormalities of eye, ear and vertebrae. It presents with congenital lid coloboma, vertebral column anomalies, preauricular skin tags and limbal dermoid.

Pierre Robin Anomaly

1. Pierre Robin anomaly is characterized by cleft palate, glossoptosis and micrognathia.
2. It can lead to respiratory distress as a result of obstruction of the airway by the tongue.

Meningoencephalocele

1. Meningoencephalocele is the herniation of the brain along with the meninges as a result of congenital defects in the cranial sutures.
2. It presents as pulsating mass medial to medial canthus and the mass typically shows bulging on performing Valsalva maneuver or coughing.

GIST BOX 14.2

- The congenital anomalies of orbit are usually associated with anomalies of the surrounding bones of the skull and face.
- Premature closure or fusion of the bony sutures of the skull resulting in abnormal shape of the head is called craniosynostosis.
- Crouzon's syndrome is a craniofacial dysostosis and it shows brachycephaly and maxillary hypoplasia.
- Apert's syndrome is a craniofacial dysostosis and it is involves oxycephaly associated with syndactyly of fingers and toes.
- Treacher Collins syndrome is characterized by mandibulofacial dysostosis. The ocular features are antimongoloid slant, coloboma of lower eyelid, ptosis and inferior punctal agenesis.
- Hypertelorism is defined as a condition in which the distance between the orbits is increased. Normal distance between the orbits is about 15 mm at birth and 25 mm in adults.
- Goldenhar syndrome is a variant of hemifacial microsomia presenting with unilateral abnormalities of eye, ear and vertebrae. It presents with congenital lid coloboma, vertebral column anomalies, preauricular skin tags and limbal dermoid.

CHAPTER

14.3 Inflammatory Diseases of Orbit

ORBITAL INFLAMMATIONS*

The orbit tends to be involved in both infective and non-infective inflammatory diseases. The orbital inflammations are classified as:

- Acute orbital inflammation
- Chronic specific orbital inflammation
- Chronic non-specific orbital inflammation.

Acute Orbital Inflammations

Acute orbital inflammations are classified as:

- Preseptal cellulitis
- Orbital cellulitis
- Subperiosteal abscess
- Orbital abscess
- Cavernous sinus thrombosis.

Preseptal Cellulitis

Definition

Preseptal cellulitis is defined as infection of soft tissues anterior to orbital septum (Fig. 14.3.1).

Orbital Septum

It is a fibrous membrane, which arises from orbital rim and inserts into the tarsal plate of the eyelids. It acts as a barrier and prevents deeper extension of the infection into the orbit.

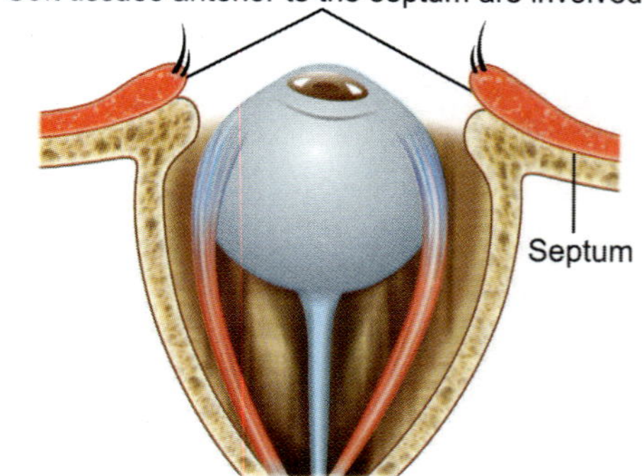

FIG. 14.3.1: Preseptal cellulitis

Etiopathogenesis

Preseptal cellulitis is also called periorbital cellulitis the infection is limited to the anterior part of the orbit.

Trauma, insect bites, infection of the surrounding structures such as sinusitis, upper respiratory tract infection, inflammations of glands of eyelids, for example, hordeolum externum or internum and infections of the cutaneous structures of the eyelids are the usual sources of infection.

- Both preseptal cellulitis and orbital cellulitis are more common in children than in the adults.
- Sinusitis is the most common source of infection.

Streptococcus pneumoniae (*S. pneumoniae*), *Staphylococcus aureus* and *Haemophilus influenzae* (*H. influenzae*) are the most common causative organisms.

Haemophilus influenzae was the commonest cause of preseptal cellulitis, especially in children in the past and it usually used to follow upper respiratory tract infection. With the introduction of *Haemophilus* vaccine, the incidence has come down drastically.

Clinical features

Redness and swelling of the periorbital area with mild to moderate pain of the affected eye are the usual presenting symptoms.

It can be differentiated from orbital cellulitis by the absence of proptosis and presence of normal vision and extraocular movements.

Differential diagnosis

Preseptal cellulitis has to be differentiated from orbital cellulitis and other causes of lid edema such as allergic lid edema, dacryoadenitis, etc.

Treatment

It is done by oral broad-spectrum antibiotics and anti-inflammatory drugs. Follow-up is advised to look for orbital cellulitis and treatment for the same if it develops.

*Orbital Cellulitis****

Definition

Orbital cellulitis is defined as infection of soft tissues of the orbit posterior to the orbital septum (Fig. 14.3.2).

Etiopathogenesis

1. Extension of infection from the surrounding structures is the most common mode of infection. Sinusitis from the surrounding paranasal sinuses is the most common source of infection accounting for about 85% of infections. The other sources of infection are from the infections of the eye, lacrimal sac, face, ears, teeth, etc.
2. Exogenous infections following penetrating injuries, surgeries on the orbit are the second most common mode of infection.

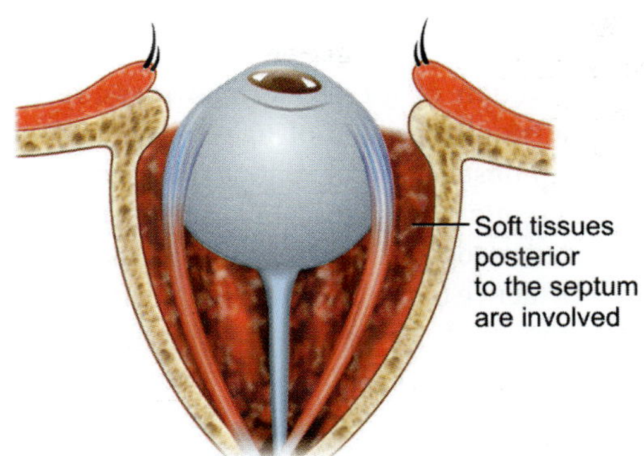

FIG. 14.3.2: Orbital cellulitis

3. Endogenous infections from distant source of infection like abscess involving the other organs are a relatively rare mode of infection.

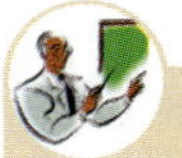

The reasons for sinusitis being the most common source of infection for orbital cellulitis are:

- Anatomical proximity.
- Ethmoidal sinusitis is the most common type of sinusitis associated with sinus-related preseptal cellulitis or orbital cellulitis. This is because of the fact that orbit is separated from ethmoidal sinus by the presence of lamina papyracea, a thin bone, which offers least resistance to the spread of infection.
- The presence of dehiscences in the lamina papyracea, ophthalmic veins communicating between the orbit and sinuses are the other factors responsible for spread of infection from the surrounding paranasal sinuses to orbit.

Streptococcus pneumoniae, Staphylococcus aureus and *H. influenzae* are the most common causative organisms in children.

In adults, the common causative organisms are *Staphylococcus aureus, S. pneumoniae, S. pyogenes, Pseudomonas aeruginosa, Escherichia coli* and anaerobes. *Mucor* and *Aspergillus* are the common fungi associated with orbital cellulitis.

Pathology of orbital cellulitis

Orbital cellulitis differs from inflammations at other sites and results in rapid necrosis of the tissue because of:

1. Absence of lymphatic supply, thus limiting the role of protective factors.
2. Elevation of the intraorbital pressure because of presence of tight compartments and obstruction of venous flow secondary to septic thrombophlebitis leading to localization to form abscess, thus increasing the virulence of the causative organisms.
3. Spread of infection as thrombophlebitis through the vascular communications resulting in easy spread of infection to cavernous sinus and intracranial extension.

Clinical features

Symptoms

- Severe pain, swelling of the eyes, proptosis, limitation of eye movements
- Visual symptoms such as double vision, diminution of vision and loss of vision
- General symptoms such as fever, malaise, headache, etc.

Signs

- Tenderness of the eyelids
- Chemosis of conjunctiva
- Proptosis and limitation of eye movements
- Diminution of vision of various grades depending on the severity of infection and the stage of infection.

Stages of orbital cellulitis

The disease usually passes through five stages as described below:

1. Stage of inflammation of preseptal soft tissues: The symptoms are minimal with mild pain and swelling of the eyes, and the signs include chemosis of conjunctiva.
2. Stage of inflammation of orbital soft tissues: The symptoms include moderate-to-severe pain, painful eye movements and signs show moderate-to-severe chemosis of conjunctiva.
3. Stage of subperiosteal abscess: It is the accumulation of pus in the subperiosteal space between the orbital bone and the periosteum. It presents with displacement of the globe and limitation of eye movements in the direction of abscess.
4. Stage of orbital abscess: It is the collection of pus within the orbital soft tissues. It presents with proptosis, ophthalmoplegia and marked diminution of vision.
5. Stage of complications involving the spread of infection to cavernous sinus: It presents with loss of vision, proptosis, ophthalmoplegia, involvement of the other eye and central nervous system (CNS) symptoms, for example, disorientation, etc.

Complications

1. Ocular complications include exposure keratopathy secondary to proptosis, diplopia secondary to ophthalmoplegia and loss of vision because of optic atrophy or central retinal artery occlusion.
2. Orbital complications, for example, formation of subperiosteal abscess or orbital abscess (Fig. 14.3.3).
3. Intracranial extension of infection resulting in cavernous sinus thrombosis, meningitis, etc.

Differential diagnosis

1. Orbital cellulitis should be differentiated from preseptal cellulitis (Table 14.3.1).

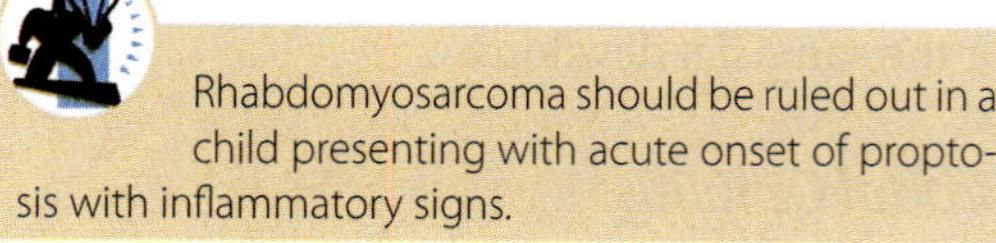

Rhabdomyosarcoma should be ruled out in a child presenting with acute onset of proptosis with inflammatory signs.

2. Orbital cellulitis should be differentiated from pseudotumor of orbit, thyroid oph-

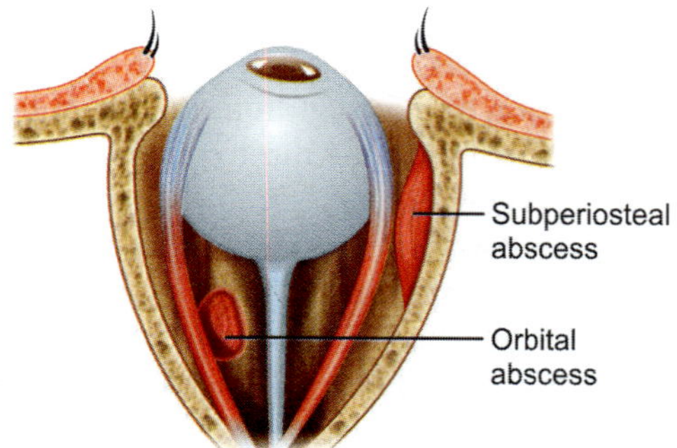

FIG. 14.3.3: Subperiosteal abscess and orbital abscess

TABLE 14.3.1: Differences between preseptal cellulitis and orbital cellulitis	
Preseptal cellulitis	*Orbital cellulitis*
Inflammation of the soft tissues anterior to the orbital septum	Inflammation of the soft tissues posterior to the orbital septum
Mild inflammation	Moderate-to-severe inflammation
Mild-to-moderate pain, swelling and redness of the eyes	Moderate-to-severe pain, marked swelling and chemosis
Proptosis is absent, vision is normal and extraocular movements are normal and full without any limitation	Proptosis is present with diminution or loss of vision and ophthalmoplegia

thalmopathy, necrotic retinoblastoma or malignant melanoma, Wegener's granulomatosis involving orbit, etc.

Investigations

1. Complete hemogram shows increased white blood cell count with leukocytosis.
2. Ultrasound examination can show complications such as subperiosteal abscess and orbital abscess.
3. Imaging studies such as computed tomography (CT) scan and magnetic resonance imaging (MRI) show the extent of inflammation, differentiate orbital cellulitis from preseptal cellulitis and also show the associated sinusitis as a source of infection for orbital cellulitis.
4. Bacterial cultures from nasal and conjunctival swab to find out the causative organisms.

Treatment

Broad-spectrum intravenous antibiotics are the treatment of choice for orbital cellulitis. Later, the antibiotics can be changed according to the culture and sensitivity report. Since the patient requires intravenous antibiotics and close watch to look for complications, patient is hospitalized.

Medical line of treatment

Ceftazidime or cefotaxime 100–150 mg/kg/day are the preferred antibiotics for treatment of orbital cellulitis. The antibiotics are continued for 10–14 days followed by oral antibiotics for another 2–3 weeks. Metronidazole and vancomycin are considered in resistant cases. Anti-inflammatory drugs are indicated for symptomatic relief.

Surgical treatment

Surgical intervention in the form of incision and drainage is indicated in cases of:

- Worsening of proptosis
- Progressive visual loss
- Orbital abscess or subperiosteal abscess
- No response to medical treatment after 24–48 hours.

*Cavernous Sinus Thrombosis***

Definition

Cavernous sinus thrombosis is thrombosis of the cavernous sinus as a result of spread of infection from the drainage area (Figs 14.3.4 and 14.3.5).

Etiopathogenesis

Cavernous sinus thrombosis usually occurs as a complication of the drainage area, most com-

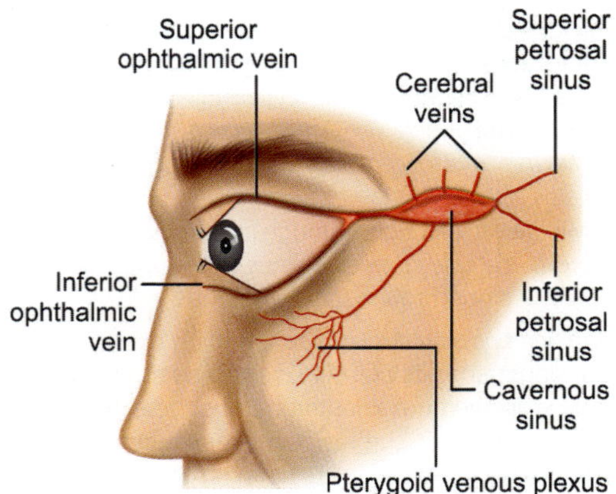

FIG. 14.3.4: Cavernous sinus communications

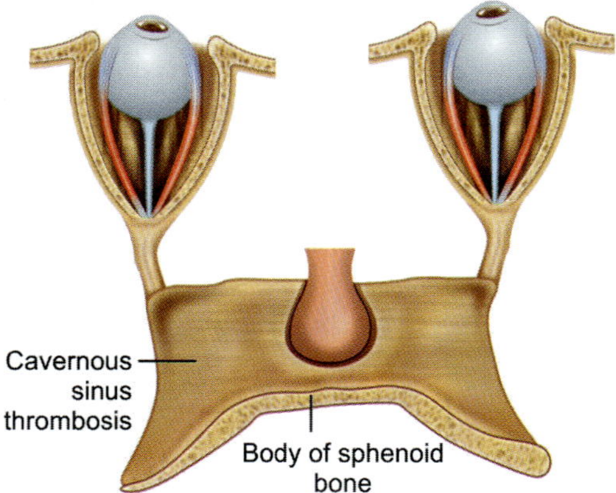

FIG. 14.3.5: Cavernous sinus

monly involving the upper lip and lower part of nose, called dangerous zone of face.

Clinical Anatomy of Cavernous Sinus**

Cavernous sinus is a dural venous sinus situated in the middle cranial fossa on either side of the body of sphenoid bone.

Cavernous sinus communicates superiorly with cerebral veins, inferiorly with pterygoid venous plexus, anteriorly with superior and inferior ophthalmic veins, posteriorly with lateral sinus. Cavernous sinuses of both the sides are in communication with each other by transverse sinus. Because of these communications, infections can reach cavernous sinus. The common infections leading to cavernous sinus thrombosis are:

- Infections from face including infections of eyes, eyelids, orbit, nose, sinus-related infections through ophthalmic veins.
- Meningitis and cerebral abscess through cerebral veins.
- Middle ear infections through lateral sinus.
- From one side cavernous sinus to the opposite cavernous sinus through transverse sinus.

Structures passing through the cavernous sinus: Cavernous sinus transmits vital nerves and arteries, and hence in case of cavernous sinus thrombosis, these vital structures are affected. The structures passing through the lateral wall of the sinus are oculomotor nerve, trochlear nerve, ophthalmic and maxillary divisions of trigeminal nerve. The structures passing through the cavernous sinus are internal carotid artery and abducens nerve.

Infections of ear, eyes, teeth and septicemia are some of the causes for infectious cavernous sinus thrombosis.

Staphylococcus aureus is the most common organism responsible for cavernous sinus thrombosis. The other causative organisms are *S. pneumoniae* and anaerobes.

Dangerous Zone of Face

Upper lip and lower part of face is called dangerous zone of face as infections in this area can easily spread to cavernous sinus resulting in cavernous sinus thrombosis. The infection spreads from facial vein, which drains into superior ophthalmic vein that in turn drains into cavernous sinus.

Clinical features

1. It presents with periorbital edema, proptosis, chemosis and severe eye pain often associated with systemic symptoms such as headache, fever, vomiting, etc.
2. Initially, it is unilateral, but invariably becomes bilateral because of spread of infection as a result of communication between the two cavernous sinuses.
3. Edema in the mastoid region because of thrombosis of the emissary veins is one of the pathognomonic sign in the initial stages.
4. Palsies of oculomotor nerve, trochlear nerve, ophthalmic and maxillary divisions of trigeminal nerve and abducens nerve leading to ophthalmoplegia, ptosis, dilated non-reacting pupil and corneal anesthesia are seen in later stages.
5. Fundoscopy shows dilated and tortuous retinal veins and papilledema.

Complications

- Intracranial extension of infection leading to meningitis, brain abscess, etc.
- Delirium, coma and death.

Differential diagnosis

Cavernous sinus thrombosis has to be differentiated from the following causes by the fact that, cavernous sinus thrombosis, which is a severe inflammation, usually bilateral with presence of systemic symptoms, signs of raised intracranial tension, limitation of extraocular movements, cranial nerve palsies.

Preseptal cellulitis: It is mild inflammation with presence of normal eye movements and normal anterior segment findings.

Orbital cellulitis: It is moderate-to-severe inflammation, but systemic symptoms and signs of raised intracranial tension are absent, and it is unilateral condition.

Panophthalmitis: It is severe inflammation of all the three coats of the eye and the intraocular cavities. Anterior segment shows pus in the anterior chamber with hazy cornea. It is also a unilateral condition with absence of signs of raised intracranial tension and cranial nerve palsies.

Investigations

Imaging studies such as CT scan and MRI are helpful for confirmation of diagnosis and to differentiate it from orbital cellulitis and preseptal cellulitis.

Treatment

Cavernous sinus thrombosis is a potentially dangerous disease with high risk of mortality and hence requires aggressive treatment to prevent development of intracranial complications:

1. Treatment is by intravenous antibiotics; third-generation cephalosporins such as ceftazidime and cefotaximo are the preferred antibiotics. Antibiotic treatment is continued for 3–4 weeks.
2. Use of anticoagulant treatment by using heparin is still controversial and not followed routinely.
3. Steroids are used under cover of antibiotics in cases associated with cerebral edema.

Chronic Specific Orbital Inflammations

Chronic specific orbital inflammations include fungal infections and parasitic infections.

Fungal Infections of Orbit

Fungal infections of orbit are commonly seen in patients with systemic diseases, for example, diabetes or with immunodeficiency or renal failure.

The common fungi associated with infections of orbit are *Mucor* and *Aspergillus*. Fungal infections of the paranasal sinuses extending into the orbit are the common source of infection.

Mucor infections present with rapidly progressive orbital cellulitis, as the infection spreads rapidly as necrotizing vasculitis. The infection becomes rapidly complicated by the development of orbital apex syndrome resulting in proptosis, painful ophthalmoplegia, loss of vision, etc.

Aspergillus presents with slowly progressive orbital mass with minimal inflammatory symptoms. Vision is preserved till late in the disease and visual involvement is seen in cases with orbital apex syndrome.

The treatment is by surgical debridement and intravenous antifungals like amphotericin B and other appropriate antifungal drugs.

Parasitic Infections of Orbit

Orbital cysticercosis and echinococcosis leading to orbital hydatid cyst are the common parasitic infections of orbit.

Orbital cysticercosis

Etiopathogenesis

Orbital cysticercosis is caused by cestode *Taenia solium*. Pigs are the intermediate host for larvae of *T. solium*. Human beings acquire infection by ingestion of pork or by ingestion of the eggs in water or vegetables.

Clinical features

Orbital cysticercosis usually involves the anterior orbit commonly involving the extraocular muscles, conjunctiva and eyelids.

The clinical features depend on the location of the cysticercosis cyst; proptosis is seen in posteriorly located cysts and anteriorly located cysts present as a cystic swelling. Involvement of the extraocular muscles leads to diplopia and restriction of eye movements.

A ruptured cyst leads to severe inflammation because of release of toxins and similarly, a cyst with dead cysticercus cellulosae causes inflammation because of release of toxins. A live cyst will not produce any inflammatory reaction.

Investigations

Radiological investigations, for example, CT scan/MRI or B-scan are required for confirmation of diagnosis. B-scan shows a cyst with high-internal reflectivity corresponding to scolex.

Treatment

Medical management is by oral anthelmintic drugs such as albendazole or praziquantel. Albendazole is given in a dose of 15 mg/kg for 2–4 weeks with oral steroids 1 mg/kg for 4–6 weeks.

Surgical treatment in the form of excision of the cyst is rarely required in cases not responding to medical treatment. The cyst has to be removed in total without causing rupture, as rupture leads to severe orbital inflammation.

Hydatid cyst of orbit

Etiopathogenesis

Hydatid cyst is caused by *Echinococcus.*

Clinical features

The clinical features are similar to that of cysticercosis cyst in the form of proptosis and limitation of extraocular movements.

Investigations

Radiological investigations such as CT scan or MRI or B-scan are required for confirmation of diagnosis.

Treatment

Surgical treatment in the form of excision of the cyst is the treatment of choice. The cyst has to be removed in total without causing rupture, as rupture leads to severe orbital inflammation.

Chronic Non-specific Orbital Inflammations

*Idiopathic Orbital Inflammatory Syndrome***

Definition

Idiopathic orbital inflammatory syndrome is a non-neoplastic idiopathic inflammation of the orbit.

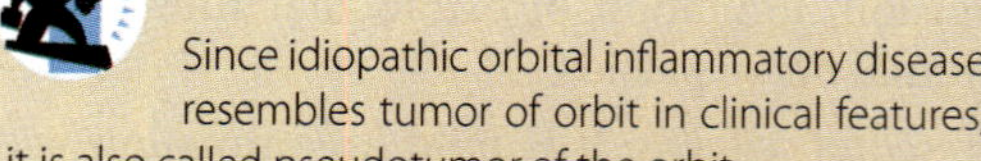

Since idiopathic orbital inflammatory disease resembles tumor of orbit in clinical features, it is also called pseudotumor of the orbit.

It is the third most common orbital disease followed by Graves' disease and lymphoproliferative disorders.

Etiopathogenesis

Idiopathic orbital inflammatory disease is commonly seen in middle age. It is characterized by the absence of ocular or systemic cause for inflammation and hence, it is a diagnosis of exclusion.

The pathogenesis is characterized by non-specific inflammation with infiltration by lymphocytes, plasma cells, macrophages, neutrophils and eosinophils. Depending on the type of histopathological cellular infiltration, pseudotumor is classified as:

- Cellular/Granulomatous
- Eosinophilic
- Vasculitic
- Sclerosing.

The exact etiology is unknown and the proposed etiological factors include infections, autoimmune and genetic factors.

Clinical features

Idiopathic orbital inflammatory disease presents with acute or subacute or chronic features.

The acute presentation is the most common type of presentation. Acute pseudotumor presents with proptosis, diplopia, ocular pain, ophthalmoplegia, chemosis, etc. Visual loss is seen in involvement of the optic nerve.

It commonly presents as acute recurrent unilateral disease. Bilateral involvement is commonly seen in children. Idiopathic orbital inflammatory syndrome can be diffused involving multiple structures or localized. The localized variety can be:

- Myositis with predominant involvement of the extraocular muscles
- Dacryoadenitis with involvement of the lacrimal gland
- Idiopathic sclerosing orbital inflammation characterized by presence of fibrosis as seen on histopathology.

The diffuse type of orbital inflammatory syndrome always offers diagnostic challenges and it has to be differentiated from systemic diseases and thyroid eye disease.

Differential diagnosis

Idiopathic orbital inflammatory syndrome has to be differentiated from orbital cellulitis, thyroid eye disease, orbital tumors and systemic diseases such as Wegener's granulomatosis, lymphoma, leukemia, sarcoidosis, amyloidosis, etc.

Investigations

Idiopathic orbital inflammatory syndrome can be differentiated from:

1. Orbital cellulitis by the absence of signs of infection, e.g. fever, etc.
2. Thyroid eye disease by the absences of thyroid lid signs.
3. Systemic diseases by laboratory investigations such as antinuclear antibody, anti-neutrophil cytoplasmic antibodies, etc.
4. Radiological investigations such as CT scan, MRI show enlargement of the extraocular muscles with involvement of the tendons, thus differentiating it from thyroid orbitopathy in which the tendons of extraocular muscles are typically spared.
5. Fine-needle aspiration biopsy for histological confirmation of diagnosis.

Treatment

1. Corticosteroids are the treatment of choice; oral steroids 1–2 mg/kg, tapered slowly over 4–6 weeks are the mainstay of treatment.

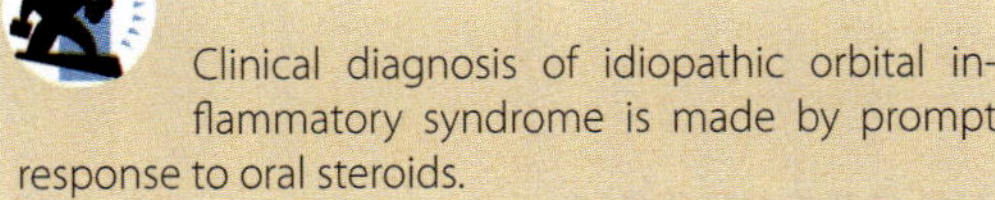

Clinical diagnosis of idiopathic orbital inflammatory syndrome is made by prompt response to oral steroids.

2. Immunosuppressants such as cyclophosphamide, cyclosporine, methotrexate, etc. are used in cases showing recurrence to steroids or in cases with no response to steroids or as steroid-sparing drugs in case of complications to steroids.
3. Immunomodulators and radiotherapy are the other treatment options.

GIST BOX 14.3

- Preseptal cellulitis is defined as infection of soft tissues anterior to orbital septum.
- Orbital cellulitis is defined as infection of soft tissues of the orbit posterior to the orbital septum.
- Cavernous sinus thrombosis is thrombosis of the cavernous sinus as a result of spread of infection from the drainage area.
- Orbital cysticercosis and echinococcosis leading to orbital hydatid cyst are the common parasitic infections of orbit.
- Idiopathic orbital inflammatory syndrome is a non-neoplastic idiopathic inflammation of the orbit.

CHAPTER

14.4 Proptosis

EYE PROPTOSIS***

Definition

Proptosis is defined as abnormal forward displacement of eyeball beyond the orbital margins.

The word exophthalmos though indicates abnormal forward displacement of the eyeball; it is used to indicate proptosis caused by endocrine dysfunction as in thyroid eye disease. Hence, exophthalmos is defined as proptosis or forward displacement of the eyeball caused by thyroid eye disease. It is the commonest cause for proptosis.

Proptosis indicates passive protrusion of the eye and exophthalmos indicates active protrusion of the eye.

Etiopathogenesis

Proptosis is because of mass lesions pushing the eyeball forwards. The direction of displacement depends on the direction of mass lesion. It can be axial proptosis due to retrobulbar space occupying lesions, eccentric proptosis due to mass lesion in the peribulbar space or surrounding structures (eyeball will be pushed in opposite direction to that of mass occupying lesion, e.g. mass in maxillary sinus will cause proptosis in upward direction).

Classification

Acute Proptosis

Acute proptosis is characterized by sudden onset of proptosis and the common causes of acute proptosis are:

- Orbital infections such as orbital cellulitis, fungal infections of the orbit
- Orbital emphysema
- Orbital hemorrhage
- Idiopathic orbital inflammatory syndrome
- Thyroid orbitopathy
- Systemic diseases such as Wegener's granulomatosis, lymphoma, leukemia and polyarteritis nodosa.

Acute Proptosis in Children*

The common causes for acute proptosis in children are:

- Rhabdomyosarcoma.
- Neuroblastoma.
- Orbital cellulitis.
- Orbital emphysema.
- Orbital hemorrhage.
- Idiopathic orbital inflammatory syndrome.
- Capillary hemangioma.
- Lymphangioma.

Intermittent Proptosis

Intermittent proptosis is characterized by presence of transitory proptosis. The causes for intermittent proptosis are:

- Orbital varices
- Recurrent orbital hemorrhage and orbital emphysema.

Orbital varices are the most common cause of intermittent proptosis. It is characterized by intermittent proptosis on bending the head forward or by Valsalva maneuver.

Chronic Proptosis

Chronic proptosis is characterized by insidious slowly progressive proptosis. The causes for chronic proptosis are:

- Congenital lesions, e.g. dermoid
- Lacrimal gland tumors
- Hamartomas such as cavernous hemangioma, lymphangioma
- Primary tumors such as optic nerve glioma, optic nerve sheath meningioma
- Secondary tumors such as retinoblastoma, malignant melanoma
- Metastatic tumors such as lymphoma and leukemia.

Pulsating Proptosis

Pulsating proptosis is characterized by the presence of pulsations synchronously with the arterial pulse. True pulsating proptosis is seen in:

- Carotid cavernous fistula
- Aneurysm of internal carotid artery.

Transmitted cerebral pulsations in proptosis are seen in:

- Congenital conditions with absence of orbital roof as in meningocele, meningoencephalocele
- Acquired conditions with destruction of the orbital roof as in neurofibroma.

Evaluation

History

All cases of proptosis are evaluated by history to find out the type of proptosis and associated symptoms, which will give clue toward the diagnosis. The history should include:

- Age
- Mode of onset
- Duration
- Progression
- Associated symptoms
- Symptoms of thyroid dysfunction
- Any other systemic illness or malignancy.

Clinical Examination

Inspection: The following things are noted in inspection:

- Proptosis or pseudoproptosis
- Axial or eccentric proptosis (Figs 14.4.1A and B)
- Unilateral or bilateral proptosis (Fig. 14.4.2)
- Pulsating proptosis
- Inflammatory signs
- Ocular examination to note vision, anterior segment, pupillary response, extraocular movements and fundus.

Unilateral Proptosis*

- Congenital causes such as dermoid cyst, orbital teratoma.
- Traumatic causes such as orbital hemorrhage, orbital emphysema.
- Inflammations such as orbital cellulitis, pseudotumor.
- Vascular malformations such as orbital varices, carotid cavernous fistula.
- Cysts of the orbit.
- Tumors such as hemangioma, rhabdomyosarcoma, optic nerve glioma, lymphoma, metastatic tumors, etc.

Bilateral Proptosis*

- Anomalies of skull, e.g. craniofacial dysostosis.
- Systemic diseases such as histiocytosis, amyloidosis, etc.
- Inflammations, e.g. cavernous sinus thrombosis.
- Tumors such as lymphoma, leukemia, secondaries from neuroblastoma, nephroblastoma.
- Exophthalmos.

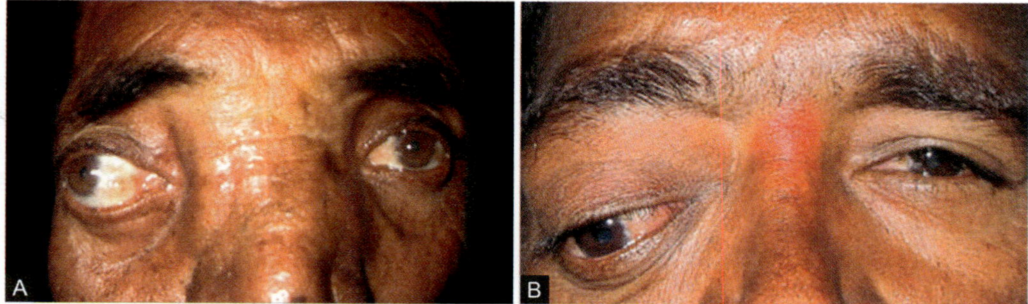

FIGS 14.4.1A and B: Eccentric proptosis of right eye

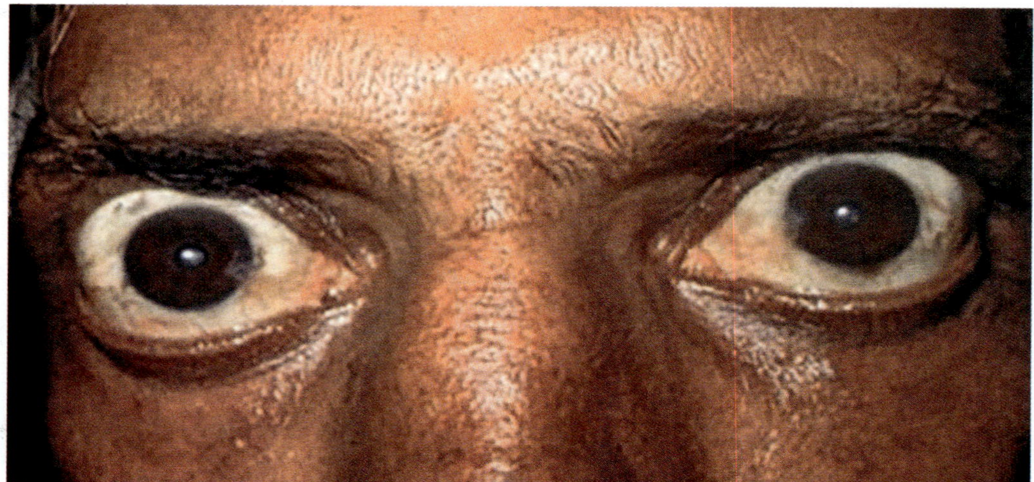

FIG. 14.4.2: Bilateral axial proptosis

Palpation: It is done to find out the retrodisplacement of the globe, compressibility of the lesion, feeling for pulsations and regional lymph nodes.

Exophthalmometry: Measurement of proptosis/exophthalmos is called exophthalmometry:

1. By plastic scale: A plastic scale is placed tightly on the lateral orbital margin and the level of the apex of the cornea is read from the scale:
   - Normal 16 mm
   - Borderline 16–20 mm
   - Proptosis > 21 mm or difference of more than 2 mm between two eyes.
2. Instruments to measure proptosis Luedde's exophthalmometer, Hertel's exophthalmometer.

Investigations

- Blood investigations including thyroid function tests, complete hemogram, etc.
- Ear, nose and throat (ENT) examination to rule out lesions of nose or paranasal sinuses
- Stool examination for cysts and ova of parasites
- To rule out systemic diseases by investigations, for example, antinuclear antibodies, etc.
- Radiological investigations including X-ray, orbital ultrasonography, computed tomography (CT) scan, magnetic resonance imaging (MRI), etc.
- Orbital venography and carotid angiography
- Fine-needle aspiration biopsy, incisional biopsy and excisional biopsy.

PSEUDOPROPTOSIS*

Pseudoproptosis is defined as a condition in which the eyeball appears to be proptosed, but there is no displacement of the eyeball. The common causes for pseudoproptosis are:

- Enlargement of the eyeball as in pathological myopia, buphthalmos, staphylomas, etc.
- Causes in the eyelid, e.g. lid retraction
- Causes resulting in false impression of proptosis in the contralateral eye as in unilateral ptosis, microphthalmos, phthisis bulbi, enophthalmos and globe retraction.

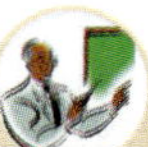

Enophthalmos*

- It is defined as posterior displacement or inward displacement of the eyeball.
- It is because of decrease in the contents of the orbit. The causes for enophthalmos are:
  - Blowout fractures leading to loss of orbital contents.
  - Atrophy of the orbital contents following irradiation, trauma, infection, cicatrizing carcinomas, aging, etc.

GIST BOX 14.4

- Proptosis is defined as abnormal forward displacement of eyeball beyond the orbital margins.
- Exophthalmos is defined as proptosis or forward displacement of the eyeball caused by thyroid eye disease; it is the commonest cause for proptosis.
- Proptosis can be acute, chronic, intermittent, pulsating, unilateral or bilateral.
- Pseudoproptosis is defined as a condition in which the eyeball appears to be proptosed, but there is no displacement of the eyeball.

CHAPTER

14.5 Thyroid Eye Diseases

DEFINITION***

Thyroid eye disease indicates ocular changes seen in the orbit and periorbital tissues in association with dysthyroid states. It is also known as thyroid orbitopathy, Graves' ophthalmopathy, endocrine exophthalmos, etc.

The association of ophthalmopathy in patients with thyroid abnormalities was noticed by Robert Graves.

ETIOPATHOGENESIS

Thyroid eye disease is most commonly seen in association with Graves' disease characterized by hyperthyroidism. Eye manifestations can also be seen in hypothyroidism or euthyroidism.

Thyroid eye diseases are more common in females compared to males. Smoking has got strong association with development of thyroid orbitopathy.

Graves' disease is an autoimmune disease characterized by the presence of thyroid-stimulating immunoglobulins giving rise to hyperthyroidism.

The pathogenesis of thyroid ophthalmopathy is explained by immunological mechanism. The orbital fibroblasts are the main target sites, which may express thyroid-stimulating hormone (TSH) receptors. The cellular infiltration and proliferation of the fibroblasts leads to protrusion of the eye as a result of increase in the retrobulbar tissue.

CLINICAL FEATURES**

The ocular features of thyroid eye disease are as follows.

Exophthalmos

Exophthalmos indicates proptosis caused by endocrine dysfunction as in thyroid eye disease. The word exophthalmos is almost synonymous with thyroid ophthalmopathy. It is caused by increased volume of retrobulbar fat and enlargement of the extraocular muscles (Figs 14.5.1A and B).

Eyelid Signs

Lid retraction is the most common eyelid sign seen in thyroid ophthalmopathy. It is caused by increased sensitivity of the Müller's muscle of the eyelid to adrenaline secondary to increased levels of thyroid hormones and fibrosis of the inferior rectus muscle leading to secondary overaction of superior rectus and levator muscle.

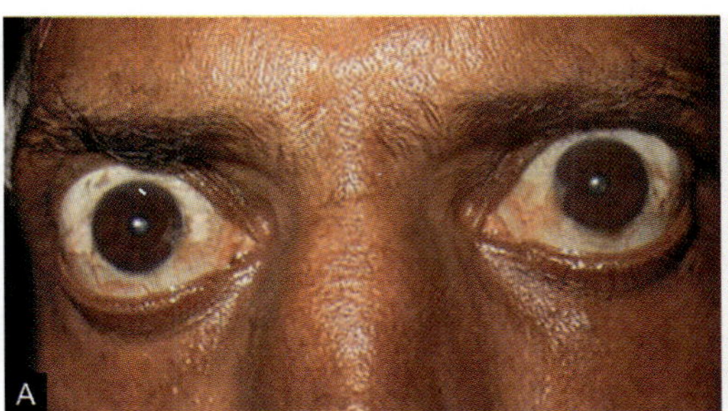

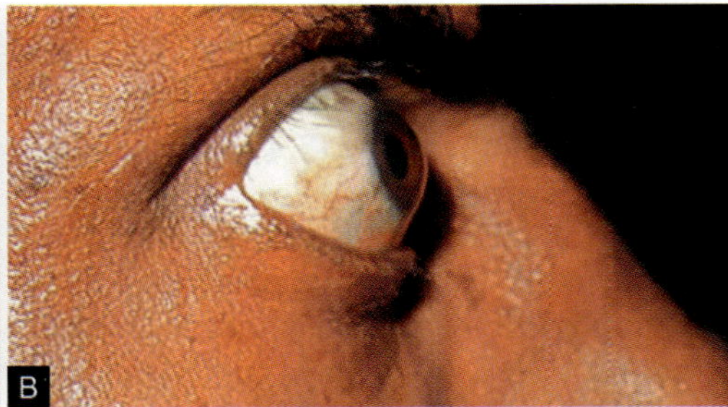

FIGS 14.5.1A and B: Exophthalmos

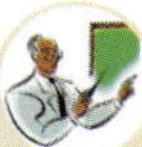

Ocular Signs in Exophthalmos

- Dalrymple's sign: Lid retraction.
- Von Graefe sign: Upper lid lag on downgaze.
- Grove sign: Resistance of upper lid to downward traction.
- Gifford sign: Difficult to evert upper eyelid.
- Griffith sign: Lower lid lags behind the globe on upgaze.
- Kocher's sign: Staring look of eyes.
- Rosenbach sign: Tremors of closed eyelid.
- Stellwag sign: Infrequent blinking.
- Jellinek sign: Increased pigmentation of upper eyelid.
- Joffroy's sign: Decreased wrinkling on forehead on upgaze.
- Enroth sign: Fullness of eyelids.
- Riesman's sign: Bruit over the eyelid.
- Mobius sign: Convergence weakness.

Extraocular Muscle Involvement

Enlargement of the extraocular muscles is seen in thyroid orbitopathy because of infiltration of the extraocular muscles and deposition of the mucopolysaccharides. Inferior rectus is the most common muscle involved resulting in limitation of abduction and diplopia in upgaze.

Intraocular pressure is elevated in upgaze because of fibrosis of the inferior rectus and this variation of intraocular pressure in upgaze is one of the confirmatory tests for thyroid ophthalmopathy.

Medial rectus, superior rectus and lateral rectus are involved in decreasing order following inferior rectus. Oblique muscles are rarely involved. In thyroid ophthalmopathy, typically non-tendinous part of the extraocular muscles are involved.

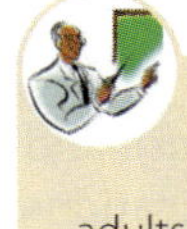

Thyroid orbitopathy is the most common cause unilateral or bilateral proptosis in adults.

COMPLICATIONS

Thyroid orbitopathy is largely a self-limiting disease, but complications are encountered secondary to exophthalmos.

The complications leading to diminution of vision and vision loss are:

- Corneal complications in the form of exposure keratitis leading to corneal ulcer and other complications
- Optic neuropathy secondary to increased intraorbital pressure.

American Thyroid Association and Werner SC have classified thyroid ophthalmopathy into six grades, which can be remembered by the NOSPECS (Table 14.5.1).

TABLE 14.5.1: NOSPECS grading

Grade	*Symptoms*
Grade 0	**N**o symptoms or signs
Grade 1	**O**nly signs no symptoms (signs limited to upper lid retraction with or without lid lag or proptosis)
Grade 2	**S**oft tissue involvement
Grade 3	**P**roptosis
Grade 4	**E**xtraocular muscle involvement
Grade 5	**C**orneal involvement
Grade 6	**S**ight loss because of optic neuropathy

INVESTIGATIONS

- Thyroid function tests in the form of estimation of triiodothyronine (T_3), thyroxine (T_4) and TSH levels
- Testing for TSH-receptor antibodies
- Orbital imaging in the form of computed tomography (CT) scan or magnetic resonance imaging (MRI). CT scan is more sensitive and it shows enlargement of the non-tendinous part of the extraocular muscles.

TREATMENT**

Thyroid eye disease is self-limiting disease and treatment is required to prevent complications in the acute episode:

1. The treatment of the thyroid abnormality by use of antithyroid drugs is required in all the cases.
2. Treatment of eyelid retraction:
   a. Eyelid retraction is treated by guanethidine 5% eyedrops.
   b. Artificial tears are used in cases associated with exposure keratopathy.
   c. Surgical procedures such as tarsorrhaphy or recession of levator and Müller's muscle and injection of botulinum toxin in cases with moderate-to-severe exposure, which may result in exposure keratopathy.
3. Treatment of thyroid myopathy: Thyroid myopathy with involvement of the extraocular muscles is treated by recession surgery on the fibrotic muscle.
4. Treatment of progressive proptosis:
   a. Systemic steroids, immunosuppressive drugs or radiotherapy are indicated in cases of progressive exophthalmos associated with inflammatory signs, chemosis and orbital edema.
   b. Surgical orbit decompression is considered in cases with optic nerve compression resulting in optic neuropathy.

GIST BOX 14.5

- Thyroid eye disease indicates ocular changes seen in the orbit and periorbital tissues in association with dysthyroid states; it is also known as thyroid orbitopathy, Graves' ophthalmopathy, endocrine exophthalmos, etc.
- Thyroid eye disease is most commonly seen in association with Graves' disease characterized by hyperthyroidism.
- The clinical features of thyroid eye disease are exophthalmos, eyelid signs and extraocular muscle involvement.
- Lid retraction is the most common eyelid sign seen in thyroid ophthalmopathy.
- American Thyroid Association and Werner SC have classified thyroid ophthalmopathy into six grades, which can be remembered by the NOSPECS.

CHAPTER

14.6 Orbital Trauma

Orbit is a bony cavity, which protects the eyeball from injuries by acting as a bony socket, which encloses the eyeball. Orbit is involved in different types of trauma and it prevents the injury to the eyeball, especially in blunt injuries.

Blunt injury of the orbit leads to orbital contusion, orbital hemorrhage and orbital fractures. Penetrating injuries of the orbit leads to intraorbital foreign bodies.

ORBITAL CONTUSION

Orbital contusion is because of rupture of the blood vessel in the periorbital structure and results in ecchymosis of the periorbital structures. A simple orbital contusion is usually limited to periorbital tissues and eyelids. It is called black eye.

> The submuscular areolar tissue of upper eyelids is in continuity with subaponeurotic space of scalp allowing easy passage of fluid and blood to the upper eyelids. Hence, black eye or ecchymosis of upper eyelids is common in cases of injuries to the head and face above the level of the eyebrows.

Clinical Features

Orbital contusion presents as swelling and ecchymosis of the periorbital tissues.

Investigations

Orbital contusion should be evaluated to look for associated orbital hemorrhage, orbital fracture by radiological investigations such as X-ray and computed tomography (CT) scan.

Treatment

The treatment of simple orbital contusion is by cold compression by using ice packs and use of anti-inflammatory drugs.

ORBITAL HEMORRHAGE**

Orbital hemorrhage is because of bleeding into the retrobulbar space behind the globe. It is also called retrobulbar hemorrhage (Figs 14.6.1A to C).

Retrobulbar hemorrhage leads to increase in intraorbital pressure resulting in compression of the vital structures including optic nerve, which can lead to loss of vision.

Clinical Features

Orbital hemorrhage presents with sudden onset of increasing proptosis, pain, limitation of the extraocular movements, elevation of intraocular pressure and subconjunctival hemorrhage with extension of the hemorrhage behind the globe (posterior limit cannot be made out).

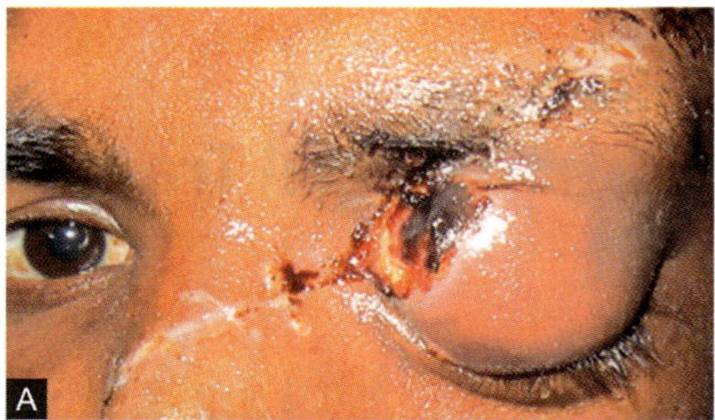

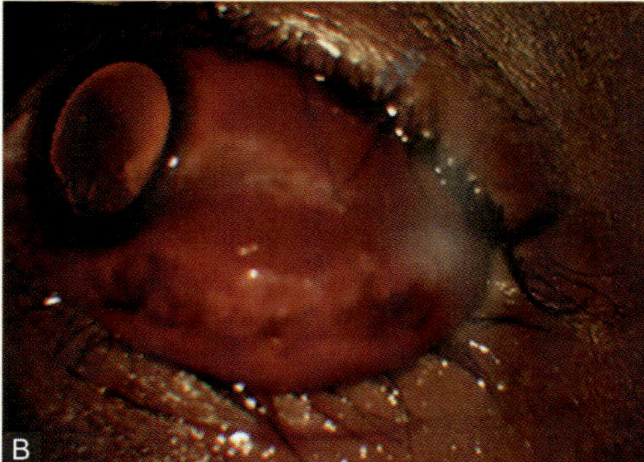

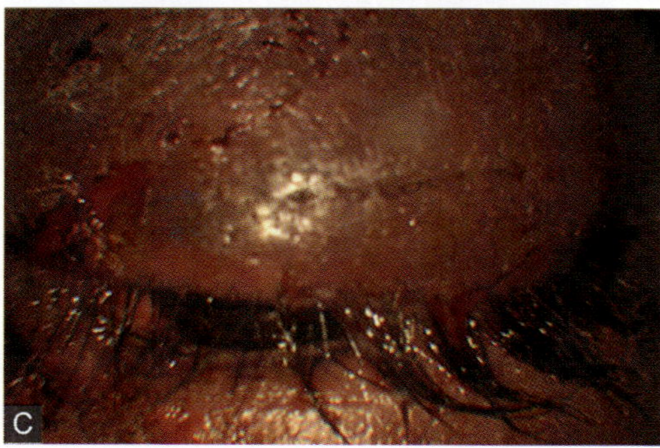

FIGS 14.6.1A to C: Orbital hemorrhage

Investigations

Orbital hemorrhage should be evaluated to look for associated orbital fracture by radiological investigations such as X-ray and CT scan.

Treatment

The treatment of orbital hemorrhage is an emergency to prevent optic nerve compression. The treatment is by reduction of intraocular pressure by using intraocular pressure lowering agents, for example acetazolamide or topical antiglaucoma medications.

Retrobulbar hemorrhage with elevated intraorbital pressure threatening vision is treated by emergency lateral canthotomy to decrease the intraorbital pressure. Cold compression by using ice packs and anti-inflammatory drugs are used for pain relief.

ORBITAL FRACTURES

Orbital fractures are commonly seen in injuries involving the face and the head. Orbital fractures are seen in the Le Fort fractures II and III.

Orbital fracture may involve the orbital rim, orbital walls or the orbital apex involving the optic canal or superior orbital fissure.

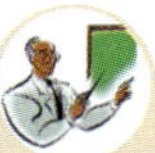

Le Fort Fracture

The fractures involving the face are described by Le Fort and they are classified as:

- Le Fort I: It is the fracture involving the lower part of the face involving the lower part of the maxilla above the level of the teeth.
- Le Fort II: It is a fracture of pyramidal configuration involving the lacrimal, nasal and maxilla.
- Le Fort III: It is a fracture, which causes craniofacial disjunction with fracture line passing through nasofrontal suture, maxillofrontal suture, orbital wall and zygomatic arch.

Orbital Blowout Fractures**

Definition

Orbital blowout fractures are isolated comminuted fractures and they occur as a result of sudden increase in the intraorbital pressure following blunt trauma leading to fracture of the one or more orbital walls.

Etiopathogenesis

Orbital fractures are usually caused by blunt injury by objects larger than the size of the eye such as human fist, cricket ball, etc.

Blowout fractures involving the walls of the orbit are the most common type of orbital fractures.

The mechanism of orbital fractures is explained by two theory:

1. The hydraulic theory states that increased intraorbital pressure results in fracture at the weakest point in the orbital wall, thus acting as a decompensation mechanism. Blowout fractures thus act as a decompensating mechanism against the raised intraorbital pressure, thus preventing damage to the vital orbital contents.
2. The buckling theory states that transmission of the force of injury from the orbital rim results in buckling and fracture of the orbital wall.

Orbital floor and medial wall of the orbit are the weak points in the orbital wall, hence orbital blowout fractures most commonly involve the orbital floor and medial wall.

Classification

Orbital blowout fractures are classified into:

- Pure blowout fractures indicate blowout fracture of the orbital wall without involvement of the orbital rim
- Impure blowout fractures indicate blowout fracture of the orbital wall with involvement of the orbital rim.

Clinical Features

The clinical features in the early stages are periorbital edema, ecchymosis, emphysema and paresthesia and numbness of the skin of the cheek because of involvement of the infraorbital nerve.

After the acute phase with resolution of the edema, enophthalmos of variable degree and diplopia are seen:

1. Enophthalmos is because of decrease in the orbital contents as a result of escape of the orbital contents into the maxillary antrum and entrapment of the inferior rectus muscle causing posterior traction of the eyeball.
2. Diplopia is because of entrapment of the inferior rectus or inferior oblique into fracture site in case of orbital floor fracture or because of injury to the nerves supplying the extraocular muscles (Figs 14.6.2 and 14.6.3).

All cases with orbital fractures should be evaluated to look for associated eye injuries and traumatic optic neuropathy. Though orbital fractures act as decompensating mechanism to prevent injury to the eyeball, significant ocular damage is seen in about 15–30% of cases.

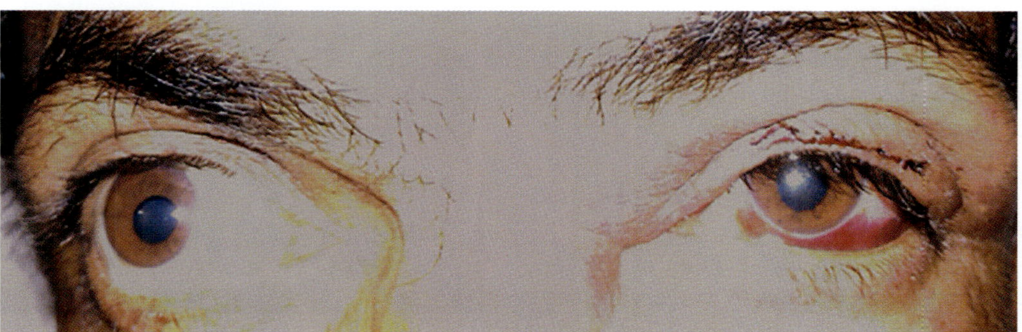

FIG. 14.6.2: Orbital floor fracture

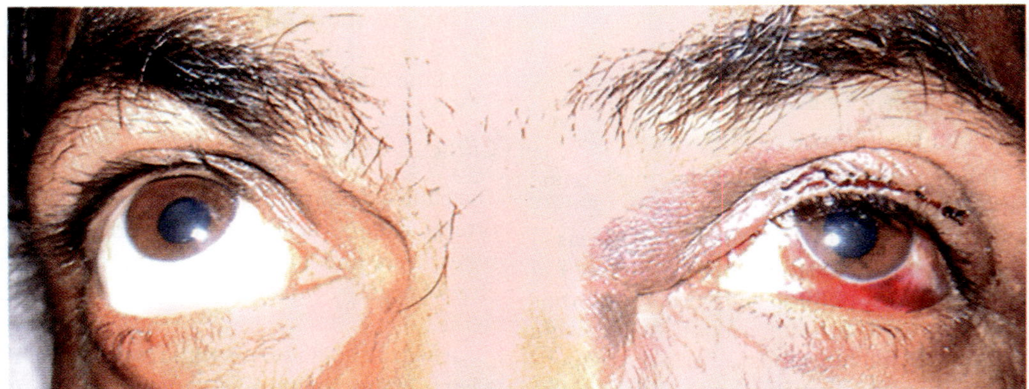

FIG. 14.6.3: Limitation of elevation because of orbital floor fracture with entrapment of inferior rectus

Investigations

Radiological investigations such as X-ray and CT scan are valuable in assessing the extent and severity of fracture.

Radiological investigations show haziness extending into the maxillary antrum from the orbit as a result of herniation of the orbital fat. This is called teardrop sign (Fig. 14.6.4).

Treatment

The treatment in the acute phase following injury is by use of anti-inflammatory drugs, antibiotics and cold compression.

The definitive treatment of orbital blowout fracture is by surgical repair. The surgery is usually done once the periorbital edema is decreased by the end of 2nd week. The indications for surgery are:

- Diplopia
- Significant enophthalmos (enophthalmos of more than 2 mm).

Open reduction and fixation of the fractured fragments is done by surgery. In cases with large fractures, the defect is filled by using autologous bone graft or by using alloplastic agents, for example, Teflon.

Blowout Fracture of Medial Wall of Orbit

- It involves the lamina papyracea and lacrimal bones.
- The mechanism and clinical features are similar to blowout fracture of the orbital floor except for horizontal diplopia because of entrapment of the medial rectus muscle.
- The treatment is similar to blowout fracture of the orbit.

INTRAORBITAL FOREIGN BODY

Intraorbital foreign body is commonly seen in association with penetrating and perforating injuries. Intraorbital foreign bodies can reach the

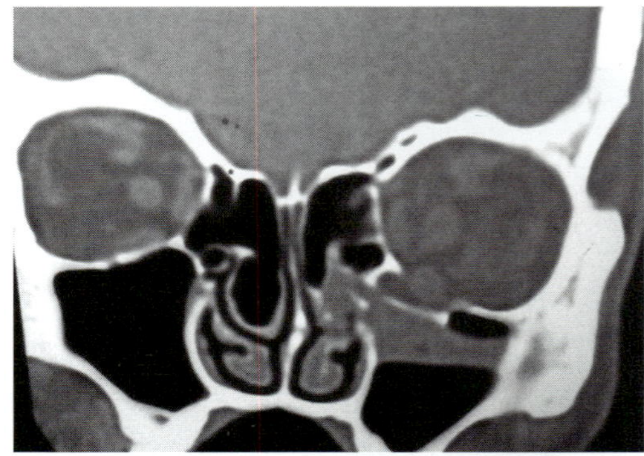

FIG. 14.6.4: Computed tomography scan showing inferior orbital fracture in the same patient with teardrop sign.

orbit or retro-orbital space by perforating the eye or the periorbital tissues.

The clinical features and treatment are similar to those of intraocular foreign bodies.

GIST BOX 14.6

- Orbital contusion is because of rupture of the blood vessel in the periorbital structure and results in ecchymosis of the periorbital structures. A simple orbital contusion is usually limited to periorbital tissues and eyelids. It is called black eye.
- Orbital hemorrhage is because of bleeding into the retrobulbar space behind the globe. It is also called retrobulbar hemorrhage.
- Orbital fractures are commonly seen in injuries involving the face and the head. Orbital fractures are seen in the Le Fort fractures II and III.
- Orbital blowout fractures are isolated comminuted fractures and they occur as a result of sudden increase in the intraorbital pressure following blunt trauma leading to fracture of the one or more orbital walls. Orbital floor and medial wall of the orbit are the weak points in the orbital wall; hence, orbital blowout fractures most commonly involve the orbital floor and medial wall.

CHAPTER

14.7 Cysts and Tumors of Orbit

CYSTS OF ORBIT

Orbital cysts include:

1. Congenital and developmental cysts such as dermoid cyst, epidermoid cyst, teratoma, congenital cystic eyeball, etc.
2. Acquired cysts such as parasitic cysts, hematic cysts, etc.

Dermoid cyst is the most common orbital tumor seen in children and it is described under tumors of the eyelids.

Cysticercosis cyst and orbital hydatid cyst are the common parasitic cysts of the orbit and they are described under parasitic infections of the orbit.

TUMORS OF ORBIT

Classification

Tumors of the orbit are classified into primary orbital tumors, secondary orbital tumors and metastatic tumors (Figs 14.7.1A and B).

Primary Orbital Tumors

Primary orbital tumors arise from the orbital structures and are subclassified into:

- Congenital and developmental such as dermoid cyst, epidermoid cyst and teratoma
- Vascular tumors such as capillary hemangioma, cavernous hemangioma and lymphangioma

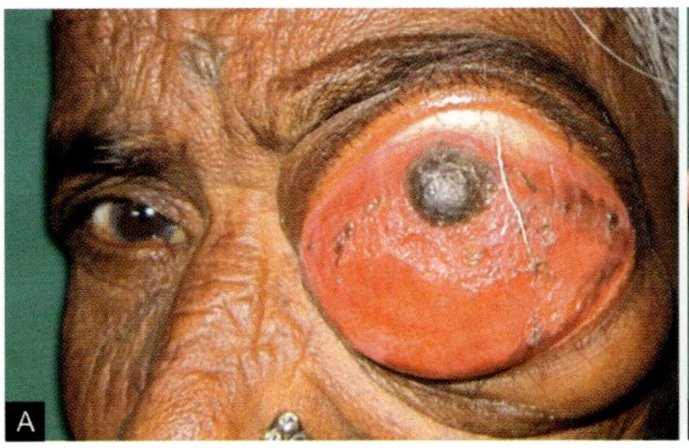

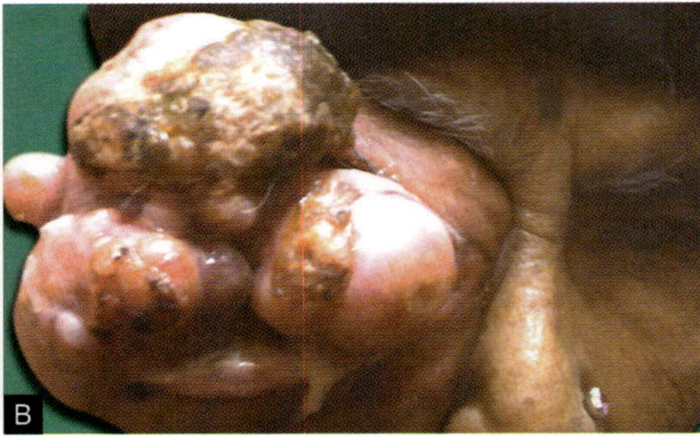

FIGS 14.7.1A and B: Tumors of orbit

- Neural tumors such as neurofibromatosis and neurofibroma
- Soft tissue tumors, for example, rhabdomyosarcoma
- Fibro-osseous tumors such as fibroma, osteoma, fibrous dysplasia, osteoblastoma and osteosarcoma.

Secondary Orbital Tumors

Secondary orbital tumors arise from surrounding structures of the orbit such as paranasal sinuses, nasopharynx, intracranial cavity or from eye and its adnexal structures and involve the orbit by extension.

Metastatic Orbital Tumors

Metastatic include tumors arising from the distant organs and reaching the orbit by hematogenous spread. The common sites for metastasis to orbit are carcinomas of breast, lungs and prostate, neuroblastoma, malignant melanoma, leukemia, etc.

Congenital and developmental tumors, and vascular tumors are described under tumors of the eyelids.

Rhabdomyosarcoma**

Etiopathogenesis

Rhabdomyosarcoma is the most common soft tissue sarcoma in children. Head and neck is the most common site for occurrence of rhabdomyosarcoma. The other sites of occurrence of the tumor are pelvis, extremities, trunk and orbit.

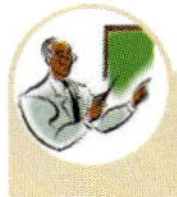

Rhabdomyosarcoma is the most common primary orbital malignant tumor.

Orbital rhabdomyosarcoma arises from primitive muscle cells and in orbit, it arises from extraocular muscles. Orbital rhabdomyosarcoma is seen in children below 15 years with a mean age of 7 years.

Rhabdomyosarcoma is associated with maternal exposure to X-rays or use of tobacco, cocaine and marijuana. It is associated with neurofibromatosis, basal cell nevus syndrome and mutation in the *p53* tumor suppressor gene on chromosome 17.

Clinical Features

Orbital rhabdomyosarcoma most commonly presents as rapidly progressive proptosis of sudden onset. It commonly involves the superonasal quadrant of the orbit. It can also present as subconjunctival mass or ptosis. The mass is usually firm with erythema and chemosis, but other inflammatory signs are absent.

Histopathology

1. Embryonal type is the most common pathological subtype and it has got favorable prognosis.
2. Alveolar subtype is the most malignant variety and it is associated with worst prognosis.
3. Pleomorphic, spindle cell and botryoid are the other histopathological subtypes of rhabdomyosarcoma.

Differential Diagnosis

Rhabdomyosarcoma has to be differentiated from:

- Orbital cellulitis
- Orbital inflammatory syndrome
- Lymphoma
- Capillary hemangioma
- Metastatic disease.

Investigations

Radiological investigations such as computed tomography (CT) scan, magnetic resonance imaging (MRI) show mass arising from the extraocular muscles.

Treatment

Radiotherapy and chemotherapy are the common modes of treatment. Surgical treatment in the form of exenteration is required in advanced cases for debulking the tumor.

GIST BOX 14.7

- Orbital cysts include congenital and developmental cysts such as dermoid cyst, epidermoid cyst, teratoma, congenital cystic eyeball, etc. and acquired cysts such as parasitic cysts, hematic cysts, etc.
- Tumors of the orbit are classified into primary orbital tumors, secondary orbital tumors and metastatic tumors.
- Rhabdomyosarcoma is the most common soft tissue sarcoma in children.

FREQUENTLY ASKED QUESTIONS (FAQs)

*Short Answers

1. Anatomy of walls of orbit.
2. Contents of orbit.
3. Apertures of orbit.
4. Surgical spaces of orbit.
5. Craniosynostosis.
6. Hypertelorism.
7. Classify orbital inflammations.
8. Mention the causes of acute proptosis in children.
9. Mention the causes of unilateral proptosis.
10. Mention the causes for bilateral proptosis.
11. Pseudoproptosis.
12. Enophthalmos.

**Short Essays

1. Cavernous sinus thrombosis.
2. Pseudotumor of the orbit (idiopathic orbital inflammatory syndrome).
3. Clinical anatomy of cavernous sinus.
4. Clinical features of thyroid ophthalmopathy.
5. Describe the treatment of thyroid ophthalmopathy.
6. Orbital hemorrhage.
7. Blowout fractures of orbit.
8. Rhabdomyosarcoma.

***Long Essays

1. Describe the etiopathogenesis, clinical features and treatment of orbital cellulitis.
2. Define proptosis. Discuss etiology, classification and evaluation of eye proptosis.
3. Describe the etiopathogenesis, clinical features and treatment of thyroid eye disease.

BIBLIOGRAPHY

1. Dutta LC. Modern Ophthalmology, vol. 7, 3rd edition. New Delhi: Jaypee Brothers Medical Publishers (P) Ltd; 2005.
2. Gordon LK. Orbital inflammatory disease: a diagnostic and therapeutic challenge. Eye. 2006;20(10):1196-206.
3. Maheshwari R, Weis E. Thyroid associated orbitopathy. Indian J Ophthalmol. 2012;60(2):87-93.
4. Srinivasan R, Gulnar D. Orbital pseudotumor. Kerala J Ophthalmol. 2009;21(2):127-31.
5. Werner SC. A new classification of the eye changes of Graves' disease. Arch Ophthalmol. 1969;82(3):421-3.
6. Wulc AE, Edmonson BC. Orbital infections. Duane's Clinical Ophthalmology, vol 2.
7. Yen MT, Flaharty PM, Anderson RL. Congenital and developmental anomalies of the orbit. In: William T, Edward AJ (Eds). Duane's Clinical Ophthalmology, vol 2. Philadelphia: Lippincott Williams & Wilkins; 2006.

SECTION 15

Strabismus

CHAPTER

15.1 Anatomy and Physiology of Ocular Movements

ANATOMY OF EXTRAOCULAR MUSCLES

Extraocular muscles control the eye movements. There are six pairs of extraocular muscles and they consist of four rectus muscles including superior rectus, inferior rectus, medial rectus and lateral rectus, and two oblique muscles superior oblique and inferior oblique (Fig. 15.1.1).

RECTUS MUSCLES*

Origin

The four rectus muscles have common origin arising from the common tendinous ring called annulus of Zinn attached to the apex of the orbit.

Insertion

The rectus muscles are inserted into the sclera anterior to the equator by flat tendons. The distance of insertion of the rectus muscles from the limbus is:

- Medial rectus 5.5 mm medial to the limbus
- Lateral rectus 6.5 mm lateral to the limbus
- Inferior rectus 6.9 mm inferior to the limbus
- Superior rectus is 7.7 mm superior to the limbus.

Nerve Supply*

Superior rectus, inferior rectus and medial rectus are supplied by oculomotor nerve and III cranial nerve. Lateral rectus is supplied by abducent nerve and VI cranial nerve.

Blood Supply*

Blood supply is from muscular branches of the ophthalmic artery. Medial muscular branches supply medial rectus and inferior rectus. Lateral muscular branches supply lateral rectus and superior rectus.

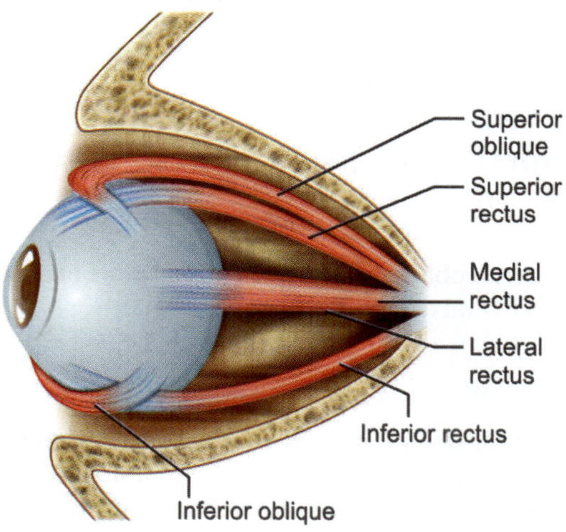

FIG. 15.1.1: Extraocular muscles

OBLIQUE MUSCLES*

Superior Oblique

Origin

Superior oblique arises from body of the sphenoid bone above and medial to the optic foramen.

Course

The superior oblique muscle runs forward between the roof and medial wall of the orbit to reach the trochlea or pulley. It passes through the pulley becoming tendinous and passes downward, backward and laterally.

Insertion

The superior oblique gets inserted into superotemporal quadrant of the globe posterior to the equator.

Nerve Supply

Superior oblique is supplied by trochlear nerve and the IV cranial nerve.

Blood Supply

Blood supply is from lateral muscular branch of the ophthalmic artery.

Inferior Oblique*

Origin

Inferior oblique arises from orbital plate of maxilla lateral to lacrimal fossa.

Course

Inferior oblique passes backwards and laterally parallel to the tendon of the superior oblique between the inferior rectus and floor of the orbit.

Insertion

Inferior oblique gets inserted into inferior part of the posterolateral quadrant of the globe.

Nerve Supply

Inferior oblique is supplied by oculomotor nerve and III cranial nerve.

Blood Supply

Blood supply is from medial muscular branch of the ophthalmic artery.

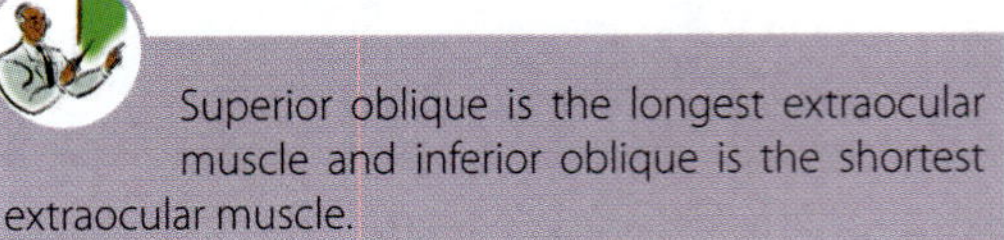

Superior oblique is the longest extraocular muscle and inferior oblique is the shortest extraocular muscle.

ACTIONS OF EXTRAOCULAR MUSCLES*

The actions of extraocular muscles are given in Table 15.1.1.

TABLE 15.1.1: Actions of extraocular muscles

Muscle	*Primary action*	*Secondary action*	*Tertiary action*
Medial rectus	Adduction	–	–
Lateral rectus	Abduction	–	–
Superior rectus	Elevation	Intorsion	Adduction
Inferior rectus	Depression	Extorsion	Adduction
Superior oblique	Intorsion	Depression	Abduction
Inferior oblique	Extorsion	Elevation	Abduction

OCULAR MOVEMENTS

The eyes show a wide range of ocular movements and the ocular movements are because of rotation of globe and this rotation occurs around a center of rotation. This is explained by Listing's plane and Fick's axes.

The Fick's axes include X, Y and Z axis. X axis is transverse axis responsible for vertical movements. Y axis is sagittal axis responsible for torsional movements. The Z axis is vertical axis responsible for horizontal movements. Listing's plane is an equatorial plane, which contains the center of rotation, and X and Z axes with Y axis being perpendicular to the plane. The ocular movements include uniocular movements and also binocular movements.

Uniocular Movements

The uniocular movements are also called ductions (Table 15.1.2).

TABLE 15.1.2: Uniocular movements

Movement	*Description*
Abduction	Lateral movement
Adduction	Medial movement
Supraduction	Elevation or upward movement
Infraduction	Depression or downward movement
Incycloduction	Intorsion or rotatory movement with superior limbus rotating medially
Excycloduction	Extorsion or rotatory movement with superior limbus rotating laterally

Binocular Movements*

The binocular movements include versions and vergences.

Versions

Versions are also called conjugate movements and include binocular symmetric movements with both eyes moving in same direction (Table 15.1.3 and Figs 15.1.2A to H).

Vergences

Vergences are also called disconjugate movements and include binocular symmetric movements with both eyes moving in opposite directions (Table 15.1.4 and Figs 15.1.3A and B).

POSITIONS OF GAZE

There are nine positions of gaze. They are classified as detailed in Table 15.1.5.

TABLE 15.1.3: Versions

Version	*Direction*
Dextroversion	Both eyes toward right side
Levoversion	Both eyes toward left side
Supraversion	Both eyes upward
Infraversion	Both eyes downward
Dextroelevation	Both eyes toward right side and upward
Levoelevation	Both eyes toward left side and upward
Dextrodepression	Both eyes toward right side and downward
Levodepression	Both eyes toward left side and downward
Dextrocycloversion	Both eyes show rotatory movement with superior limbus rotating medially
Levocycloversion	Both eyes show rotatory movement with superior limbus rotating laterally

TABLE 15.1.4: Vergences

Vergence	*Direction*
Convergence	Both eyes moving inwards
Divergence	Both eyes moving outwards

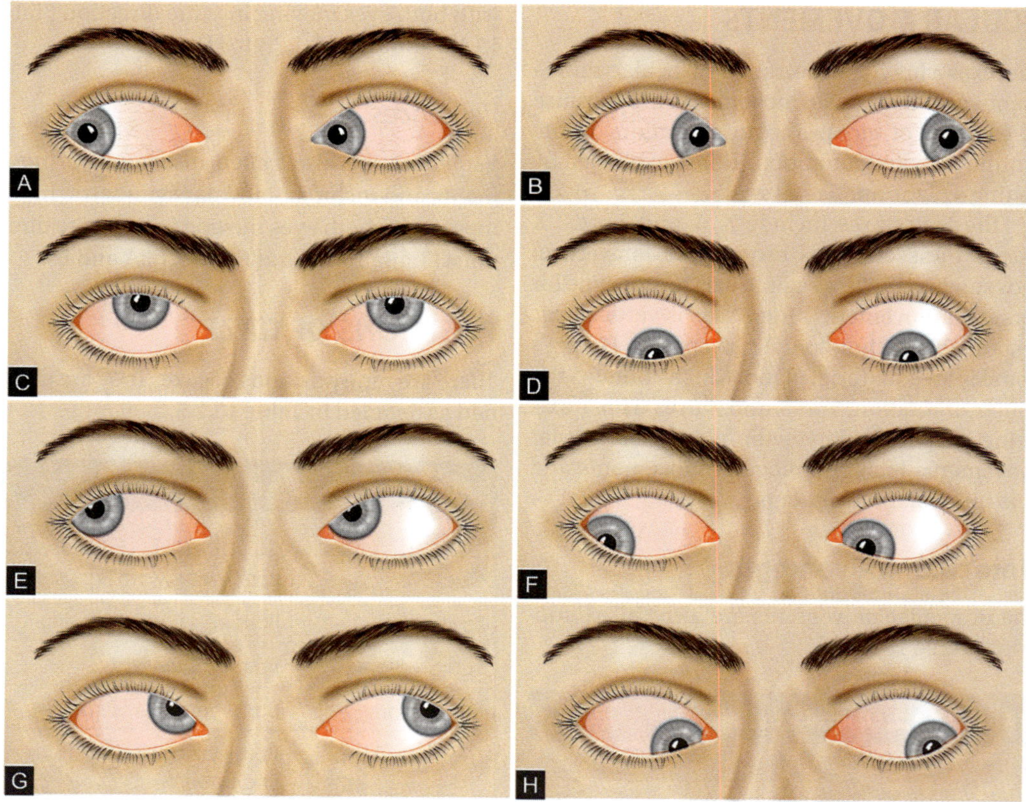

FIGS 15.1.2A to H: Versions. **A.** Dextroversion; **B.** Levoversion; **C.** Supraversion; **D.** Infraversion; **E.** Dextroelevation; **F.** Dextrodepression; **G.** Levoelevation; **H.** Levodepression.

TABLE 15.1.5: Positions of gaze

Position	*Description*
Primary position	Primary position with the eyes looking straight ahead
Secondary positions	They include dextroversion, levoversion, supraversion and infraversion
Tertiary positions	They include dextroelevation, levoelevation, dextrodepression and levodepression
Cardinal positions	They include dextroversion, levoversion, dextroelevation, levoelevation, dextrodepression and levodepression

LAWS OF OCULAR MOVEMENTS (Table 15.1.6)

Sherrington's Law

Sherrington's law states that increased innervation to an extraocular muscle is associated with reciprocal decrease in innervation to antagonist of the agonist.

Hering's Law*

Hering's law states that during conjugate eye movements such as versions equal innervations flows to yoke muscles.

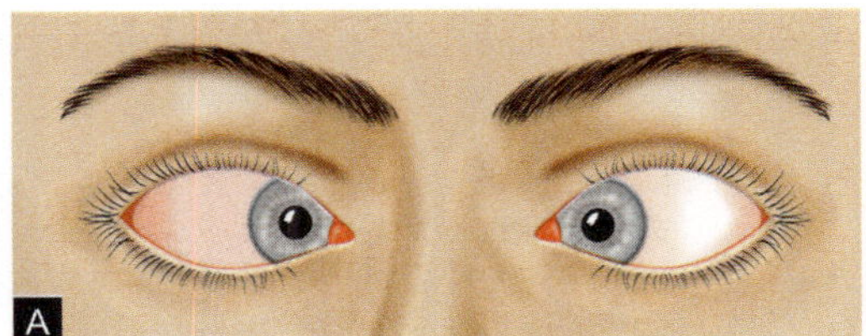

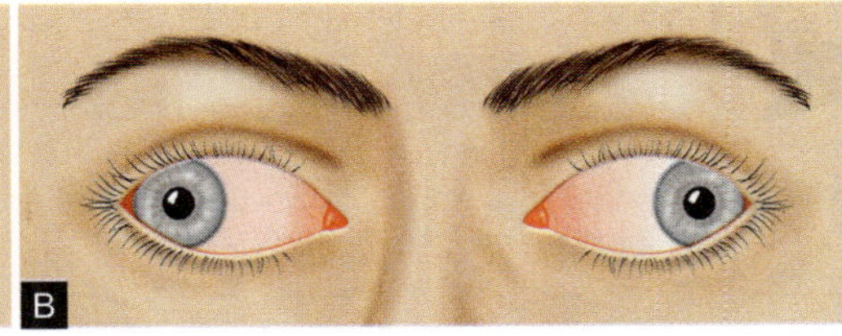

FIGS 15.1.3A and B: Vergences. **A.** Convergence; **B.** Divergence.

TABLE 15.1.6: Laws of ocular movements

Laws	*Description*
Agonist	A muscle, which moves the eye in the direction of action
Antagonist	A muscle, which opposes the action of the agonist in the same eye
Synergist	A muscle, which aids the action of the agonist in the same eye
Yoke muscles	They are called contralateral synergists and represent one muscle from each eye, which produce conjugate eye movements

Agonist, Synergist and Antagonist (Table 15.1.7)

TABLE 15.1.7: Agonist, synergist and antagonist of muscles

Agonist	*Synergist*	*Antagonist*
Medial rectus	Superior rectus Inferior rectus	Lateral rectus Superior oblique Inferior oblique
Lateral rectus	Superior oblique Inferior oblique	Medial rectus Superior rectus Inferior rectus
Superior rectus	Medial rectus Inferior oblique	Inferior rectus Superior oblique
Inferior rectus	Medial rectus Superior oblique	Superior rectus Inferior oblique
Superior oblique	Lateral rectus Inferior rectus	Superior rectus Inferior oblique
Inferior oblique	Superior rectus Lateral rectus	Inferior rectus Superior oblique

Yoke Muscles (Table 15.1.8)

TABLE 15.1.8: Yoke muscle pairs

Version	*Description*
Dextroversion	Right lateral rectus and left medial rectus
Levoversion	Right medial rectus and left lateral rectus
Dextroelevation	Right superior rectus and left inferior oblique
Dextrodepression	Right inferior rectus and left superior oblique
Levoelevation	Right inferior oblique and left superior rectus
Levodepression	Right superior oblique and left inferior rectus

Hering's law governs the binocular eye movements and explains the versions whereas Sherrington's law governs uniocular ductions. The clinical application of Hering's law explains the secondary changes in the extraocular muscles as a consequence of paralysis. The changes seen following paralysis of the extraocular muscle are overaction of the contralateral synergist, underaction of the ipsilateral antagonist and secondary inhibitional palsy of the contralateral antagonist. This explains the reason secondary angle of deviation is greater than primary angle of deviation in case of paralytic squint.

GIST BOX 15.1

- Extraocular muscles control the eye movements. There are six pairs of extraocular muscles and they consist of four rectus muscles including superior rectus, inferior rectus, medial rectus and lateral rectus, and two oblique muscles, superior oblique and inferior oblique.
- The four rectus muscles have common origin arising from the common tendinous ring called annulus of Zinn attached to the apex of the orbit. The rectus muscles are inserted into the sclera anterior to the equator by flat tendons.
- Superior rectus, inferior rectus and medial rectus are supplied by oculomotor nerve, III cranial nerve. Lateral rectus is supplied by abducent nerve and VI cranial nerve.
- Superior oblique arises from body of the sphenoid bone above and medial to the optic foramen. It gets inserted into superotemporal quadrant of the globe posterior to the equator. It is supplied by trochlear nerve, the IV cranial nerve.
- Inferior oblique arises from orbital plate of maxilla lateral to lacrimal fossa. It gets inserted into inferior part of the posterolateral quadrant of the globe, and it is supplied by oculomotor nerve and III cranial nerve.
- The ocular movements include uniocular movements and binocular movements. The uniocular movements are also called ductions and include abduction, adduction, supraduction, infraduction, incycloduction and excycloduction. The binocular movements include versions and vergences.
- Hering's law states that during conjugate eye movements such as versions equal innervation flows to yoke muscles.
- Sherrington's law states that increased innervation to an extraocular muscle is associated with reciprocal decrease in innervation to antagonist of the agonist.

CHAPTER

15.2 Binocular Single Vision

DEFINITION*

The coordinated use of both the eyes to produce a single vision is called binocular single vision.

DEVELOPMENT OF BINOCULAR SINGLE VISION

Though we have two eyes and image formation occurs in both the eyes separately, we perceive a single unified image and this occurs because of presence of binocular single vision.

Binocular single vision is absent at birth and it is acquired after birth as a conditioned reflex.

At birth, both the eyes move randomly; there is no central fixation and the visual acuity at birth is about 6/60.

By 6 weeks of age the fixation reflex appears and it develops completely by 6 months. Binocular single vision is achieved by 6 years of age and the visual acuity becomes 6/6 by this age.

Hence, 6 months to 6 years is the vital period in the development of visual acuity and any disease of the eye affecting the visual pathway will lead to disorders of binocular single vision.

GRADES OF BINOCULAR SINGLE VISION*

Binocular single vision is of three grades:

1. Simultaneous macular perception: It is the ability of the eyes to see two dissimilar images simultaneously and to superimpose them.
2. Fusion: It is the ability of the eyes to superimpose two images, which are slightly dissimilar and incomplete and make complete image by fusing them.
3. Stereopsis: It is the ability of the eyes to have depth perception and to form a three dimension image.

ANOMALIES OF BINOCULAR SINGLE VISION*

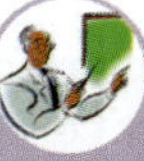

The anomalies of binocular single vision are:

- Suppression.
- Amblyopia.
- Diplopia.
- Anomalous retinal correspondence.

Suppression

Suppression is defined as cortical inhibition of the image formed on the squinting eye to avoid confusion formed as a result of image falling on the fovea in the normal eye and extrafoveal point in the squinting eye.

The suppression can be detected by Worth 4-dot test. Suppression when not corrected will lead to development of amblyopia.

Amblyopia**

The word amblyopia is derived from Greek word and it means dull eye or lazy eye.

Definition

Amblyopia is defined as unilateral or bilateral reduction in visual acuity caused by abnormal binocular interaction during the period of visual development between 6 months and 6 years.

*Classification**

Depending on the cause, amblyopia is classified into:

- Anisometropic amblyopia
- Stimulus deprivation amblyopia
- Strabismic amblyopia
- Meridional amblyopia
- Isoametropic amblyopia
- Organic amblyopia.

Anisometropic amblyopia

Anisometropic amblyopia develops as a result of ammetropia because of constantly blurred image in the ammetropic eye. It is most commonly seen in case of hypermetropia. Mild-to-moderate myopia rarely causes amblyopia as the myopic eye is used for near vision.

Stimulus deprivation amblyopia

Stimulus deprivation amblyopia develops as a result of diseases, which obstruct the light rays as in congenital corneal opacity, moderate-to-severe congenital ptosis, congenital and developmental cataract, congenital diseases of the retina, etc.

Strabismic amblyopia

Strabismic amblyopia develops as a result of constant unilateral squint as a result of suppression of the squinting eye.

Meridional amblyopia

Meridional amblyopia develops as a result of uncorrected astigmatism as a result of constant blurring of vision in one meridian.

Isoametropic amblyopia

Isoametropic amblyopia develops as a result of high ammetropia. It differs from anisometropic amblyopia by the fact that it is bilateral and it is seen in cases of high ammetropia of both the eyes. It is commonly seen in bilateral high hypermetropia.

Organic amblyopia

Organic amblyopia develops as a result of organic diseases of the visual pathway, e.g. nutritional and hereditary optic neuropathies, toxic amblyopia, etc. Unlike the other types of amblyopia, this can be seen in any age.

*Clinical Features**

1. Visual acuity is decreased.
2. Visual acuity is typically better on checking the visual acuity by single optotypes, but this decreases on checking with multiple letter charts. This is termed as crowding phenomenon.
3. Improvement or no change in visual acuity on viewing through the neutral density filter is seen in amblyopic eye, whereas the visual acuity decreases in the normal eye on viewing through the neutral density filter. This occurs because neutral density filter decreases the luminance thus affecting the central visual acuity. Since the amblyopic eye does not use central visual acuity, the neutral density filter does not affect it.
4. Eccentric fixation is observed in cases of severe amblyopia.

*Treatment**

Treatment of amblyopia is done by:

1. Treatment of the cause in cases in which it can be corrected, e.g. surgical treatment of congenital cataract, congenital corneal opacities, congenital ptosis, etc.
2. Optical correction of the underlying refractive errors.
3. Stimulation of the amblyopic eye is done by occlusion therapy. The occlusion therapy can be total or partial. Total occlusion is indicated in severe amblyopia and it is done by occluding the normal eye and forcing the child to use the amblyopic eye. Partial occlusion is indicated in mild-to-moderate amblyopia and it is done by causing blurring of vision in the normal eye by use of coated glasses. The other methods of stimulation of the amblyopic eye is by penalization of the normal eye by using atropine eyedrops to the normal eye or by use of complementary and alternative medicine (CAM) stimulator to stimulate the amblyopic eye by asking the child to view the rotating drum with stripes, etc.
4. Use of medical drugs such as levodopa to stimulate the amblyopic eye.

Diplopia

Diplopia occurs because of formation of image on the fovea in one eye and formation of image in the extrafoveal point in another eye.

Anomalous Retinal Correspondence

Anomalous retinal correspondence is characterized by the correspondence of fovea of one eye with the extrafoveal point of the other eye. It is seen in mild squint. The presence of anomalous retinal correspondence is tested by Worth 4-dot test.

GIST BOX 15.2

- The coordinated use of both the eyes to produce a single vision is called binocular single vision.
- Binocular single vision is absent at birth and it is acquired after birth as a conditioned reflex. Simultaneous macular perception, fusion and stereopsis are the grades of binocular single vision. Suppression, amblyopia, diplopia and anomalous retinal correspondence are the anomalies of binocular single vision.
- Amblyopia is defined as unilateral or bilateral reduction in visual acuity caused by abnormal binocular interaction during the period of visual development between 6 months and 6 years.

CHAPTER

15.3 Strabismus

DEFINITION

Strabismus is defined as a group of clinical conditions characterized by misalignment of the visual axes of the two eyes. It is also called crossed eyes or squint.

CLASSIFICATION*

Strabismus is broadly classified into:

- Latent strabismus/squint or heterophoria
- Manifest strabismus/squint or heterotropia.

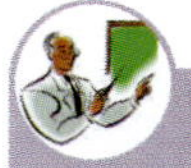

Strabismus can be classified depending on the various factors are:

- Based on the time of onset:
  - Congenital.
  - Acquired.
- Based on the direction of deviation:
  - Horizontal including medial deviation (esophoria or esotropia) and lateral deviation (exophoria or exotropia).
  - Vertical deviation hyperphoria/hypertropia.
  - Cyclotorsional including cyclophoria/cyclotropia.
- Based on the association with extraocular movements:
  - Concomitant squint or non-paralytic squint: It is characterized by normal extraocular movements and constant degree of squint in all the directions of gaze.
  - Incomitant squint or paralytic squint: It is characterized by limited extraocular movements in the direction of action of the paralyzed muscle and varying degree of squint in different directions of gaze.
- Based on the nature:
  - Constant squint.
  - Intermittent squint.

LATENT STRABISMUS/ HETEROPHORIA**

Latent squint/Heterophoria is defined as a clinical condition in which the alignment of the eyes is maintained by the fusional reflexes, hence the latent squint becomes manifest when the fusion of the two eyes is disrupted.

Etiology

Heterophoria is very common in clinical practice and it is estimated that up to 70% of people have some degree of latent strabismus. The causes for latent strabismus are:

1. Anatomical factors such as orbital asymmetry, variations in the interpupillary distance and optical axis, faulty insertion of extraocular muscles, etc.
2. Physiological factors such as accommodation and convergence, with increased accommodation and convergence resulting in esophoria, and decreased accommodation and convergence resulting in exophoria.
3. Neurogenic factors such as diseases affecting the motor neuron with upper motor neuron disease causing comitant squint and lower motor neuron diseases causing incomitant squint.

Classification

Depending on the direction of deviation, heterophoria is classified as follows.

Esophoria: It is characterized by heterophoria with tendency of the eyes to deviate inward. It is of three types:

1. Convergence excess esophoria, which increases on near fixation.
2. Divergence weakness esophoria, which decreases on near fixation.
3. Basic type with no change in esophoria on near fixation.

Exophoria: It is characterized by heterophoria with tendency of the eyes to deviate outward. It is of three types:

1. Convergence weakness exophoria, which increases on near fixation.
2. Divergence excess exophoria, which decreases on near fixation.
3. Basic type with no change in exophoria on near fixation.

Hyperphoria: It is characterized by heterophoria with tendency of the eyes to deviate upward or downward in the vertical direction.

Cyclophoria: It is characterized by heterophoria with tendency of the eyes to deviate along the anteroposterior axis. It can be:

1. Incyclophoria in which the upper limbus rotates nasally.
2. Excyclophoria in which the upper limbus rotates temporally.

Clinical Features

Heterophoria may be:

1. Asymptomatic, when the fusional reserve can compensate for the phoria called compensated phoria.
2. Symptomatic, when the fusional reserve cannot compensate for the phoria called decompensated phoria.

The risk factors for decompensated phoria are increasing age leading to weakness of fusion, stress, general debilitating conditions, etc. The clinical features seen in decompensated phoria are:

- Symptoms of muscle fatigue, e.g. headache, eye strain, difficulty in focusing, etc.
- Symptoms of loss of binocular single vision, e.g. diplopia, crowding of words, while reading, etc.
- Symptoms of defective postural sensations, e.g. difficulty to identify moving objects, etc.

Evaluation

Evaluation of heterophoria is done by:

- Assessment of visual acuity and refractive error
- Cover-uncover test
- Prism-bar cover test
- Maddox rod test
- Maddox wing test
- Measurement of fusional reserves, accommodation and convergence
- Assessment of binocular vision
- Synoptophore test.

Treatment

The treatment of heterophoria is done by:

1. Optical correction of the underlying refractive error if any or correction of any abnormalities of the accommodative convergence and accommodation.

2. Orthoptic exercises for improving convergence insufficiency or divergence weakness. Orthoptic exercises are done using synoptophore.
3. Surgical treatment is indicated in cases with:
   a. Manifest squint or tropia lasting longer than phoria or tropia lasting longer than 50% of the waking hours.
   b. Increase in the degree of deviation.
   c. Complications such as diplopia, anomalous retinal correspondence, suppression, etc.
4. Surgical treatment, when required is done on similar guidelines as that of tropia.

MANIFEST STRABISMUS/ HETEROTROPIA

Manifest squint is characterized by the presence of misalignment of the visual axes always. It is broadly classified into:

- Comitant squint or non-paralytic squint
- Incomitant squint or paralytic squint.

Comitant Squint***

Definition

Comitant squint is a type of squint characterized by normal extraocular movements and constant degree of squint in all the directions of gaze.

Etiopathogenesis

Binocular vision and coordinated ocular movements are absent at birth and they develop between 6 months and 6 years of age. Any disruptions, which occur in this period lead to development of squint. The causes can be:

1. Sensory problems, e.g. refractive error, cataract, corneal opacity, etc. These lead to squint by preventing the formation of clear image.
2. Motor problems, e.g. abnormalities of extraocular muscles, abnormalities of accommodation and convergence, etc. These lead to squint by preventing the proper alignment of the eyes.
3. Central problems, e.g. defective fusion, abnormalities in the cortical control of extraocular movements, etc.

Comitant squint can be esotropia, exotropia or hypertropia depending on the direction of deviation.

*Esotropia***

Definition

Convergent strabismus with eye deviated nasally is called esotropia (Fig. 15.3.1).

The word esotropia is derived from Greek and it means to turn inward.

Clinical types

The common clinical types of esotropia are:

- Accommodative esotropia
- Non-accommodative esotropia
- Secondary esotropia.

Accommodative esotropia

Accommodative esotropia is because of increased convergence associated with accommodation reflex. It is of three subtypes:

1. Refractive accommodative esotropia: It is associated with high hypermetropia. It is treated by correction of the refractive error.
2. Non-refractive accommodative esotropia: It is associated with high accommodative convergence/accommodation (AC/A) ratio with minimal refractive error or no refractive error. It is treated by giving near addition to overcome the high AC/A ratio.
3. Mixed accommodative esotropia: It is combination of both refractive and non-refractive accommodative esotropia.

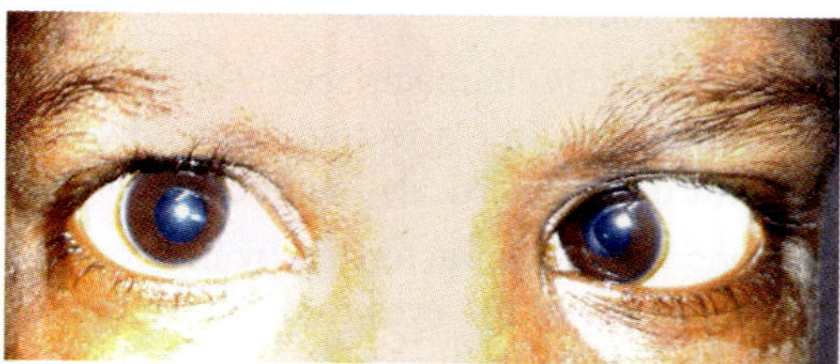

FIG. 15.3.1: Esotropia

Non-accommodative esotropia

Non-accommodative esotropia includes:

1. Congenital or essential infantile esotropia.
2. Acquired esotropia including basic esotropia, convergence excess esotropia, divergence insufficiency esotropia, acute esotropia and cyclic esotropia.

Congenital or infantile esotropia

Definition: Congenital esotropia, the esotropia present at birth is relatively less common. Infantile esotropia defined as large angle constant esotropia with onset before 6 months of age is more common.

Etiopathogenesis: The proposed mechanisms of development of congenital or infantile esotropia are:

1. Congenital absence of cortical fusion potential—Worth's theory.
2. Primary motor misalignment and poor binocular status—Chavasse theory.

Clinical features: It presents as a large angle constant esotropia with onset within 6 months of age:

1. Infantile esotropia of longer duration is associated with significant amblyopia.
2. Refractive error usually in the form of hypermetropia is associated with significant number of cases.
3. Inferior oblique overaction, dissociated vertical deviation and latent nystagmus are the common motor abnormalities associated with infantile esotropia.

Treatment: The treatment of congenital or infantile esotropia is usually by surgery. Surgery is indicated as early as by the age of 12 months after correction of the amblyopia and correction of the refractive error, if any.

Acquired esotropia

Basic esotropia: It is called essential esotropia of late onset. It is similar to infantile esotropia, except for the fact that the age of onset is > 6 months.

Acute esotropia: It is defined as esotropia of sudden onset in a person with previously normal binocular vision. It is usually associated with sudden onset of diplopia. The common causes for acute esotropia are systemic diseases, e.g. diabetes, hypertension, atherosclerosis, intracranial aneurysms, head injury, intracranial tumors, etc.

Cyclic esotropia: It is a rare type of esotropia characterized by cyclic episodes of esotropia with periods of normal alignment of eyes in between. It is a slowly progressive condition ultimately resulting in constant esotropia.

Secondary esotropia

Secondary esotropia includes:

1. Sensory deprivation esotropia: It results from primary visual deprivation as a result of monocular diseases, e.g. cataract, etc. which limit the sensory fusion resulting in development of secondary esotropia.
2. Consecutive esotropia: It results from surgical overcorrection of exotropia.

Exotropia

Definition

Divergent strabismus with eye deviated temporally is called exotropia (Fig. 15.3.2).

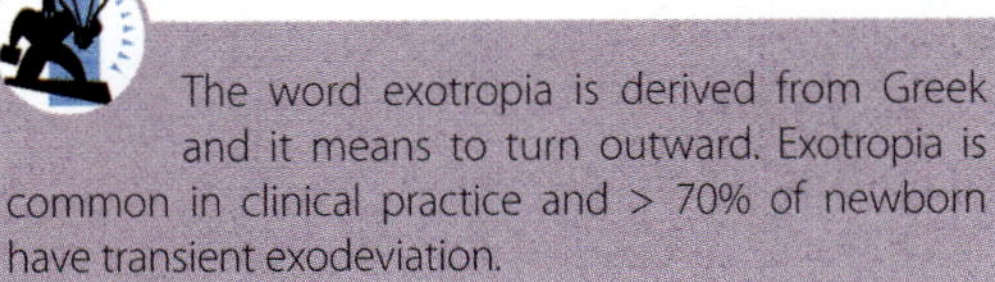

The word exotropia is derived from Greek and it means to turn outward. Exotropia is common in clinical practice and > 70% of newborn have transient exodeviation.

Clinical types

Infantile exotropia

Infantile exotropia represents essential exotropia with onset before 6 months of age. It is less common than infantile esotropia.

Primary exotropia

Primary exotropia includes basic exotropia, convergence weakness exotropia and the divergence

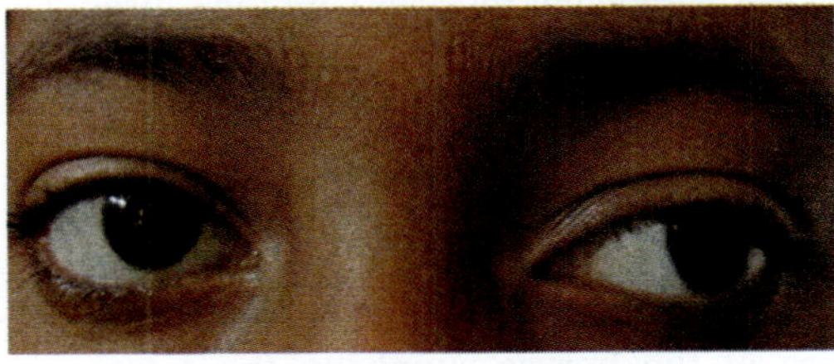

FIG. 15.3.2: Exotropia

excess exotropia. Primary exotropia is more commonly intermittent in nature.

Secondary exotropia
Secondary exotropia includes sensory deprivation exotropia and consecutive exotropia.

Hypertropia**

Hypertropia is characterized by vertical misalignment of eyes with upward deviation of the squinting eye. Hypotropia is characterized by vertical misalignment of the eyes with downward deviation of the squinting eye.

The common causes for hypertropia are:
- Trochlear nerve (cranial nerve IV) palsy
- Thyroid eye disease
- Duane's retraction syndrome
- Brown's syndrome.

Incomitant Squint***

Definition

Incomitant squint is characterized by limited or restricted extraocular movements and varying degree of squint in different directions of gaze. It includes:
- Paralytic squint
- Restrictive squint.

Paralytic Squint

Definition
Paralytic squint is characterized by limited extraocular movements in the direction of action of the paralyzed muscle and varying degree of squint in different directions of gaze.

Etiopathogenesis
Paralytic squint is caused by paralysis or paresis of the extraocular muscles with the causes classified as:
- Neurogenic
- Myogenic
- Neuromuscular junction.

Neurogenic causes
The neurogenic causes are congenital anomalies of the nerves supplying the extraocular muscles, inflammatory diseases affecting the nerves, e.g. cavernous sinus thrombosis, meningitis, trauma (head injury), neoplastic conditions (brain tumors), cerebrovascular accidents (cerebral hemorrhage), thrombosis, aneurysms, etc.

Myogenic causes
The myogenic causes such as congenital anomalies of the extraocular muscles, traumatic causes and diseases affecting the extraocular muscles, e.g. thyroid myopathy, etc.

Neuromuscular causes
The diseases affecting the neuromuscular junction, e.g. myasthenia gravis, etc.

Clinical features

Symptoms
1. Diplopia is the main distressing symptom of paralytic squint. It is more marked toward the action of the paralyzed muscle.
2. Vertigo, nausea, vomiting and false projection of the object are the other symptoms of paralytic squint.

Signs
On examination:
1. Primary deviation is the deviation of the squinting eye when the normal eye fixates is less than secondary deviation, i.e. deviation of the normal eye when the squinting eye fixates.
2. Limitation of the ocular movements in the direction of action of the paralyzed muscle.
3. Compensatory head posture to neutralize diplopia.

Clinical types
All types of paralytic squint show involvement of one or more muscles of the eye. The common clinical variants seen are:
- Oculomotor nerve palsy
- Trochlear nerve palsy
- Abducent nerve palsy
- Total ophthalmoplegia
- Internal ophthalmoplegia
- Internuclear ophthalmoplegia.

All the above conditions are described under neurophthalmology.

Investigations

Presence of paralytic squint warrants a neurological examination and requires radiological investigations such as computed tomography (CT) or magnetic resonance imaging (MRI) to find out the underlying cause. The ocular tests carried out are as follows.

Diplopia charting

Diplopia charting is done by dissociating the eyes by placing the red glass in front of right eye and green glass in front of left eye. A streak of light is moved in all the six positions of gaze and the patient is instructed to tell the gaze where separation of images is maximum and this will be seen in the direction of action of the paralyzed muscle.

Hess screen test

Hess screen test is done by asking the patient to read the Hess chart after dissociating the eyes by placing the red glass in front of right eye and green glass in front of left eye. It provides information regarding the secondary changes in the extraocular muscles as a consequence of paralysis. The changes seen following paralysis of the extraocular muscle are overaction of the contralateral synergist, underaction of the ipsilateral antagonist and secondary inhibitional palsy of the contralateral antagonist.

Worth 4-dot test

Worth 4-dot test is done by asking the patient to read four dots in the Snellen's visual chart after dissociating the eyes by placing the red glass in front of right eye and green glass in front of left eye. The patient sees two red lights and three green lights and hence shows diplopia.

Forced duction test

Forced duction test is done to differentiate the paralytic squint caused by paralysis of a muscle from restrictive squint. It is done under topical anesthesia. It is done by holding the muscle by a fixation forceps and eyeball is moved in the field of action of the paralyzed muscle. If the eyeball can be moved easily, it indicates that the test is negative and the cause is paralytic squint. The positive test as indicated by unable to move the eye indicates a positive test and the cause is restrictive squint.

Treatment

Treatment is done by:

1. Treating of the underlying cause.
2. Treatment of diplopia is done by temporary occlusion of the affected eye or by prismatic correction or by decentration of the lenses of spectacles.
3. Surgical intervention, if required is done after a waiting period of 6 months in patients in whom there is no significant improvement. Surgical treatment is by recession and resection muscle surgeries. Injection of botulinum toxin to cause chemodenervation is used as adjunctive or alternative procedure to surgery.

*Restrictive Squint***

Definition

Restrictive squint is characterized by restriction of the extraocular movements with small deviation in the primary position of gaze and a positive forced duction test.

Etiology

Restrictive squint is usually caused by the fibrosis of the extraocular muscle or by restriction of the movement of the extraocular muscle.

The common clinical syndromes presenting with restrictive squint are:

- Brown's syndrome or superior oblique tendon sheath syndrome
- Strabismus fixus
- Duane's retraction syndrome.

Brown's syndrome

Brown's syndrome is a type of restrictive strabismus characterized by the restriction of elevation in adduction. It is named after Harold W Brown, who first described the disease. This disease is also known as superior oblique tendon sheath syndrome.

It is of two types, congenital or true Brown's syndrome caused by congenital in elastic superior oblique muscle tendon complex and acquired Brown's syndrome caused by inflammation of the trochlea associated with sinusitis or rheumatoid arthritis and trauma either surgical or mechanical.

Diplopia in upgaze is the most common clinical feature. Inflammatory signs such as orbital pain and tenderness in the superonasal quadrant are also seen in inflammatory Brown's syndrome. Limitation of elevation in adduction and positive forced duction test in adduction on trying elevation of the globe in adduction are the consistent signs of Brown's syndrome.

Medical treatment in the form of steroids is indicated in treatment of inflammatory Brown's syndrome. Surgical treatment in the form of recession of superior oblique muscle is indicated in restrictive causes.

Strabismus fixus

Strabismus fixus is a rare type of restrictive squint characterized by fibrosis of medial rectus muscles of both the eyes resulting in strabismus with eyes fixed in convergent position.

*Duane's syndrome**

Duane's syndrome is a congenital syndrome characterized by fibrosis of lateral rectus or medial rectus or both. Depending on the muscle involved Duane's syndrome is classified as follows.

Type I: It is characterized by limitation of abduction, narrowing of palpebral fissure and retraction of the globe on attempted adduction and widening of the palpebral fissure on attempted abduction. It is the most common type of Duane's syndrome.

Type II: It is characterized by limitation of adduction, narrowing of palpebral fissure and retraction of the globe on attempted abduction.

Type III: It is characterized by limitation of both abduction and adduction, narrowing of palpebral fissure and retraction of the globe on attempted adduction.

The treatment is by recession of the involved muscle.

The differences between comitant and incomitant squint are given in Table 15.3.1.

Pseudostrabismus/Pseudosquint*

It is a condition characterized by false or pseudoappearance of squint in presence of normal alignment of the visual axis. It is seen in conditions such as epicanthal folds, hypertelorism and orbital asymmetry.

Pseudoesotropia is seen in conditions associated with prominent epicanthal fold covering the normal nasal part of the globe and in negative angle kappa.

Pseudoexotropia is seen in hypertelorism and in positive angle kappa. Pseudohypertropia is seen in orbital asymmetry.

'A' and 'V' Pattern Heterotropia

Horizontal squint can be associated with varying amount of deviation in upward or downward gaze and it may commonly follow 'A' and 'V' pattern. This is commonly because of dysfunction of the oblique muscles. 'V' pattern is associated with inferior oblique overaction and 'A' pattern is associated with superior oblique overaction.

'A' pattern esotropia is labeled for esotropia, which increases in upward gaze and 'A' pattern exotropia is labeled for exotropia, which decreases in downward gaze. 'V' pattern esotropia is labeled for esotropia, which decreases in upward gaze and 'V' pattern exotropia is labeled for exotropia, which increases in downward gaze.

Evaluation of Heterotropia**

Evaluation of heterotropia is done by the following (refer Chapter 5 Diagnostic Tests in Ophthalmology in Author's textbook *'Clinical Methods in Ophthalmology'*):

- Assessment of visual acuity and refractive error
- Hirschberg corneal reflex test

TABLE 15.3.1: Differences between comitant and incomitant squint**

Comitant squint	*Incomitant squint*
Positive family history and most cases are developmental	Usually caused by trauma or diseases affecting the nerves, muscles or neuromuscular junction
Insidious in onset	Sudden in onset
Symptoms, e.g. diplopia, nausea, etc. are absent	Symptoms, e.g. diplopia, vertigo, nausea and vomiting, and false projection are present
Abnormal head posture is absent	Abnormal head posture is present
Primary angle of deviation is equal to secondary angle of deviation	Secondary angle of deviation is greater than primary angle of deviation
Extraocular movement are normal	Extraocular movements are limited in direction of gaze of action of the paralyzed muscle
Amblyopia may be present	Amblyopia is absent
Secondary changes are absent	Secondary changes are seen following paralysis of the extraocular muscle and involve overaction of the contralateral synergist, underaction of the ipsilateral antagonist and secondary inhibitional palsy of the contralateral antagonist
Treatment involves optical correction, orthoptic exercises and squint surgery	Treatment is by treating of the underlying disease

- Cover test
- Cover-uncover test
- Alternate cover test
- Prism bar cover test
- Krimsky corneal reflex test
- Maddox rod test
- Maddox wing test
- Measurement of fusional reserves, accommodation and convergence
- Assessment of binocular vision
- Synoptophore test.

Treatment of Heterotropia

The treatment of heterotropia is done by:**

1. Optical correction of the underlying refractive error if any or correction of any abnormalities of the accommodative convergence and accommodation.
2. Orthoptic exercises for improving convergence insufficiency or divergence weakness. Orthoptic exercises are done using synoptophore.
3. Occlusion therapy is indicated in cases associated with amblyopia.

*Surgical Treatment***

The basic principle of squint surgery is to weaken or recess the overacting muscle and to strengthen or resect the underacting muscle.

Recession: It is done by making the muscle slackening the muscle by shifting the insertion of the muscle posteriorly toward its origin.

Resection: It is done by making the muscle taut by shortening the muscle.

Hence in esotropia, the surgery done is recession of medial rectus and resection of lateral rectus and in exotropia, the surgery done is resection of medial rectus and recession of lateral rectus.

The amount of recession and resection depends on the degree of squint. Each millimeter recession will approximately correct 2–3 prism diopters of squint.

The surgeries for weakening the muscle are:

- Recession
- Myotomy
- Tenotomy.

Surgeries for strengthening the muscle are:

- Resection
- Tucking
- Transposition.

Treatment Options

The treatment options in esotropia are:

1. Recession of medial rectus and resection of lateral rectus of the eye with squint.
2. Recession of medial rectus of both the eyes.

The treatment options in exotropia are:

1. Recession of lateral rectus and resection of medial rectus of the eye with squint.
2. Recession of lateral rectus of both the eyes.

Transposition of the horizontal rectus muscles or oblique muscle surgery is indicated in cases of heterotropia associated with 'A' and 'V' patterns.

GIST BOX 15.3

- Strabismus is defined as a group of clinical conditions characterized by misalignment of the visual axes of the two eyes. It is also called crossed eyes or squint.
- Latent squint/Heterophoria is defined as a clinical condition in which the alignment of the eyes is maintained by the fusional reflexes; hence, the latent squint becomes manifest when the fusion of the two eyes is disrupted.
- Manifest squint is characterized by the presence of misalignment of the visual axes always. It is classified into comitant squint or non-paralytic squint and incomitant squint or paralytic squint.
- Comitant squint is a type of squint characterized by normal extraocular movements and constant degree of squint in all the directions of gaze. It can be esotropia, exotropia or hypertropia depending on the direction of deviation.
- Incomitant squint is characterized by limited or restricted extraocular movements and varying degree of squint in different directions of gaze. It includes paralytic squint and restrictive squint.

CHAPTER

15.4 Nystagmus

DEFINITION**

Nystagmus is defined as involuntary rapid, regular, rhythmic oscillatory movements of the eye.

> Nystagmus is often associated with decreased vision. Nystagmus often leads to nodding of the head to compensate the rapid eye movements. The word nystagmus is derived from Greek word nystagmus meaning nodding.

ETIOPATHOGENESIS

Nystagmus occurs because of disturbances in the sensory motor system controlling the eye movements. The disturbances can be seen in sensory visual pathway, midbrain, cerebellum and vestibular system.

CLASSIFICATION

Nystagmus can be classified based on the type of movements, direction of movements and the cause for nystagmus. Based on the type of involuntary movements, nystagmus is classified into:

1. Pendular nystagmus: It is characterized by eye movements, which are equal in velocity and amplitude in each direction.
2. Jerky nystagmus: It is characterized by eye movements, which are unequal in velocity and amplitude in each direction with slow movement in one direction and fast jerk movement in another direction.

Based on the direction of involuntary movements, nystagmus is classified into:

- Horizontal nystagmus
- Vertical nystagmus
- Rotatory nystagmus.

Based on the etiology, nystagmus is classified into:

- Physiological nystagmus
- Pathological nystagmus.

Physiological Nystagmus

Optokinetic Nystagmus

Optokinetic nystagmus is a jerky nystagmus induced by drifting visual stimuli. It is used for testing visual acuity in children by optokinetic nystagmus test.

It is tested by presenting, moving a target such as rotating drum with stripes and it occurs as a result of effort of the motor system to keep the moving image stationary on the fovea. This reflex develops completely by 6 months and the presence of this indicates good visual acuity.

End-gaze Nystagmus

The nystagmus associated with extreme positions of gaze is called end-gaze nystagmus. It is a fine jerk nystagmus with the fast phase being in the direction of the gaze.

Vestibular Nystagmus

Vestibular nystagmus is produced by the vestibulo-ocular reflex. This reflex is seen in cases of head movement and it is responsible for formation of clear retinal image by producing compensatory eye movements.

Physiological vestibular nystagmus can be induced by caloric test. If ear is irrigated with cold water it results in development of jerky nystagmus of the opposite side eye and if warm water is irrigated into ear, it results in development of jerky nystagmus of the same side eye.

Pathological Nystagmus

Pathological nystagmus can be of various types as described below.

Congenital Nystagmus

Congenital nystagmus is also called infantile nystagmus syndrome and presents as an inherited genetic condition. This presents within the first 6 months of life and is associated with normal eyes and normal neurological development. The diagnosis is made by presence of mild nystagmus with absence of ocular or neurological anomalies.

Sensory Deprivation Nystagmus

Sensory deprivation nystagmus occurs as a result of ocular anomaly or visual pathway anomaly resulting in sensory deprivation.

This is seen in congenital and developmental abnormalities of the eyes, e.g. cataract, corneal opacity, aniridia, albinism, retinopathy of prematurity, retinal dystrophies, Leber's congenital amaurosis, macular hypoplasia, etc.

Neurological Nystagmus

Neurological nystagmus occurs as a result of neurological anomalies and diseases, and is usually associated with developmental delay and neurological problems. The common causes are neurodegenerative disorders, brain tumors, etc.

Vestibular Nystagmus

Vestibular nystagmus occurs as a result of altered input from the vestibular nuclei to the horizontal gaze center. It can be peripheral nystagmus or central nystagmus.

The peripheral vestibular nystagmus is caused by diseases of the inner ear such as labyrinthitis and Ménière's disease, and is associated with symptoms, e.g. deafness, tinnitus, etc.

The central vestibular nystagmus is caused by diseases of the brainstem, e.g. cerebrovascular diseases, multiple sclerosis, etc. The central vestibular nystagmus can be:

1. Upbeat nystagmus: This is a jerk nystagmus with fast component upward. It is seen in cerebellar diseases and commonly as an adverse effect to anticonvulsant drugs such as phenytoin.
2. Downbeat nystagmus: This is a jerk nystagmus with fast component downward. It is seen in diseases of the cervicomedullary junction, tumors of foramen magnum, brainstem lesions, etc.
3. Periodic alternating nystagmus: This is a jerk nystagmus, which changes in the rhythm and amplitude at periodic intervals. This is seen in demyelinating diseases of the brainstem.

Miner's Nystagmus

Miner's nystagmus is seen in mine workers as a result of fixation difficulties in dim illumination. It presents as rapid rotatory nystagmus.

See-saw Nystagmus

See-saw nystagmus is seen in chiasmal lesions, and is characterized by elevation and intorsion of one eye and depression and extorsion of another eye.

Latent Nystagmus

Latent nystagmus is characterized by the presence of nystagmus on covering one eye. It is absent when the both the eyes are open and presents as bilateral jerky nystagmus with fast component toward the uncovered eye on covering one eye. It is usually associated with congenital or infantile esotropia.

EVALUATION OF A PATIENT WITH NYSTAGMUS

1. This involves a complete history regarding age of onset and associated ocular and neurological diseases.
2. Ocular examination to look for sensory deprivation.
3. Neurological examination.

TREATMENT

Medical Treatment

1. Optical treatment in the form of glasses, contact lenses and prisms.
2. Pharmacological treatment is by benzodiazepines such as clonazepam, gamma-aminobutyric acid (GABA) agonists and baclofen. Baclofen is recommended for use in periodic alternating nystagmus.

Surgical Treatment

Surgical treatment is usually indicated in infantile or congenital nystagmus. It is in the form of Anderson-Kestenbaum procedure to move the eyes into null zone to correct the abnormal head posture.

NYSTAGMOID MOVEMENTS

The involuntary abnormal eye movements, which appear such as nystagmus are called nystagmoid movements. The common nystagmoid movements are:

1. Opsoclonus: Involuntary, rapid eye movements are called opsoclonus. Opsoclonus is usually associated with myoclonic movements of extremities. They differ from nystagmus by the fact that they are not regular and rhythmic as compared to nystagmus. It occurs in opsoclonus myoclonus syndrome, encephalitis, etc.
2. Ocular flutter: Involuntary horizontal repetitive, irregular eye movements are called ocular flutter. They are seen in cerebellar lesions.
3. Ocular bobbing: Involuntary abnormal vertical eye movements are called ocular bobbing. They are seen in pontine lesions.

GIST BOX 15.4

- Nystagmus is defined as involuntary rapid, regular, rhythmic oscillatory movements of the eye. Nystagmus occurs because of disturbances in the sensory motor system controlling the eye movements.
- The involuntary abnormal eye movements, which appear such as nystagmus are called nystagmoid movements.

FREQUENTLY ASKED QUESTIONS (FAQs)

*Short Answers

1. Mention the origin and insertions of rectus muscles of the eye.
2. Mention the origin and insertions of oblique muscles of the eye.
3. Mention the actions of extraocular muscles of eye.
4. Mention the nerve supply and blood supply of extraocular muscles of the eye.
5. Mention the binocular movements of the eye.
6. Mention the laws governing the ocular movements of the eye.
7. Define binocular single vision. Mention the grades of binocular single vision.
8. Mention the anomalies of binocular single vision.
9. Classify amblyopia.
10. Mention the clinical features of amblyopia.
11. Treatment of amblyopia.
12. Classify squint.
13. Pseudosquint/Pseudostrabismus.
14. Duane's syndrome.

**Short Essays

1. Amblyopia.
2. Heterophoria.
3. Esotropia.
4. Hypertropia.
5. Treatment of manifest squint.
6. Mention the tests for clinical evaluation of heterotropia.
7. Squint surgeries.
8. Restrictive squint.
9. Mention the differences between comitant and incomitant squint.
10. Nystagmus.

***Long Essays

1. Describe the clinical features and management of comitant squint.
2. Describe the clinical features and management of incomitant squint.

BIBLIOGRAPHY

1. Agarwal S, Agarwal A, Buratto L, et al. Text Book of Ophthalmology, vol. 1. New Delhi: Jaypee Brothers Medical Publishers (P) Ltd; 2002.
2. Agarwal A. Handbook of Ophthalmology. New Jersey: Slack Incorporated; 2006.
3. Dutta LC. Modern Ophthalmology, vol. 7, 3rd edition. New Delhi: Jaypee Brothers Medical Publishers (P) Ltd; 2005.
4. Harley RD, Nelson LB, Olitsky SE. Harley's Pediatric Ophthalmology. Philadelphia: Lippincott Williams & Wilkins; 2005.
5. Wright KW, Spiegel PH. Pediatric Ophthalmology and Strabismus, 2nd edition. New York: Springer-Verlag; 2002.

SECTION 16

Neurophthalmology

CHAPTER

16.1 Diseases of Visual Pathway

VISUAL PATHWAY

The visual pathway is the path along which the visual sensations from retina reach the visual cortex. It involves the optic nerve, optic chiasm, two optic tract, lateral geniculate body, optic radiation and visual cortex.

Anatomy of Visual Pathway

The anatomy of visual pathway (Fig. 16.1.1) is described under physiology of eye and vision.

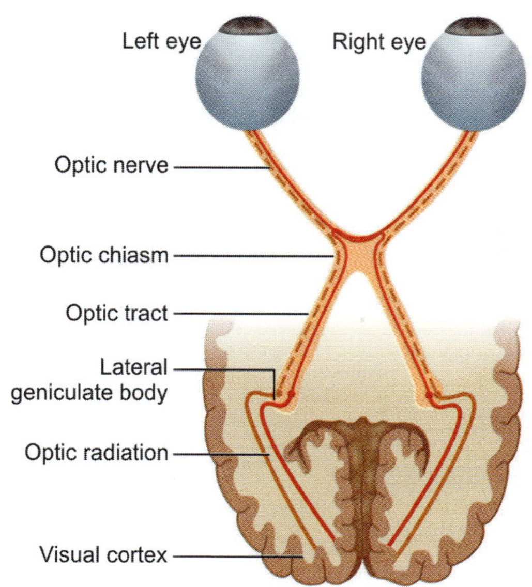

FIG. 16.1.1: Anatomy of visual pathway

VISUAL FIELD

Visual field is defined as an area of surroundings that can be seen while fixating an object with both the eyes kept open. The normal visual field extends 50° superiorly, 60° nasally, 70° inferiorly and 90° temporally.

Visual field and retina have got inverse relationship because of the effect of the dioptric apparatuses of the eye, which project image from visual field onto the opposite part of the retina corresponding to it:

- The image of the object in the nasal part of visual field is projected onto the temporal part of the retina.
- The image of the object in the temporal part of the field is projected onto the nasal part of the retina.
- The image of object in the upper half of visual field is projected onto the lower part of the retina.
- The image of object in the lower half of visual field is projected onto the upper part of the retina.

Right visual field projects onto the nasal field of the right eye and the temporal field of the left eye. Left visual field projects onto the temporal field of right eye and the nasal field of the left eye.

Hence, the visual information from the right visual field is in left optic tract and the visual information from the left visual field is present in right optic tract because of decussation of nasal fibers to opposite side at the optic chiasm.

Since the image formed on the retina is inverted, the right optic tract carries the information from the right visual field and left optic tract from the left visual field.

Traquair has defined visual field as an island of vision in a sea of blindness. The island contains a peak and a bottomless pit. The peak of the island is represented by fovea, the point with highest visual acuity and the bottomless pit is represented by blind spot, optic disk.

Visual Field Defects**

Visual field defect is loss of a part of visual field and it occurs because of lesions of the visual pathway (Table 16.1.1):

1. *Scotoma:* It is defined as an area of decreased visual function in the visual field.
2. *Quadrantanopia:* It is defined as visual defect involving one quadrant.
3. *Hemianopia:* It is defined as visual defect involving the two adjacent quadrants.
4. *Homonymous hemianopia:* It is a type of hemianopia characterized by involvement of the same side of the visual field in each eye.
5. *Heteronymous hemianopia:* It is a type of hemianopia characterized by involvement of the opposite side of the visual field in each eye.
6. *Congruous hemianopia:* It indicates symmetrical loss of visual field.
7. *Incongruous hemianopia:* It indicates asymmetrical loss of visual field.

PUPIL AND PUPILLARY ABNORMALITIES

Pupil is called gateway to brain as the pupillary reactions are controlled by autonomous nervous system, a part of central nervous system; hence, the diseases of the nervous system influence the pupillary reflexes.

TABLE 16.1.1: Visual field defects

Site of lesion	*Visual defect*	*Common causes*
Optic nerve (Fig. 16.1.2A) Proximal part of optic nerve (Fig. 16.1.2B)	Total blindness of the affected eye with absence of direct reflex and presence of near reflex Ipsilateral blindness and contralateral hemianopia or quadrantanopia	Optic atrophy
Sagittal lesions of the optic chiasm (Fig. 16.1.2C)	Bitemporal hemianopia with loss of pupillary reflexes	Pituitary gland tumors, craniopharyngioma, suprasellar aneurysms
Lateral chiasmal lesions (Fig. 16.1.2D)	Binasal hemianopia with loss of pupillary reflexes	Atheroma of the carotids
Optic tract (Fig. 16.1.2E)	Incongruous homonymous hemianopia with pupils showing Wernicke's pupillary reaction	Aneurysms of superior cerebellar or posterior cerebral artery, syphilitic meningitis, tubercular meningitis
Lateral geniculate body (refer Fig. 16.1.2E)	Incongruous homonymous hemianopia with sparing of pupillary reflexes	Vascular lesions, trauma and tumors
Optic radiations	Congruous homonymous hemianopia Inferior quadrantic hemianopia called pie on the floor is seen in parietal lobe lesions (Fig. 16.1.2F) and superior quadrantic hemianopia called pie in the sky is seen in temporal lobe lesions (Fig. 16.1.2G)	Vascular lesions, trauma and tumors
Visual cortex (Fig. 16.1.2H)	Congruous homonymous hemianopia sparing the macula with normal pupillary reactions	Vascular lesions of posterior cerebral artery

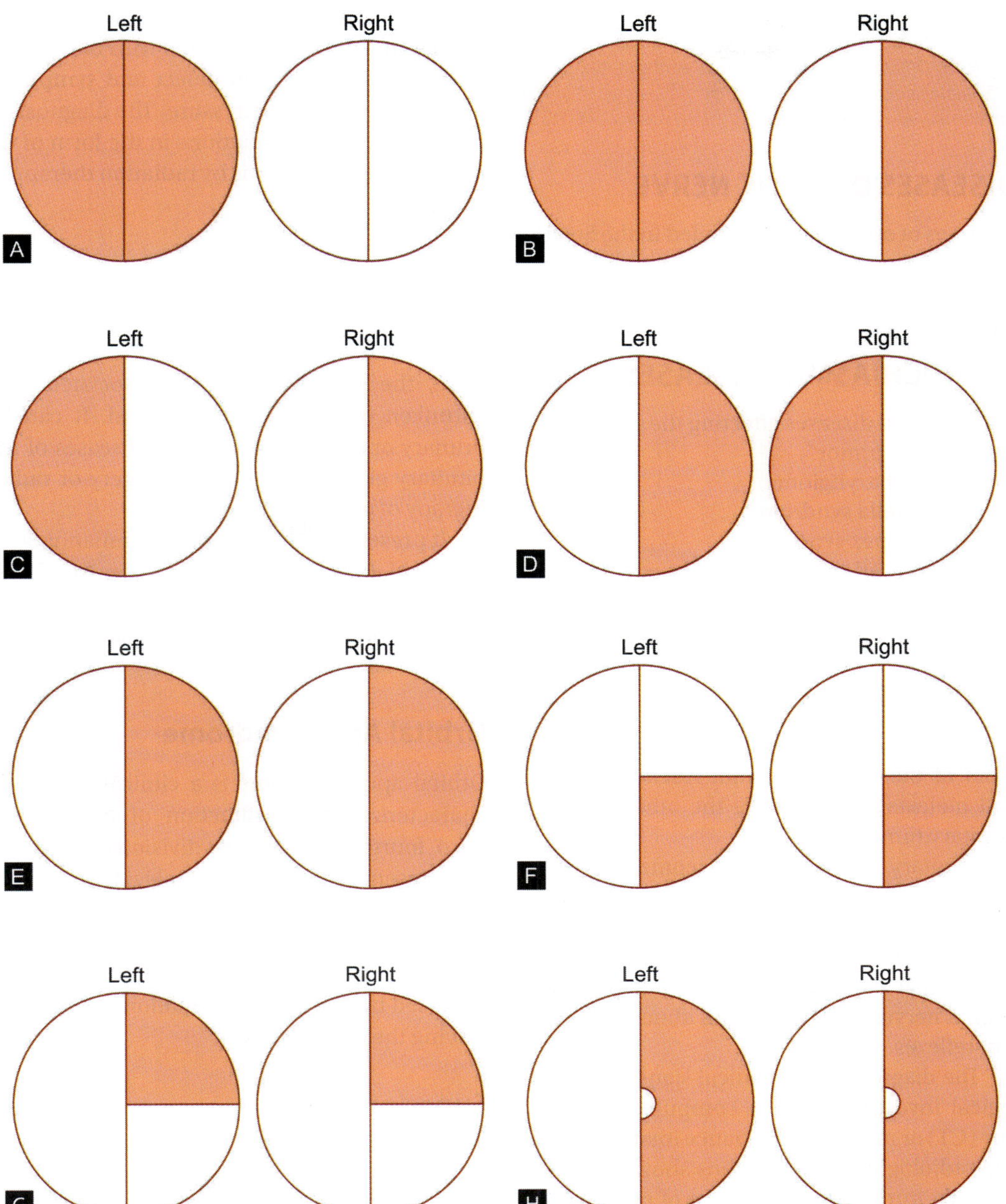

FIGS 16.1.2A to H: Visual defects in lesions of visual pathway. **A.** Lesion: Optic nerve of right eye; **B.** Lesion: Proximal part of optic nerve of right eye; **C.** Lesion: Sagittal lesion of the optic chiasm (bitemporal hemianopia); **D.** Lesion: Lateral chiasmal lesion (binasal hemianopia); **E.** Lesion: Optic tract and lateral geniculate body (homonymous hemianopia); **F.** Lesion: Optic radiation in parietal lobe lesion involving superior fibers (inferior quadrantic hemianopia); **G.** Lesion: Optic radiation in temporal lobe involving inferior fibers (superior quadrantic hemianopia); **H.** Lesion: Visual cortex (homonymous hemianopia sparing macula).

Pupil and its abnormalities are described detail in Chapter 2 'Ocular Examination' in Author's textbook *'Clinical Methods in Ophthalmology'.*

DISEASES OF OPTIC NERVE

Diseases of optic nerve is detailed in the Section 12 'Optic Nerve'.

CHIASMAL AND RETROCHIASMAL DISEASES

The common diseases affecting the chiasm are:

- Pituitary tumor
- Craniopharyngioma
- Empty sella syndrome
- Orbital apex syndrome
- Superior orbital fissure syndrome
- Cavernous sinus syndrome
- Tolosa-Hunt syndrome.

Pituitary Tumor

Pituitary adenomas are the most common tumors of the pituitary gland. Adenocarcinoma and metastatic tumors are the other common pituitary tumors.

Pituitary adenomas most commonly present with hormone abnormalities resulting in signs of hyperpituitarism, bitemporal hemianopia visual field defect and symptoms of raised intracranial pressure manifesting as palsies of cranial nerves III, IV or VI and abnormal pupillary reflexes.

The diagnosis is by clinical signs and radiological investigations, i.e. computed tomography (CT) or magnetic resonance imaging (MRI). The radiological investigations show erosion of the sella turcica. The treatment of pituitary adenoma is by radiation therapy or by surgery.

Craniopharyngioma

Craniopharyngioma is a benign tumor arising from the stomatodeum, an embryonic tissue, which gives rise to pituitary gland. It is commonly seen in children. It presents with bitemporal hemianopia visual field defect and symptoms of raised intracranial pressure. The diagnosis is by radiological examinations in the form of CT or MRI. The treatment is by radiation therapy or by surgery.

Empty Sella Syndrome

Empty sella syndrome is a clinical syndrome characterized by enlargement of the pituitary fossa, the sella turcica. It is associated with shrunken or small pituitary gland. It can be primary or secondary following diseases of the pituitary gland, i.e. following surgery or radiotherapy of pituitary gland tumors.

It presents with bitemporal hemianopia visual field defect and symptoms of raised intracranial pressure. The diagnosis is by radiological examinations in the form of CT or MRI. The symptomatic cases are treated by surgery.

Orbital Apex Syndrome*

Orbital apex syndrome is a clinical syndrome characterized by dysfunction of the second, third, fourth, sixth and first division of the nerve V. It presents with ophthalmoplegia, ptosis, loss of corneal sensation and optic nerve involvement in the form of edema of the optic nerve head and optic atrophy. Orbital apex syndrome is caused by trauma, inflammation or tumor involving the orbital apex.

Superior Orbital Fissure Syndrome*

Superior orbital fissure syndrome is characterized by dysfunction of the third, fourth, sixth and first division of the nerve V. It presents with ophthalmoplegia, ptosis and loss of corneal sensation. Optic nerve involvement seen in orbital apex syndrome is absent in superior orbital fissure syndrome.

Cavernous Sinus Syndrome*

Cavernous sinus syndrome is characterized by dysfunction of the third, fourth, sixth, first and second divisions of the nerve V. The common causes for cavernous sinus syndrome are cavernous sinus thrombosis and aneurysm of the internal carotid artery.

Tolosa-Hunt Syndrome*

Tolosa-Hunt syndrome is a granulomatous vasculitis involving the cavernous sinus and/or superior orbital fissure. It presents with features of cavernous sinus syndrome or superior orbital fissure syndrome.

AMAUROSIS FUGAX**

Definition

Amaurosis fugax is defined as transient painless partial or complete uniocular, or binocular loss of vision, which lasts for few seconds to several minutes and returns back to normal even without treatment.

The word amaurosis fugax is derived from Greek word 'amaurosis,' meaning darkness and the Latin word 'fugax,' meaning fleeting, thus indicating transient darkness.

Etiopathogenesis

Etiopathogenesis occurs because of vascular or circulatory disturbances affecting the retina and visual pathway. The common causes are:

1. Vascular causes such as thromboembolism, hypoperfusion, vasculitis, carotid artery stenosis, coagulation disorders, hyperviscosity disorders, giant cell arteritis, migraine, etc.
2. Ocular causes such as intermittent attacks of angle closure glaucoma leading to intermittent elevation in intraocular pressure, orbital tumors, posterior vitreous detachment, intraocular hemorrhage, etc.
3. Neurological causes such as papilledema, intracranial tumors, etc.

Clinical Features

The patient typically presents with transient painless partial or complete uniocular, or binocular loss of vision, which lasts for few seconds to several minutes and returns back to normal even without treatment.

Investigations

All patients with amaurosis fugax require evaluation to prevent serious vascular events such as stroke, myocardial infarction or irreversible blindness.

The investigations include thorough laboratory workup to rule out underlying vascular and neurological in addition to ocular examination.

The investigations include carotid Doppler to rule out carotid artery stenosis; echocardiography to rule out cardiac emboli; blood investigations such as erythrocyte sedimentation rate (ESR) and C-reactive protein to rule out giant cell arteritis; coagulation profile to rule out coagulation disorders and hyperviscosity syndromes.

Treatment

The treatment depends on the underlying cause such as carotid artery endarterectomy for carotid artery stenosis, treatment of giant cell arteritis by steroids, treatment of migraine.

GIST BOX 16.1

- The visual pathway is the path along which the visual sensations from retina reach the visual cortex. It involves the optic nerve, optic chiasm, two optic tracts, lateral geniculate body, optic radiation and visual cortex.
- Visual field is defined as area of surroundings that can be seen while fixating an object with both the eyes kept open. The normal visual field extends 50° superiorly, 60° nasally, 70° inferiorly and 90° temporally.
- Visual field defect is loss of a part of visual field and it occurs because of lesions of the visual pathway.
- Amaurosis fugax is defined as transient painless partial or complete uniocular, or binocular loss of vision, which lasts for few seconds to several minutes and returns back to normal even without treatment.

CHAPTER

16.2 Diseases of Ocular Motility

The extraocular muscles are supplied by cranial nerves III, IV, and VI, and are responsible for extraocular movements.

CRANIAL NERVE III**

The III nerve supplies the superior rectus, medial rectus, inferior rectus and inferior oblique muscles. It also supplies the levator palpebrae superioris and parasympathetic innervation to sphincter pupillae and ciliary muscles.

Etiology

The common causes for III nerve palsy are:

- Vascular diseases, e.g. diabetes and hypertension
- Aneurysms of the posterior communicating artery
- Head injury with subdural hematoma
- Tumors
- Vasculitis
- Idiopathic.

Clinical Features

The clinical features of III nerve palsy are:

- Ptosis because of involvement of levator palpebrae superioris
- Limitation of adduction because of involvement of medial rectus
- Limitation of elevation because of involvement of superior rectus and inferior oblique
- Limitation of depression because of involvement of inferior rectus
- Dilated pupil and defective accommodation because of parasympathetic palsy
- The eye remains downward and outward position because of unopposed action of lateral rectus and superior oblique respectively (Figs 16.2.1A and B).

The oculomotor nerve can be involved in syndromes because of involvement of the fasciculus part of the oculomotor nerve as mentioned in Table 16.2.1.

Localizing the Site of Lesion in Oculomotor Nerve Palsy

The associated clinical features help in localizing the site of lesion. The cranial nerve III can be affected anywhere along the course of the nerve. The course of the oculomotor nerve can be considered under nucleus, fasciculus, basilar, intracavernous and intraorbital parts.

Oculomotor Nucleus

1. The oculomotor nerve starts from the nucleus situated in the midbrain at the level of the superior colliculi. The oculomotor nucleus consists of single central levator subnucleus, paired superior rectus subnucleus, which

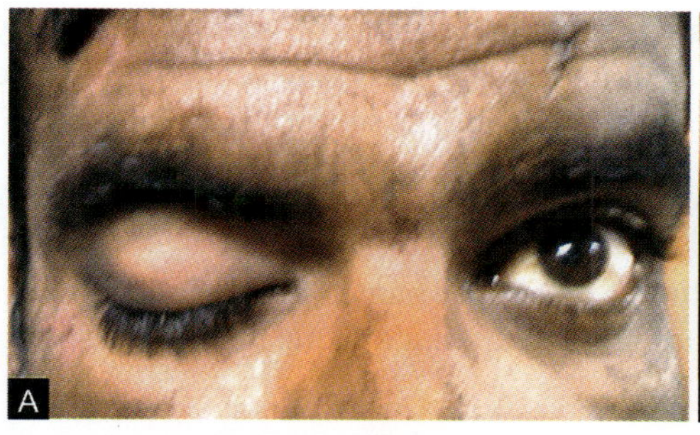

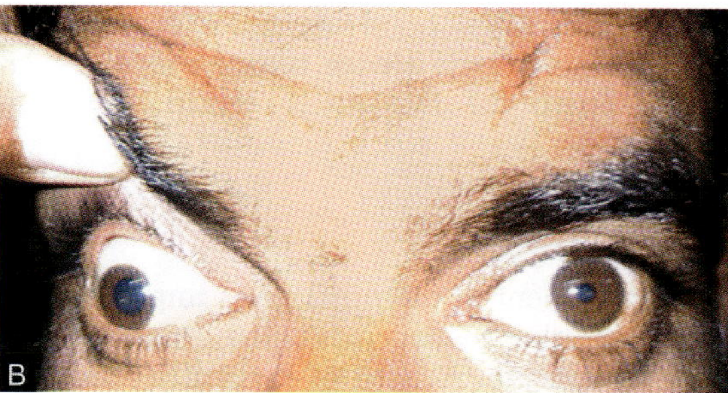

FIGS 16.2.1A and B: Oculomotor nerve palsy of right side. **A.** Complete ptosis of right eye; **B.** On lifting the eyelid, the eyeball is deviated downward and outward with dilatation of the pupil.

innervates the contralateral superior rectus and paired medial rectus, inferior rectus and inferior oblique subnuclei, which innervate the ipsilateral muscles.

2. Vascular diseases and tumors are the common causes for nuclear lesions of the oculomotor nerve.
3. The nuclear causes of III nerve palsy are characterized by bilateral ptosis, since there is one central levator subnucleus supplying both the sides of levator muscle.

Fasciculus

Fasciculus consists of the nerve fibers, which leave the oculomotor nucleus through the red nucleus. The common causes involving this part are ischemic lesions and tumors.

Basilar Part

1. Basilar part includes the peripheral nerve in the subarachnoid space. The common causes affecting the nerve are aneurysm of the posterior communicating artery and head injury.
2. The pupil will be usually involved in these lesions and the III nerve palsy is usually acute and painful.

Cavernous Part

1. Cavernous part includes the part of the nerve in the cavernous sinus. It presents as a part of cavernous sinus syndrome.
2. Cavernous sinus syndrome characterized by dysfunction of the third, fourth, sixth, first and second divisions of the V nerve.

Orbital Part

Orbital part includes the part of the nerve in the orbit. In the orbit, the oculomotor nerve divides into superior branch, which supplies superior rectus and levator palpebrae superioris and inferior branch, which supplies inferior rectus,

TABLE 16.2.1: Syndrome associated with III nerve palsy

Syndrome	*Features*	*Site*
Weber's syndrome	Ipsilateral III nerve palsy and contralateral hemiparesis	Cerebral peduncle
Benedikt's syndrome	Ipsilateral III nerve palsy and contralateral extrapyramidal signs	Red nucleus
Nothnagel syndrome	Ipsilateral III nerve palsy and cerebellar ataxia	Superior cerebellar peduncle
Claude's syndrome	It shows features of both Benedikt's syndrome and Weber's syndrome	

medial rectus, inferior oblique, sphincter pupillae and ciliary muscle. Hence, selective involvement of one of the divisions is seen in orbital lesions.

Investigations

The involvement of the pupil gives important clues for further management. The lesions involving pupil are because of surgical lesions, whereas the lesions, which spare the pupil are usually because of medical causes such as diabetes and hypertension.

> Pupillary fibers are superficial in location, whereas the motor fibers are located deep inside the trunk of the oculomotor nerve and are supplied by vasa nervorum. The microangiopathy caused by vascular diseases such as diabetes, hypertension, will involve the vasa nervorum, thus affecting the motor fibers sparing the pupillary fibers. The superficially located pupillary fibers are usually damaged by the surgical compressive lesions.

The investigations whether are usually based on the pupillary involvement or not and in cases without pupillary involvement, investigations are done to find out the underlying medical disease by:

- Blood pressure
- Random blood sugar or fasting blood sugar
- Venereal Disease Research Laboratory (VDRL) test or fluorescent treponemal antibody absorption (FTA-ABS) test for syphilis
- Antinuclear antibody (ANA).

Radiological investigations such as magnetic resonance imaging (MRI), angiography are advised in:

- Oculomotor nerve palsy with pupillary involvement
- Presence of neurological signs
- No signs of recovery even after 3 months
- Oculomotor nerve palsy in younger people.

Treatment

Oculomotor palsy because of ischemia caused by diabetes or hypertension usually resolves by 3–6 months. The treatment of the underlying cause is required in cases of surgical causes. Treatment of the paralytic squint caused by oculomotor nerve palsy is described under the treatment of paralytic squint.

CRANIAL NERVE IV**

The IV nerve is also named trochlear nerve and it supplies the superior oblique muscle of the eye.

> The trochlear nerve is the thinnest and has got longest intracranial course among all the cranial nerves. Thus, head injury is the common cause for acquired IV nerve palsy.
>
> It differs from other cranial nerves by the fact that it is the only cranial nerve, which emerges from the dorsal aspect of the brain and crosses over completely to the opposite side; thus, innervating the superior oblique muscle of the opposite side.

Etiology

The common causes for IV nerve palsy are:

- Head injury
- Vascular diseases such as diabetes and hypertension
- Tumors
- Vasculitis
- Aneurysms
- Congenital.

Clinical Features

The clinical features of IV nerve palsy are because of involvement of the superior oblique muscle, which causes depression, intorsion and abduction of the globe. The clinical features are:

- Presence of vertical or torsional diplopia worse in the downgaze
- Compensatory head tilt toward the contralateral side
- The unilateral cases show hypertropia of the involved eye, which increases on tilting the head to the ipsilateral side
- The bilateral cases show V-pattern esotropia and hypertropia of right eye on left gaze and hypertropia of left eye on right gaze.

Clinical Evaluation of IV Nerve Palsy

Parks-Bielschowsky Head Tilt Test

Parks-Bielschowsky 3 step test is helpful in finding the paretic muscle in cases of hypertropia/ vertical diplopia. It is performed in three steps.

Step 1

Observe for the presence of hypertropia in either of the eyes. The presence of hypertropia in right eye is caused by underaction of depressors of right eye (right inferior rectus or right superior oblique) or underaction of elevators of left eye (left superior rectus or left inferior oblique).

Step 2

Ask the patient to look in right gaze and left gaze and look for the gaze in which the hypertropia increases. Since the vertical recti muscles have got their maximum action in abduction position and oblique muscles have their maximum action in adduction position:

- Hypertropia of right eye increasing in right gaze (right inferior rectus or left inferior oblique)
- Hypertropia of right eye increasing in left gaze (right superior oblique or left superior rectus)
- Hypertropia of left eye increasing in left gaze (right inferior oblique or left inferior rectus)
- Hypertropia of left eye increasing in right gaze (right superior rectus or left superior oblique).

Step 3

Ask the patient to tilt the head. Look for the side of head tilt having the hypertropia. Hypertropia increasing by tilt of the head to same side is caused by oblique muscle, whereas hypertropia increasing by tilt of the head to the opposite side is caused by vertical rectus muscle:

- Hypertropia of right eye increasing in right head tilt (left inferior oblique)
- Hypertropia of right eye increasing in left head tilt (left superior rectus)
- Hypertropia of left eye increasing in left head tilt (right inferior oblique)
- Hypertropia of left eye increasing in right head tilt (right superior rectus).

Double Maddox Rod Test

Double Maddox rod test is done to diagnose cyclotropia. Two Maddox rods are placed one each in front of each eye with the axis horizontal so that the subject sees two vertical lines on viewing handheld light. Routinely, white Maddox rod is placed in front of left eye and red Maddox rod is placed in front of right eye. Normal subjects see the lines parallel to each other; in incyclotropia, 12 O'clock position of the line is seen turned nasally and in excyclotropia the line is turned temporally. The subject is asked to rotate the Maddox rods till the lines are parallel. If the subject rotates the vertical axis for more than 10° temporally, then it indicates bilateral superior oblique palsy.

Investigations

- Blood pressure, random blood sugar or fasting blood sugar to rule out microvascular diseases
- Magnetic resonance imaging brain is indicated in acquired IV nerve palsies with non-microvascular causes.

Treatment

1. Diplopia is treated by prisms or occlusion of the affected eye.
2. Surgical treatment is indicated in long-standing cases without improvement and surgery is in the form of strengthening of the superior oblique or weakening of inferior oblique. Knapp's procedure or Harada procedure is usually done.

CRANIAL NERVE VI**

The VI nerve is also named abducent nerve and it supplies the lateral rectus muscle of the eye.

Etiology

The common causes for VI nerve palsy are:

- Head injury
- Vascular diseases such as diabetes and hypertension
- Tumors
- Vasculitis
- Demyelinating conditions
- Congenital.

Clinical Features

The clinical features of VI nerve palsy are:

- Esotropia in primary position with limitation of abduction
- Horizontal diplopia on gaze toward the action of the paralyzed muscle.

Localizing the Site of Lesion in Abducent Nerve Palsy

The associated clinical features help in localizing the site of lesion.

Abducent Nucleus

Abducent nucleus is located in the pons and is closely associated with horizontal gaze center and fasciculus of the facial nerve; hence, lesions involving the abducent nucleus are usually associated with failure of horizontal gaze and lower motor neuron facial nerve palsy.

Fasciculus

Fasciculus consists of fibers, which leave the brainstem at the pontomedullary junction. The lesions at this level usually involve the pontine paramedian reticular formation (PPRF) and pyramidal tract resulting in two syndromes (Table 16.2.2).

TABLE 16.2.2: Syndrome associated with VI nerve palsy

Syndrome	*Features*
Foville's syndrome	It is characterized by involvement of cranial nerves V, VI, VII, and VIII with horizontal gaze palsy because of involvement of the pontine paramedian reticular formation
Millard-Gubler syndrome	It is characterized by ipsilateral VI nerve palsy with contralateral hemiplegia because of involvement of pyramidal tract

Basilar Part

Raised intracranial pressure, nasopharyngeal tumors and cerebellopontine angle tumors, i.e. acoustic neuroma are the common causes for involvement of the abducent nerve in this part. These are usually associated with involvement of cranial nerves V, VII and VIII.

The VI nerve palsy is a classic example for false localizing sign occurring as a result of raised intracranial pressure. The proposed mechanism is stretching of the nerve against the ridge of the petrous temporal bone secondary to raised intracranial pressure.

Cavernous Part

Cavernous part presents as a part of cavernous sinus syndrome.

Management

Management is on similar lines of paralytic squint. Diplopia in the initial stages is treated by prisms or occlusion of the affected eye. Cases with no improvement even after waiting for 6 months are treated by surgeries. The surgery done is resection of lateral rectus or recession of medial rectus or transposition of the vertical rectus.

GIST BOX 16.2

- The extraocular muscles are supplied by III, IV and VI cranial nerves, and are responsible for extraocular movements.
- The common causes for III nerve palsy are vascular diseases such as diabetes and hypertension, aneurysms of the posterior communicating artery, head injury with subdural hematoma, etc.
- The clinical features of III nerve palsy are ptosis because of involvement of levator palpebrae superioris, dilated pupil and defective accommodation because of parasympathetic palsy, limitation of elevation, adduction, depression, and the eye remains in downward and outward position because of unopposed action of lateral rectus and superior oblique respectively. The involvement of the pupil gives important clues for further management. The lesions involving pupil are because of surgical causes, whereas the lesions, which spare the pupil, are usually because of medical causes, i.e. diabetes and hypertension.
- Oculomotor palsy because of ischemia caused by diabetes or hypertension usually resolves by 3–6 months. The treatment of the underlying cause is required in cases of surgical causes.
- The trochlear nerve is the thinnest and has got longest intracranial course among all the cranial nerves. Thus, head injury is the common cause for acquired IV nerve palsy.
- The clinical features of IV nerve palsy are because of involvement of the superior oblique muscle resulting in vertical or torsional diplopia worse in the downgaze and compensatory head tilt toward the contralateral side.
- The VI nerve supplies the lateral rectus muscle of the eye.
- The clinical features of VI nerve palsy are esotropia in primary position with limitation of abduction and horizontal diplopia on gaze toward the action of the paralyzed muscle.
- The VI nerve palsy is a classic example for false localizing sign occurring as a result of raised intracranial pressure.

FREQUENTLY ASKED QUESTIONS (FAQs)

*Short Answers

1. Orbital apex syndrome.
2. Cavernous sinus syndrome.
3. Superior orbital fissure syndrome.
4. Tolosa-Hunt syndrome.

**Short Essays

1. Visual field defects in the lesions of the visual pathway.
2. Amaurosis fugax.
3. Third cranial nerve palsy.
4. Fourth cranial nerve palsy.
5. Sixth cranial nerve palsy.

BIBLIOGRAPHY

1. Agarwal A. Handbook of Ophthalmology, Slack Incorporated; 2006.
2. Bacigalupi M. Amaurosis fugax—a clinical review. The Internet Journal of Allied Health Sciences and Practice. 2006;4(2).
3. Dutta LC. Modern Ophthalmology, 3rd edition. New Delhi: Jaypee Brothers Medical Publishers (P) Ltd; 2005.
4. Gerstenblith AT, Rabinowitz MP. The Wills Eye Manual: Office and Emergency Room Diagnosis and Treatment of Eye Disease. Lippincott Williams & Wilkins.
5. Kanski JJ. Clinical Ophthalmology, 5th edition. London: Butterworth-Heinemann; 2003.

SECTION 17

Intraocular Tumors

CHAPTER

17.1 Uveal Tumors

Uveal tumors include tumors of the iris, ciliary body and choroid. The common benign tumors of the uvea include nevus of iris, nevus of choroid and choroidal hemangioma.

The nevi of iris appear as flat-pigmented lesion. It is a benign lesion with very little malignant potential. The choroidal nevi also appear as flat-pigmented lesion. The nevi of iris and choroid can be seen in association with neurofibromatosis and they become apparent at or near puberty.

The choroidal nevus has got malignant potential; hence, they have to be examined at regular intervals. The risk of malignant change into choroidal melanoma is seen in cases associated with increasing size, increasing pigmentation and serous detachment.

MALIGNANT MELANOMA**

Malignant melanoma is a malignant tumor seen in the uveal tract arising from neuroectodermal melanocytes.

Uveal melanoma is the most common primary intraocular malignancy in adults.

Etiopathogenesis

Malignant melanoma is more common in Caucasians and white races, and less common in African blacks. Exposure to ultraviolet (UV) rays is regarded as a risk factor. It is seen in middle age or elderly aged people and is rare below 30 years of age. Ocular melanocytosis and dysplastic nevus syndrome are the known predisposing conditions.

Clinical Features

Clinical features of malignant melanoma depend on the location of melanoma.

Malignant Melanoma of Choroid

Malignant melanoma is common among the uveal melanomas.

Clinical Features

The clinical features of malignant melanoma of the choroid depend on the stage of the disease.

Quiescent stage: The tumor remains asymptomatic in this stage and noted on fundus examination. Choroidal melanoma appears as dark brown mass and it is associated with exudative retinal detachment in case of involvement of the retinal pigment epithelium by breaking through the Bruch's membrane.

Stage of glaucoma: It is characterized by onset of secondary glaucoma because of obstruction of the aqueous outflow by forward displacement of the lens-iris diaphragm or compression of the vortex veins as a result of growth of tumor or by invasion of the angle of anterior chamber by the tumor cells.

Stage of extraocular extension: It is characterized by the spread of the tumor outside the globe involving the orbit.

Stage of metastasis: It is characterized by the hematogenous spread to distant sites, e.g. liver.

Pathology

Melanomas show anaplastic melanocytic cells. Based on the type of cells present in the tumor, it is further classified into:

- Spindle cell melanoma
- Epithelioid cell melanoma
- Mixed cell melanoma.

Investigations

1. Ultrasonography by brightness (B)-scan shows a solid biconvex mass.
2. Computed tomography (CT) and magnetic resonance imaging (MRI) give more details regarding the extension of the tumor.
3. Fundus fluorescein angiography can differentiate choroidal melanomas from other lesions such as choroidal hemorrhage, choroidal hemangioma, etc.

Differential Diagnosis

Choroidal melanoma has to be differentiated from the following:

- Choroidal nevus
- Metastatic carcinoma
- Choroidal hemangioma.

Treatment

Choroidal melanomas are classified by Collaborative Ocular Melanoma Study (COMS) as follows. Treatment is based on the type.

Small melanomas: The melanomas measuring < 5 mm in diameter are included in this group. The treatment of tumors in this group is by follow-up and observation. Treatment, if required is done by laser photocoagulation or by photodynamic therapy.

Medium melanomas: The melanomas measuring between 5 and 16 mm in diameter are included in this group. The treatment of tumors in this group is by microsurgical resection, radiotherapy or enucleation.

Large melanomas: The melanomas measuring > 16 mm in diameter are included in this group. The treatment of tumors in this group is by enucleation or exenteration depending on the stage of tumor following initial radiotherapy. Chemotherapy is not very effective in treatment of melanomas; hence, it is not a popular method for treatment of melanomas.

Malignant Melanoma of Ciliary Body

Malignant melanoma of the ciliary body is a relatively rare tumor arising from the ciliary body. Malignant melanoma of the ciliary body presents as dilated episcleral sentinel blood vessel. Clinical features and treatment are similar to that of choroidal melanoma.

Malignant Melanoma of Iris

Malignant melanoma of iris presents as an iris nodule with variable pigmentation associated with secondary features such as ectropion uveae and neovascularization of iris. Malignant melanoma of iris has to be differentiated from iris nevus, leiomyoma and metastatic carcinoma of iris.

Treatment

Treatment is by observation and excision of the iris in the initial stages. Radiotherapy and enucleation are indicated in advanced cases.

GIST BOX 17.1

- Uveal tumors include tumors of the iris, ciliary body and choroid. The common benign tumors of the uvea include nevus of iris, nevus of choroid and choroidal hemangioma.
- Uveal melanoma is the most common primary intraocular malignancy in adults.
- Malignant melanoma of choroid is common among the uveal melanomas.
- Malignant melanoma arises from neuroectodermal melanocytes.
- Malignant melanoma is more common in Caucasians and white races, and less common in African blacks. Ocular melanocytosis and dysplastic nevus syndrome are the known predisposing conditions.

CHAPTER 17.2

Retinal Tumors

Tumors of the retina are relatively rare except retinoblastoma, the most common primary malignant neoplasm of the eye in childhood.

RETINOBLASTOMA***

Retinoblastoma is the most common primary intraocular malignancy in children.

Etiology

- The incidence of retinoblastoma is from 1:15,000 to 1:20,000
- About 70% of the cases are unilateral, whereas bilateral involvement is seen in about 30% of cases
- Median age of diagnosis is 12 months in the bilateral cases and 24 months in the unilateral cases
- Race and sex predisposition is not found.

Pathogenesis

1. Retinoblastoma arises from immature retinal cells, primitive precursor cells of the photoreceptors.
2. Retinoblastoma most commonly occurs as a sporadic condition in about 93–94% cases with most of them presenting with unilateral and unifocal involvement.
3. A positive family history is seen in about 6–7% of cases, mode of inheritance is autosomal dominant pattern with most of them being bilateral and multifocal.
4. Hereditary retinoblastoma is associated with loss of gene on the long arm of chromosome 13 called 13q deletion syndrome. The pathogenesis of hereditary retinoblastoma is explained by Knudson's two-hit hypothesis. The first hit called germinal mutation and is found in all cells. The second hit called somatic mutation when occurs in the retinal cells gives rise to retinoblastoma.
5. Knudson's two-hit hypothesis explains the occurrence of non-ocular tumors, e.g. osteosarcoma, soft tissue sarcoma, etc. in hereditary retinoblastoma.

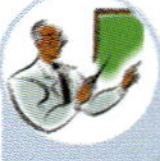

Secondary Malignancies Associated with Retinoblastoma

Secondary malignancies are seen in survivors of hereditary type of retinoblastoma because of presence of germinal mutation in all the cells of the body. This risk is increased in children who have received radiation therapy as treatment for retinoblastoma.

The common secondary malignancies seen are osteosarcoma, rhabdomyosarcoma and other soft tissue sarcomas, melanoma, chondrosarcoma, brain tumors, lymphoma, etc.

Trilateral Retinoblastoma

Bilateral retinoblastoma with intracranial primitive neuroectodermal tumor in the pineal or suprasellar region, e.g. pineoblastoma is called trilateral retinoblastoma.

Clinical Features*

1. Leukocoria, white pupillary reflex is the most common clinical presentation of retinoblastoma. About 60% of cases of retinoblastoma present as leukocoria.
2. Strabismus is the second common clinical presentation accounting for 20% of cases.
3. Proptosis, secondary glaucoma, orbital cellulitis, hyphema, heterochromia iridis, white spots on the iris, failure to thrive and nystagmus are the types of clinical presentations of retinoblastoma.

Depending on the clinical features and ocular involvement retinoblastoma can be divided into four stages:

1. *Quiescent stage:* It is the initial stage of retinoblastoma and it usually extends from 6 months to 1 year. On examination by indirect ophthalmoscopy, the tumor appears as yellowish white fluffy mass of the retina with dilated and tortuous retinal vessels feeding the tumor. Advanced lesions show either endophytic growth with tumor mass filling the vitreous cavity or exophytic growth of the tumor into the retina causing retinal detachment. The patient is usually symptom free, but presents with leukocoria or strabismus.
2. *Glaucomatous stage:* It is because of extension of the tumor leading to distension of the globe or involvement of the angle of the anterior chamber by the tumor cells resulting in rise of intraocular pressure and secondary glaucoma. The patient presents with pain, redness, watering because of secondary glaucoma. Hyphema, pseudohypopyon and raised intraocular pressure are seen in this stage.
3. *Extraocular extension:* It is because of growth of the tumor involving the orbit and optic nerve. The patient presents with fungating extraocular mass, proptosis and orbital cellulitis.
4. *Metastasis:* The tumor undergoes metastasis by lymphatics spread and hematogenous spread. Lymphatic spread results in involvement of the preauricular and cervical lymph nodes. Hematogenous spread results in spread of tumor to bone and liver commonly. Intracranial extension of the tumor is common and it occurs more commonly by extension along the optic nerve.

Classification**

Retinoblastoma is classified by different systems to predict the prognosis of the retinoblastoma and to advice the treatment modality. The commonly accepted treatment modalities are:

- Reese-Ellsworth classification system
- International Classification of Retinoblastoma (ICRB).

Reese-Ellsworth Classification System

Reese-Ellsworth classification system was proposed to predict the prognosis of retinoblastoma after treatment with external beam radiation. It classifies retinoblastoma into five groups as follows:

1. *Group 1:* Very favorable:
   - Solitary tumor < 4 disk diameter in size at or behind equator
   - Multiple tumors, none over 4 disk diameter in size, all at or behind the equator.
2. *Group 2:* Favorable:
   - Solitary tumor, 4–10 disk diameter in size, at or behind equator
   - Multiple tumors, 4–10 disk diameter in size, behind the equator.
3. *Group 3:* Doubtful:
   - Any tumor extending anterior to equator
   - Solitary tumor larger than 10 disk diameter behind equator.
4. *Group 4:* Unfavorable:
   - Multiple tumors, some larger than 10 disk diameter in size
   - Any tumor extending anteriorly to the ora serrata.
5. *Group 5:* Very unfavorable:
   - Massive tumors involving over half part of the retina
   - Vitreous seeding.

International Classification of Retinoblastoma

International classification of retinoblastoma was proposed to predict the prognosis of retinoblastoma after treatment with focal treatment modalities such as laser photocoagulation, thermotherapy, chemotherapy, etc. It classifies retinoblastoma into five groups:

1. *Group A:* Small intraretinal retinoblastoma < 3 mm.
2. *Group B:* Retinoblastoma > 3 mm located within 3 mm of fovea or within 1.5 mm of optic disk or subretinal fluid < 3 mm from the tumor margin.
3. *Group C:* Retinoblastoma with the focal subretinal or vitreous seeding within 3 mm of tumor.
4. *Group D:* Retinoblastoma with the diffuse subretinal or vitreous seeding > 3 mm from the tumor.
5. *Group E:* Extensive retinoblastoma occupying $> 50\%$ of globe or retinoblastoma associated with neovascular glaucoma or involving the postlaminar optic nerve, choroid, sclera and orbit.

Pathology**

Gross Pathology

The tumor mass appears as chalky white mass with foci of calcification.

Histopathology

Retinoblastoma arises from undifferentiated neuroectodermal cells that are the precursors of retinal neuroepithelium. Microscopically, retinoblastoma consists of small, round tumor cells with large hyperchromatic nuclei.

Histopathologically, retinoblastoma is classified into:

- Well-differentiated retinoblastoma
- Poorly differentiated retinoblastoma.

Well-differentiated retinoblastoma

Well-differentiated retinoblastoma shows tumor cells arranged in the form of rosettes and fleurettes.

Rosettes: It indicates typical arrangement of tumor cells around a cavity resembling to the petals of rose.

Flexner-Wintersteiner rosette: They consist of arrangement of the cuboidal or columnar tumor cells around a clear central lumen. This is highly specific of retinoblastoma. This is also seen in medulloepithelioma (Fig. 17.2.1).

Homer-Wright rosette: They consist of radial arrangement of tumor cells around a central tangle of neural fibers. These are also seen in neuroblastoma and medulloblastoma (Fig. 17.2.2).

Fleurettes: They consist of tumor cells projecting through fenestrated membrane with pear-shaped eosinophilic processes.

> The presence of rosettes and fleurettes indicates tumor cells showing differentiation toward formation of photoreceptors and is supposed to be associated with good prognosis.

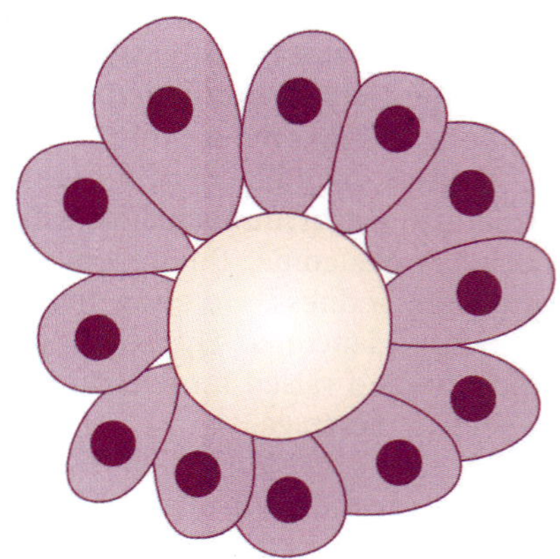

FIG. 17.2.1: Flexner-Wintersteiner rosette

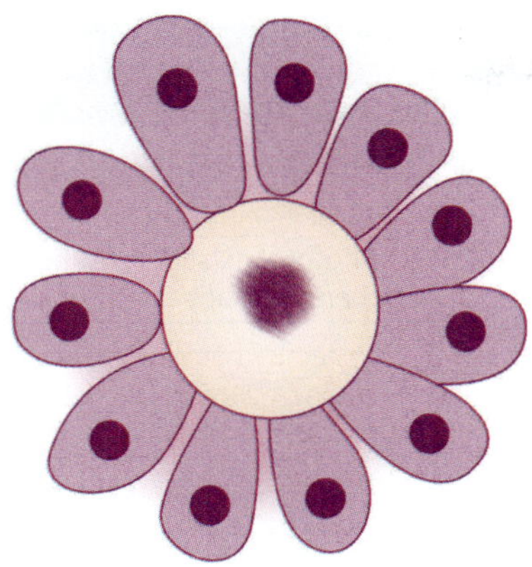

FIG. 17.2.2: Homer-Wright rosette

Poorly differentiated retinoblastoma

Poorly differentiated retinoblastoma shows small, round tumor cells with large hyperchromatic nuclei and scanty cytoplasm with mitotic figures and areas of necrosis. Poorly differentiated retinoblastoma shows pseudorosette. Pseudorosette indicates arrangement of the tumor cells around the lumen of blood vessels.

Differential Diagnosis

Retinoblastoma has to be differentiated from other causes of leukocoria and other retinal tumors.

Leukocoria in Children***

The common causes of leukocoria in children are classified as retinoblastoma and pseudoretinoblastoma or pseudoglioma.**

The causes for pseudoretinoblastoma are:

- Coats' disease.
- Retinopathy of prematurity.
- Persistent hyperplastic primary vitreous.
- Congenital cataract.
- Choroidal coloboma.
- Toxocariasis.
- Retinal dysplasia.
- Hereditary conditions, e.g. Norrie's disease, incontinentia pigmenti.

Retinoblastoma has to be differentiated from other retinal tumors, they are:

- Retinal astrocytoma
- Medulloepithelioma
- Retinal hemangiomas.

Investigations

Radiological investigations such as X-rays, computed tomography (CT), magnetic resonance imaging (MRI) and ultrasonography are very sensitive for diagnosis of retinoblastoma:

- X-rays show calcification and erosion of the optic foramen
- Computed tomography scan shows calcification and intraocular extension of the tumor within the eye and extraocular extension of the tumor
- Magnetic resonance imaging is helpful in the cases with optic nerve and intracranial involvement
- B-scan shows high internal reflectivity of the tumor mass because of calcification.

Laboratory tests by increased level of lactate dehydrogenase in the aqueous humor are rarely used.

In patients with suspected metastasis, bone scan, bone marrow aspiration and lumbar puncture for cerebrospinal fluid (CSF) analysis are carried out.

Treatment**

The treatment modalities available for retinoblastoma are as follows.

Laser photocoagulation: This is indicated in tumors measuring < 4 mm in diameter situated in the posterior pole. It is done by using xenon arc or argon laser.

Cryotherapy: This is indicated in tumors measuring < 4 mm in diameter situated in the equatorial region or in the periphery of the retina.

Thermotherapy: This is indicated in tumors measuring < 4 mm in diameter situated in the posterior pole as an alternative treatment to laser photocoagulation.

Plaque brachytherapy: This is indicated in tumors measuring < 16 mm in diameter and situated 3 mm away from the optic nerve and fovea. It is done by placing the radioactive implant over the sclera.

External beam radiotherapy: This is indicated in bilateral retinoblastoma or in unilateral advanced retinoblastoma.

Systemic chemotherapy: This is indicated in advanced bilateral or unilateral retinoblastoma for chemoreduction and in treatment of metastasis. Vincristine, etoposide and carboplatin are the most common chemotherapeutic agents used for chemotherapy.

Periocular chemotherapy: This is done by subconjunctival injections of chemotherapeutic agents, e.g. carboplatin.

Enucleation: It was the most popular and the only definitive treatment of retinoblastoma. But with the advent of the recent treatment modalities, enucleation is reserved for eyes in which the vision cannot be restored.

Orbital exenteration: It is considered in cases with orbital extension not responding to radiotherapy or chemotherapy. The treatment depends on the stage of the disease and the recent treatment guidelines are as per the ICRB (Table 17.2.1).

Prognosis

With the recent advances in diagnosis and treatment of retinoblastoma, the mortality has come down drastically. The cure rate is almost 95% in developed countries. Untreated retinoblastoma invariably leads to death by intracranial extension by 2 years of diagnosis of retinoblastoma.

Optic nerve involvement, undifferentiated tumor, choroidal invasion and late presentation in the advanced stage are associated with poor prognosis.

TABLE 17.2.1: Treatment modalities for retinoblastoma

Group	*Treatment modalities*
Group A	Focal therapy by laser photocoagulation/cryotherapy/thermotherapy
Group B and C	Systemic chemotherapy for chemoreduction followed by plaque brachytherapy
Group D	• Unilateral tumors are treated by enucleation • Bilateral tumors are treated by chemotherapy and radiotherapy
Group E	• Unilateral tumors are treated by enucleation • Bilateral tumors are treated by chemotherapy and radiotherapy, followed by enucleation of the worse eye • Orbital exenteration is considered in cases with orbital involvement

Follow-up

Follow-up is essential to detect recurrence of the tumor or development of secondary tumor. First follow-up is done 3–4 weeks after the treatment. The next examinations are done once in 3 months for 2 years, once in 6 months for next 3 years and once in a year later.

Genetic Counseling*

Genetic counseling is the most important aspect of management of retinoblastoma (Table 17.2.2).

TABLE 17.2.2: Genetic counseling

Laterality	*Negative family history*	*Positive family history*
Unilateral retinoblastoma	Siblings (1%) Offspring (8%)	Siblings (40%) Offspring (40%)
Bilateral retinoblastoma	Siblings (6%) Offspring (40%)	Siblings (40%) Offspring (40%)

RETINAL ASTROCYTOMA

1. It is a relatively rare benign tumor of the retina and optic nerve head. The tumor arises from retinal astrocytes.
2. It appears as a yellowish white retinal mass involving the superficial layers of the retina. It remains asymptomatic and detected on retinal examination by ophthalmoscopy; visual impairment is seen in cases involving the macula and in cases with complications, e.g. retinal detachment.
3. Bilateral and multifocal retinal astrocytomas are usually associated with the tuberous sclerosis.
4. Since most of the retinal astrocytomas are benign, they may not require treatment. Treatment is advised in cases with macular involvement and is done by laser photocoagulation, cryotherapy or radiotherapy.

RETINAL HEMANGIOMAS

Hemangiomas are benign tumors arising from blood vessels. Retinal hemangiomas are of two subtypes as follows:
1. Capillary hemangioma.
2. Cavernous hemangioma.

Capillary Hemangioma

1. It is a rare benign, but sight threatening tumor arising from retinal vasculature or optic disk vessels.
2. Capillary hemangioma appears as round lesion, orange-red in color with dilated and tortuous retinal blood vessels.
3. Capillary hemangiomas are usually associated with intraretinal and subretinal exudation leading to complications such as exudative retinal detachment.
4. Bilateral and multifocal capillary hemangiomas are usually associated with von Hippel-Lindau disease.
5. Treatment modalities are photocoagulation, cryotherapy or radiation therapy.
6. Photodynamic therapy and antivascular endothelial growth factors are the recent modes of treatment.

Cavernous Hemangioma

1. It is a rare condition. If it occurs, it will be unilateral in most of the cases. Rarely it causes visual impairment unlike capillary hemangioma.
2. It presents as cluster of vascular saccules in the sensory retina with normal appearance of the retinal blood vessels, thus differentiating it from capillary hemangioma, which appears as a round, orange-red lesion with dilated and tortuous retinal blood vessels.
3. It rarely causes visual impairment because of recurrent or massive vitreous hemorrhage.
4. Treatment is by cryotherapy or by surgical excision done in cases associated with nonresolving vitreous hemorrhage.

Retinal Pigment Epithelial Tumors

Congenital hypertrophy of the retinal pigment epithelium:
1. It is a benign congenital condition affecting the retinal pigment epithelium.
2. It presents as a grayish black lesion of the retina. It presents in two varieties:
   a. Typical variety presenting as solitary pigmented lesion.
   b. Atypical variety presenting as multiple pigmented plaques. Atypical variety is often associated with familial colonic adenomatous polyposis.
3. It is a benign condition and does not require treatment.

Adenoma and adenocarcinoma of the retinal pigment epithelium are the other tumors of the retinal pigment epithelium.

GIST BOX 17.2

- Retinoblastoma is the most common primary intraocular malignancy in children.
- Retinoblastoma arises from immature retinal cells, primitive precursor cells of the photoreceptors.
- Retinoblastoma most commonly occurs as a sporadic condition in about 93–94% cases with most of them presenting with unilateral and unifocal involvement.
- Leukocoria, white pupillary reflex is the most common clinical presentation of retinoblastoma. Strabismus is the second common clinical presentation.
- Retinoblastoma arises from undifferentiated neuroectodermal cells that are the precursors of retinal neuroepithelium. Well-differentiated retinoblastoma shows tumor cells arranged in the form of rosettes and fleurettes.
- Retinoblastoma has to be differentiated from other causes of leukocoria and other retinal tumors.
- Computed tomography scan shows calcification and intraocular extension of the tumor within the eye and extraocular extension of the tumor.
- The treatment modalities available for retinoblastoma are laser photocoagulation, cryotherapy, thermotherapy, plaque brachytherapy, external beam radiotherapy, systemic chemotherapy, periocular chemotherapy, enucleation and orbital exenteration.

FREQUENTLY ASKED QUESTIONS (FAQs)

*Short Answers

1. Clinical features of retinoblastoma.
2. Genetic counseling in retinoblastoma.

**Short Essays

1. Malignant melanoma.
2. Classification of retinoblastoma.
3. Histopathology of retinoblastoma.
4. Treatment of retinoblastoma.
5. Pseudoglioma.

***Long Essays

1. Describe the etiology, clinical features and management of retinoblastoma.
2. Describe the differential diagnosis of leukocoria in children. Describe the stages and management of retinoblastoma.

BIBLIOGRAPHY

1. Abramson DH, Frank CM, Susman M, et al. Presenting signs of retinoblastoma. J Pediatr. 1998;132:505-8.
2. Abramson DH, Schefler AC, Dunkel IJ, et al. Adult ophthalmic oncology: ocular diseases.
3. Dutta LC. Modern Ophthalmology, 3rd edition. New Delhi: Jaypee Brothers Medical Publishers (P) Ltd.
4. Ryan SJ. Retinoblastoma. St. Louis: Mosby-Year Book Inc; 2006.
5. Rodriguez-Galindo C, Wilson MW. Retinoblastoma, New York: Springer; 2010.
6. Yanoff M, Duker JS. Ophthalmology, 3rd edition. St. Louis, Mo: Mosby Elsevier; 2008.

SECTION 18

Ocular Trauma

CHAPTER

18.1 Mechanical Injuries

CAUSES FOR MECHANICAL INJURIES

The usual causes for mechanical injuries are:

- Occupational hazards or workplace injuries
- Road traffic accidents
- Sports and recreational activities
- Assault/Fighting.

> Ocular damage caused by trauma is one of the most common causes of ocular morbidity and mortality worldwide.
>
> Ocular trauma is the most common cause of uniocular blindness worldwide.
>
> Mechanical injuries account for the most common type of ocular trauma.

CLASSIFICATION OF OCULAR TRAUMA

The Birmingham Eye Trauma Terminology System definitions and classifications are commonly used for classification of ocular trauma. According to this, the outermost layer of the eyeball involving cornea and sclera is called eye wall. Ocular trauma is classified depending on the presence of partial thickness or full-thickness wound in the eye wall into:

- Closed globe injury
- Open globe injury.

Closed Globe Injury

Closed globe injury is a type of ocular injury characterized by partial thickness wound in the eye wall.

Based on the mode of injury, closed globe injury is further classified into:

1. *Contusion:* It is a type of closed globe injury caused by blunt trauma.
2. *Lamellar laceration:* It is a type of closed globe injury caused by sharp object.

Open Globe Injury

Open globe injury is a type of ocular injury characterized by full-thickness wound in the eye wall.

Based on the mode of injury, open globe injury is further classified into:

1. *Rupture:* It is a type of open globe injury caused by blunt object.
2. *Laceration:* It is a type of open globe injury caused by sharp object.

Laceration injury is further classified into:

1. *Penetrating injury:* It is a type of laceration injury characterized by single laceration injury through the eye wall.

2. *Penetrating injury with intraocular foreign body:* It is a type of penetrating injury associated with retained intraocular foreign body.
3. *Perforating injury:* It is a type of laceration injury characterized by presence of two lacerating injuries, one entry and another exit wound caused by same object.

BLUNT OCULAR INJURY***

Blunt injury can lead to open globe or closed globe injury.

Mechanisms of Blunt Injury*

Coup injury: It occurs at the site of impact because of the force caused by the trauma.

Contrecoup injury: It occurs away from the site of impact because of shock waves produced by the force caused by the trauma.

Anteroposterior compression and equatorial expansion: It occurs because of anteroposterior compression and equatorial expansion resulting in distortion of the ocular structures.

Indirect injury: It results from the globe hitting against the orbital bony walls.

The blunt injury can lead to damage to globe or to adnexal structures and the damage to globe can be in the form of open globe injury or closed globe injury.

Closed Globe Injury

Cornea

Corneal abrasion: It is because of epithelial damage of the cornea. The treatment is by pad and bandage after applying antibiotic eye ointment to prevent secondary infection of the epithelial defect.

Traumatic corneal ulcer: It is because of secondary infection of epithelial defect. Treatment is similar to treatment of corneal ulcer.

Corneal edema: It is because of rupture of Descemet's membrane and entry of aqueous into corneal stroma.

Partial-thickness corneal tear: The treatment of the condition is by use of antibiotics to prevent secondary infection, and pad and bandage. Large partial thickness tears can be sutured.

Sclera

Partial-thickness scleral tear: The treatment of the condition is similar to treatment of partial-thickness corneal tear.

Anterior Chamber

Angle of the anterior chamber and ciliary body angle recession: It is defined as separation of circular and longitudinal fibers of the ciliary muscle as a result of blunt trauma to the eye.

Hyphema**

Definition: Collection of blood/red blood cells (RBCs) in the anterior chamber is called hyphema (Figs 18.1.1A and B).

Etiology

- Trauma including blunt injury, penetrating injury and surgical trauma is the most common cause for hyphema.
- The causes for spontaneous hyphema are following intraocular surgeries, rubeosis iridis, bleeding disorders, tumors such as melanoma, retinoblastoma, side effects of anticoagulants, etc.
- The source of bleeding is from either branches of major/minor arterial circle of iris or radial vessels at the root of the iris.

Pathogenesis: Blunt injury is the most common mode of injury leading to hyphema. The common cause for hyphema is tears in the ciliary body and root of the iris leading to bleeding into anterior chamber.

Contd...

Contd...

Clinical features: The clinical features depend on the degree and grade of hyphema. Hyphema is graded as:

- *Grade I:* Hyphema filling less than one third of anterior chamber.
- *Grade II:* Hyphema filling one third to half of anterior chamber.
- *Grade III:* Hyphema filling more than half to near total of anterior chamber.
- *Grade IV:* Hyphema filling complete anterior chamber. It is also called eight ball black hyphema.
  Hyphema of grade more than II present with defective vision along with the signs of injury.

Treatment: The treatment of hyphema is by:

- Bedrest with head-end elevation.
- Topical steroids and cycloplegic drugs to treat associated uveitis.
- Antiglaucoma medications such as timolol eyedrops or oral acetazolamide for cases presenting with increased intraocular pressure (IOP).
- Surgical drainage of the hyphema is indicated in cases with elevated IOP not responding to treatment with IOP of more than 50 mm Hg for 5 days or 35 mm Hg for 7 days, corneal blood staining and non-resolving hyphema of more than 10 days.

Complications: Secondary glaucoma and corneal blood staining are the two common complications leading to loss of vision following hyphema:

- Cases with rebleeding, which commonly occurs between 2nd and 5th day are treated by aminocaproic acid, an antifibrinolytic agent either by topical or oral route.
- Patients with sickle cell disease need cautious management as the sickle red cells, which are rigid than normal RBCs clog the trabecular meshwork and cause secondary glaucoma. Hence, surgical drainage is indicated in cases of hyphema with sickle cell disease for IOP of more than 25 mm Hg of 1 day duration.

Gonioscopy is performed after 4–6 weeks of traumatic hyphema and those presenting with angle recession are follow-up to look for angle recession glaucoma.

Initially, it causes hypotony, but as the angle structures heal, it leads to fibrosis and synechial closure of the angle of the anterior chamber causing glaucoma called 'angle-recession glaucoma'. It is described in detail under secondary glaucoma.

Iris

Iridodialysis: It is defined as separation of root of the iris from its attachment at the ciliary body. It presents with irregular pupil or most commonly D-shaped pupil with torn iris from ciliary body

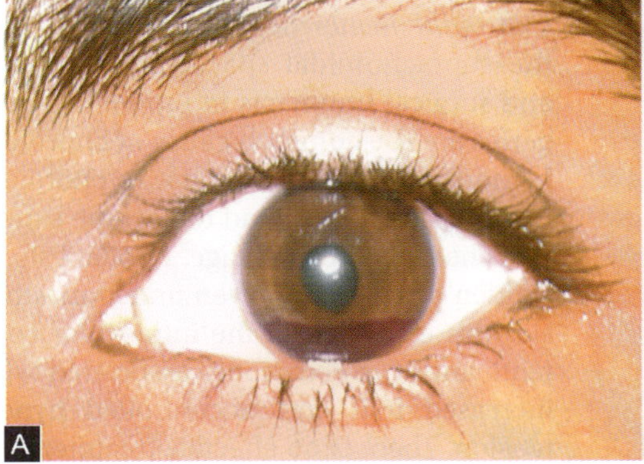

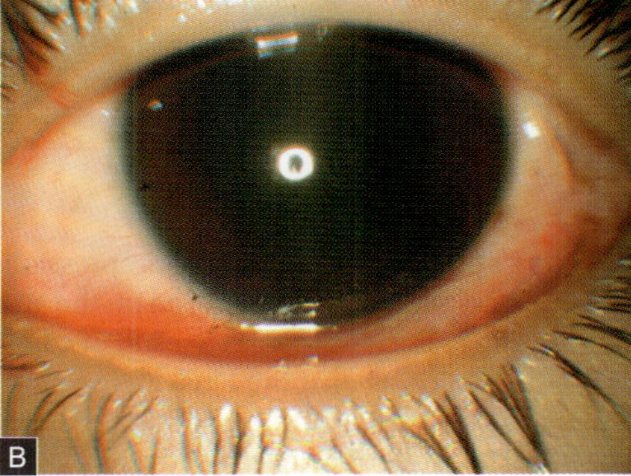

FIGS 18.1.1A and B: Hyphema

in the periphery resulting in double pupil. Secondary glaucoma can occur as a complication because of associated hyphema, traumatic iritis and injury to structures of the angle of the anterior chamber. Surgical repair of the iridodialysis is indicated in large dialysis resulting in uniocular double vision.

Anteflexion of iris: It is seen associated with iridodialysis in which the detached portion of the iris is anteflexed with the posterior pigmented layer of the iris facing anteriorly.

Retroflexion of iris: It is also seen in association with iridodialysis in which the detached portion of the iris is retroflexed onto the ciliary body.

Iridermia: It is traumatic separation of the whole of the iris resulting in aniridia. The iris is completely torn from the ciliary body attachment and is found floating in the anterior chamber. It is usually associated with hyphema.

Traumatic iridocyclitis: It is inflammation of the iris, or ciliary body and iris together, because of trauma. The treatment is by using cycloplegic drugs and steroids.

Pupil*

Traumatic miosis: It is constriction of pupil as a result of spasm of the sphincter pupillae because of irritation of ciliary nerves.

Traumatic mydriasis: It is dilatation of the pupil because of injury to the sphincter pupillae resulting in tears in the muscle.

Sluggish reaction of the pupil: It is because of either traumatic miosis or mydriasis.

D-shaped pupil: It is seen in iridodialysis.

Lens*

Vossius ring: It is circular pigmentary impression of the pupillary margin of the iris seen on the anterior capsule of the lens seen as a result of compression of the iris against the lens. It is seen as pigmentary impression of the pupillary margin of the iris on the anterior capsule of the lens.

Subluxation or dislocation of lens: It is because of anteroposterior compression and equatorial expansion following blunt injury resulting in zonular dehiscence. The clinical features and treatment are described under ectopia lentis.

Concussion Cataract*

Traumatic cataract seen because of blunt injury, is called concussion cataract. It is because of entry of aqueous into the lens cortex through the tears in the anterior capsule of the lens produced secondary to blunt injury.

The lens opacity typically involves the sutures of the lens and assumes a star shape along the suture lines and hence it is called rosette- or star-shaped cataract.

The management of traumatic cataracts is similar to senile cataract; however, all cases of traumatic cataracts require careful evaluation to look for the associated features such as subluxation of cataract, zonular dehiscences, etc. the presence of which will alter the corse of surgery or postoperative visual prognosis.

The other causes for traumatic cataract are penetrating injury, exposure to radiation, electric shock, etc.

Vitreous

- Vitreous detachment
- Vitreous hemorrhage
- Vitreous liquefaction.

These are described under the Section 10 'Vitreous'.

Choroid

1. *Choroidal hemorrhage:* Is bleeding into the suprachoroidal space. Blunt trauma and surgical trauma as in intraocular surgeries are the common cause of choroidal hemorrhage. The intraoperative choroidal hemorrhage may extend to become expulsive choroidal hemorrhage. It manifests as sudden onset of pain even under anesthesia with expulsion of the intraocular contents and it is commonly associated with increased IOP, and uncontrolled hypertension. There is no effective treatment for

Commotio Retinae (Fig. 18.1.2)*

It is defined as opacification of the retina following concussion injury to the retina following blunt trauma.

*Berlin's Edema**

Commotio retinae involving the posterior pole of the retina is called Berlin's edema. It was first described by Rudolf Berlin. But Berlin's edema is not edema of the retina, but it is the opacification of retina involving the posterior pole of the retina.

Etiopathogenesis: Commotio retinae follows blunt injury and it develops within few hours following injury. It is the result of damage to the outer retinal layers resulting from concussion shock waves and hence, the mode of injury is by contrecoup mechanism. Disruption of the outer segments of the photoreceptors and damage to retinal pigment epithelium resulting in opacification of the retina is the most common mechanism of injury.

Clinical Features: Defective vision is seen following injury and it may recover spontaneously over 3–4 weeks and hence has good visual prognosis. Berlin's edema results in the development of cherry-red spot at the macula.

Treatment: There is no effective treatment for commotio retinae and Berlin's edema, and it usually resolves completely without any permanent visual sequelae. The poor visual prognosis is seen in macular involvement and permanent visual loss is seen in cases associated with retinal pigment epithelial changes, macular hole, and choroidal neovascular membrane.

massive choroidal hemorrhage and usually leads to irreversible loss of vision.

2. *Choroidal rupture:* Are defined as breaks in the choroid because of blunt injury. Choroidal ruptures may be anterior involving the ora serrata or posterior occurring concentric to the optic disk. The choroidal ruptures involving macula can lead to poor vision in the initial stages because of associated macular edema and in later stages because of complications such as choroidal neovascularization membrane formation.
3. Choroidal detachment.

Retina

1. *Traumatic retinal tear:* A retinal break caused by dynamic vitreoretinal traction following trauma is called retinal tear. Giant retinal tear defined as tears extending more than 90° of the circumference of the globe are more common following trauma.
2. *Traumatic retinal detachment:* It is retinal detachment following trauma and described under retina.
3. *Traumatic macular hole:* It can follow Berlin's edema or commotio retinae, or choroidal rupture. The clinical features and treatment are similar to idiopathic macular hole.
4. Commotio retinae.

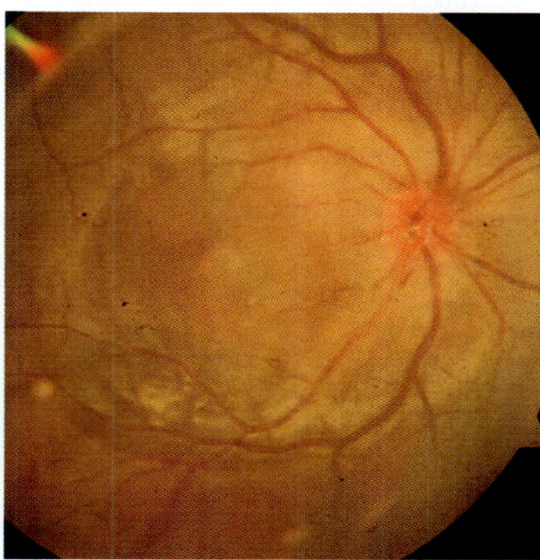

FIG. 18.1.2: Commotio retinae

Optic Nerve

- Avulsion of optic nerve
- Traumatic optic neuropathy.

These are described under Section 12 'Optic Nerve.'

Adnexal Lesions seen in Blunt Trauma

Eyelids

Ecchymosis of eyelids—black eye (Figs 18.1.3A and B): Black eye is common following blunt injury to eyes or part of the head above the eyes. The factors responsible for ecchymosis of eyelids are:*

1. Skin of the eyelids is the thinnest in body. It does not have a subcutaneous fatty layer.
2. Layer of the loose subcutaneous tissue gets distended easily by blood in case of injuries to head.
3. The submuscular areolar tissue of upper eyelids is in continuity with subaponeurotic space of scalp allowing easy passage of fluid and blood to the upper eyelids leading to black eye or ecchymosis of upper eyelids in cases of head injuries.

The treatment of the condition is by cold compress and use of antiedema drugs such as serratiopeptidase.

Lid tear (Figs 18.1.4A and B): It is common following blunt injury and laceration injury and treatment is by repairing the tear by suturing.

Conjunctiva

- Subconjunctival hemorrhage
- Chemosis of conjunctiva
- *Conjunctival tear:* Small conjunctival tears can be left alone, whereas the large tears are sutured.

Subconjunctival hemorrhage and chemosis of conjunctiva are commonly seen following blunt trauma and they are discussed under Section 3 'Conjunctiva.'

Orbit

- Orbital hemorrhage
- Orbital fractures.

These are described in the Section 14 'Orbit.'

Lacrimal Apparatus

1. Injury to lacrimal gland.
2. Injury to lacrimal drainage system: These are common following blunt injury or lacerating injury. Injuries involving the lacrimal canaliculi are repaired by identifying the cut ends of lacrimal canaliculi and silicone tube intubation to maintain the patency of lacrimal drainage system.

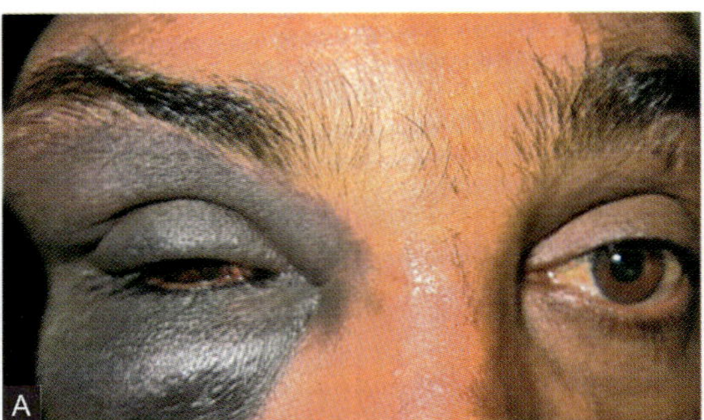

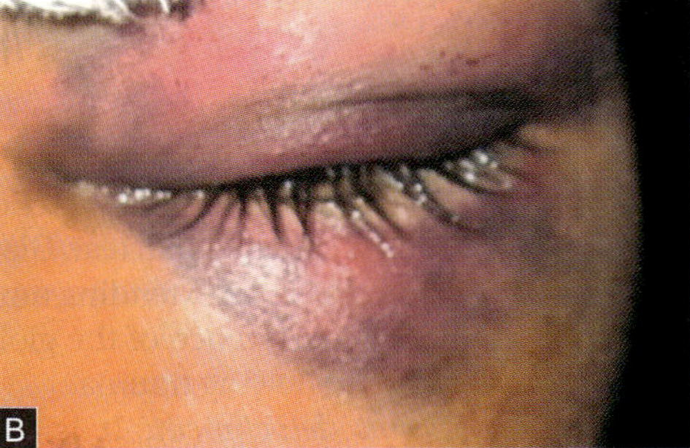

FIGS 18.1.3A and B: Ecchymosis of eyelids—black eye

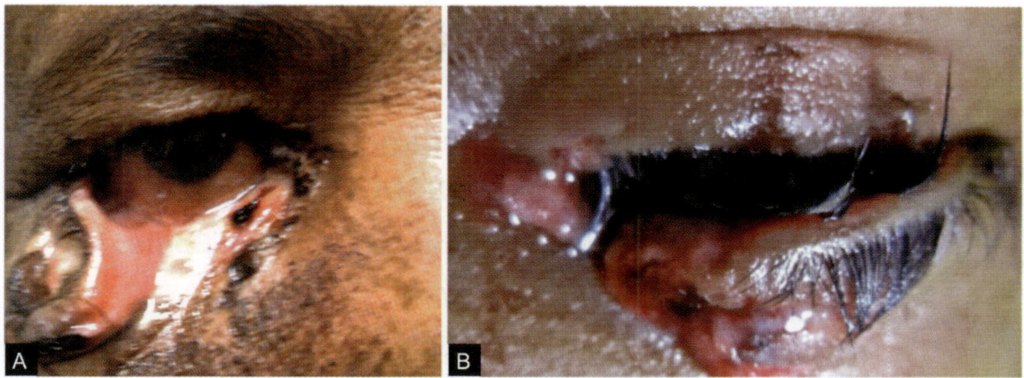

FIGS 18.1.4A and B: Lid tear

Open Globe Injury

Open globe injury involves full-thickness defect in the eye wall and open globe injury following blunt injury is called globe rupture.

*Globe Rupture***

Definition: Globe rupture is an open globe injury involving full-thickness defect in the eye wall caused by blunt trauma (Figs 18.1.5A and B).

Etiopathogenesis: Globe injury follows severe degree of blunt injury. The mechanism of injury is detailed as follows.

Coup injury: It occurs at the site of impact because of the force caused by the trauma.

Contrecoup injury: It occurs away from the site of impact because of shock waves produced by the force caused by the trauma. It is commonly seen involving the superior limbus or superonasal limbus as inferior or inferotemporal limbus is most commonly involved in the blunt trauma, as this part has least protection from the orbital walls.

Anteroposterior compression and equatorial expansion: It occurs because of anteroposterior compression and equatorial expansion resulting in giving away at the weakest point in the eye wall. This is usually the site of incision in people who have undergone cataract surgery or it may involve the limbus.

Indirect injury: It results from the globe hitting against the orbital bony walls.

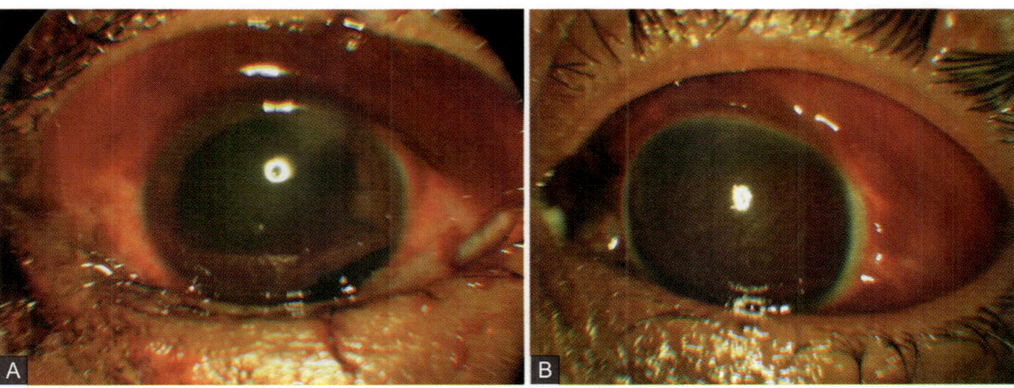

FIGS 18.1.5A and B: Globe rupture

Clinical features: Globe rupture often leads to gross diminution of vision and the severity of visual loss depends on the severity of injury and extent of damage to the intraocular structures. The clinical features depend on the severity of injury and the extent of damage to the intraocular structures. Globe rupture leads to full-thickness defect in the eye wall, which leads to prolapse of uveal tissue, angle recession, hyphema, damage to lens in the form of cataract or dislocation of lens, or expulsion of lens from the eye, vitreous loss, vitreous hemorrhage, ciliochoroidal detachment, retinal detachment, etc.

Treatment: Globe ruptures without extensive damage to the eye are managed by repairing the defect in the sclera or cornea with reposition or excision of the prolapsing uveal tissue.

Following repair posterior segment evaluation is done by B-scan imaging and appropriate treatment is done accordingly.

Bad globe ruptures with extensive damage to the intraocular structures with no visual prognosis are better managed by enucleation to prevent sympathetic ophthalmitis in the normal eye. Evisceration should not be done as this will not protect against the development of sympathetic ophthalmitis, as the surgery will not remove all the uveal pigments.

LACERATION/PENETRATING/ PERFORATING OCULAR INJURY

Laceration injury is caused by sharp object and it can lead to open globe or closed globe injury.

The closed globe injury from laceration involves lamellar lacerations involving the cornea or sclera, or lacerations involving the eyelids, eyebrows and conjunctiva.

The open globe injuries following laceration involve corneal laceration or corneal tears (Fig. 18.1.6), scleral tears and corneoscleral tears.

The treatment is by repair of the laceration/ tear by suturing. Evaluation is done to rule out posterior segment injuries and retained intraocular foreign bodies by B-scan and other radiological modalities.

Badly injured eyes are better treated by enucleation to prevent sympathetic ophthalmitis in the other eye similar to globe rupture.

EXTRAOCULAR AND INTRAOCULAR FOREIGN BODIES

Extraocular Foreign Bodies

Etiology

Presence of extraocular foreign bodies is of very common occurrence and the common foreign bodies seen are dust particles, small iron particles, small insects, vegetative matter, etc. Extraocular foreign bodies are most commonly seen in people working in workshops, agricultural workers, drivers, etc.

Clinical Features

Foreign bodies produce redness, watering and irritation/foreign body sensation of the eyes. The common sites for lodging of foreign bodies are cornea followed by conjunctiva (Fig. 18.1.7). Sulcus subtarsalis in the upper palpebral conjunctiva is one of the common sites of lodgment of foreign body. A foreign body in the sulcus subtarsalis can cause recurrent corneal epithelial defect; hence, sulcus subtarsalis has to be examined to rule out corneal foreign body in cases presenting with recurrent or persistent corneal epithelial defects by double eversion of the upper eyelid.

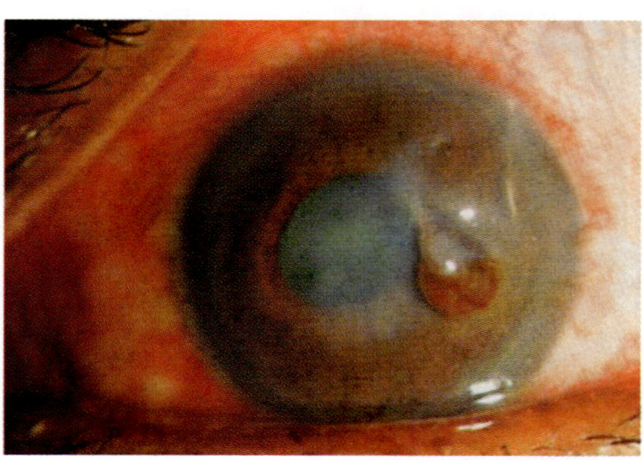

FIG. 18.1.6: Corneal tear with iris prolapse

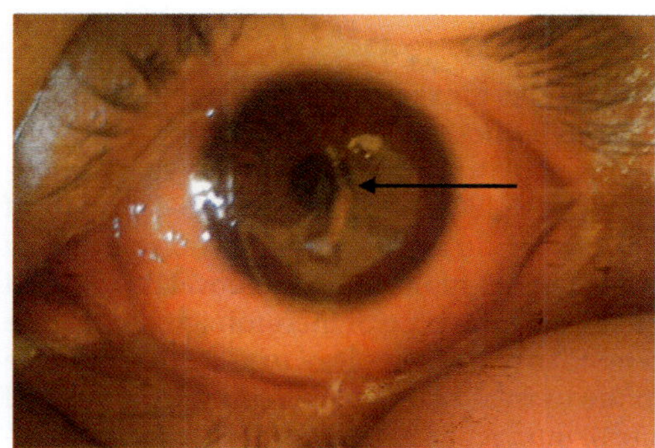

FIG. 18.1.7: Corneal foreign body

Treatment

Treatment is done by removal of the foreign body under slit lamp. Conjunctival foreign bodies are removed by forceps, cotton bud or by a hypodermic needle. Corneal foreign bodies are best removed by a hypodermic needle under slit lamp or operating microscope (Fig. 18.1.8). Antibiotic eyedrops or eye ointments are used prophylactically to prevent secondary infections.

Complications

Foreign bodies left without removal can lead to secondary infection resulting in conjunctivitis, foreign body granuloma, corneal epithelial defects, corneal ulcer, etc.

Intraocular Foreign Bodies**

Etiopathogenesis

Intraocular foreign bodies are commonly associated with penetrating and perforating injuries. In fact, all cases of penetrating injuries occurring as a result of high-speed mechanical activities should be evaluated for presence of intraocular foreign bodies.

The intraocular foreign bodies can be present anywhere in the eye from anterior chamber to retina. It is not uncommon to find intraocular foreign bodies perforating the eye to be seen in the orbit or in the retrobulbar space. Based on the nature of intraocular foreign bodies, they are broadly classified into three types as follows.

Inert intraocular foreign bodies: They include glass, gold, silver, aluminum, sand, stone, etc. These are well tolerated and do not cause specific reaction.

Irritant intraocular foreign bodies: They include copper, iron and their alloys, which cause specific toxic reaction such as chalcosis bulbi and siderosis bulbi. They have to be removed because of damage to the eye and toxic reaction caused by them.

Vegetative intraocular foreign bodies: They include wooden or vegetative matter and they are associated with the highest risk of infective endophthalmitis.

Clinical Features

The clinical features are similar to those of penetrating injury and the diminution of vision loss in the initial period depends on the severity of ocular damage caused by the perforating injury.

Presence of intraocular foreign bodies is suspected in cases showing perforating injuries arising as a result of high-speed mechanical activities with eyes showing corneal or scleral perforation, iris hole, opaque track in the lens, vitreous hemorrhage, etc.

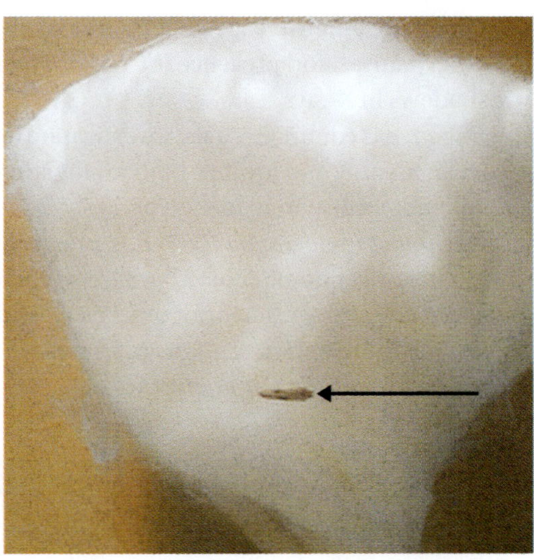

FIG. 18.1.8: Foreign body removed from cornea

Investigations

Radiological investigations are required for identifying the presence and location of the intraocular foreign body. The commonly employed radiological investigations are as follows:

1. *X-ray:* It was extensively used in the past for localization of metallic radiopaque foreign bodies. Now it is not very popular because of availability of better radiological modes of examination. Anteroposterior views and lateral views are taken and if a radiopaque foreign body is found, limbal ring method is used for its localization.

   Limbal ring method is done after suturing a limbal ring at the limbus and taking X-rays in different positions with the patient looking upwards, downwards, etc. The localization of the foreign body is done by assessment of the position of the radiopaque shadow in relation to the limbus. This can differentiate an intraocular foreign body from an orbital foreign body, as the former moves with the movement of the eyeball, while the latter does not move.

   Intraocular calcifications, retinoblastoma, hypermature cataract with calcification of the anterior capsule are some of the other causes for presence of radiopaque shadows in X-rays.
2. *B-scan:* It is commonly used investigation as it can identify and localize both radiopaque and radiotransparent foreign bodies.
3. *Computed tomography (CT):* It is presently the investigation of choice because of high specificity and sensitivity for diagnosing and localizing the intraocular foreign bodies.
4. *Magnetic resonance imaging (MRI).*

> Magnetic resonance imaging should be avoided when the presence of intraocular metallic foreign bodies is suspected.

Treatment

Indications for removal of intraocular foreign bodies

Removal of the intraocular foreign body whenever possible is the best option because of risk of specific reactions or infection caused by them. Observation without removal is indicated in cases of presence of inert foreign bodies, the removal of which may lead to more damage. The mode of treatment depends on the nature and site of intraocular foreign bodies.

Magnetic foreign bodies are removed by handheld magnet, whereas non-magnetic foreign bodies are removed by forceps:

1. Intraocular foreign bodies in the anterior chamber are removed by a corneal or limbal incision by handheld magnet or by forceps depending on the type of foreign body.
2. Intraocular foreign bodies in the iris are removed by sector iridectomy or by forceps.
3. Intraocular foreign bodies in the lens are removed by lens extraction, as presence of intraocular foreign bodies or attempts of removal can lead to cataract.
4. Intraocular foreign bodies in vitreous and retina are removed by pars plana vitrectomy and by either magnet or by forceps.

> The risk of endophthalmitis following intraocular foreign body is as high as 30%. Gram-positive organisms such as staphylococci and streptococci are the most common causative organisms responsible for endophthalmitis, whereas *Bacillus cereus,* a gram-positive organism responsible for the rapidly spreading endophthalmitis.
>
> Hence, all cases of intraocular foreign bodies particularly in the posterior segment are treated by administration of intravitreal antibiotics. 0.1 mL each of intravitreal vancomycin (1 mg/mL) and ceftazidime (2.25 mg/mL) are the most commonly administered antibiotics covering both gram-positive and gram-negative organisms.

RADIATIONAL INJURIES

The radiational injuries seen in the eye are:

- Photophthalmia seen because of exposure to ultraviolet (UV) rays

- Photoretinitis seen because of exposure to infrared rays and UV rays
- Glass blowers cataract because of exposure to infrared rays
- Radiation retinopathy, radiation kerato-conjunctivitis, radiation-induced cataract are seen on exposure to ionizing radiation.

ELECTRICAL INJURIES

The electrical injuries seen in the eye are:

- Keratitis
- Iridocyclitis
- Electric cataract.

THERMAL INJURIES

The thermal injuries commonly involve the eyelids and rarely involve the eye proper because of lid reflex. Eyelid thermal burns are treated similar to skin burns depending on the grading of burns, first- and second-degree burns are treated by medical management by using antibiotic eye ointment and third-degree burns are treated by skin grafting.

Burns involving the cornea and conjunctiva are treated by antibiotics, lubricating agents and bandage soft contact lenses.

GIST BOX 18.1

- Closed globe injury: It is a type of ocular injury characterized by partial-thickness wound in the eye wall. This includes contusion and lamellar laceration. Contusion is a type of closed globe injury caused by blunt trauma. Lamellar laceration is a type of closed globe injury caused by sharp object.
- Open globe injury: It is a type of ocular injury characterized by full-thickness wound in the eye wall. This includes rupture and laceration. Rupture is a type of open globe injury caused by blunt object. Laceration is a type of open globe injury caused by sharp object.
- Blunt injury can lead to open globe or closed globe injury. The mechanisms of blunt injury are coup injury, contrecoup injury, anteroposterior compression and equatorial expansion, and indirect injury.
- Globe rupture is an open globe injury involving full-thickness defect in the eye wall caused by blunt trauma.
- Traumatic cataract seen because of blunt injury is called concussion cataract. The lens opacity typically involves the sutures of the lens and assumes a star shape along the suture lines and hence it is called rosette cataract or star-shaped cataract.
- Penetrating injury is a type of laceration injury characterized by single laceration injury through the eye wall.
- Perforating injury is a type of laceration injury characterized by presence of two lacerating injuries, one entry and another exit wound caused by same object.
- Intraocular foreign bodies are commonly associated with penetrating and perforating injuries. In fact, all cases of penetrating injuries occurring as a result of high-speed mechanical activities should be evaluated for presence of intraocular foreign bodies.

CHAPTER

18.2 Chemical Injuries

Chemical injuries of the eye represent one of the ocular emergencies requiring immediate treatment, as delay in treatment can lead to extensive ocular damage resulting in irreversible visual impairment.***

ETIOPATHOGENESIS

Chemical injuries occur in industrial accidents, agriculture-related activities and chemical attacks. Chemical injuries are basically classified into alkali injuries and acid injuries.

Alkali vs Acid Injuries

Alkali injuries are more dangerous than acid injuries.

Alkalis Cause

- Saponification of fatty acids present in cell membranes resulting in destruction of cells and facilitating deeper penetration.
- Interaction with stromal collagen and glycosaminoglycans resulting in softening and further facilitating deeper penetration.

Acids Cause

- Protein denaturation and coagulation, thus preventing deeper penetration and limiting the ocular damage.
- Thus, alkalis are more dangerous, as they can penetrate deeper and cause more ocular damage (Figs 18.2.1A and B).

The common alkalis and acids resulting in chemical injuries are detailed in Tables 18.2.1 and 18.2.2.

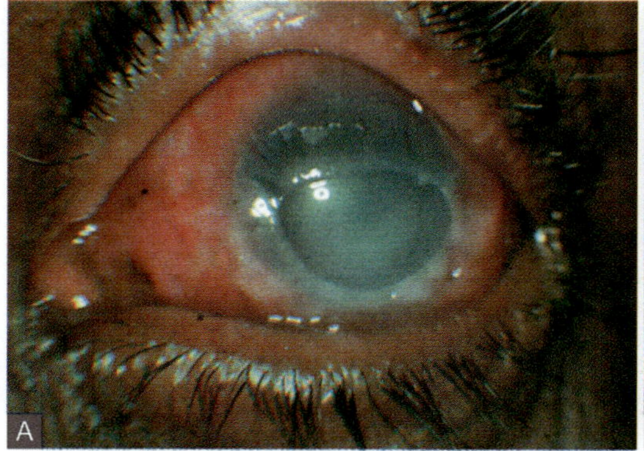

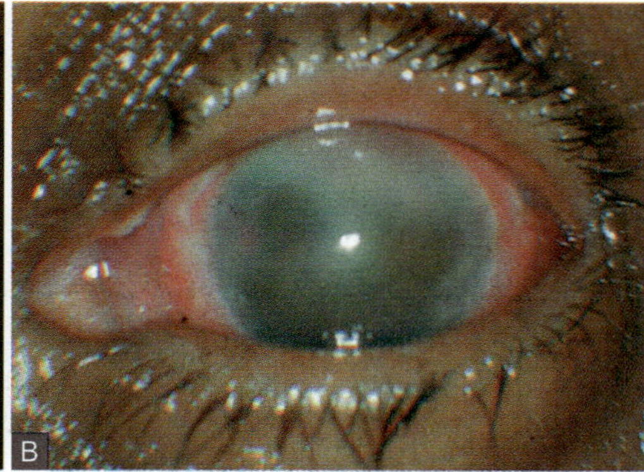

FIGS 18.2.1A and B: Alkali burns

TABLE 18.2.1: Common alkalis

Alkali	*Source of exposure*
Calcium hydroxide	Plaster, mortar, white cement, lime
Sodium hydroxide	Drain cleaners
Potassium hydroxide	Drain cleaners
Aluminum hydroxide/ Ammonia	Fertilizers

TABLE 18.2.2: Common acids

Acid	*Source of exposure*
Hydrofluoric acid	Glass cleaners
Sulfuric acid	Car batteries, toilet cleaners
Hydrochloric acid	Water treatment plants
Nitric acid	Explosives, fertilizers

CLINICAL FEATURES

The clinical features depend on the type, pH of chemical and duration of exposure to the chemical. The clinical manifestations run in three phases:

1. *Acute phase:* It starts immediately following exposure to chemical and it extends up to 3 days. It is characterized by acute ischemic necrosis of the ocular surface and rapid penetration of the chemicals.

   The clinical manifestations seen in acute phase are:
   a. *Conjunctiva:* It shows chemosis, congestion and limbal ischemia in severe cases.
   b. *Cornea:* It shows epithelial defects and corneal edema.
   c. *Anterior chamber:* It shows anterior chamber reaction and signs of iridocyclitis.
2. *Intermediate phase:* It starts from 3 days and extends till 7 days. It is characterized by active inflammation with infiltration by polymorphonuclear leukocytes (PMNLs) resulting in stromal ulceration. In intermediate phase, conjunctiva and cornea show vascularization and infiltration by PMNLs.
3. *Late phase:* It extends from the end of 1st week to several months and is characterized by scarring and cicatrization. Late phase shows complications such as symblepharon of conjunctiva, scarring of cornea, dry eye, etc.

The severity of chemical injuries is classified into four stages by Hughes Roper-Hall as given in Table 18.2.3.

CLINICAL COURSE OF CHEMICAL BURNS

Chemical burns can lead to corneal ulceration and perforation, thus leading to loss of vision. The cause of corneal ulceration is related to collagenolytic activity, which starts by 2nd week of healing. The use of steroids, which will enhance collagenolytic activity should be avoided in 2nd week.

Intraocular pressure is known to increase following chemical burns as a result of collagen

TABLE 18.2.3: Hughes Roper-Hall classification

Grade	*Clinical features*	*Prognosis*
I	Cornea shows epithelial damage No limbal ischemia	Good
II	Cornea is hazy, but iris details can be made out Limbal ischemia less than one third	Good
III	Cornea shows total corneal epithelial defect with stromal haziness with blurring of the iris details Limbal ischemia one third to half	Guarded
IV	Cornea is opaque with no view of iris details Limbal ischemia more than half	Poor

shrinkage leading to alterations in the trabecular meshwork in the initial stages of chemical burns and later as a result of release of inflammatory prostaglandins.

TREATMENT OF CHEMICAL BURNS*

The treatment depends on the phase of the chemical burns.

The treatment in acute phase is by:

1. Immediate and thorough wash with saline or water till the pH becomes normal, or near normal.
2. Mechanical removal of the chemical matter.
3. Medical treatment is by use of:
   a. Cycloplegics, e.g. atropine 1% eye ointment for pain relief by preventing ciliary spasm.
   b. Antibiotic eyedrops/ointment to prevent secondary bacterial infection.
   c. Artificial tears eyedrops.
   d. Topical corticosteroid eyedrops for control of inflammation.
   e. Antiglaucoma medications such as oral acetazolamide or topical beta blockers for control of intraocular pressure.
   f. Vitamin C and oral doxycycline/tetracycline to augment synthesis of collagen.
   g. Collagenase inhibitor, e.g. acetyl cysteine to prevent degradation of collagen.
   h. Bandage soft contact lenses are applied in case of total corneal epithelial damage to promote quick healing of corneal epithelium.
   i. Glass rod application is done to prevent development of symblepharon.

Treatment in the Intermediate Phase

The treatment in the intermediate phase is by the medical treatment as in acute phase is continued except for steroids. Corticosteroids are stopped from 2nd week/8th day onwards as collagen synthesis starts by this time and steroids can cause collagenolysis.

Treatment in the Late Phase

The treatment in the late phase is by:

1. Artificial tear supplement eyedrops are continued till the corneal epithelium heals and treatment is aimed at treatment of complications such as:
   a. Symblepharon by excision and mucosal membrane graft.
   b. Treatment of secondary glaucoma.
   c. Corneal opacity by keratoplasty, limbal stem cell transplantation and keratoprosthesis.

GIST BOX 18.2

- Chemical injuries of the eye represent one of the ocular emergencies requiring immediate treatment, as delay in treatment can lead to extensive ocular damage resulting in irreversible visual impairment.
- Alkali injuries are more dangerous than acid injuries.
- The clinical features of chemical injuries depend on the type, pH of chemical and duration of exposure to the chemical.
- The clinical manifestations run in three phases with acute phase for first 3 days, characterized by acute ischemic necrosis of the ocular surface and rapid penetration of the chemicals; intermediate phase for 3 days and extending till 7 days, characterized by active inflammation with infiltration by polymorphonuclear leukocytes resulting in stromal ulceration; and late phase extending from the end of 1 week to several months and is characterized by scarring and cicatrization.
- The severity of chemical injuries is classified into four stages by Hughes Roper-Hall classification depending on the severity of limbal ischemia.

CHAPTER

18.3 Specific Inflammations Following Ocular Trauma

SYMPATHETIC OPHTHALMITIS**

Sympathetic ophthalmitis is described in detail under the Section 7 'Uvea'; few important points are mentioned below:

1. Sympathetic ophthalmitis is defined as a bilateral granulomatous panuveitis, which occurs typically following trauma to one eye.
2. It is most common following penetrating ocular trauma with an incidence of 0.5%, whereas its incidence following surgical trauma is about 0.1%.
3. It is more commonly seen following penetrating injuries involving the ciliary zone (hence, the ciliary zone is called dangerous zone) and in injuries with incarceration of uveal tissue in the wound. The incidence is more common in males probably because of more incidence of trauma in males as compared to females.
4. Trauma leads to drainage of antigen from the eye via lymphatics, leading to development of delayed hypersensitivity resulting in granulomatous inflammation of the uveal tract. The antigen responsible is presumed to be retinal S-antigen.
5. Photophobia and diminution of vision for near in the normal eye are the earliest symptoms of sympathetic ophthalmitis. Aqueous flare in the normal eye is the earliest sign of sympathetic ophthalmitis. Bilateral granulomatous panuveitis is present in established cases of sympathetic ophthalmitis.
6. With the availability of microsurgical techniques and meticulous repair of the penetrating injuries, the incidence of sympathetic ophthalmitis has come down drastically.
7. Sympathetic ophthalmitis is prevented by early enucleation of the badly injured eye with no visual prognosis.
8. Sympathetic ophthalmitis is treated by corticosteroids and refractory cases are treated with immunosuppressive drugs.
9. Role of evisceration over enucleation to prevent sympathetic ophthalmitis in badly injured eyes is still controversial, as evisceration may not remove the uveal tissue completely.

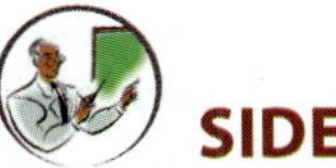

SIDEROSIS BULBI**

Definition

Pigmentary and degenerative changes in the eye following retained intraocular iron foreign body are called siderosis bulbi.

Etiopathogenesis

The corrosion of the iron occurs in the eye as it comes in contact with the ocular fluids causing electrolytic dissociation and dissemination of ferrous ions throughout the eye. These ions combine with the intracellular proteins resulting in pigmentary and degenerative changes.

The iron particles preferentially affect the epithelial structures.

The common sites of deposition of the iron ions are lens epithelium, non-pigmented ciliary epithelium, sphincter pupillae, dilator pupillae, pars plana, trabecular meshwork, corneal epithelium and retinal pigment epithelium.

Clinical Features

- Deposition of rusty patches over the anterior capsule of lens in a ring-like pattern is one of the earliest manifestations of siderosis bulbi
- Heterochromia iridis
- Complicated cataract
- Pupillary abnormalities
- Secondary glaucoma
- Corneal depositions
- Pigmentary retinal degeneration leading to the night blindness initially and total blindness later
- Reduced response on electroretinography (ERG) in the form of decreased amplitude of B-wave.

Treatment

Treatment is by early removal of intraocular foreign body containing iron. If removal of suspected iron intraocular foreign body is deferred, the cases require monitoring by ERG to look for changes and the beginning of ERG changes should be followed by removal of the intraocular foreign body.

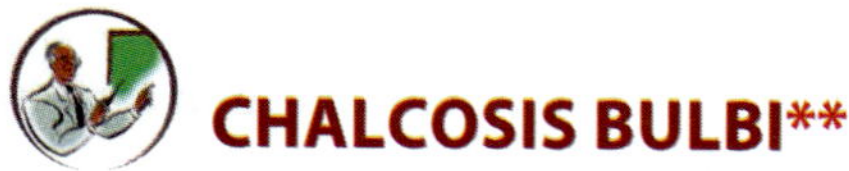

CHALCOSIS BULBI**

Definition

Pigmentary changes in the eye following retained intraocular copper alloy foreign body are called chalcosis bulbi.

Pure copper produces suppurative reaction resulting in toxic endophthalmitis, whereas copper alloys containing 85–95% lead to chronic pigmentary changes called chalcosis bulbi.

Copper alloys containing less than 85% usually will not lead to any changes.

Etiopathogenesis

Copper undergoes electrolytic dissociation and dissemination throughout the eye. The copper ions do not combine with the intracellular proteins, hence will not lead to degenerative changes such as iron and thus, visual prognosis is favorable in chalcosis bulbi compared to siderosis bulbi.

The common sites of deposition of the copper ions are anterior lens epithelium, Descemet's membrane of cornea and internal limiting membrane of retina.

Clinical Features

Examination of the eye shows:

1. Kayser-Fleischer ring in cornea as a result of deposition of iron in Descemet's membrane appearing as golden brown ring.
2. Sunflower cataract as a result of deposition of copper under the capsule of lens. It is called so because of resemblance of the golden green color opacity to petals of sunflower.
3. Golden plaques in the retina as a result of deposition of the copper in retina.
4. Visual loss is seen rarely and if seen, it is because of involvement of macula by the deposits.

Prognosis

Visual prognosis is good as compared to chalcosis bulbi.

Specific Inflammations Caused by Metallic Intraocular Foreign Bodies

- Glass, gold, silver, aluminum: No reaction
- Copper, zinc, nickel, mercury: Suppurative reaction
- Iron: Siderosis bulbi
- Copper alloys: Chalcosis bulbi.

GIST BOX 18.2

- Sympathetic ophthalmitis is defined as a bilateral granulomatous panuveitis, which occurs typically following trauma to one eye.
- Pigmentary and degenerative changes in the eye following retained intraocular iron foreign body are called siderosis bulbi.
- Pigmentary changes in the eye following retained intraocular copper alloy foreign body are called chalcosis bulbi.

FREQUENTLY ASKED QUESTIONS (FAQs)

*Short Answers

1. Mention the mechanisms of ocular damage in blunt injury.
2. Mention the effects of blunt injury on lens.
3. Mention the effects of blunt injury on pupil.
4. Concussion cataract.
5. Commotio retinae.
6. Berlin's edema.
7. Black eye.
8. Mention the treatment of intraocular foreign bodies.
9. Management of alkali injuries of eyes.

**Short Essays

1. Hyphema.
2. Globe rupture.
3. Intraocular foreign bodies.
4. Sympathetic ophthalmitis.
5. Siderosis bulbi.
6. Chalcosis bulbi.

***Long Essays

1. Classify ocular trauma. Describe the ocular manifestations of blunt ocular injury.
2. Describe the etiopathogenesis, clinical features and treatment of chemical injuries of eyes.

BIBLIOGRAPHY

1. Ballantyne JF. Siderosis bulbi. Br J Ophthalmol. 1954;38(12):727-33.
2. Chu XK, Chan CC. Sympathetic ophthalmia: to the twenty-first century and beyond. J Ophthalmic Inflamm Infect. 2013;3(1):49.
3. Catalano RA, Belin M. Ocular Emergencies. WB Saunders company; 1992.
4. John DA, Moroi SE, Stein JD. Ophthalmic Pearls: Management of an intraocular foreign body. Eye Net; 2009. pp. 31-2.
5. Kuhn F, Pieramici DJ. Ocular Trauma. Italy: Thieme Publications; 2002.
6. Kuhn F, Morris R, Witherspoon CD, et al. The Birmingham Eye Trauma Terminology system (BETT). J Fr Ophtalmol. 2004;27(2):206-10.
7. Kuhn F, Morris R, Witherspoon CD, et al. A standardized classification of ocular trauma. Ophthalmology. 1996;103(2):240-3.

SECTION 19

Community Ophthalmology

CHAPTER

19.1 Community Ophthalmology and Blindness

Community ophthalmology is the application of techniques of clinical ophthalmology in combination with the methodologies of community medicine to promote ocular health and to prevent blindness.

The five levels of prevention and control of a disease described in community medicine are employed in community ophthalmology (Table 19.1.1).

The study of community ophthalmology helps to know the most common ocular diseases prevalent in a particular area, prevalence of blindness; thus helps to formulate the preventive, promotive and curative strategies.

BLINDNESS**

Clinically, the condition in which a person is not able to perceive light is called as blindness.

However, the definition of blindness varies worldwide and for the purpose to ensure uniform data collection; World Health Organization (WHO) has proposed a uniform definition and has defined low vision and blindness.

Best-corrected visual acuity in the better eye less than 3/60 (or its equivalent) or field of vision less than 10° is referred as blindness.

Low Vision

Best-corrected visual acuity in the better eye in the range of 6/18–6/60 or its equivalent, or field of vision between 20° and 30° is referred as low vision grade I or mild visual impairment.

Best-corrected visual acuity in the better eye in the range of 6/60–3/60 or its equivalent, or field of vision between 10° and 20° is referred as low vision grade II, or severe visual impairment.

TABLE 19.1.1: Five levels of prevention and control of eye disease

Sl No	*Levels of prevention*	*Method of prevention*
1.	Positive health promotion	By appropriate health education
2.	Specific prevention of diseases	Vitamin A supplementation to prevent vitamin A deficiency
3.	Early diagnosis and treatment	Treatment of corneal ulcer early to prevent blindness
4.	Disability control	By treatment and regular follow-up of diseases such as glaucoma to limit progression of blindness
5.	Rehabilitation	By visual rehabilitation of blind people using low visual aids

The definition of blindness includes the following terminologies.

Best-corrected Visual Acuity

It is the visual acuity after appropriate treatment or standard refraction and correction by glasses.

Better Eye

The eye with relatively good vision among the two eyes is taken into consideration and it is labeled as better eye, and the other eye is labeled as worse eye and it is not considered in defining blindness, and low vision.

Categories of Visual Impairment (Table 19.1.2)**

Legal Blindness*

Best-corrected visual acuity in the better eye less than 6/60 or field of vision less than 20° is called 'legal blindness'. It is the level of visual acuity required to become eligible for disability benefits given by government.

Economic Blindness*

It is same as legal blindness. Best-corrected visual acuity in the better eye less than 6/60 or field of vision less than 20° is called 'economic blindness'. It is the level of visual acuity less than which will affect a person's profession or work, thus causing financial or economic burden.

Social Blindness*

Best-corrected visual acuity in the better eye less than 3/60 or field of vision less than 10° is called 'social blindness'. It is the level of visual acuity less than which will affect day-to-day social life.

Blindness Statistics

According to the recent statistics worldwide, there are 314 million people with visual impairment, of which 45 million come under blindness category and 269 million come under low- vision category.

In India, 12 million people come under visual impairment category and 7 million come under blindness category.

Avoidable Blindness*

Avoidable blindness is the blindness, which can be avoided by either appropriate treatment (curable blindness, e.g. blindness because of cataract can be treated by cataract surgery) or by ensuring proper preventive measures (preventable blindness, e.g. vitamin A supplementation to prevent keratomalacia and corneal blindness).

Avoidable blindness accounts for up to 80% of total blindness and 90% of the visually impaired people live in developing countries.

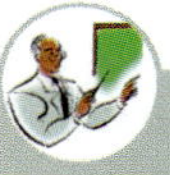

Leading Causes for Blindness in India*

Cataract: 62.6%
Refractive errors: 19.7%
Glaucoma: 5.8%
Posterior segment disorders: 4.7%
Surgical complication: 1.2%
Corneal blindness: 0.9%
Posterior capsular opacification: 0.9%
Other causes: 4.19%

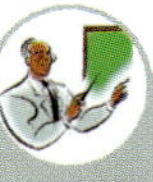

Leading Causes for Global Blindness

Cataract: 39%
Refractive errors: 18%
Glaucoma: 10%
Age-related macular degeneration: 7%
Corneal scar: 4%
Diabetic retinopathy: 4%
Trachoma: 3%
Onchocerciasis: 0.7%
Other causes: 11%

TABLE 19.1.2: Categories of visual impairment

Grades of visual impairment	*Categories of visual impairment*	*Best-corrected visual acuity in the better eye and visual field*
Grade 0	Normal	6/6–6/18
Grade I	Low vision: Mild visual impairment	6/18–6/60 or field of vision between 20° and 30°
Grade II	Low vision: Severe visual impairment (legal blindness and economic blindness)	6/60–3/60 or field of vision between 10° and 20°
Grade III	Blindness (social blindness)	3/60–1/60 or field of vision between 5° and 10°
Grade IV	Blindness (total blindness)	1/60–PL (perception of light) or field of vision less than 5°
Grade V	Blindness (total blindness)	No PL

National Programme for Control of Blindness**

The National Programme for Control of Blindness (NPCB) was launched in the year 1976 as a 100% Central Government sponsored program. It was launched with the goal to reduce the prevalence of blindness to be less than 0.3% by the year 2020.

*Objectives**

1. Establishment of eye care facilities for population of every 5 lakhs.
2. Establishment of eye care services at primary health center (PHC) and community health center (CHC).
3. Improvement of the quality of eye care services by ensuring participation of private sector.

Strategies

1. Strengthening of eye care service delivery.
2. Development of manpower for eye care services.
3. Creating public awareness about diseases of eye.
4. Development of institutional capacity for treatment of eye diseases.

Revised Strategies after 11th Five Year Plan

1. To include causes of blindness other than cataract such as corneal blindness, refractive errors, glaucoma under NPCB.
2. To improve the quality of cataract surgeries by shifting from eye camp surgeries to hospital or institutional surgeries.
3. Development of infrastructure for eye care services throughout the country by construction of eye ward, eye operation theaters, training of eye surgeons in modern cataract surgery at district level.
4. Involvement of non-government organization (NGO) and improving the performance of government organizations at medical college, and district hospitals to ensure better coverage of eye care services.

Activities under National Programme for Control of Blindness

1. Construction of eye wards, eye operation theaters at district levels with assistance from World Bank.
2. Training of eye surgeons and ophthalmic assistants.

3. Distribution of ophthalmic instruments such as slit lamp, microscope, ophthalmoscope, intraocular lenses, etc. to district blindness units in all states.
4. Involvement of NGOs by giving funds for organizing eye camps, conducting cataract surgeries and establishment of eye banks.

*Levels of Eye Care**

Eye care is given at three levels such as primary, secondary and tertiary level.

Primary level: Eye care at the this level is given by a paramedical ophthalmic assistant at the level of PHC and subcenters who carry out vision assessment and screening for some common eye diseases such as cataract on refractive error.

Secondary level: Eye care at the this level is given by an ophthalmologist at the CHC and district hospitals. Here, treatment is given for common conditions such as cataract, glaucoma, etc.

Tertiary level: Eye care at the this level is given at medical college hospitals and Regional Institute of Ophthalmology and it includes treatment of the complicated diseases such as retinal detachment, corneal opacity, etc.

Apex institute: Dr Rajendra Prasad Centre for Ophthalmic Sciences, All India Institute of Medical Sciences (AIIMS) is the Apex Institute and it provides overall supervision to carry out the activities of NPCB.

Vision 2020: The Right to Sight**

Global

Vision 2020 is a global initiative by the WHO and the International Agency for the Prevention of Blindness (IAPB).

It was launched on February 18, 1999 by the WHO and IAPB, to eliminate avoidable blindness by the year 2020 by effective global cooperation by involving NGOs like Christoffel-Blindenmission (Germany), Sightsavers International (United Kingdom), etc. It aims at performing 20 million cataract surgeries annually till 2010 and 32 million cataract surgeries annually till the year 2020.

In India

Vision 2020 is the initiative to bring government, national and international NGOs to work jointly to achieve the goal of eliminating avoidable blindness by the year 2020, to have India free of avoidable blindness; so that every citizen enjoys the gift of sight and every visually challenged will have improved quality of life as a right.

Members of Vision 2020 (India)

International non-governmental organizations: Christoffel-Blindenmission (Germany), Sightsavers International (United Kingdom), Orbis International (USA), Operation Eyesight Universal (Canada), Seva Foundation (USA), Lions Clubs International Foundation (USA).

National non-governmental organizations: LV Prasad Eye Institute, Hyderabad, Andhra Pradesh and Aravind Eye Care System, Madurai, Tamil Nadu.

National governmental organizations: Dr Rajendra Prasad Institute for Ophthalmic Sciences, New Delhi.

District Blindness Control Society/ District Health Society**

District Blindness Control Society (DBCS) was formed in 1994–1995 under NPCB for effective implementation of the NPCB at district level. A District Program Manager (DPM) is incharge of DBCS and is responsible for its functioning. The main function of DBCS is to monitor and implement NPCB at each district.

*Aims and Objectives**

1. To assess the magnitude of blindness in the district level.
2. To conduct eye camps and cataract surgeries with the help of NGOs and district mobile ophthalmic units.
3. To procure and distribute the drugs and other consumables required for cataract surgery to various government hospitals and district mobile ophthalmic units.

4. To provide financial assistance to NGOs to perform cataract surgeries.
5. To promote eye donation and to monitor the utilization of the eyes collected by eye collection centers and eye banks.
6. To monitor the implementation of the NPCB at district level.
7. To arrange for school eye screening for detection of refractive errors in children and distribution of spectacles.

*Composition of District Blindness Control Society**

Chairman: Deputy Commissioner/District Magistrate.

Vice chairman: District Health Officer.

Member secretary: District Program Manager.

Technical advisor: Head of the Department of Ophthalmology/Chief Ophthalmic Surgeon.

Members: Medical Superintendent/District Surgeon, District Education Officer, representatives of NGOs.

Due to formation of National Rural Health Mission (NRHM) under 11th Five Year Plan, DBCS under NPCB has been merged with District Health Society (DHS) under NRHM.

National Trachoma Control Programme*

The program was started in the year 1963 and it was merged with the NPCB by the year 1976.

The surgery, antibiotics, facial cleanliness and environment hygiene (SAFE) strategy and intermittent treatment as described under the treatment of trachoma are the strategies employed under National Trachoma Control Program.

GIST BOX 19.1

- Community ophthalmology is the application of techniques of clinical ophthalmology in combination with the methodologies of community medicine to promote ocular health and to prevent blindness.
- Blindness: Best-corrected visual acuity in the better eye less than 3/60 (or its equivalent) or field of vision less than 10° is referred as blindness.
- Low vision: Best-corrected visual acuity in the better eye in the range of 6/18–6/60 or its equivalent, or field of vision between 20° and 30° is referred as low vision.
- According to the recent statistics, worldwide there are 314 million people with visual impairment, of which 45 million come under blindness category and 269 million come under low vision category. In India, 12 million people come under visual impairment category and 7 million come under blindness category.
- Avoidable blindness is the blindness, which can be avoided by either appropriate treatment (curable blindness, e.g. blindness because of cataract can be treated by cataract surgery) or by ensuring proper preventive measures (preventable blindness, e.g. vitamin A supplementation to prevent keratomalacia and corneal blindness).
- The National Programme for Control of Blindness was launched in the year 1976 as a 100% Central Government sponsored program. It was launched with the goal to reduce the prevalence of blindness to less than 0.3% by the year 2020.
- Vision 2020: The Right to Sight is a global initiative by the World Health Organization (WHO) and the International Agency for the Prevention of Blindness (IAPB). It was launched on February 18, 1999 by WHO and IAPB to eliminate avoidable blindness by the year 2020 by effective global cooperation by involving nongovernmental organizations like Christoffel-Blinden Mission (Germany), Sightsavers International (United Kingdom), etc.
- District Blindness Control Society was formed in 1994–1995 under National Programme for Control of Blindness (NPCB) for effective implementation of the NPCB at district level.

CHAPTER

19.2 Nutritional Blindness and Childhood Blindness

NUTRITIONAL BLINDNESS**

The diseases of the eye due to vitamin A deficiency, which will lead to blindness are included under nutritional blindness.

Xerophthalmia**

A Greek word meaning dry eyes, i.e. 'xero', means 'dry'; 'ophthalmia', means 'eyes'. It is defined as a condition in which cornea and conjunctiva become dry due to deficiency of vitamin A. Xerophthalmia is one of the leading causes of childhood blindness worldwide, particularly in developing countries.

It includes a wide spectrum of conditions starting from mild varieties, e.g. night blindness and conjunctival xerosis, and severe varieties, e.g. corneal xerosis to keratomalacia.

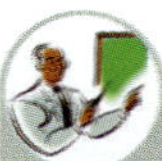

Vitamin A

Vitamin A is an essential micronutrient; it plays an important role in vision, immune function, skin health and normal growth in human beings.

It is a fat-soluble vitamin also called 'retinol'. Its high sources are fish, meat, egg and dairy products.

Carotenoids precursor form of vitamin A is present in green leafy vegetables, carrot, orange and other yellow fruits.

*Classification of Xerophthalmia (Table 19.2.1)**

Night blindness: It is the earliest manifestation of vitamin A deficiency. Scotopic vision is a function of rods affected since vitamin A is an essential component of rhodopsin, pigment present in rods. Normal night vision usually returns back within 3 days of supplementing vitamin A.

Conjunctival and corneal xerosis: It is due to keratinization occurring in the epithelial surfaces of mucous membranes. Keratinizing metaplasia occurs in the epithelial surfaces due to deficiency of vitamin A, which is responsible for maintenance of normal epithelial architecture.

TABLE 19.2.1: Classification of xerophthalmia

Symbol	*Type*
XN	Night blindness
X1A	Conjunctival xerosis
X1B	Bitot's spots
X2	Corneal xerosis
X3A	Corneal ulceration/keratomalacia involving less than one third of cornea
X3B	Corneal ulceration/keratomalacia involving less than one third of cornea
XF	Xerophthalmic fundus
XS	Corneal scars secondary to xerophthalmia

Bitot's spots are defined as collections of foamy material over an area of conjunctival xerosis consisting of desquamated keratinized epithelial cells and saprophytic bacilli. Their presence indicates conjunctival xerosis. Bitot's spots along with night blindness indicate significant vitamin A deficiency. Bitot's spots usually disappear within 2 weeks of starting treatment by vitamin A. However in few, they may persist for an indefinite time, usually in the temporal quadrant of the conjunctiva because of the persisting keratinizing metaplasia caused by vitamin A deficiency.

Corneal ulceration/keratomalacia: It is because of liquefactive necrosis of the cornea. Corneal ulcers in vitamin A deficiency show sharply demarcated punched out ulcers situated usually in the periphery of the cornea.

Fundus xerophthalmic: It is characterized by the presence of yellowish dots in the periphery of the fundus representing the loss of pigment from retinal pigment epithelium. They may cause blind spots or scotomas. It usually responds within 2 weeks of supplementing vitamin A.

Treatment of Vitamin A Deficiency (Table 19.2.2)*

Women of reproductive age with vitamin A deficiency should have a daily dose of 10,000 IU for 2 weeks. Large doses of vitamin A are contraindicated in women of reproductive age as they are contraindicated in pregnancy.

Prophylaxis of Vitamin A Deficiency*

1. Dietary modification by promoting adequate intake of vitamin A rich foods such as green leafy vegetables.
2. Fortification of foods such as dairy products with vitamin A.
3. Supplementation of single large doses of vitamin A on periodic basis scheduled as follows (Table 19.2.3).

Three doses of vitamin A 200,000 IU on day 1, day 2 and day 8 are given immediately after birth of child to women to ensure a good supply of vitamin A in her breast milk.

CHILDHOOD BLINDNESS**

According to the WHO, worldwide there are 1.4 million children who are blind; two third of them live in the developing countries. The causes for blindness vary between various countries.

Causes for Childhood Blindness

The causes can be classified based on etiology as:

1. Genetic and hereditary causes such as familial cataract, retinal dystrophies, retinoblastoma, congenital glaucoma, etc.
2. Intrauterine causes such as infections during pregnancy—toxoplasmosis, rubella, cytomegalovirus, herpes simplex, etc.

TABLE 19.2.2: Treatment of vitamin A deficiency

Schedule	*In children aged > 1 year*	*In children < 1 year or weight < 8 kg*	*In children with severe vomiting or diarrhea*
Immediately on diagnosis	Oral vitamin A 200,000 IU	Oral vitamin A 100,000 IU	Water miscible retinyl palmitate 100,000 IU can be used instead of first dose
Next day	Oral vitamin A 200,000 IU	Oral vitamin A 100,000 IU	
2–4 week later	Oral vitamin A 200,000 IU	Oral vitamin A 100,000 IU	

TABLE 19.2.3: Supplementation of single large doses of vitamin A

Schedule	*Dose*
First dose at 9 month with measles vaccination	100,000 IU
Second dose at 18 month with booster dose of DPT*/OPV†	200,000 IU
Third dose at 24 month	200,000 IU
Fourth dose at 30 month	200,000 IU
Fifth dose at 36 month	200,000 IU

*DPT, diphtheria, pertussis, tetanus; †OPV, oral polio vaccine.

3. Neonatal causes like ophthalmia neonatorum, retinopathy of prematurity, etc.
4. Infantile and childhood causes like uncorrected refractive errors, vitamin A deficiency, injuries and infections of eye, etc.

Childhood Blindness in India

In India, the major causes of childhood blindness are uncorrected refractive errors followed by corneal blindness due to vitamin A deficiency and amblyopia following cataract surgery. Prevention of childhood blindness is included in NPCB under 11th Five Year Plan. Under NPCB, following activities are carried out with the aim to prevent childhood blindness:

1. School eye screening to detect refractive errors and provision of free spectacles.
2. Administration of vitamin A drops under universal immunization program.
3. Provision of grants for establishment of eye banks and eye donation centers for treatment of corneal blindness.
4. Creating awareness to prevent eye injuries and eye infections.

GIST BOX 19.2

- The diseases of the eye due to vitamin A deficiency, which will lead to blindness are included under nutritional blindness.
- Xerophthalmia is defined as a condition in which cornea and conjunctiva become dry due to deficiency of vitamin A. It is one of the leading causes of childhood blindness worldwide, particularly in developing countries.
- According to the WHO, worldwide there are 1.4 million children who are blind; two third of them live in the developing countries.
- In India, the major causes of childhood blindness are uncorrected refractive errors followed by corneal blindness due to vitamin A deficiency and amblyopia following cataract surgery.

FREQUENTLY ASKED QUESTIONS (FAQs)

*Short Answers

1. Legal blindness.
2. Social blindness.
3. Economic blindness.
4. Avoidable blindness.
5. Mention the leading causes of blindness in India.
6. Mention the aims and objectives of National Programme for Control of Blindness (NPCB).
7. Levels of eye care under NPCB.
8. Mention the aims and objectives of District Blindness Control Society (DBCS).
9. Mention the composition of DBCS.
10. National Trachoma Control Programme.
11. Treatment of vitamin A deficiency.
12. Prophylaxis for vitamin A deficiency.

**Short Essays

1. Blindness.
2. Categories of visual impairment.
3. National Programme for Control of Blindness (NPCB).
4. District Blindness Control Society (DBCS).
5. Vision 2020.
6. Nutritional blindness.
7. Xerophthalmia.
8. Childhood blindness.

BIBLIOGRAPHY

1. About Vision 2020: The Right to Sight—India Forum.
2. Dandona R, Dandona L. Childhood blindness in India: a population based perspective. Br J Ophthalmol. 2003;87(3):263-5.
3. Foster A, Gilbert C, Johnson G. Changing patterns in global blindness: 1988-2008. Community Eye Health. 2008;21(67):37-9.
4. Gilbert C, Hernandez-Duran LA, Kotiankar S, et al. Prevention of childhood blindness. International Centre for Eye Health. 1998.
5. Jose R, Rathore AS, Rajshekar V, et al. Salient features of the National Program for Control of Blindness during the XIth five-year plan period. Indian J Ophthalmol. 2009;57(5):339-40.
6. Jose R, Rathore AS, Sachdeva S. Community ophthalmology: revisited. Indian J Community Med. 2010;35(2):356-8.
7. Jose R, Sachdeva S. Community rehabilitation of disabled with a focus on blind persons: Indian perspective. Indian J Ophthalmol. 2010;58(2):137-42.
8. National Programme for Control of Blindness. Revised guidelines for DBCS. 2005.
9. National Institute of Health and Family Welfare documentation services. National Programme for Control of Blindness.
10. National Programme for Control of Blindness. Guidelines for State Health Society & District Health Society. Revised 11th Five Year Plan 2009.

11. Pradhan KB, Banerjee P. Community ophthalmology-dimensions. Community Ophthalmology. 2001;1:17-21.
12. Resnikoff S, Pascolini D, Mariotti SP, et al. Global magnitude of visual impairment caused by uncorrected refractive errors in 2004. Bull World Health Organ. 2008;86(1):63-70.
13. van Dijk K. Definition: visual impairment. New Vision.
14. World Health Organization. Vision 2020: The right to sight. Global initiative for the elimination of avoidable blindness. Action Plan 2006-2011. Geneva: WHO; 1999.
15. West KP, Sommer A. Delivery of oral doses of vitamin A deficiency and nutritional blindness: a state-of-the-art review. Nutrition policy discussion paper No. 2.
16. World Health Organization. Global initiative for the elimination of avoidable blindness. Programme for the Prevention of Blindness and Deafness. Geneva: WHO; 1997.
17. World Health Organization. Preventing blindness in children: report of WHO/IAPB scientific meeting. Programme for the Prevention of Blindness and Deafness, and International Agency for Prevention of Blindness. Geneva: WHO; 2000.

SECTION 20

Systemic Ophthalmology

CHAPTER

20.1 Systemic Ophthalmology

Systemic ophthalmology deals with the study of ocular manifestations in systemic diseases and systemic manifestations of ocular diseases.

> The ocular manifestations may be the presenting feature of underlying systemic disease and ocular diseases can be associated with systemic diseases; hence, the knowledge of systemic ophthalmology helps ophthalmologists in proper diagnosis and appropriate treatment.

The ocular manifestations are seen in most of the types of systemic diseases. The ocular manifestations are seen in:

- Metabolic diseases
- Infective diseases
- Diseases of the skin and mucous membranes
- Diseases of the central nervous system
- Hematological diseases
- Vascular diseases
- Nutritional diseases
- Inborn errors of metabolism
- Diseases of the musculoskeletal system
- Collagen vascular diseases
- Traumatic disorders.

METABOLIC DISEASES

Diabetes

The association of diabetes with various ocular manifestations is well evident and screening for eye examination is compulsory in all patients with diabetes.

Diabetes can affect all parts of the eye; the common ocular manifestations seen in diabetes from anterior to posterior are:**

1. *Eyelids:* Recurrent hordeolum and chalazion.
2. *Conjunctive:* Telangiectasia and tortuous conjunctival blood vessels, and recurrent subconjunctival hemorrhage.
3. *Cornea:* Increased incidence of infective keratitis, decreased corneal sensation and delayed epithelial healing.
4. *Iris:* Uveitis and rubeosis iridis.
5. *Lens:* Diabetic cataract and early onset of senile cataract.
6. *Vitreous:* Hemorrhage vitreous.
7. *Retina:* Diabetic retinopathy and diabetic papillopathy.
8. *Extraocular muscles:* Increased incidence of ophthalmoplegia.
9. *Intraocular pressure:* Increased incidence of primary open-angle glaucoma and neovascular glaucoma.
10. *Vision and refraction:* Hyperglycemia results in myopia and hypoglycemia results in hypermetropia. Diabetic retinopathy, diabetic papillopathy, diabetic cataract, vitreous hemorrhage, primary open-angle glaucoma, neovascular glaucoma, etc. are some of the common causes for poor vision in diabetes.

The ocular manifestations seen in other metabolic diseases are described in the Table 20.1.1.

TABLE 20.1.1: Metabolic diseases

Disease	*Ocular manifestation*
Gout	Episcleritis, scleritis and uveitis
Galactosemia	Metabolic cataract

INFECTIVE DISEASES

Bacterial, viral, fungal and parasitic infective diseases, all are associated with the ocular manifestations.

Bacterial Diseases (Table 20.1.2)

TABLE 20.1.2: Bacterial diseases

Disease	*Ocular manifestation*
Tuberculosis*	• Tubercles of the eyelids, conjunctiva, sclera and uveal tract • Granulomatous conjunctivitis • Phlyctenular conjunctivitis, phlyctenular keratitis • Granulomatous uveitis, choroiditis, choroidal granuloma • Retinal periphlebitis, Eales' disease
Syphilis*	• Chancre of conjunctiva • Interstitial keratitis • Iridocyclitis • Chorioretinitis • Neuroretinitis • Argyll Robertson pupil
Leprosy*	Madarosis, lagophthalmos, entropion, ectropion, trichiasis, dacryocystitis, neurotrophic keratitis, granulomatous uveitis, interstitial keratitis, episcleritis, scleritis and cataract
Diphtheria	Membranous conjunctivitis, keratitis
Gonorrhea	Ophthalmia neonatorum, purulent conjunctivitis, corneal ulcer
Cat scratch disease (caused by *Bartonella henselae*)	Parinaud's oculoglandular syndrome, uveitis, neuroretinitis

Viral Diseases (Table 20.1.3)

TABLE 20.1.3: Viral diseases

Disease	*Ocular manifestation*
Measles	Keratitis, conjunctivitis, choroiditis, macular edema, optic neuritis, Koplik's spots on conjunctiva
Mumps	Commonest is dacryoadenitis; other ocular features are conjunctivitis, keratitis, scleritis, episcleritis, retinitis and optic neuritis
Rubella	Congenital rubella syndrome characterized by eye manifestations such as congenital cataract, microphthalmos and chorioretinitis
Herpes simplex virus	Primary herpes causes vesicular eruptions involving the skin of eyelids, acute follicular conjunctivitis, corneal lesions such as punctate epithelial keratitis, etc. Recurrent ocular herpes are: • Epithelial keratitis manifesting as punctate epithelial keratitis, dendritic keratitis and geographical keratitis • Stromal keratitis manifesting as disciform keratitis and necrotizing stromal keratitis • Endotheliitis manifesting as diskiform endotheliitis, diffuse endotheliitis and linear endotheliitis • Neurotrophic keratopathy
Herpes zoster virus	Blepharitis, conjunctivitis, corneal involvement in the form of punctate epithelial keratitis, pseudodendritic ulcer, diskiform keratitis, etc. episcleritis, scleritis, uveitis, acute retinal necrosis and progressive outer retinal necrosis
Human immunodeficiency virus (HIV)	Opportunistic infections, HIV retinopathy, tumors, e.g. Kaposi's sarcoma

*Acquired Immunodeficiency Syndrome and Eye***

Acquired immunodeficiency syndrome (AIDS) caused by human immunodeficiency virus (HIV) has become recent pandemic and is present worldwide. Ocular manifestations in AIDS are well known and are as follows.

Eyelids: Kaposi's sarcoma of eyelids, molluscum contagiosum, herpes zoster ophthalmicus, recurrent stye or chalazion, etc.

Conjunctiva: Ocular surface squamous neoplasia, Kaposi's sarcoma of conjunctiva, etc.

Cornea: Increased incidence of infective keratitis.

Iris and uveal tract: Anterior uveitis and immune recovery uveitis.

Posterior segment including retina and optic nerve: Acute retinal necrosis, HIV retinopathy, progressive outer retinal necrosis, endogenous endophthalmitis, cytomegalovirus retinitis, toxoplasma retinochoroiditis, etc.

Orbit: Fungal infections of the orbit, Kaposi's sarcoma and lymphoma.

Fungal Diseases

Systemic fungal infections can lead to the fungal corneal ulcer and endogenous endophthalmitis.

Parasitic Diseases

The common systemic parasitic diseases with ocular involvement are cysticercosis, toxoplasmosis, onchocerciasis, toxocariasis and echinococcosis.

DISEASES OF THE SKIN AND MUCOUS MEMBRANES (Table 20.1.4)

TABLE 20.1.4: Diseases of the skin and mucous membranes

Disease	*Ocular manifestation*
Atopic dermatitis	Blepharoconjunctivitis, cataract, keratoconus
Acne rosacea	Marginal keratitis, blepharitis, conjunctivitis
Psoriasis	Uveitis, blepharitis
Xeroderma pigmentosum	Destruction of the eyelids, symblepharon and carcinoma of the eyelids and conjunctiva
Stevens-Johnson syndrome	Trichiasis, distichiasis, blepharitis, symblepharon, ankyloblepharon, cicatrizing conjunctivitis, corneal ulcer, corneal opacity, corneal perforation and dry eye

DISEASES OF THE CENTRAL NERVOUS SYSTEM (Table 20.1.5)

TABLE 20.1.5: Diseases of the central nervous system

Disease	*Ocular manifestation*
Intracranial infections, e.g. meningitis, encephalitis, etc.	Papilledema, ophthalmoplegia, optic atrophy
Intracranial hemorrhages	Papilledema, cranial nerve palsies
Intracranial space occupying lesions	Papilledema, cranial nerve palsies
Demyelinating diseases	Optic neuritis, nystagmus, ophthalmoplegia
Head injury	Papilledema, Hutchinson's pupil, traumatic optic neuropathy

HEMATOLOGICAL DISEASES (Table 20.1.6)

TABLE 20.1.6: Hematological diseases

Disease	*Ocular manifestation*
Anemia	Retinopathy characterized by venous tortuosity, cotton-wool spots, flame-shaped retinal hemorrhages, retinal edema and white-centered hemorrhages called Roth's spots
Leukemia	Retinopathy characterized by retinal hemorrhages, white-centered retinal hemorrhages, cotton-wool spots, venous tortuosity, optic nerve infiltration, sea-fan neovascularization affecting the peripheral retina, etc. Choroidal deposits appearing as leopard skin is seen in chronic leukemias
Sickle cell disease	Proliferative retinopathy, vitreous hemorrhage, retinal detachment

VASCULAR DISEASES (Table 20.1.7)

TABLE 20.1.7: Vascular diseases

Disease	*Ocular manifestation*
Hypertension	Hypertensive retinopathy, vascular occlusions of retina
Thromboembolic diseases	Vascular occlusions of retina, amaurosis fugax

NUTRITIONAL DISEASES (Table 20.1.8)

TABLE 20.1.8: Nutritional diseases

Disease	*Ocular manifestation*
Vitamin A	Xerophthalmia
Vitamin B_1	Optic neuropathy, retrobulbar neuritis
Vitamin B_2	Angular conjunctivitis, corneal vascularization
Vitamin B_3, B_6, B_{12}	Nutritional optic neuropathy
Vitamin C	Dry eye, subconjunctival hemorrhage
Vitamin D	Zonular cataract, age-related macular degeneration

INBORN ERRORS OF METABOLISM (Table 20.1.9)

TABLE 20.1.9: Inborn errors of metabolism

Disease	*Ocular manifestation*
Homocystinuria	Ectopia lentis
Hyperornithinemia	Gyrate atrophy
Mucopolysaccharidoses	Corneal clouding, papilledema, optic atrophy, retinopathy

DISEASES OF MUSCULOSKELETAL SYSTEM (Table 20.1.10)

TABLE 20.1.10: Diseases of musculoskeletal system

Disease	*Ocular manifestation*
Myotonic dystrophy	Ptosis, cataract
Myasthenia gravis*	Intermittent ptosis, intermittent diplopia
Oculopharyngeal dystrophy	Ptosis, chronic progressive ophthalmoplegia

COLLAGEN VASCULAR DISEASES/ AUTOIMMUNE DISEASES (Table 20.1.11)

TABLE 20.1.11: Collagen vascular diseases

Disease	*Ocular manifestation*
Rheumatoid arthritis	Marginal keratitis, keratoconjunctivitis sicca, uveitis, scleritis
Ankylosing arthritis	Uveitis
Giant cell arteritis	Ischemic optic neuropathy, amaurosis fugax
Systemic lupus erythematosus	Marginal keratitis, keratoconjunctivitis sicca, uveitis and scleritis
Polyarteritis nodosa	Scleritis, retinitis
Wegener's granulomatosis	Marginal keratitis, uveitis, scleritis, optic neuritis

TRAUMATIC DISORDERS

- Terson's syndrome
- Purtscher's retinopathy
- Shaken baby syndrome
- Valsalva retinopathy.

Terson's Syndrome*

1. Terson's syndrome is characterized by the presence of intraocular hemorrhages associated with intracranial hemorrhage.
2. Ruptured cerebral aneurysm is the commonest cause for Terson's syndrome. The other causes are trauma, tumors and postoperative causes.
3. The pathogenesis is sudden rise of intracranial pressure resulting in intraocular hemorrhages.
4. It presents as bilateral superficial retinal hemorrhages, intraretinal hemorrhages, preretinal hemorrhages and vitreous hemorrhage associated with neurological manifestations because of intracranial bleeding.
5. Most of the times, the intraocular hemorrhages clearup spontaneously; non-resolving vitreous hemorrhages may require vitrectomy.

Purtscher's Retinopathy*

1. Purtscher's retinopathy is an ischemic retinopathy characterized by the presence of cotton-wool spots and retinal hemorrhages.
2. It is most commonly seen following head injury, chest injury or injuries to the extremities involving the long bones. The other causes are acute pancreatitis, fat embolism syndrome, etc.
3. The proposed pathogenesis is vascular occlusion caused by fat embolism, air embolism, angiospasm, etc.
4. It presents as unilateral or bilateral ischemic retinopathy characterized by the presence of cotton-wool spots and retinal hemorrhages.
5. Though the retinal hemorrhages and cotton wool spots resolve overtime, it is associated with poor visual prognosis because of ischemia of the fovea.

Shaken Baby Syndrome

1. Shaken baby syndrome is characterized by the presence of intracranial and intraocular hemorrhages as a result of vigorous shaking of infants.
2. It occurs as a result of acceleration and deceleration forces causing damage to the blood vessels of the brain and eye.
3. It presents similar to Terson's syndrome with bilateral superficial retinal hemorrhages, intraretinal hemorrhages, preretinal hemorrhages and vitreous hemorrhage associated with neurological manifestations because of intracranial bleeding.

Valsalva Retinopathy

1. Valsalva retinopathy is characterized by the presence of intraocular hemorrhages associated with Valsalva maneuver.
2. It is because of raised intrathoracic pressure and intra-abdominal pressure, which is transmitted as sudden rise of intraocular pressure as occurs in Valsalva maneuver resulting in intraocular hemorrhages.
3. It is usually seen following straining, weightlifting, violent coughing, vomiting, blowing, etc.
4. It presents with unilateral or bilateral retinal hemorrhages, preretinal hemorrhages and vitreous hemorrhages.

GIST BOX 20.1

- Systemic ophthalmology deals with the study of ocular manifestations in systemic diseases and systemic manifestations of ocular diseases.
- The ocular manifestations are seen in metabolic diseases, infective diseases, diseases of the skin and mucous membranes, diseases of the central nervous system, hematological diseases, vascular diseases, nutritional diseases, inborn errors of metabolism, diseases of the musculoskeletal system, collagen vascular diseases and traumatic disorders.

FREQUENTLY ASKED QUESTIONS (FAQs)

*Short Answers

1. Mention the ocular manifestations of tuberculosis.
2. Mention the ocular manifestations of syphilis.
3. Mention the ocular manifestations of leprosy.
4. Mention the ocular manifestations of myasthenia gravis.
5. Purtscher's retinopathy.
6. Terson's syndrome.

**Short Essays

1. Mention the ocular manifestations of diabetes.
2. Mention the ocular manifestations of acquired immunodeficiency syndrome.

BIBLIOGRAPHY

1. Dutta LC. Modern Ophthalmology, vol. III, 3rd edition. New Delhi: Jaypee Brothers Medical Publishers (P) Ltd; 2005.
2. Kanski JJ. Clinical Ophthalmology, 5th edition. Butterworth: Heinemann; 2003.

SECTION 21

Ocular Pharmacology and Ocular Therapeutics

CHAPTER

21.1 Ocular Pharmacology

Ocular pharmacology deals with the study of pharmacodynamics and pharmacokinetics of the drugs used in ophthalmology. The application of the pharmacological knowledge of a drug in treating a disease is called pharmacotherapeutics and it is the basis of pharmacological treatment.

ROUTES OF ADMINISTRATION OF DRUGS (Table 21.1.1)

TABLE 21.1.1: Results of drug administration

Topical	*Periocular*	*Intraocular*	*Systemic*
Eyedrops Eye ointment Gel Ocuserts Soft contact lenses	Subconjunctival injection Sub-Tenon's injection Peribulbar injection Retrobulbar injection	Intracameral Intravitreal	Oral Intramuscular Intravenous

Topical Administration

Topical administration is one of the most convenient methods of drug administration. Administration as eyedrops, eye ointments and eye gels are the commonest mode of topical administration of drugs. Administration as ocuserts and soft contact lenses are not commonly used.

Eyedrops

Application in the form of eyedrops is the commonest and easiest method of administration of drugs in ophthalmology. Eyedrops are also called gutta, a Latin word, which means drops.

Eyedrops can be solutions with the drug completely dissolved or suspensions with the drug suspended as fine particles. Eyedrops are best instilled into the lower conjunctival fornix after asking the patient to look upward and pulling the lower eyelid downward. One drop has to be instilled at once as the capacity of the conjunctival cul-de-sac is about 30 μL and the volume of one drop is about 30 μL. If two or more eyedrops have to be instilled then a gap of 5–10 minutes is desired to prevent overflow and dilution.

The corneal epithelium is lipophilic and acts as a barrier for hydrophilic drugs, and the corneal stroma is hydrophilic and acts as a barrier for the lipophilic drugs. Hence, to achieve high-intraocular penetration, the drug has to be both lipid soluble and water soluble.

Advantages

Eyedrops are the safest and easiest mode of administration of drug to treat superficial eye infections.

Disadvantages

1. The intraocular penetration is limited by the barrier effect of cornea to prevent intraocular penetration.

2. The duration of action is shorter because of dilution of the drug by the tears.
3. The systemic absorption via nasolacrimal duct and nasal mucosa is responsible for systemic side effects. Applying pressure over lacrimal sac area to prevent systemic absorption via the nasolacrimal duct reduces the systemic side effects.

Eye Ointments

Advantages

- They are retained in the conjunctival sac for longer time as they resist dilution by the tears because of presence of a lipid base
- The systemic absorption is less; hence, the systemic side effects are less.

Disadvantages

- Because of the presence of lipid base, ointments tend to cause blurring of vision, hence are better applied during bedtime.

Eye Gels

Eye gels combine the advantages of eyedrops and eye ointments. Most commonly lubricant eyedrops are applied as eye gels.

Ocuserts and Soft Contact Lenses

Ocuserts and soft contact lenses soaked in drugs provide sustained release of drugs and are usually used in treatment of conditions, e.g. glaucoma.

Periocular Administration

Periocular administration is commonly used for providing anesthesia and injecting anesthetic agents. Subconjunctival and sub-Tenon's injections are also used in treatment of uveitis.

Intraocular Injections

1. Intracameral injections involve injecting the drug into the anterior chamber. It is done in intracameral anesthesia and for injections of antibiotics in bacterial corneal ulcer and for intracameral injection of antifungal drugs such as amphotericin B in treatment of fungal corneal ulcer.
2. Intravitreal injections involve injecting the drug into vitreous chamber. Intravitreal injections of steroids, anti-vascular endothelial growth factor (anti-VEGF) agents, etc. is commonly used in vascular diseases of retina, diabetic retinopathy with macular edema, age-related macular degenerations, etc.

Systemic Administration

Systemic administration has got poor intraocular penetration because of presence of blood-retinal barrier and blood-aqueous barrier. Hence, systemic administration is not very effective for treatment of ocular diseases. Fluoroquinolones and cephalosporins have got relatively better intraocular penetration.

GIST BOX 21.1

- Ocular pharmacology deals with the study of pharmacodynamics and pharmacokinetics of the drugs used in ophthalmology.
- The application of the pharmacological knowledge of a drug in treating a disease called pharmacotherapeutics and it is the basis of pharmacological treatment.
- Topical administration in the form of eyedrops, eye ointments, gels, ocuserts and soft contact lenses, periocular injections in the form of subconjunctival injection, sub-Tenon's injection, peribulbar injection and retrobulbar injection, intraocular injection in the form of intracameral and intravitreal injections and systemic administration in the form of oral, intramuscular and intravenous routes are the various routes of administration employed in ocular pharmacotherapeutics.

CHAPTER

21.2 Ocular Therapeutics

LASERS IN OPHTHALMOLOGY**

Lasers are widely used in ophthalmology for therapeutic and diagnostic purposes.

The word LASER stands for light amplification by stimulated emission of radiation. The principle of lasers is stimulated emission of photons from excited atoms.

Classification of Lasers Used in Ophthalmology

Photocoagulative Lasers

Photocoagulative lasers act by causing coagulation of the target tissues by rise of temperature and causing a thermal effect. Argon laser, krypton laser, diode laser and frequency-doubled neodymium-yttrium-aluminum-garnet (Nd-YAG) laser are the common photocoagulative lasers.

The photocoagulative lasers are used in anterior as well as posterior segment. The indications for use of photocoagulative lasers in posterior segment are:

- Panretinal photocoagulation for proliferative diabetic retinopathy, central retinal vein occlusion, vascular diseases such as Eales disease, retinopathy of prematurity, etc.
- Focal laser photocoagulation for macular diseases such as diabetic maculopathy, age-related macular degeneration (ARMD) and central serous retinopathy
- Treatment of retinal breaks, retinal tears or peripheral retinal degenerations
- Treatment of tumors of retina and choroid.

The indications for use of photocoagulative lasers in anterior segment are:

- Treatment of vascular lesions of eyelid, i.e. hemangioma
- Treatment of corneal vascularization
- Iridotomy, iridoplasty, trabeculoplasty and cyclophotocoagulation in treatment of glaucoma.

Photodisruptive Lasers

Photodisruptive lasers act by causing removal of the electrons from their nuclei, producing a physical state of matter called plasma and breakdown of this leads to disruption of the tissue.

The Nd-YAG laser and femtosecond laser act by photodisruptive mechanism.

The Nd-YAG laser is used in:

- Posterior capsule capsulotomy in the treatment of after cataract
- YAG laser vitreolysis for treatment of floaters of vitreous and in vitreous block pupillary block glaucoma.

Femtosecond laser is used in:
- IntraLase laser-assisted in situ keratomileusis (LASIK) for making the corneal flap
- Femtosecond laser-assisted cataract surgery for making the capsulorhexis, construction of the corneal incision and lens fragmentation.

Photoablative Lasers

Photoablative lasers act by causing disruption of the chemical bonds in the tissue, thus resulting in removal of the target tissue by ablation.

Excimer laser acts by producing photoablation. Argon fluoride laser, which produces electromagnetic energy with a wavelength of 193 nm is the most commonly used excimer laser.

Excimer laser is used in:
- Refractive laser surgeries such as photorefractive keratectomy, laser-assisted subepithelial keratectomy (LASEK), customized LASIK, IntraLase LASIK, LASEK, etc.
- Treatment of corneal opacities by phototherapeutic keratectomy.

CRYOTHERAPY IN OPHTHALMOLOGY

- Cryotherapy means use of cold to destroy a tissue as a treatment
- It involves the use of cryoprobe to produce a freezing temperature of -40° to -100° to destroy the tissue
- Cryotherapy causes tissue injury by destruction of the cell membranes as a result of ice crystal formation
- Cryotherapy can also produce tissue adhesion by freezing and thawing.

Uses*

The uses of cryotherapy are:
- To perform cryopexy in treatment of retinal breaks
- To perform cyclocryotherapy to destroy the ciliary processes in treatment of neovascular glaucoma and absolute glaucoma
- Treatment of retinal tumors, tumors of eyelids, etc.
- It was used in intracapsular cataract extraction for cryoextraction of the lens.

ANTIVASCULAR ENDOTHELIAL GROWTH FACTORS IN OPHTHALMOLOGY**

Antivascular endothelial growth factors (Anti-VEGF) are one of the newer therapeutic modalities and have come as a big hope for many retinal diseases.

Mechanism of Action

Anti-VEGF act by inhibiting the angiogenesis by inhibiting the VEGF.

Uses

Anti-VEGF used in treatment of wet ARMD, choroidal neovascularization, diabetic retinopathy, retinal vein occlusion, etc.

Adverse Effects

- The ocular side effects are usually because of the intravitreal injection and include secondary glaucoma, retinal detachment, endophthalmitis, etc.
- The systemic side effects of use of anti-VEGF drugs are thromboembolic events, cerebrovascular accidents, cardiovascular events, etc.

Commonly used Anti-VEGF Drugs

Anti-VEGF drugs are usually administered by the intravitreal route. The commonly used Anti-VEGF drugs are detailed below.

Bevacizumab

Bevacizumab is a recombinant humanized monoclonal antibody directed against the VEGF. It is widely used as an off-label drug for treatment of ARMD, diabetic retinopathy, vein occlusions of retina, etc.

> Bevacizumab is popularly called by its trade name Avastin. It is accepted for its use in colorectal cancer, non-squamous non-small cell lung cancer of lungs along with the chemotherapy to prevent the rapid growth of the tumor by inhibiting the angiogenesis.

Ranibizumab

Ranibizumab is popularly known by its trade name Lucentis. It is a monoclonal antibody fragment, which inhibits VEGF-A. It is recommended for use in eye and is used in treatment of ARMD, diabetic retinopathy, vein occlusions of retina, etc.

Pegaptanib Sodium

Pegaptanib sodium is available in the brand name of Macugen. It is an antagonist of VEGF. It is used in the treatment of ARMD.

ANTIMETABOLITES IN OPHTHALMOLOGY**

The 5-fluorouracil and mitomycin C are most commonly used antimetabolites in ophthalmology.

5-fluorouracil

The 5-fluorouracil is an antimetabolite drug. Being a pyrimidine analog, it acts by inhibition of thymidylate synthase resulting in failure of deoxyribonucleic acid (DNA) synthesis.

Mechanism of Action

The 5-fluorouracil is used in ophthalmology because of its ability to prevent fibroblastic proliferation and scarring.

It can be used intraoperatively during surgery or postoperatively by subconjunctival injections of 0.1 mL (5 mg).

Uses

The 5-fluorouracil is used in:

- Trabeculectomy
- Pterygium surgery
- Dacryocystorhinostomy
- Vitreoretinal surgery to prevent proliferative vitreoretinopathy
- Treatment of ocular surface squamous neoplasia.

Complications

The 5-fluorouracil is toxic to corneal epithelium and it can cause corneal epithelial defects or corneal epithelial erosions. Conjunctival wound leak resulting in overfiltration and hypotony when applied for trabeculectomy are among the other complications.

Mitomycin C*

Mitomycin C is an antibiotic with antimetabolite actions.

Mechanism of Action

Mitomycin C acts by affecting the DNA synthesis by preventing the cross-linking between the adenine and guanine.

It can be used intraoperatively during surgery or postoperatively by topical application. The dosage is 0.2 mg/mL in the concentration of 0.02%.

Uses

Mitomycin C is used in:

- Trabeculectomy
- Pterygium surgery
- Dacryocystorhinostomy
- Corneal refractive surgeries
- Treatment of ocular surface squamous neoplasia
- Conjunctival melanoma.

Complications

Mitomycin C is toxic to corneal endothelium and it can cause corneal endothelial decompensation on inadvertent entry into anterior chamber. Scleral necrosis on application for pterygium surgery and conjunctival wound leak resulting in overfiltration and hypotony when applied for trabeculectomy are the other complications.

DRUGS USED IN OPHTHALMOLOGY

Please refer Chapter 8 'Drugs Used in Ophthalmology' in Author's textbook *'Clinical Methods in Ophthalmology'* *for more details (also for Q. No. 3–13 in Short Answers and Q. No. 4–6 in Short Essays refer the same).*

GIST BOX 21.2

- Lasers are widely used in ophthalmology for therapeutic and diagnostic purposes.
- Photocoagulative lasers act by causing coagulation of the target tissues by rise of temperature and causing a thermal effect. Argon laser, krypton laser, diode laser and frequency-doubled neodymium-yttrium-aluminum-garnet (Nd-YAG) laser are the common photocoagulative lasers.
- Photodisruptive lasers act by causing removal of the electrons from their nuclei producing a physical state of matter called plasma and breakdown of this leads to disruption of the tissue. Nd-YAG and femtosecond laser act by photodisruptive mechanism.
- Photoablative lasers act by causing disruption of the chemical bonds in the tissue, thus resulting in removal of the target tissue by ablation. Excimer laser acts by producing photoablation.
- Antivascular endothelial growth factors (Anti-VEGF) are one of the newer therapeutic modalities and have come as a big hope for many retinal diseases. They act by inhibiting the angiogenesis by inhibiting the vascular endothelial growth factor. They are used in treatment of wet age-related macular degeneration (ARMD), choroidal neovascularization, diabetic retinopathy, retinal vein occlusion, etc.

FREQUENTLY ASKED QUESTIONS (FAQs)

*Short Answers

1. Mention the uses of cryotherapy in ophthalmology.
2. Uses of mitomycin C in ophthalmology.
3. Timolol.
4. Pilocarpine.
5. Latanoprost.
6. Hyperosmotic agents.
7. Mention the uses of atropine in ophthalmology.
8. Mention the uses of mydriatics and cycloplegics in ophthalmology.
9. Mention the uses of steroids in ophthalmology.
10. Acyclovir.
11. Mention the uses of non-steroidal anti-inflammatory drugs.
12. Mention the different types of anesthesia used in ophthalmology.
13. Mention the different types of lasers used in ophthalmology.

**Short Essays

1. Lasers in ophthalmology.
2. Anti-VEGF in ophthalmology.
3. Antimetabolites in ophthalmology.
4. Antiglaucoma drugs.
5. Cycloplegics.
6. Antifungal drugs used in ophthalmology.

BIBLIOGRAPHY

1. Abraham LM, Selva D, Casson R, et al. The clinical applications of fluorouracil in ophthalmic practice. Drugs. 2007;67(2):237-55.
2. Abraham LM, Selva D, Casson R, et al. Mitomycin: clinical applications in ophthalmic practice. Drugs. 2006;66(3):321-40.
3. Dutta LC. Modern Ophthalmology, vol 2, 3rd edition. New Delhi: Jaypee Brothers Medical Publishers (P) Ltd; 2005.
4. Moo-Young GA. Lasers in ophthalmology. West J Med. 1985;143(6):745-50.

Cornea (Table 22.1.3)

TABLE 22.1.3: Cornea

Infection	*Pathogen*
Bacterial corneal ulcer	Gram-positive cocci such as *Staphylococcus aureus (S. aureus), Staphylococcus epidermidis, Streptococcus pyogenes, Streptococcus pneumoniae, Pneumococci*, etc. Gram-negative cocci, e.g. *Neisseria gonorrhoeae (N. gonorrhoeae)* and *Neisseria meningitidis*, etc. Gram-positive bacilli, e.g. *Corynebacterium diphtheriae, Bacillus cereus, Clostridium, Listeria monocytogenes*, etc. Gram-negative bacilli, e.g. *Pseudomonas aeruginosa, Escherichia Coli, Proteus, Moraxella, Haemophilus aegyptius*, etc.
Hypopyon corneal ulcer*	*Pneumococcus*
Corneal ulcer with hypopyon*	*Pseudomonas*, staphylococci, streptococci
Fungal corneal ulcer	Filamentous fungi such as *Aspergillus, Fusarium* and yeast, e.g. *Candida*
Parasitic keratitis	*Acanthamoeba, Onchocerca*, microsporidia
Viral keratitis	Herpes simplex virus, herpes zoster virus

Uvea (Table 22.1.4)

TABLE 22.1.4: Uvea

Infection	*Pathogen*
Anterior uveitis	Pyogenic bacteria, e.g. streptococci, staphylococci, pneumococci, etc. bacteria causing granulomatous inflammation such as *Mycobacterium tuberculosis (M. tuberculosis), Mycobacterium leprae, Treponema pallidum*, etc. Viruses, e.g. herpes simplex, herpes zoster, cytomegalovirus, etc. Fungi, e.g. *Candida, Histoplasma*, etc. Parasites, e.g. *Toxoplasma, Toxocara*, etc. *Rickettsia*
Posterior uveitis	Parasitic causes include toxoplasmosis, toxocariasis, cysticercosis, onchocerciasis, etc. Viral causes include herpes zoster virus, herpes simplex type 1 and type 2 virus, and cytomegalovirus Bacterial causes include syphilis, tuberculosis, etc. Fungi, e.g. *Candida*
Panuveitis	Tuberculosis, syphilis
Acute postoperative endophthalmitis*	*Staphylococcus aureus (S. aureus), Streptococcus* species
Chronic endophthalmitis	*Propionibacterium acnes, Staphylococcus epidermidis, Corynebacterium* species, fungi, etc.
Traumatic endophthalmitis	*Streptococcus* species, *Bacillus* species
Endogenous endophthalmitis	*Candida* species, *Escherichia coli (E. coli)*
Panophthalmitis	*Staphylococcus, Streptococcus, Pseudomonas, E. coli*

Optic Nerve (Table 22.1.5)

TABLE 22.1.5: Optic nerve

Infection	*Cause*
Optic neuritis	Infectious causes such as syphilis, tuberculosis, cat-scratch fever, Lyme disease, cryptococcal meningitis in patients with acquired immunodeficiency syndrome (AIDS), sinus-related infections, etc. Parainfectious causes following viral infections such as mumps, measles or following immunization against measles, rubella, etc.

Lacrimal Sac (Table 22.1.6)

TABLE 22.1.6: Lacrimal sac

Infection	*Pathogen*
Chronic dacryocystitis	Bacteria are the most common causative agents; common bacteria causing dacryocystitis are *Staphylococcus epidermidis, Staphylococcus aureus (S. aureus), Pseudomonas, Pneumococcus, Propionibacterium* and *Escherichia coli.* Granulomatous inflammations, e.g. tuberculosis, syphilis and fungi such as *Aspergillus, Candida* are rare cause of dacryocystitis
Acute dacryocystitis	*Streptococcus pyogenes, pneumococci* and *S. aureus*
Acute dacryoadenitis	Viral infections such as mumps, measles, influenza, mononucleosis, herpes and cytomegalovirus Bacteria such as *S. aureus, Neisseria gonorrhoeae, Haemophilus influenzae, Chlamydia trachomatis*, etc.
Chronic dacryoadenitis	Tuberculosis, syphilis, etc.
Canaliculitis	*Actinomyces israelii*, gram-positive anaerobic bacteria are the most common causes and other causes include *Fusarium, Candida*, herpes simplex and *Propionibacterium*

Orbit (Table 22.1.7)

TABLE 22.1.7: Orbit

Infection	*Pathogen*
Preseptal cellulitis*	*Streptococcus pneumoniae (S. pneumoniae), Staphylococcus aureus (S. aureus)* and *Haemophilus influenzae*
Orbital cellulitis*	*S. aureus, S. pneumoniae, Streptococcus pyogenes, Pseudomonas aeruginosa, Escherichia coli* and fungi such as *Mucor* and *Aspergillus*

MICROBIOLOGICAL INVESTIGATIONS IN OPHTHALMOLOGY

The common methods of collection of specimens in ophthalmology are:

- Lid swab
- Conjunctival swab
- Corneal scrapings
- Anterior chamber tap
- Vitreous tap.

The common investigations performed and their uses are listed in Table 22.1.8.

TABLE 22.1.8: Microbiological investigation

Microbes	*Investigations*
Bacteria	Staining with Gram stain and Giemsa's stain Culture on blood agar
Fungi	Potassium hydroxide mount Gram stain, periodic acid-Schiff stain, calcofluor white stain, Gomori methenamine silver stain Culture on Sabouraud agar
Acanthamoeba	Calcofluor white, Giemsa, lactophenol cotton blue stains can show cysts and trophozoites of *Acanthamoeba* Potassium hydroxide mount, Gram staining, periodic acid-Schiff can identify *Acanthamoeba* cysts Culture on *Escherichia coli* enriched non-nutrient agar
Chlamydia	Detection of inclusion bodies (Halberstaedter and Prowazek bodies) by Giemsa stain, iodine stain and immunofluorescent stains in conjunctival smears Isolation of the *Chlamydia* by inoculation of conjunctival scrapings into tissue culture or yolk sac of embryonated eggs; detection of specific antibodies by using complement fixation, microimmunofluorescence, enzyme-linked immunosorbent assay (ELISA) and polymerase chain reaction (PCR)
Viruses	Viral culture from the infected specimens; antigen detection by immunofluorescence method or ELISA and PCR

GIST BOX 22.1

- Ocular microbiology deals with the application of microbiology for diagnosing and treatment of ocular infections.
- The knowledge of ocular microbiology helps in diagnosing and treatment of ocular infections, collection of the specimens from infective conditions, sterilization techniques of the operation theater, prevention of the postoperative infections, opportunistic infections of the eye and prevention of transmission of infection in ophthalmic practice.
- The common methods of collection of specimens in ophthalmology are lid swab, conjunctival swab, corneal scrapings, anterior chamber tap and vitreous tap.

FREQUENTLY ASKED QUESTIONS (FAQs)

*Short Answers

1. Normal conjunctival flora.
2. Mention the microbes causing ophthalmia neonatorum.
3. Mention the bacteria, which can penetrate intact corneal epithelium.
4. Mention the causative agents for corneal ulcer with hypopyon and hypopyon corneal ulcer.
5. Mention the causative agents for different types of endophthalmitis.
6. Mention the causative agents for preseptal cellulitis and orbital cellulitis.

BIBLIOGRAPHY

1. Karimsab D, Razak SK. Study of aerobic bacterial conjunctival flora in patients with diabetes mellitus. Nepal J Ophthalmol. 2013;5(1):28-32.
2. Therese KL, Madhavan HN. Microbiological procedures for diagnosis of ocular infections. [online]. Available from www.ijmm.org

Index

Page numbers followed by *f* refer to figure, *t* refer to table and *b* refer to box

A

B

C

D

E

F

G

H

I

J

K

L

M

N

O

P

Q

R

S

 T

 U

W

X

Y

Z